Histamine Research in the New Millennium

Histamine Research in the New Millennium

Proceedings of the International Sendai Histamine
Symposium held in Sendai, Japan, 22–25 November 2000

Editors:

Takehiko Watanabe
Department of Pharmacology
Tohoku University School of Medicine
Japan

Henk Timmerman
Leiden/Amsterdam Center for Drug Research
Division of Medical Chemistry
Vrije Universiteit
Amsterdam, The Netherlands

Kazuhiko Yanai
Department of Pharmacology
Tohoku University School of Medicine
Sendai, Japan

2001

ELSEVIER

Amsterdam – London – New York – Oxford – Paris – Shannon – Tokyo

ELSEVIER SCIENCE B.V.
Sara Burgerhartstraat 25
P.O. Box 211, 1000 AE Amsterdam, The Netherlands

First edition 2001

Library of Congress Cataloging in Publication Data
A catalog record from the Library of Congress has been applied for.

International Congress Series No. 1224
ISBN: 0-444-50582-2
ISSN: 0531-5131

⊘ The paper used in this publication meets the requirements of ANSI/NISO Z39.48-1992 (Permanence of Paper).

Printed in the Netherlands

Preface

The International Sendai Histamine Symposium was held from November 22 to 25, 2000, in Sendai, Japan, as the fifth in a series of International Meetings on Histamine. Prof. Kenji Tasaka, Okayama University, Japan organized the first one, in 1981 as a Satellite Symposium of the International Conference of the IUPHAR (International Union of Pharmacology) Congress. The following three meetings were held as the similar satellites. The second, third and fourth were organized by Prof. Jean-Charles Schwartz, Paris, (France), Prof. Henk Timmerman, Amsterdam, (The Netherlands), and Prof. Lorne Brandes, Winnipeg, (Canada) in 1984, 1990 and 1993, respectively. Since then, there has been no international histamine meeting on the occasion of the following IUPHAR Conferences. Therefore, we decided to organize an international symposium on histamine in 2000, the last year of 20th century. There was another reason for the meeting: As The Japanese Histamine Research Society has organized and held Annual Meetings in the autumn since 1996, to celebrate the 5th anniversary, we planned this as an international meeting.

In the 2000 Symposium, 69 oral and 71 poster sessions were presented; and the number of attendants was about 300 from 25 countries. These figures were higher than we had expected. We would like to thank many companies for their financial support, without which the Symposium would not have been possible, as it has been.

It is amazing that histamine, discovered almost 100 years ago, still attracts the interests of many scientists working in different fields, i.e., in clinics, pharmacology, medicinal chemistry, physiology, histology, biochemistry, molecular biology, immunology, etc. The reason, in our opinion, is that histamine plays very important role in popular diseases such as type I allergic diseases (asthma, allergic rhinitis, urticaria) and peptic ulcers. Many of the roles of histamine, especially also in the central nerve system, remain to be elucidated.

In this latter respect, the cloning of the H_3 receptor and developments of H_3 ligands and drugs as well as the productions of knockout mice of genes related to histamine will be very helpful. In the Symposium, the cloning of H_4 receptors and H_3 receptor subtypes were reported. It is not our intention to review the new findings here. However, we are confident that histamine will further prove to be a very important chemical mediator: many new drugs will be developed to increase the QOL of people in the world. We expect that the complete physiological roles of histamine will be disclosed in the new Millennium.

It is our great pleasure to be able to publish the Proceeding of the Symposium within a year after the Symposium, and in the year in which the 400th Anniversary of friendship between Japan and the Netherlands, the opening of the trade through a small island near Nagasaki, Dejima was celebrated. We thank all the vi

contributors for their kind cooperation. Last but not at least, we appreciate the members of Japanese Histamine Research Society and the local organizing committee, and especially Dr. Eiko Sakurai for her extraordinary secretarial contribution, without her help this Symposium would not have been completed.

The Editors
Takehiko Watanabe
Henk Timmerman
Kazuhiko Yanai

Acknowledgements

The following companies and individuals have made major contribution to International Sendai Histamine Symposium.

SUPPORTED BY

THE COMMEMORATIVE ASSOCIATION FOR THE JAPAN WORLD EXPOSITION (1970)

SENDAI TOURISM & CONVENTION BUREAU
INOUE FOUNDATION FOR SCIENCE
INTELLIGENT COSMOS ACADEMIC FOUNDATION
THE NOVARTIS FOUNDATION
DAINIPPON PHARMACEUTICAL CO., LTD.
NIPPON BOEHRINGER INGELHEIM CO., LTD.
TAIHO PHARMACEUTICAL CO., LTD.
UCB JAPAN CO., LTD.
OTSUKA PHARMACEUTICAL CO., LTD.
ELI LILLY JAPAN K.K.
ASAHI CHEMICAL INDUSTRY CO., LTD
AVENTIS PHARMA LTD.
IWAKI SEIYAKU CO., LTD.
EISAI CO., LTD.
SSP CO., LTD
KAKEN PHARMACEUTICAL CO., LTD.
KANEBO, LTD.
KISSEI PHARMACEUTICAL CO., LTD.
KYORIN PHARMACEUTICAL CO., LTD.
KYOWA HAKKO KOGYO CO., LTD.
KIRIN BREWERY CO., LTD.
GLAXO WELLCOME K.K.
GRELAN PHARMACEUTICAL CO., LTD.
SATO PHARMACEUTICAL CO., LTD.
SANKYO CO., LTD.
DAIICHI PHARMACEUTICAL CO., LTD.
TAISHO PHARMACEUTICAL CO., LTD.
CHUGAI PHARMACEUTICAL CO., LTD.SS
TSUMURA & CO.
TEIKOKU HORMONE MFG. CO., LTD.
TEIJIN LIMITED
TERUMO CORPORATION, JAPAN
TOYAMA CHEMICAL CO., LTD.
TORII PHARMACEUTICAL CO., LTD.
NIKKEN CHEMICALS CO., LTD.
NICHIIKO PHARMACEUTICAL CO., LTD.
NIPPON KAYAKU CO., LTD.
NIHON PHARMACEUTICAL CO., LTD.
NIPPON ROCHE K.K.
WYETH LEDARLE JAPAN,LTD.
NOVARTIS PHARMACEUTICALS CORPORATION
BANYU PHARMACEUTICAL CO., LTD.
PFIZER PHARMACEUTICALS, INC.
MITSUBISHI-TOKYO PHARMACEUTICALS, INC.
MINOPHAGEN PHARMACEUTICAL CO.
MEIJI SEIKA KAISHA, LTD.
MOCHIDA PHARMACEUTICAL CO., LTD.
YAMANOUCHI PHARMACEUTICAL CO., LTD.
WAKAMOTO PHARMACEUTICAL CO., LTD.
ASTRAZENECA K.K.
AZWELL CO., LTD
WELFIDE CORPORATION
OTSUKA PHARMACEUTICAL FACTORY, INC.
ONO PHARMACEUTICAL CO., LTD.
KOWA COMPANY, LTD.
SAWAI PHARMACEUTICAL CO., LTD.
SANTEN PHARMACEUTICAL CO., LTD.
SCHERING-PLOUGH K.K.
SHIONOGI CO., LTD.
SHIN-NIHON PHARMACEUTICAL CO., LTD.
SUMITOMO PHARMACEUTICALS
TAKEDA CHEMICAL INDUSTRIES, LTD.
TANABE SEIYAKU CO., LTD.
TOWA PHARMACEUTICAL CO., LTD.
NIPPON SHINYAKU CO., LTD.
NIHON SCHERING'S
NIPPON ZOKI PHARMACEUTICAL CO., LTD.
BAYER, LTD.
HISHIYAMA PHARMACEUTICAL CO., LTD.
FUJISAWA PHARMACEUTICAL CO., LTD.
FUSO PHARMACEUTICAL INDUSTRIES, LTD.
MARUISHI PHARMACEUTICAL CO., LTD.
MARUHO CO., LTD.
MERCK HOEI, LTD.
ROHTO PHARMACEUTICAL CO., LTD.
JAPAN TOBACCO INC. CORPORATE RABITON INST., INC.
BLOCK DRUG JAPAN
NIPPON ORGANON K.K.
TEO PHARMACY
SMITHKLINE BEECHAM CO., LTD.
KYOTO PHARMACEUTICAL INDUSTRIES, LTD.
YAMADA BEE FARM
OGAWA & CO., LTD.
DAIICHI RADIOISOTOPE LAB., LTD.
SANYO MARUNAKA CO., LTD.
SEGAMI MEDICS
SHIBATA INTECH CO., LTD.
EIKEN CHEMICAL CO., LTD.
MEDICAL & BIOLOGICAL LABORATORIES CO., LTD.
CEREBOS PACIFIC LTD.
YAYOI MEMORIAL FUND
DEPARTMENT OF PHARMACOLOGY, TOHOKU UNIVERSITY SCHOOL OF MEDICINE

Contents

4. Histamine H_1 antagonists

5. Safety and efficiency of histamine H_1 antagonists

6. Signal transduction

16. Signal transduction

17. Mast cells

Plenary lectures

Histamine Research in the New Millennium
T. Watanabe, H. Timmerman and K. Yanai (Editors)

Regulation of mast cell differentiation

Yukihiko Kitamura, Eiichi Morii, Hideki Ogihara, Tomoko Jippo, and Akihiko Ito

Department of Pathology, Osaka University Medical School, Yamada-oka 2-2, Suita, Osaka, 565-0871, Japan

We used various mouse mutants for studying regulation of mast cell differentiation. Their bone marrow origin was shown using giant granules of beige mice as a marker. We found the mast cell deficiency of W/W^v and Sl/Sl^d mice. The W locus encodes the c-*kit* receptor tyrosine kinase, and the *Sl* locus a lignad of c-*kit* that is the most important growth factor for development of mast cell, stem cell factor. The *mi* locus encodes a member of the basic helix-lop-helix-leucine zipper protein family of transcription factor (MITF), and mast cells of *mi/mi* mice showed various phenotypic abnormalities. Mast cells of *mi/mi* mice synthesized the mutant *mi*-MITF in normal amount, and the *mi*-MITF showed inhibitory effect on the transcription of various mast cell-specific genes. On the other hand, mice of *tg/tg* possess the transgene insertional mutation at the 5' flanking region of the *mi* gene and do not express any MITFs. The comparison between phenotypes of *mi/mi* mast cells and those of *tg/tg* mast cells gave some insights on the regulation of mast cell phenotypes by transcription factors.

1. DEVELOPMNTAL PROCESSES

We started studying mast cell differentiation by identifying their bone marrow origin. We kept beige Chediak-Higashi syndrome mice, and by chance we saw a paper in the library that described the giant granules of beige-type mast cells. We attempted to examine the bone marrow origin of mast cells using the giant granules as a marker. Transplantation of bone marrow cells from beige mice to irradiated normal control (+/+) mice resulted in the development of beige-type mast cells with giant granules [1]. In addition to beige mice, we found that two mouse mutants, W/W^v and Sl/Sl^d, genetically lack mast cells [2,3]. Afterwards, the W locus was identified to encode the c-*kit* receptor tyrosine kinase, and the *Sl* locus to encode the ligand of a c-*kit* receptor, stem cell factor (SCF).

When we found mast cell deficiency in *W/W^v* and *Sl/Sl^d* mice, some people considered that these mutant mice possessed mast cell but that their mast cells were not stained with dyes conventionally used for identifying mast cells. Yamatodani et al [4] showed that histamine content was remarkably deficient in tissues of these mutant mice. This brought most people over our opinion that *W/W^v* and *Sl/Sl^d* mice really lack mast cells. In addition to mast cell-deficient mice, we found mast cell-deficient *Ws/Ws* rats that have a small deletion in the tyrosine kinase domain of the c-*kit* gene [5].

By using *W/W^v* mice as recipients, we demonstrated that mast cells are the progeny of the multipotential hematopoietic stem cell. Most of the progeny of the multipotential stem cell such as erythrocytes, platelets, neutrophils, eosinophils, and basophils leave the bone marrow after they differentiate. However, mast cells do not complete their differentiation in the hematopoietic tissue. Precursors of mast cells leave the bone marrow, migrate in blood and invade connective or mucosal tissue, proliferate and differentiate into mast cells [6].

Although most of the progeny from the multipotential stem cell lose their proliferation potential when they differentiate fully, some morphologically identifiable mast cells have an appreciable proliferation potential. Neutrophils, eosinophils and basophils appear to die after functioning. In contrast, when highly degranulated mast cells were injected into the skin of *W/W^v* mice, the proporion of injection sites at which mast cell clusters appeared was comparable to the value observed when morphologically intact mast cells were injected, indicating that the proliferation potential of mast cells is not reduced by their degranulation [6].

2. GAIN-OF-FUNCTION MUTATION OF c-*kit*

Double gene dose of the loss-function-mutation of c-*kit* resulted in mast cell deficiency in mice and rats. A human patient that might be a probable homozygote of the c-*kit* loss-of-function mutation has been reported as well. In contrast, gain-of-function mutation of c-*kit* gene has been found not only in human mast cell tumors directly obtained from patients but also in human (HMC-1), mouse (P-815) and rat (RBL-2H3) tumor mast cell lines. Interestingly, a particular aspartic acid in the tyrosine kinase domain changes to valine (HMC-1) or tyrosine (P-815 and RBL-2H3). The mutant c-*kit* proteins were activated without SCF [7].

Differentiation-inducing activity of c-*kit* was shown using the gain-of-function mutation. IC-2 is a murine mast cell line that does not show significant differentiation. When the cDNA encoding the gain-of-function mutation of c-*kit* was introduced into IC-2 cells, they showed not only malignant transformation but also remarkably differentiated phenotype.

3. MICE OF *mi/mi* GENOTYPE

Decrease of mast cells had been described in the skin of *mi/mi* mice. Although *W/Wᵛ* and *Sl/Slᵈ* mice practically lack mast cells, the mast cell deficiency of *mi/mi* mice was not so severe. The number of mast cells in the skin of 3 week-old *mi/mi* mice was about 40% that of the control +/+ mice. Since the mast cell deficiency was more remarkable in *mi/mi* embryos, the mast cell deficiency of *mi/mi* mice appeared to be age-dependent. Mice of *mi/mi* genotype also show other abnormalities, microphthalmia, depletion of pigment in both hair and eyes, osteopetrosis and deficiency in natural killer activity.

Using transgenic insertional mutant at the *mi* locus, which was discovered among transgenic mice originally developed to study the vasopressin promoter, Hodgkinson et al [8] succeeded in cloning the *mi* gene. The *VGA-9-tg/tg* homozygous transgenic mice exhibited symptoms similar to that of *mi/mi* mice due to the disruption of the promoter region of the *mi* gene. The *mi* gene encodes a novel member of the basic-helix-loop-helix-leucine zipper family of transcription factors. The *mi* transcription factor (hereafter MITF) encoded by the mutant *mi* allele deletes 1 of 4 consecutive arginines in the basic domain. The *mi* mutant MITF (*mi*-MITF) is defective in DNA binding activity and nuclear localization potential and does not transactivate the target genes.

4. PHENOTYPIC ABNORMALITY OF MAST CELLS

In addition to the decrease in number, we found the phenotypic abnormality in mast cells of *mi/mi* mice. First we noticed that the counted number of mast cells in the skin of *mi/mi* mice was dependent on dyes used for staining. Skin pieces of *mi/mi* and control +/+ mice were stained with alcian blue and berberine sulfate. In the skin of +/+ mice, the number of alcian blue-positive mast cells was comparable to that of berberine sulfate-positive mast cells. In contrast, the number of berberine-positive mast cells was only 6% that of alcian blue-positive mast cells in the skin of *mi/mi* mice. Berberine sulfate has been reported to bind heparin. When heparin content per skin mast cell was evaluated, the value in *mi/mi* mast cell was 34% that of +/+ mast cell [9]. Molecular mechanism of reduced heparin content will be described later.

Cultured mast cells (CMCs) derived from the spleen of *mi/mi* mice are deficient in the expression of genes encoding c-*kit* receptor tyrosine kinase, p75 nerve growth factor receptor, integrin α-4 subunit, mouse mast cell protease (mMCP)-2, 4, 5, 6, 7 and 9, granzyme B, and cathepsin G.

Since mMCPs are strongly expressed by CMCs, they are useful to investigate the mechanism of transcriptional regulation by MITF. MITFs have both enhancing and suppressing effects on the transcription of mMCPs. For examples, we show the enhancing effect of +-MITF on the transcription of mMCP-6 and the suppressing effect of *mi*-MITF on the transcription of mMCP-7.

5. ENHANCING EFFCT OF +-MITF

Expression of mMCP-6 gene is severely reduced in CMCs and skin mast cells of not only *mi/mi* but also *tg/tg* mice. Since practically any MITFs were not expressed by *tg/tg* CMCs, the presence of +-MITF appeared to be indispensable for the expression of mMCP-6 gene. In the promoter region of mMCP-6 gene, there are a GACCTG motif and two CANNTG motifs, all of which were recognized and bound by +-MITF. Binding of +-MITF remarkably enhanced the transcription of the mMCP-6 gene [10].

Most transcription factors do not work alone, but function in cooperation with other transcription factors. MITF cooperates with polyomavirus enhancer binding protein 2 (PEBP2) in the transacativation of MMCP-6 gene. The simultaneous transfecton of MITF and PEBP2 cDNAs synergistically increased the MMCP-6 promoter activity. The above-mentioned GACCTG motif recognized by MITF partly overlapped the motif which was recognized by PEBP2, TGTGGTC.

6. SUPPRESSING EFFECT OF *mi*-MITF

The transcription of mMCP-2, mMCP-4, mMCP-5, mMCP-6 and mMCP-9 was severely impaired in both *mi/mi* and *tg/tg* CMCs [11]. On the other hand, the transcription of mMCP-7 gene was markedly reduced in *mi/mi* CMCs, but the reduction was significantly smaller in *tg/tg* CMCs [12]. The presence of *mi*-MITF appeared to inhibit the expresion of mMCP-7 gene. Similar inhibitory effect of *mi*-MITF was also observed on the transactivation of c-*kit*, tryptophan hydroxylase (TPH) and granzyme B genes in CMCs

Both mMCP-6 and mMCP-7 are tryptase and genes encoding each of them reside on chromosome 17. Although the coding region of the mMCP-7 gene is highly homologous with that of mMCP-7 gene, the mechanism of transactivation appeared to be different. MITF-binding site was not present in the promoter region which was essential for transcription of mMCP-7 gene. On the other hand, an AP-1 binding motif was present and biding of c-Jun to this region was important for the transactivation.

Either +-MITF or *mi*-MITF may bind c-Jun. Binding of +-MITF enhanced the transcriptional activity of c-Jun, but that of *mi*-MITF suppressed the activity of c-Jun [12].

CMCs of *mi/mi* mice expressed *mi*-MITF whereas CMCs of *tg/tg* mice did not express any MITFs. To investigate the function of *mi*-MITF generally, mRNAs obtained from *mi/mi* CMCs or *tg/tg* CMCs were subtracted from cDNA library of +/+ CMCs, and the (+/+ -*mi/mi*) and (+/+ - *tg/tg*) subtraction libraries were obtained. When the number of clones that hybridized more efficiently with +/+ CMC cDNA probe than with *mi/mi* or *tg/tg* CMC cDNA probe was compared by Southern analysis, the number was significantly greater in the (+/+ -*mi/mi*) library than in (+/+ -*tg/tg*) library. The presence of *mi*-MITF rather than the absence of +-MITF shows an inhibitory effect on the expression of many target genes [13].

7. CONTENTS OF HISTAMINE AND SEROTONIN IN *mi/mi* MICE

Histamine content in the skin of *mi/mi* mice was 7% that of control +/+ mice. Since the number of mast cells was also decreased in the skin of *mi/mi* mice to 40% that of control +/+ mice, the relative histamine content per mast cell was 18% that of +/+ mice [9]. We expected that content of histamine was decreased in *mi/mi* CMCs as well. However, this was not the case. The histamine content of *mi/mi* CMCs was comparable to that of +/+ CMCs. The mRNA expression of histidine decarboxylase gene was also comparable between *mi/mi* CMCs and +/+ CMCs. The decrease of histamine content in *mi/mi* skin mast cells may be due to a defect of histamine production but to a defect of histamine storage. The histamine content of +/+ CMCs is known to be 1% that of +/+ peritoneal mast cells [14], indicating a remarkable increase of histamine content during the differentiation to connective tissue-type mast cells. Only connective tissue-type mast cells such as skin mast cells and peritoneal mast cells contain heparin. Therefore, low heparin content of *mi/mi* skin mast cells may explain the storage defect. N-deacetylase/N-sulfotransfersase-2 (NDST-2) is essential for the synthesis of heparin. We recently found the inhibitory effect of *mi*-MITF on the transcription of the NDST-2 gene. Transcription of NDST-2 was deficient in *mi/mi* CMCs but not in *tg/tg* CMCs (Morii et al, unpublished data). The deficient transcription of the NDST-2 gene may be a cause of low histamine content in *mi/mi* skin mast cells.

In contrast to normal histamine content in *mi/mi* CMCs, serotonin content was significantly reduced in *mi/mi* CMCs. Since the transcription of the gene encoding TPH is somewhat reduced in *tg/tg* CMCs, +-MITF appeared to play a role for the transcription of TPH. However, the tanscripton of TPH gene was impaired more severely in *mi/mi* CMCs than in *tg/tg* CMCs [12]. The *mi*-MITF appeared to have inhibitory effect on the transcription of the TPH gene. Although MITF affects the contents of both histamine and serotonin in mast cells, our results suggested that the mechanisms are different.

REFERENCES

1. Y. Kitamura, M. Shimada, K. Hatanaka, and Y. Miyano, Nature 268 (1977) 442-443.
2. Y. Kitamura, S. Go, and K. Hatanaka, Blood 52 (1978) 447-452.
3. Y. Kitamura, and S. Go, Blood 53 (1979) 492-497.
4. A. Yamatodani, K. Maeyama, T. Watanabe, H. Wada, and Y. Kitamura, Biochem Pharmacol 31 (1982) 305-309.
5. T. Tsujimura, S. Hirota, S. Nomura, Y. Niwa, M. Yamazaki, T. Tono, E. Morii, H.M. Kim, K. Kondo, Y. Nishimune, and Y. Kitamura, Blood 78 (1991) 1942-1946.
6. Y. Kitamura, Annu Rev Immunol 7 (1989) 59-76.
7. T. Furitsu, T. Tsujimura, T. Tono, H. Ikeda, H. Kitayama, U. Koshimizu, H. Sugahara, J.H. Butterfield, L.K. Ashman, Y. Kanayama, Y. Matsuzawa, Y. Kitamura, and Y. Kanakura, J Clin Invest 92 (1993) 1736-1744.
8. C.A. Hodgkinson, K.J. Moore, A. Nakayama, E. Steingrimsson, N.G. Copeland, N.A. Jenkins, H. Arnheiter, Cell 74 (1993) 395-404.
9. T. Kasugai, K. Oguri, T. Jippo-Kanemoto, M. Morimoto, A. Yamatodani, K. Yoshida, Y. Ebi, K. Isozaki, H. Tei, T. Tsujimura, S. Nomura, M. Okayama, and Y. Kitamura, Am J Pathol 143 (1993) 1337-1347.
10. E. Morii, T. Tsujimura, T. Jippo, K. Hashimoto, K. Takebayashi, K. Tsujino, S. Nomura, M. Yamamoto, and Y. Kitamura, Blood 88 (1996) 2488-2494.
11. Y. Ge, T. Jippo, Y.M. Lee, S. Adachi, and Y. Kitamura, Am J Pathol, in press.
12. H. Ogihara, E. Morii, D.K. Kim, K. Oboki, and Y. Kitamura, Blood, in press.
13. A. Ito, E. Morii, D.K. Kim, T.R. Kataoka, T. Jippo, K. Maeyama, H. Nojima, and Y. Kitamura, Blood 93 (1999) 1189-1196.
14. T. Nakano, T. Sonoda, C. Hayashi, A. Yamatodani, Y. Kanayama, H. Asai, T. Yonezawa, Y. Kitamura, and S.J. Galli, J Exp Med 162 (1985) 1025-1043.

Histamine Research in the New Millennium
T. Watanabe, H. Timmerman and K. Yanai (Editors)

The histamine H$_3$ receptor : gene organization, multiple isoforms, constitutive activity and molecular pharmacology

J.-M. Arrang[a], S. Morisset[a], A. Rouleau[a], J. Tardivel-Lacombe[a], F. Gbahou[a], X. Ligneau[b], A. Héron[c], A. Sasse[a], H. Stark[d], W. Schunack[d], C.R. Ganellin[e] and J.-C. Schwartz[a]

[a]Unité de Neurobiologie et Pharmacologie Moléculaire (U.109) INSERM, Centre Paul Broca, 2ter rue d'Alésia, 75014 Paris, France.

[b]Laboratoire Bioprojet, 9 rue Rameau, 75002 Paris, France.

[c]Laboratoire de Physiologie, Faculté des Sciences Pharmaceutiques et Biologiques, 4 Avenue de l'Observatoire, 75006 Paris, France.

[d]Institut für Pharmazie, Freie Universität Berlin, Königin-Luise-Strasse 2+4, 14195 Berlin, Germany

[e]Department of Chemistry,University College London, 20 Gordon Street, London WC1H 0AJ, UK.

We show by genomic DNA analysis that the coding region of the rat H$_3$ receptor comprises three exons interrupted by two introns located in the second transmembrane domain and second intracellular loop, respectively. We have identified several isoforms of the receptor by cDNA cloning. Four variants, termed H$_{3(445)}$, H$_{3(413)}$, H$_{3(410)}$ and H$_{3(397)}$ and generated by pseudo-intron retention/deletion at the level of the third intracellular loop, display rather similar pharmacological profiles but differential tissue expression. Two short variants, termed H$_{3(nf1)}$ and H$_{3(nf2)}$ and corresponding to frame shift and stop codon interposition, are presumably non functional. We have assigned the human H$_3$ receptor gene to the telomeric region of the q arm of chromosome 20 and shown that the organization of the coding region of the human and rat H$_3$ receptor genes is similar. Whereas the two deduced proteins differ by only five amino acids at the level of the transmembrane domains, we show that some ligands display distinct affinities for the recombinant rat and human H$_3$ receptors, a difference that we assign to two aminoacids in TM3. Finally, we show that the recombinant H$_3$ receptor displays high constitutive activity and, having identified a neutral antagonist, we use it to demonstrate that native H$_3$ autoreceptors also display high constitutive activity in their control of histaminergic neuron activity *in vitro* and *in vivo*.

1. INTRODUCTION

The histamine H$_3$ receptor (H$_3$R) was initially characterized as an autoreceptor regulating histamine synthesis and release in brain [1,2]. Since then, numerous studies, mainly performed in the rat, have established its presynaptic and postsynaptic localisations, signalling mechanisms and detailed pharmacology, and a possible molecular heterogeneity of the receptor has been suggested [3]. However, it is only recently that a cDNA encoding the human H_3R was identified [4].

Starting from the human H_3R sequence, we have established the organization of the rat and human H_3R genes and evidenced the existence of multiple isoforms of the receptor. We have identified ligands displaying distinct apparent affinities at the rat and human H_3Rs and identified the amino acid residues responsible for such differences in species pharmacological profiles. Finally, we show that the recombinant H_3R displays high constitutive activity, i.e., is spontaneously active even in the absence of agonist. We have established that the constitutive activity of the native H_3R is present in brain preparations *in vitro* and that it controls histaminergic neuron activity *in vivo*.

2. GENE ORGANIZATION AND MULTIPLE ISOFORMS OF THE RAT H_3R

Starting from the published sequence of the human H_3R we have cloned the rat H_3R [5-7] and determined its encoded sequence which is in agreement with that found independently by Lovenberg et al. [8].

Nucleotide sequence analysis of genomic DNA revealed that the coding region of the rat H_3 receptor comprises three exons interrupted by two introns of ~1 kb each (Figure 1). The two introns are located at the same level as the two introns that we recently identified in the coding region of the human H_3-receptor gene [9], i.e., in the second transmembrane domain and second intracellular loop, respectively.

We have identified several isoforms of the rat H_3 receptor by cDNA cloning. Two of them, termed $H_{3(nfl)}$ and $H_{3(nf2)}$, do not contain a full length open reading frame and would correspond to truncated, i.e., presumably non functional isoforms. The $H_{3(nfl)}$ isoform is generated by the use of two potential splice donor dinucleotides (GT) at the splice junction site of intron 1. The $H_{3(nf2)}$ isoform is generated by the use of an alternative splice acceptor site within intron 2. The functional significance, if any, of their transcripts is unclear. $H_{3(nfl)}$ cDNAs were isolated from striatum and the general distribution pattern of $H_{3(nf2)}$ mRNAs analyzed by *in situ* hybridization is very similar to the pattern of H_3 receptor mRNAs, suggesting that they are expressed in the same neuronal populations and that they might be involved in the regulation of the expression and/or function of H_3 receptors.

We recently reported the deletion of a 30-amino acid fragment in the third intracellular loop of the receptor, which leads to a shorter isoform, termed H_{3S}, in the guinea pig [10].The retention/deletion of a corresponding 32-amino acid sequence at the same level of the human [9] and rat H_3 receptor also leads to the existence of H_{3L} and H_{3S} variants that we now propose to designate according to their reduced amino acid length, i.e., $H_{3(445)}$ and $H_{3(413)}$ isoforms. In addition to these previously known variants, we recently identified $H_{3(410)}$- and $H_{3(397)}$-receptor isoforms in which the fragment deleted from the third intracytosolic loop was longer, including three and sixteen additional amino acids, respectively. We also recently determined, by nucleotide sequence analysis of the human gene, that the deleted sequence is not flanked by introns [9]. The absence of flanking introns in the rat gene is supported by PCR analysis of genomic DNA, since the size of the amplified fragment spanning the third intracellular loop, was similar to that expected from the corresponding rat cDNA sequence. Moreover, nucleotide sequence analysis revealed the presence of the same consensus splice donor (5'-GTATGGG-3') together with various acceptor sites at the 5' and 3' ends of each deleted sequence, indicating that the $H_{3(413)}$, $H_{3(410)}$, and $H_{3(397)}$ isoforms are generated by deletion of a pseudo-intron, as we recently showed for the human receptor [9].

The expression pattern of the various isoforms clearly differs, among both brain regions and peripheral tissues: in the latter, only the longer ($H_{3(445)}$) isoform was observed and the relative ratios of the isoforms dramatically varied among brain areas [6]. Although the longer isoform was the more abundant in most brain regions, a significant expression level of the shorter variants was observed, except in the cerebellum where they were hardly detectable. The $H_{3(397)}$ variant was even predominant in striatum. These findings may indicate that the splicing mechanisms are regulated within the same neurons or that the various isoforms are differentially expressed among distinct neuronal populations in which they may subserve different functions.

We recently reported from functional studies that the pharmacological profiles of the rat $H_{3(445)}$ and $H_{3(413)}$ isoforms were rather similar [5]. Binding studies confirm that the various isoforms, including the $H_{3(397)}$ variant, display limited pharmacological differences (Table 1). However, these pharmacological differences of multiple variants displaying different expression patterns may partly account for the H_3-receptor heterogeneity previously reported in tissues from functional and binding studies [11-13].

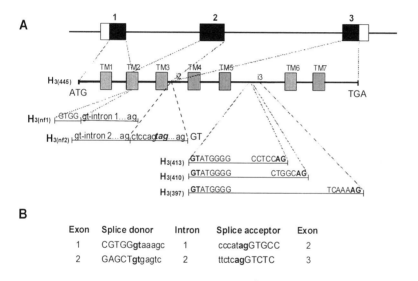

Figure 1 : Exon/intron structure of the rH_3-receptor gene and rH_3R isoforms generated by retention/deletion of pseudo-introns. A: Top, diagram of the rH_3R genomic DNA. Exons indicated by the boxes are numbered . Open boxes indicate nontranslated sequence. Bottom, structure of the $rH_{3(445)}$ receptor cDNA. Regions encoding transmembrane domains are represented by hatched boxes (TM1-TM7). i2 and i3 indicate the second and third intracytosolic loops, respectively. Deletions/insertions leading to two presumably non-functional H_3R isoforms, $H_{3(nf1)}$ and $H_{3(nf2)}$, and three functional shorter isoforms, $H_{3(413)}$, $H_{3(410)}$, and $H_{3(397)}$ are indicated. B: Exon/intron junctions within the rH_3R gene.

Table 1
Compared potencies of H_3-receptor ligands on the inhibition of $[^{125}I]$iodoproxyfan binding to H_3-receptor isoforms transfected in Cos-1 ($H_{3(397)}$) or CHO-K1 ($H_{3(413)}$ and $H_{3(445)}$) cells

	K_i (nM)		
Ligands	**$H_{3(397)}$**	**$H_{3(413)}$**	**$H_{3(445)}$**
Histamine	28 ± 4	61 ± 8	20 ± 2
Imetit	1.1 ± 0.2	1.0 ± 0.2	0.33 ± 0.04
Thioperamide	1.7 ± 0.3	4.3 ± 1.2	6.5 ± 0.2
Ciproxifan	0.8 ± 0.1	0.96 ± 0.18	3.9 ± 0.2
Clobenpropit	0.5 ± 0.1	0.44 ± 0.08	1.4 ± 0.1
FUB 465	376 ± 24	399 ± 18	132 ± 12
Proxyfan	9.6 ± 2.4	5.6 ± 0.5	2.9 ± 0.2

Each value represents the mean of 2-4 independent experiments with triplicate determinations each.

3. CHROMOSOMAL MAPPING AND ORGANIZATION OF THE HUMAN H_3R GENE

The chromosomal assignment of the human H_3R gene was performed using a human x rodent cell hybrid panel and two different sets of PCR primers amplifying nonoverlapping fragments. Analysis of the vectors obtained from the PCR results assigned the gene 12.90 cR and 16.96 cR downstream from the microsatellite marker D20S173, with the two sets of primers, respectively. This locates the H_3R gene locus within the D20S173-qTEL interval, i.e. in the telomeric region of the q arm of chromosome 20 (20qTEL) (Figure 2).

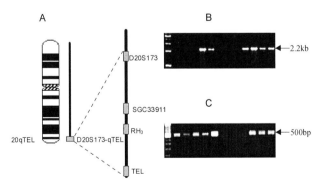

Figure 2 : Chromosomal mapping of the human H_3-receptor gene : **A:** Schematic representation of the localization of the gene on chromosome 20. **B and C:** A human x rodent somatic cell hybrid was subjected to PCR analysis using primers based on sequences of TM3 and third intracytosolic loop (B) and TM1 and intron 1 (C).

Screening of a human striatum cDNA library led to the isolation of a full-length cDNA sequence displaying a 100% identity with the human H$_3$R cDNA previously described [4]. The organization of the H$_3$-receptor gene was determined by alignment of this sequence and DNA sequences of chromosome 20. The human H$_3$R gene sequence corresponded to a 3,965-bp fragment of the dJ1005F21.02586 chromosomal sequence (accession number to the Sanger Centre AL078633). Nucleotide sequence analysis of this fragment revealed that the human H$_3$R gene is similar to that of the rat H$_3$R : it comprises three exons interrupted by two introns [9].

Furthermore the same mechanism as in the rat is responsible for the generation of multiple hH$_3$R isoforms, i.e. retention/deletion of a pseudo intron located in the third intracytoplasmic loop.

4. DISTINCT PHARMACOLOGY OF THE RAT AND HUMAN H$_3$Rs ANALYZED BY SITE-DIRECTED MUTAGENESIS

Whereas the histamine H$_3$ receptor (H$_3$R) was initially identified in the rat brain [1,2], its presence in the human brain was confirmed a few years later [14]. In both cases a functional test, the inhibition of [^{3}H]histamine release from depolarized brain slices, was used, but the pharmacological characterization of the human H$_3$R has remained preliminary since the availability of fresh brain tissues obtained during neurosurgery is limited. Nevertheless there were some indications that the pharmacology of the human and the rat H$_3$R may slightly differ [14,15 and X. Ligneau, unpublished observation].

With the recent cloning of the human H$_3$R (hH$_3$R) [4], it became feasible to determine with greater precision the apparent affinity of ligands at this receptor and assess the existence of species differences.

Using recombinant receptors expressed in different cell lines, we confirm that the H$_3$Rs can be differentiated pharmacologically in two species and we identify the area very likely responsible for this difference.

Previous indications of such species differences, mainly between the hH$_3$R and rH$_3$R, were derived from either functional or binding assays performed with fresh brain tissues. In agreement, the prototypical H$_3$R antagonist thioperamide was found to be slightly (4-fold) less potent at the H$_3$R modulating [^{3}H]histamine release from depolarised human when compared to rat brain slices, K_i values being 16 nM [14] and 4 nM [2], respectively. Other functional or binding studies performed with various ligands led to even higher K_i values for this compound at the hH$_3$R, i.e., 85-200 nM [15,16]. In the same way the antagonist ciproxifan displayed significantly higher potency at the rH$_3$R when compared to the hH$_3$R in fresh brain tissues using either functional or binding assays performed under parallel conditions [17 and X. Ligneau, unpublished observations]. Interestingly, however, both histamine and (R)α-methylhistamine were found to be nearly equipotent at the native rH$_3$R and hH$_3$R in brain [2,14,15].

Here we come to similar conclusions, i.e., thioperamide and ciproxifan are about 10-fold more potent at the rH$_3$R than at the hH$_3$R, whereas histamine, (R)α-methylhistamine and the two antagonists clobenpropit [18] and proxyfan [19] were nearly equipotent.

Moreover, we have identified one compound, the antagonist FUB 349 [20], displaying a reverse preference, i.e., being about 5-fold more potent at the human than at the rat receptor.

While this work was in progress, Lovenberg et al. [8] confirmed the higher potency of thioperamide (K_i = 4 nM) at this receptor when compared to its human counterpart (K_i = 58 nM or K_i = 20 nM in Lovenberg et al. [4]).

The identification of residues responsible for this heterogeneity was facilitated by the realization that the rH$_3$R and hH$_3$R sequences differed by only five amino acid residues, at the level of the putative TM helices where ligands are thought to bind. Among these helices, TM3 was a good candidate since, at this level, the rH$_3$R differs from the hH$_3$R by two residues located in vicinity to the aspartate residue (Asp[114]) present in all aminergic receptors and purported to salt-link the ammonium group of histamine and agonists (Figure 3). Mutation of these two residues, i.e., Ala[119] into Thr[119] and Val[122] into Ala[122], to obtain a partially "humanized" rat H$_3$ receptor led to the expected changes. In agreement i) the affinity of ligands not discriminating hH$_3$R and rH$_3$R, e.g., [^{125}I]iodoproxyfan or clobenpropit was not significantly modified, ii) in contrast the affinities of a rH$_3$R-preferring ligand, ciproxifan, was reduced, whereas that of FUB 349, a hH$_3$R-preferring ligand, was enhanced so that the affinity of these compounds did not differ anymore from corresponding values at the hH$_3$R (Figure 4).

The mutated amino acids may modify, e.g., hydrophobic interactions, which are presumed to have greater influence on the binding of lipophilic antagonists than on that of hydrophilic agonists. The purported salt link of basic compounds like histamine, (R)α-methylhistamine, and clobenpropit with Asp[114] seems to be of greater importance for these compounds than their hydrophobic interactions.

More extensive structure-activity together with modelling studies are in progress to provide more details about a possible interaction of ligands with the receptor at this level and should facilitate the rational design of novel ligands to be used as drugs in humans.

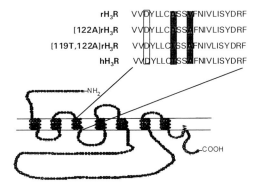

Figure 3 : Putative membrane topology of the histamine H$_3$ receptor. The amino acid sequence of the third transmembrane domain of the rat (rH$_3$R) and the human (hH$_3$R) receptor is shown. The open box indicates the position of aspartic acid 114, known to be conserved in all aminergic receptors. The grey boxes indicate the amino acids in position 119 and 122. Mutations at these positions in the rat receptor are underlined.

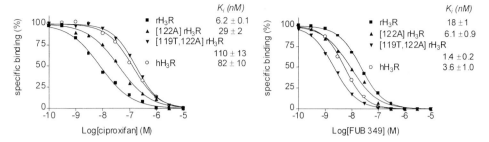

Figure 4: Inhibition of [^{125}I]iodoproxyfan binding to mutant rat receptors by ciproxifan and FUB 349. Membranes of Cos-1 cells expressing wild-type rat receptors (rH$_3$R), mutant [122A] rat receptors, mutant [119T, 122A] rat receptors or wild-type human receptors (hH$_3$R) were incubated with 25 pM [^{125}I]iodoproxyfan and ciproxifan or FUB 349 in increasing concentrations. Each point represents the mean value from two different experiments with triplicate determinations each. The K_i values (nM) of ciproxifan and FUB 349 obtained for each receptor are indicated.

5. HIGH CONSTITUTIVE ACTIVITY OF THE RECOMBINANT H$_3$R

After cloning the rat H$_3$R, we noticed that the carboxy terminus of i3 has a stretch of eight amino acids strikingly similar to the corresponding sequence of a mutated human β_2-adrenergic receptor in which the mutation confers a constitutive activity (CAM hβ_2-AR in Figure 5) that is absent in the native receptor [21]. Thus, among these eight amino acids, six (five in the mouse) are identical in the rat H$_3$ receptor and in the mutated β_2-adrenergic receptor, whereas the other two amino acids are conserved. Furthermore, this region is also critical for constitutive activity in other native or mutated heptahelical receptors.

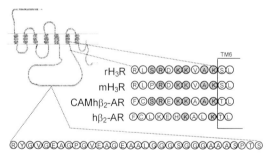

Figure 5 : Two rat H$_3$-receptor isoforms and their expression in rat brain regions. Putative seven-transmembrane topography of H$_{3S}$ and H$_{3L}$ alternatively spliced variants differing by a 32-aminoacid insertion in the i3 loop. This loop C-terminal sequence is also compared to that of the mouse (mH$_3$R), the native human β_2-adrenergic receptor (hβ_2-AR) and a constitutively active mutant (CAM hβ_2-AR) [21].

We have, therefore, assessed the constitutive activity of the H$_{3L}$ and H$_{3S}$ isoforms, i.e., H$_{3(445)}$ and H$_{3(413)}$ respectively, expressed in CHO cells at low, medium and high densities, i.e., 30-80, 300-500 and ~1,000 fmol/mg protein as determined by [^{125}I]iodoproxyfan assay

[22], respectively. The coupling changes associated with receptor expression were evaluated in two signalling pathways activated by histamine and involving G_i/G_o-proteins, i.e., adenylyl cyclase inhibition and phospholipase A_2 activation. In both pathways, constitutive activity of both the H_{3L} and H_{3S} receptors was clearly evidenced. In agreement, [³H]arachidonic acid ([³H]AA) release evoked by the Ca^{2+}-ionophore A23187 was enhanced (Figure 6) whereas forskolin-induced cAMP accumulation was reduced (in both cases in total absence of histamine) when the receptor density was enhanced. These changes were largely reversed in the presence of thioperamide, a compound so far considered as the prototypical H_3-receptor antagonist [2], but appearing here, as predicted by binding data [23], as an extremely potent inverse agonist.

Constitutive activity was slightly more pronounced with the H_{3L} isoform : there was already a tendency to spontaneous activity and a response to thioperamide at low expression levels of H_{3L} (effects that became significant at 80 fmol/mg protein, not shown), and, at intermediate levels, changes were more marked than with the H_{3S} isoform (Figure 6).

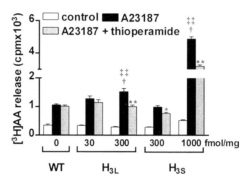

Figure 6 : Constitutive activity and pharmacology of H_{3S} or H_{3L} receptors expressed in CHO cells. Effects of thioperamide on [³H]AA release evoked by 2 µM A23187 in CHO cells expressing various densities of the two H_3-receptor isoforms. Means ± SEM of 3-10 determinations in an experiment that was replicated with similar data. *P<0.05, **P<0.001 vs A23187 alone; †P<0.001 vs wild-type cells; ‡P<0.01; ‡‡P<0.001 vs CHO(H_{3S}) cells expressing 300 fmol/mg protein (ANOVA followed by Newman-Keuls test).

These observations suggested that constitutive H_3-receptor activity was likely to occur in brain where the H_{3L} isoform predominates and where the density of [125I]iodoproxyfan binding sites [22] is presumably more than 500 fmol/mg protein in cells expressing the H_3 receptor (assuming that these cells represent less than 20% of the total). To assess this possibility, we needed to identify ligands displaying well-defined agonist, inverse agonist, and neutral antagonist properties in cell lines and, then to determine the effects of these probes at the native cerebral receptor. Neutral antagonists are not easily identified because, theoretically, they correspond to ligands displaying equal affinity for the active and inactive receptor conformations, a condition obviously difficult to achieve [24,25]. In agreement, a large number of tested antagonists (defined by their ability to block the histamine response at the autoreceptor inhibiting [³H]histamine release from synaptosomes) behaved as potent inverse agonists : they decreased [³H]arachidonic acid (AA) release from CHO cells at concentrations up to two orders of magnitude less than those required to antagonize histamine at the H_3 autoreceptor in synaptosomes. This included FUB 465 (ethyl-3-(1*H*-imidazol-4-yl)propyl ether), an antagonist with only micromolar affinity at the synaptosomal autoreceptor and exerting inverse agonist activity with an EC_{50} of ~10 nM in CHO(H_3) cells (Figure 7).

6. PROXYFAN, A NEUTRAL ANTAGONIST ON SELECTED TESTS

After testing a large variety of compounds, we identified proxyfan (3-(1*H*-imidazol-4-yl)propyl-phenylmethyl ether) as a potent (Ki ~10 nM) neutral antagonist : i) it inhibited the effects of histamine at the synaptosomal H_3 autoreceptor, ii) in CHO(H_3) cells with moderate expression, it inhibited those of the agonist imetit as well as those of the inverse agonists ciproxifan and FUB 465, without affecting [^{3}H]AA release alone, even at a 10 µM concentration (Figure 7). As expected, however, the pharmacological profile of proxyfan depended on the test system, i.e. on the equilibrium between the active and inactive conformations of the receptor and/or the stoichiometric ratio of the receptor to the various G proteins : proxyfan displayed partial inverse agonism on [^{3}H]AA release in CHO cells with high expression and partial agonism when cAMP was evaluated. Hence, the compound can be used as a neutral antagonist only after careful assessment of its effect on the test system which is selected.

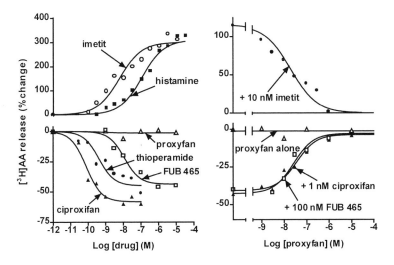

Figure 7 : Effects of H_3-receptor ligands on A23187-evoked [^{3}H]AA release from CHO cells expressing the H_{3S} receptor (500 fmol/mg protein). Release (cpm/well) evoked byA23187 was of 1281 ± 59 (over a basal value of 584 ± 28) and data are expressed in percent change of this value. Proxyfan (3-(1*H*-imidazol-4-yl)propyl-phenylmethyl ether) antagonized the effects of imetit, an agonist, and ciproxifan or FUB 465 (ethyl-3-(1*H*-imidazol-4-yl ether), two inverse agonists.

7. CONSTITUTIVE ACTIVITY OF THE NATIVE H₃R STUDIED ON BRAIN TISSUES *IN VITRO*

The constitutive activity of the H_3 autoreceptor controlling [³H]histamine release could be evidenced in cortical synaptosomes submitted to a strong depolarizing stimulus (40-55 mM K^+) in the mouse or rat. In agreement, both thioperamide and FUB 465 behaved as inverse agonists enhancing significantly the amine release, release being on the contrary reduced by the agonist imetit. Proxyfan, which alone did not affect [³H]histamine release, blocked the opposite effects of either thioperamide and FUB 465 or imetit, therefore acting again as a neutral antagonist (Figure 8). Clearly these responses could not involve endogenous histamine, and the endogenous amine level, even in the 55 mM K^+ medium, was two orders of magnitude less than its EC_{50} value as an agonist (5.3 ± 0.2 nM vs 200 ± 50 nM). That blockade of the H_3-autoreceptor stimulation by endogenous histamine does not significantly contribute to the releasing effect of drugs like thioperamide is also shown by i) the lack of releasing effect of proxyfan, acting here as a potent neutral antagonist, ii) the potent releasing effect of FUB 465, a potent inverse agonist at the H_3R mediating [³H]AA release (EC_{50}~10 nM) but weak neutral antagonist when opposed to histamine regarding the [³H]amine release (K_i = 580 nM).

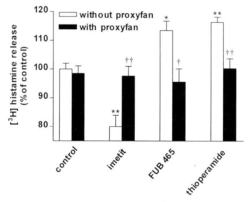

Figure 8 : Effects of H_3-receptor ligands on the K^+-induced release of [³H]histamine from mouse cortical synaptosomes. Drugs (100 nM) were added with 55 mM K^+ and, when required, 10 µM proxyfan. Means ± SEM of 12-40 determinations from four separate experiments. *P<0.01; **P<0.001 vs control; †P<0.01; ††P<0.001 vs without proxyfan (ANOVA followed by Newman-Keuls test).

In addition, binding of the guanylnucleotide analogue [³⁵S]GTPγ[S] to mouse (or rat, not shown) cerebral membranes, demonstrated the coupling of the native H_3 receptor with G proteins [26], i.e. constitutive activity (Figure 9) . Thus, specific [³⁵S]GTPγ[S] binding was significantly reduced by FUB 465, ciproxifan or thioperamide, which were acting as inverse agonists as their effects were blocked by 1 µM proxyfan. Proxyfan also blocked the increase in binding elicited by imetit, but did not itself significantly affect binding, and was therefore acting again as a neutral antagonist in this test system. In contrast with this pattern, yohimbine, an inverse agonist at overexpressed or mutated α_2-adrenergic receptors, failed to decrease [³⁵S]GTPγ[S] binding to cerebral membranes, indicating that constitutive receptor activity is not an inevitable consequence of the experimental conditions required to evaluate the binding, as previously proposed [24].

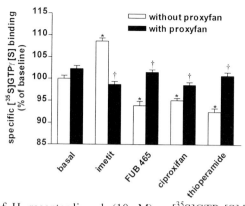

Figure 9 : Effects of H_3-receptor ligands (10 nM) on [^{35}S]GTPγ[S] binding to mouse cerebral cortical membranes in the presence or absence of 1 μM proxyfan. Means ± SEM of 9-24 determinations from four separate experiments. *P<0.001 vs basal; †P<0.01 vs without proxyfan (ANOVA followed by Newman-Keuls test).

8. CONSTITUTIVE ACTIVITY OF THE NATIVE H_3R CONTROLLING BRAIN HISTAMINERGIC NEURON ACTIVITY *IN VIVO*

Three inverse agonists markedly enhanced cerebral histamine neuron activity *in vivo*, increasing by ~80% at maximum the levels of the histamine metabolite *tele*-methylhistamine (t-MeHA), a reliable marker of this activity (Figure 10), and increasing histamine turnover as evaluated by the pargylin-induced t-MeHA accumulation in brain (not shown). This effect reflects an inverse agonist rather than the antagonist activity (towards endogenous histamine) of these ligands, as assumed so far [2, 27]. In agreement, the effect of FUB 465 obtained at a low dose (ED_{50} ~1 mg/kg, p.o.) was more consistent with its nanomolar potency as an inverse agonist than its micromolar potency as an antagonist. Moreover, the increases in t-MeHA level by FUB 465 and ciproxifan were competitively antagonized by proxyfan given at doses of ~2 mg/kg which also blocked the decrease in t-MeHA level induced by the agonist imetit. At these doses, proxyfan administered alone failed to affect significantly t-MeHA levels, indicating that it was acting as a neutral antagonist *in vivo* on a system regulated by H_3 receptors displaying constitutive activity. The small but significant increase (by ~20%) observed with proxyfan in doses above 10 mg/kg, might reflect its antagonist activity towards endogenous histamine.

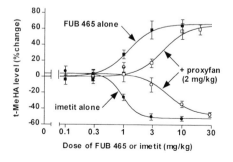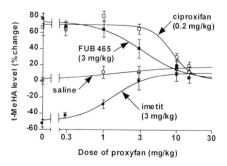

Figure 10 : Changes in brain t-MeHA levels in mice receiving H_3-receptor ligands (p.o.) and killed 90 min thereafter. Means ± SEM of 8-16 values expressed as percent change of values obtained in vehicle-treated mice (119 ± 4 ng/g).

9. CONCLUSIONS

The cloning of the H₃R gene has allowed to initiate a series of novel studies which have already brought to light a number of interesting informations and also raised new questions. The existence of variants of the H₃R were already suggested before this cloning, namely starting from the observation of complex binding data. Although this aspect was not really clarified so far, the existence of splice variants could be established. It remains to understand the functional significance, if any, of these variants.

In addition the molecular genetic studies have established two aspects of the H₃R pharmacology which have already important implications in terms of drug development. The first one is the confirmation of important pharmacological differences of the human as compared to rodent H₃Rs, at least for some antagonists. The second one is the important role of constitutive activity in the function of the H₃R as an autoreceptor, which suggests that the drugs we have to look for are full inverse agonists rather than antagonists in order to enhance cerebral histamine release and thereby improve vigilance, cognition satiety or vestibular reflexes.

REFERENCES

1. J.-M. Arrang, M. Garbarg and J.-C. Schwartz, Nature, 302 (1983) 832.
2. J.-M. Arrang, M. Garbarg, J.-C. Lancelot, J.-M. Lecomte, H. Pollard, M. Robba, W. Schunack and J.-C. Schwartz, Nature, 327 (1987) 117.
3. S.J. Hill, C.R. Ganellin, H. Timmerman, J.-C. Schwartz, N.P. Shankley, J.M. Young, W. Schunack, R. Levi and H.L. Haas, Pharmacol. Rev., 49 (1997) 253.
4. T.W. Lovenberg, B.L. Roland, S.J. Wilson, X. Piang, J. Pyati, A. Huvar, M.R. Jackson and M.G. Erlander, Mol. Pharmacol., 55 (1999) 1101.
5. S. Morisset, A. Rouleau, X. Ligneau, F. Gbahou, J. Tardivel-Lacombe, H. Stark, W. Schunack, C.R. Ganellin, J-C. Schwartz and J-M. Arrang, Nature, 408 (2000) 860.
6. S. Morisset, A. Sasse, F. Gbahou, A. Héron, X. Ligneau, J. Tardivel-Lacombe, J.-C. Schwartz and J.-M. Arrang, Biochem. Biophys. Res. Commun., (2000) in press.
7. X. Ligneau, S. Morisset, J. Tardivel-Lacombe, F. Gbahou, C.R. Ganellin, H. Stark, W. Schunack, J.-C. Schwartz, and J.-M. Arrang, Br. J. Pharmacol., 131 (2000) 1247.
8. T.W. Lovenberg, J. Pyati, H. Chang, S.J Wilson and M.G. Erlander, J. Pharmacol. Exp. Ther., 293 (2000) 771.
9. J. Tardivel-Lacombe, S. Morisset, F. Gbahou, J.-C. Schwartz and J.-M. Arrang, NeuroReport, 12 (2001) in press.
10. J. Tardivel-Lacombe, A. Rouleau, A. Héron, S. Morisset, C. Pillot, V. Cochois, J.-C Schwartz, and J.-M. Arrang, NeuroReport, 11 (2000) 755.
11. E.A. Harper, N.P. Shankley, and J.W. Black, Brit. J. Pharmacol., 128 (1999) 751.
12. E. Schlicker, M. Kathmann, H. Bitschnau, I. Marr, S. Reidemeister, H. Stark and W. Schunack, Naunyn-Schmiedeberg's Arch. Pharmacol., 353 (1996) 482.
13. R.E. West, A. Zweig, N.Y. Shih, M.I. Siegel, R.W. Egan and M.A. Clark, Mol. Pharmacol., 38 (1990) 610.
14. J.-M. Arrang, B. Devaux, J.-P. Chodkiewicz and J.-C. Schwartz, J. Neurochem., 51 (1988) 105.
15. R.E. West, R.L. Wu, M.M. Billah, R.W. Egan and J.C. Anthes, Eur. J. Pharmacol., 377 (1999) 233.

16. Y. Cherifi, C. Pigeon, M. Le Romancer, A. Bado, F. Reyl-Desmars and M.J.M. Lewin, J. Biol. Chem., 267 (1992) 25315.
17. X. Ligneau, J.-S. Lin, G. Vanni-Mercier, M. Jouvet, J.L. Muir, C.R. Ganellin, H. Stark, S. Elz, W. Schunack. and J.-C. Schwartz, J. Pharmacol. Exp. Ther. 287 (1998) 658.
18. H. Van der Goot, M.J.P. Schepers, G.H. Sterk and H. Timmerman, Eur. J. Med. Chem., 27 (1992) 511.
19. H. Stark, A. Hüls, X. Ligneau, K. Purand, H. Pertz, J.-M. Arrang, J.-C. Schwartz and W. Schunack, Arch. Pharm. Pharm. Med. Chem., 331 (1998) 211.
20. H. Stark, X. Ligneau, J.-M. Arrang, J.-C. Schwartz and W. Schunack, Bioorg. Med. Chem. Lett., 8 (1998) 2011.
21. P. Samama, S. Cotecchia, T. Costa and R.J. Lefkowitz, J. Biol. Chem., 268 (1993) 4625.
22. X. Ligneau, M. Garbarg, M.L. Vizuete, J. Diaz, K. Purand, H. Stark, W. Schunack and J.C. Schwartz, J. Pharmacol. Exp. Ther., 271 (1994) 452.
23. E.A. Clark and S.J. Hill, Brit. J. Pharmacol., 114 (1995) 357.
24. T. Costa, Y. Ogino, P.J. Munson, H.O. Onaran and D. Rodbard, Mol. Pharmacol.,41 (1992) 549.
25. G. Milligan, R.A. Bond and M. Lee, Trends Pharmacol. Sci., 16 (1995) 10.
26. E.A. Clark and S.J. Hill, Eur. J. Pharmacol., 296 (1996) 223.
27. M. Garbarg, M.D. Trung Tuong, C. Gros and J.-C. Schwartz, Eur. J. Pharmacol., 164 (1989) 1.

CNS Overviews

Histamine Research in the New Millennium
T. Watanabe, H. Timmerman and K. Yanai (Editors)

25

The discovery of potent non-imidazole H₃-receptor histamine antagonists

C. Robin Ganellin[a]*, Fabien Leurquin[a], Antonia Piripitsi[a], Jean-Michel Arrang[b], Monique Garbarg[b], Xavier Ligneau[c], Holger Stark[d], Walter Schunack[d] and Jean-Charles Schwartz[b]

[a] Department of Chemistry, University College London, Christopher Ingold Laboratories, 20 Gordon Street, London, WC1H OAJ, U.K.

[b] Unité de Neurobiologie et Pharmacologie Moléculaire (U.109) de l'INSERM, Centre Paul Broca, 2 ter rue d'Alésia, 75014 Paris, France.

[c] Laboratoire Bioprojet, 9 rue Rameau, 75002 Paris, France.

[d] Institut für Pharmazie, Freie Universität Berlin, Königin-Luise-Strasse 2+4, 14195 Berlin, Germany.

Histamine has been converted into a non-imidazole H₃-receptor histamine antagonist by addition of a 4-phenylbutyl group at the N^α - position followed by removal of the imidazole ring. The resulting compound, *N*-ethyl-N-(4-phenylbutyl)amine, remarkably has a $K_i = 1.3$ µM as an H₃ antagonist. Using this as a lead compound, a novel series of homologous O and S isosteric tertiary amines was synthesised and structure-activity studies furnished *N*-(5-phenoxypentyl)pyrrolidine ($K_i = 0.18 \pm 0.10$ µM, for [³H]histamine release from rat cerebral cortex synaptosomes) which, more importantly, was active *in vivo*. Substitution of CN into the *para* position of the phenoxy group gave N-(5-*p*-cyanophenoxypropyl)piperidine. UCL 1980 ($K_i = 19 \pm 7$ nM), $ED_{50} = 1.9 \pm 1.2$ mg/kg *per os* in mice on brain *tele*-methylhistamine levels. Further optimisation of this structure gave UCL 2138, *N*-(3-*p*-cyanophenoxypropyl)-piperidine. $K_i = 11 \pm 1.5$ nM, $ED_{50} = 0.20 \pm 0.07$ mg/kg.

1. INTRODUCTION

There is considerable interest in obtaining a potent centrally acting H₃-receptor histamine antagonist. Such a compound entering the brain would lead to an increase in histamine transmission through histaminergic pathways. It would be investigated for potential therapeutic applications such as schizophrenia, attention deficit hyperactivity disorder, age-related memory and learning deficits, Alzheimer's disease, sleep disorders (e.g. narcolepsy) and disruption in circadian sleep patterns [1,2].

The archetypal prototype H₃-antagonist is thioperamide (1) but, although it is potent *in vitro* ($K_i = 4$ nM) it has a relatively high ED_{50} of *ca* 1 mg/kg in vivo when given *per os* to the mouse [3] and assayed for its effect on *tele*-methylhistamine, the primary catabolite of histamine in the brain. Thus, although it does penetrate the blood-brain barrier it does not do so readily [4].

Passive access of molecules to the brain is dependent on their physicochemical properties which can be described [5] by equation (1). where the Brain/Blood ratio (BB) is increased by molecular contributions described by R (excess molar refraction) and V (molar volume of McGowan) but decreased by Π (dipolarity and polarisability), $\Sigma\alpha$ (sum of hydrogen-bond acidity) and $\Sigma\beta$ (sum of hydrogen-bond basicity).

(1) Thioperamide

$$\log BB = c_1 + c_2 R - c_3 \Pi - c_4 \Sigma\alpha - c_5 \Sigma\beta + c_6 V \qquad (1)$$

Thus polar groups which make hydrogen bonds have a pronounced effect in reducing drug access to the brain.

Thioperamide possesses an imidazole ring and a thiourea group and both these structural features are polar and strongly hydrogen-bonding and they have considerable negative effects on brain penetration. For over a decade, medicinal chemists have been seeking to make H_3 antagonists which do not contain these moieties.

2. GENERATION OF A LEAD COMPOUND

Table 1
Compounds where the 4(5)-substituted imidazole ring has been replaced. Comparison of H_3-antagonists activities with the 4(5)-substituted imidazole analogues [8]

UCL	Structure		$K_i{}^a$ (nM)	cf [b] (nM)
1031			3100	330
1200			1000	29
1264		R=NO$_2$	2500	29
1265		R=CF$_3$	1300	17
1282			$\gg$1000	13

[a]K$^+$-evoked [³H]histamine release assay *in vitro* on synaptosomes of rat cerebral cortex [13]; [b]K$_i$ for the corresponding 4(5)-imidazole analogue

Attempts to replace the imidazole ring by other heterocycles have led to a considerable reduction in potency [6,7] e.g. structures in Table 1 [8]. Until recently, all potent H_3-receptor ligands possessed an imidazole ring with a side chain in the 4(5)-position and no other ring substituent.

As an approach to discovering a non-imidazole compound we considered the nature of the chemical changes needed to convert an agonist into an antagonist. For example, introduction of additional groups into the molecule which can locate accessory binding sites at the receptor, and then removal of the imidazole ring to yield a non-imidazole antagonist. To start with, however, there was no obvious indications as to which groups might be effective for binding, or which positions in the histamine molecule would be the most appropriate for substitution.

Previous work has shown that methylation of histamine in the imidazole ring greatly reduces agonist activity [9] but that methylation in the side chain actually increases potency [10], presumably through increasing the affinity for the receptor. It was of interest therefore to observe that N^{α}-(4-phenylbutyl)histamine (2) was a pure antagonist of histamine at the H_3 receptor with a $K_i = \mu M$ [11] (Table 2). Removal of the imidazole ring from this structure led to the synthesis and testing of N-ethyl-N-(4-phenylbutyl)amine (3) which, remarkably, was found to have a $K_i = 1.3$ μM as an H_3-receptor histamine antagonist [12]. Thus removal of the imidazole ring had led merely to a twofold drop in affinity and had successfully produced the necessary lead to generate a non-imidazole H_3-receptor histamine antagonist.

3. STRUCTURE-ACTIVITY FINDINGS

Table 2
N^{α}-(4-Phenylbutyl)histamine provides the lead for a non-imidazole H_3-antagonist

	Structure	Action	$K_i{}^a$ (μM)
	CH₂CH₂NH₂ Histamine, HN—N	Agonist	
2	CH₂CH₂NH–(CH₂)₄–Ph, HN—N	Antagonist	0.7
3	$CH_3CH_2NH-(CH_2)_4-Ph$	Antagonist	1.3
4	$CH_3CH_2N-(CH_2)_4-Ph$, Me	Antagonist	1.1

^{a}see footnote a of Table 1

The compounds were tested for histamine antagonism at the H_3-receptor in an *in vitro* functional assay on synaptosomes of rat cerebral cortex [13] and, *in vivo*, given orally to mice for their effect on brain *tele*-methylhistamine levels [13].

In order to improve the accessibility of compounds and facilitate the structure-activity exploration, ether isosteres were examined (Table 3). The sulfur isostere (6) of 3 was not active but, surprisingly, *N*-ethylation to give the tertiary amine 8 increased affinity by nearly an order of magnitude ($K_i = 0.18$ μM). Homologues (n = 4-5) were also examined (compounds 9-12) and found to be similarly active *in vitro* and, interestingly, compound 12 (n = 5) was active *in vivo* ($ED_{50} \approx 15$ mg/kg *per os*) [14].

Similar results were obtained with the oxygen ether series, with n = 3-6. The optimum chain length appeared to be n = 5 for *in vivo* activity in both series.

The phenoxypentylamine structure was then optimised for activity with respect to the tertiary amino group (Table 4). Most of the series showed little variation in activity *in vitro*, but NPr_2 (17) and *N*-methylpiperazino (22) were distinctly less active.

Most important, however, was the finding that the pyrrolidino and piperidino compounds were active orally *in vivo*, with the former being of special interest, having an ED_{50} value of 3.4 mg/kg. It is apparent that the amino group is a determinant of *in vivo* activity; potency decreases in the order $N(CH_2)_4 > N(CH_2)_5 > N(CH_3)C_2H_5 > N(C_3H_7)C_2H_5$ but there is no obvious overall correlation, either with carbon content or size.

Substituents were then introduced into the phenoxy group of the pyrrolidine derivative 18

Table 3
Ether isosteres (O and S). Comparison of homologues as H_3 antagonists

	X	n	R	*in vitro* K_i^a (μM)	*in vivo* ED_{50}^b (mg/kg)
5	O	3	H	ca 5	n.d.^{c}
6	S	3	H	> 5	n.d.
7	O	3	C_2H_5	0.35 ± 0.01	> 10
8	S	3	C_2H_5	0.18 ± 0.04	> 10
9	O	4	C_2H_5	0.11 ± 0.02	> 10
10	S	4	C_2H_5	0.19 ± 0.03	> 10
11	O	5	C_2H_5	0.23 ± 0.06	17 ± 4
12	S	5	C_2H_5	0.34 ± 0.08	ca 15
13	O	6	C_2H_5	ca 0.2	> 10

^{a}K^+-evoked [^{3}H]histamine release assay *in vitro* on synaptosomes of rat cerebral cortex [13]; ^{b}*in vivo* assay after *per os* administration to mice, measuring the modulation of *tele*-methylhistamine level in the brain [13]; ^{c}n.d.= not determined

Table 4
Phenoxypentylamines. Comparison of different amino groups for H_3 antagonism

$O-(CH_2)_5-NR^1R^2$

	R^1	R^2	in vitro K_i^a (μM)	in vivo ED_{50}^b (mg/kg)
14	CH_3	CH_3	0.31 ± 0.10	> 10
15	CH_3	C_2H_5	0.36 ± 0.15	ca 10
16	C_2H_5	C_3H_7	0.46 ± 0.11	> 10
17	C_3H_7	C_3H_7	ca 1.5	> 10
18	$CH_2 - (CH_2)_2 - CH_2$		0.18 ± 0.10	3.4 ± 1.7
19	$CH_2 - (CH_2)_3 - CH_2$		0.14 ± 0.07	6.9 ± 3.1
20	$CH_2 - (CH_2)_4 - CH_2$		0.12 ± 0.05	> 10
21	$(CH_2)_2 - O - (CH_2)_2$		0.64 ± 0.28	> 10
22	$(CH_2)_2 - N (CH_3) - (CH_2)_2$		2.8 ± 0.7	> 10

$^{a, b}$see footnotes of Table 3

and the compounds 33-35 were tested *in vivo*. Activity was found to be in the potency order *p*-NO$_2$>*p*-COCH$_3$>*p*-CN>*p*-NH$_2$>*p*-F>*p*-Cl>*m*-Cl~*m*-NO$_2$~*m*-CN>*p*-Me. The *p*-NO$_2$, *p*-CN and *p*-COCH$_3$ compounds 28, 30 and 34, being the most potent (ED$_{50}$ = 1.1 to 1.9 mg/kg *per os*).

4. OPTIMISATION OF STRUCTURE FOR IN VIVO POTENCY

Taking the *p*-CN and *p*-COCH$_3$ phenoxy groups the structures were then altered to reoptimise them with respect to *in vivo* activity (Table 6). Now, the diethylamino (NEt$_2$) or piperidino (N(CH$_2$)$_5$ or pip.) amines were found to yield very potent compounds when n = 3 or 4 [15]. Thus UCL 2138 (R = CN, n = 3, NR^{1}R^2 = pip.) had ED$_{50}$ = 0.20 $\pm$ 0.07 mg/kg *per os* with a K_i = 10.9 $\pm$ 1.5 nM.

This represents a very important finding since this compound is approximately five times more potent than thioperamide *in vivo* although it has only about one third of the potency *in vitro*. Presumably therefore UCL 2138 has inherently less affinity for the H_3 receptor but its greater *in vivo* potency is consistent with better brain penetrability.

Subsequent to this work others have reported on non-imidazole H_3 receptor antagonists [16,17] but there is no indication that they are sufficiently active *in vivo*.

Table 5
Phenoxypentylpyrrolidines. Effect of substituents on H_3 antagonist activity

	R	in vitro K_i^a (μM)	in vivo ED_{50}^b (mg/kg)
23	4-CH$_3$	0.11 ± 0.05	ca 20
24	4-OCH$_3$	0.053 ± 0.016	> 10
25	4-F	0.11 ± 0.03	5.1 ± 1.8
26	4-Cl	0.13 ± 0.05	7.3 ± 3.4
27	3-Cl	0.21 ± 0.06	ca 10
28	4-NO$_2$	0.039 ± 0.011	1.1 ± 0.6
29	3-NO$_2$	0.10 ± 0.04	ca 10
30	4-CN	0.019 ± 0.007	1.9 ± 1.2
31	3-CN	0.073 ± 0.020	ca 10
32	4-C$_6$H$_5$	0.41 ± 0.18	2.8 ± 0.8
33	3-C$_6$H$_5$	n.d.^{c}	> 10
34	4-COCH$_3$	0.019 ± 0.003	1.5 ± 0.8
35	4-NH$_2$	0.10 ± 0.05	2.6 ± 0.9

$^{a, b, c}$see footnotes of Table 3

Table 6
H_3 -Receptor antagonist potencies of reoptimised structures

UCL	R	n	NR^{1}R^2	in vitro K_i^a (nM)	in vivo ED_{50}^b (mg/kg)
2092	CN	3	NEt$_2$	95 ± 28	0.50 ± 0.15
2138	CN	3	pip	11 ± 1.5	0.20 ± 0.07
2133	CN	4	NEt$_2$	62 ± 15	1.1 ± 0.5
2104	COCH$_3$	3	NEt$_2$	20 ± 7	0.44 ± 0.10
2180	COEt	3	pip	4.7 ± 0.8	0.60 ± 0.16

$^{a, b}$see footnotes of Table 3

REFERENCES

1. R. Leurs, P. Blandina, C. Tedford, H. Timmerman, Trends Pharmacol. Sci., 19 (1998) 177.
2. J.G. Phillips, S.M. Ali, S.L. Yates and C.E. Tedford, Ann. Rep. Med. Chem., 33 (1998) 31.
3. J.-M. Arrang, M. Garbarg, J.-C. Lancelot, J.-M. Lecomte, H. Pollard, M. Robba, W. Schunack, J.-C. Schwartz, Nature (London), 327 (1987) 117.
4. E. Sakurai, E. Gunji, Y. Iizuka, N. Hikichi, K. Maeyama, T. Watanabe, J. Pharm. Pharmacol., 46 (1994) 209.
5. H.S. Chadha, M.H. Abraham, R.C. Mitchell, BioMed. Chem. Lett., 4 (1994) 2511.
6. C.R. Ganellin, D. Jayes, Y.S. Khalaf, W. Tertiuk, J.-M. Arrang, N. Defontaine, J.-C. Schwartz, Coll. Czech. Chem. Commun., 56 (1991) 2448.
7. K. Kiec-Kononowicz, X. Ligneau, H. Stark, J.-C. Schwartz, W. Schunack, Arch. Pharm. Pharm. Med. Chem., 328 (1995) 445.
8. C.R. Ganellin, S.K. Hosseini, Y.S. Khalaf, W. Tertiuk, J.-M. Arrang, M. Garbarg, X. Ligneau and J.-C. Schwartz, J. Med. Chem., 38 (1995) 3342.
9. J.-M. Arrang, M. Garbarg, J.-C. Schwartz, Nature (London), 302 (1983) 832.
10. J-M. Arrang, M. Garbarg, J.-C. Schwartz, R. Lipp, H. Stark, W. Schunack and J-M. Lecomte, New Perspectives in Histamine Research, Birkhauser Verlag, Basel, (1991), pp. 55.
11 R. Lipp, W. Schunack, J.-M. Arrang, M. Garbarg, J.-C. Schwartz, Poster P 119, 10th EFMC International Symposium on Medicinal Chemistry, Budapest, Hungary, August (1988). H. Stark, R. Lipp, J.-M. Arrang, M. Garbarg, J.-C. Schwartz, W. Schunack, Eur. J. Med. Chem., 29 (1994) 695.
12. Y.S. Khalaf. Synthesis and Structure-Activity Studies of Novel H_3-Receptor Histamine Antagonists. Ph.D Thesis, University of London, (1990), p 101.
13. C.R. Ganellin, A. Fkyerat, B. Bang-Andersen, S. Athmani, W. Tertiuk, M. Garbarg, X. Ligneau, J.-C. Schwartz, J. Med. Chem., 39 (1996) 3806-3813.
14. C. R. Ganellin, F. Leurquin, A. Piripitsi, J.-M. Arrang, M. Garbarg, X. Ligneau, W. Schunack and J.-C. Schwartz, Arch. Pharm. Pharm. Med. Chem., 331 (1998) 395.
15. Preparation of aryloxyalkylamines as histamine H_3 receptor antagonists, Eur Patent No. 978512 (2000).
16. K. Walczynski, R. Guryn, O.P. Zuiderveld and H. Timmerman, Arch. Pharm. Pharm. Med. Chem., 332 (1999) 389.
17. I.D. Linney, I.M. Buck, E.A. Harper, S.B. Kalindjian, M.J. Pether, N.P. Shankley, G.F. Watt and P.T. Wright, J. Med. Chem., 43 (2000) 2362.

Histamine Research In the New Millennium
T. Watanabe, H. Timmerman and K. Yanai (Editors)

Histaminergic and cholinergic transmission in cognitive processes

Athineos Philippu* **, Helmut Prast*, Michaela M. Kraus

Department of Pharmacology and Toxicology, Institute of Pharmacy, University of Innsbruck, Peter-Mayr-Strasse 1, Innsbruck, Austria

The activity of histaminergic neurons is permanently modulated by neighbouring cholinergic neurons via M_1 receptors, cholinergic transmission by histaminergic neurons through H_1, H_2, H_{3A} and H_{3B} receptors. In the nucleus accumbens, glutamatergic neurons originating from the hippocampus modulate cholinergic transmission in a direct and an indirect way via stimulation of histaminergic neurons. Facilitation of memory by histamine is independent of cholinergic transmission.

1. INTRODUCTION

Histaminergic and cholinergic neurons of the brain have been implicated in cognitive processes. It has been shown that an interrelationship exists between latency in the active avoidance response and the decrease in the brain histamine level [1]. Histamine increases recall in a step-down inhibitory avoidance task when given immediately post-training [2]. Intracerebroventricular injection of histamine seems to facilitate memory in adult [3] and old rats [1]. Cognitive performance of rats in object recognition and in a passive avoidance task is strongly impaired by H_3 receptor agonists which decrease neuronal release of histamine [4]. Furthermore, histamine influences synaptic plasticity in hippocampal slices [5].

There is evidence that histaminergic neurons facilitate memory by modulating cholinergic transmission [6-8]. Dopaminergic, GABAergic and glutamatergic neurons also modulate cholinergic and histaminergic neurons thus influencing their functions. The concept "one transmitter one brain structure one function" has led, and still leads, to erroneous conclusions. The performance of a brain function necessitates the concerted agonistic and antagonistic action of more than one transmitter in more than one brain structure and is partly based on a receptor-mediated neuronal communication. In the following we will outline this neuronal cross-talk and its possible involvement in memory. Transmitter release was investigated under in vivo conditions which warrant the undisturbed engineering of neuronal processes. For this purpose we used the   push-pull   technique   for superfusion of distinct brain areas and determination of transmitters released in the superfusate [9,10]. Because of the good time resolution (11), this

*This work was supported by the Fonds zur Foerderung der wissenschaftlichen Forschung and the **Jubilaeumsfonds der Oesterreichischen Nationalbank

technique is appropriate for the simultaneous assessment of transmitter release and performance of memory or other tasks.

2. CHOLINERGIC NEURONS MODULATE HISTAMINERGIC TRANSMISSION

In vitro experiments with brain slices and synaptosomes revealed that muscarinic acetylcholine receptor agonists reduce the release of histamine, while muscarinic receptor antagonists are ineffective. Determination of turnover led to similar findings [12]. The ineffectiveness of muscarinic antagonists has been interpreted as suggesting that cholinergic neurons may not modulate histamine release in the brain [12-14]. However, the in vivo determination of histamine release in the anterior hypothalamic area by the push-pull superfusion technique has led to different conclusions.

The release of histamine in the anterior hypothalamic area is tetrodotoxin (TTX)-sensitive but compound 48/80 resistant. Thus, histamine released in the superfusate seems to be, at least to a major part, of neuronal origin [15]. The non-selective antagonist of muscarinic receptors atropine enhances the release of histamine in a concentration-dependent way. The release of histamine is also enhanced, when the hypothalamus is superfused with the selective M_1 receptor antagonist pirenzepine. Similarly, histamine release rate in the hypothalamus is enhanced on superfusion with 4-diphenylacetoxy-N-methylpiperidine (4-DAMP) that predominantly blocks M_1 and M_3 receptors. On the other hand, the selective M_2 muscarinic receptor antagonist methoctramine and the selective M_3 receptor antagonist p-fluorohexahydro-sila-difenidol (p-F-HHSiD), are ineffective.

Since hypothalamic superfusion with antagonists of the muscarinic receptors increase histamine release rate, acetylcholine released from cholinergic neurons of this brain region seems to modulate the release of histamine from neighbouring histaminergic neurons. The findings that the release of histamine is enhanced by selective antagonists of M_1 receptors, while antagonists of M_2 and M_3 receptors are ineffective, demonstrate that mainly M_1 muscarinic receptors, located as heteroreceptors on histaminergic neurons, are involved in the modulation of histamine transmission by cholinergic neurons in the anterior hypothalamus [15].

3. HISTAMINERGIC NEURONS MODULATE CHOLINERGIC TRANSMISSION

Because of the relatively low concentration of acetylcholine in the hypothalamic superfusate [16], effects on the release of acetylcholine by fluoromethylhistidine (FMH), that inhibits biosynthesis of histamine [17], histamine receptor ligands and other receptor ligands were studied in the nucleus accumbens (ventral striatum) that possesses a high density of cholinergic neurons.

Superfusion of the nucleus accumbens with histamine increases the acetylcholine release rate in a concentration-dependent way [18]. The release of acetylcholine elicited by histamine is attenuated in the presence of the D_1 receptor antagonist (±)-7-bromo-8-hydroxy-3-methyl-1-phenyl-2,3,4,5-tetrahydro-1H-3-

benzazepine hydrochloride (SKF-83566) and the $D_{2/3}$ agonist quinpirole. When combined, these compounds remove the dopaminergic modulation of acetylcholine release [18-19]. Thus, the effect of histamine on acetylcholine outflow is partly mediated through dopaminergic neurons.

Besides dopaminergic neurons, GABAergic neurons also modulate acetylcholine release because, in the nucleus accumbens, acetylcholine outflow is greatly enhanced by the $GABA_A$ receptor antagonist bicuculline [18,20].

The release by histamine of acetylcholine indicates that histaminergic neurons modulate the release of acetylcholine. This idea is supported by the finding that superfusion with FMH elicits a gradual, long-lasting decrease in the release of ace-tylcholine. The decrease in acetylcholine release elicited by FMH is due to the progressive inhibition of histamine synthesis in this brain region [18]. The data obtained with FMH and histamine show that cholinergic neurons of the ventral striatum are permanently modulated by histamine released from neighbouring histaminergic neurons. The question arises now, which histamine receptors are in-volved in the modulation of acetylcholine release by histamine.

3.1. H_1 receptors

In the nucleus accumbens superfusion with the H_1 receptor agonist 2-thiazolylethylamine (TEA) elevates acetylcholine outflow, while the H_1 receptor antagonist triprolidine elicits the opposite effect. Moreover, triprolidine abolishes the TEA- and histamine-induced release of acetylcholine [19]. These results suggest that in the striatum cholinergic neurotransmission is modulated by neighbouring histaminergic neurons via H_1 receptors. Since removal of the dopaminergic modulation in the presence of quinpirole and SKF-83566 does not influence the inhibition of acetylcholine release elicited by triprolidine, the H_1 receptors seem to be located on cholinergic neurons and to possess functional importance to acetylcholine release.

3.2. H_2 receptors

H_2 receptors are also involved in the modulation of acetylcholine release [19]. In the nucleus accumbens, the outflow of the neurotransmitter is enhanced by the H_2 receptor antagonists famotidine and ranitidine, while the H_2 agonist impromidine exerts the opposite effect. However, the H_2 agonist dimaprit promotes acetylcholine outflow; this effect is not influenced by FMH but is strongly enhanced by the $GABA_A$ receptor antagonist bicuculline. The releasing effect of famotidine is abolished by FMH and SKF-83566 combined with quinpirole. In the presence of bicuculline the releasing effect of famotidine is reversed to a reduced release.

3.3. H_3 receptors

The H_3 receptor antagonists thioperamide and clobenpropit enhance the release rate of acetylcholine. The releasing effect of thioperamide is abolished, when the striatum is presuperfused with FMH thus indicating the dependence on endogenous histamine. The release of acetylcholine elicited by thioperamide is greatly diminished in the presence of SKF-83566 and quinpirole [18]. Acetylcholine release is also increased on superfusion with the H_3 agonists imetit and immepip. However, the releasing effects of these drugs are FMH-resistant.

The findings show that H_1, H_2 and H_3 receptors are involved in the modulation of cholinergic transmission. Histamine released from histaminergic neurons enhances cholinergic transmission by stimulating H_1 receptors located on cholinergic neurons. This seems to be the dominating effect. Via H_2 receptors histamine inhibits dopaminergic and GABAergic activity thus modulating indirectly cholinergic transmission. By acting on H_2 receptors located on cholinergic neurons, histamine either promotes, or inhibits acetylcholine release probably via stimulating of H_2 receptor subtypes. Furthermore, histamine modulates its own release via H_3 autoreceptors (site of action of thioperamide) and cholinergic activity through H_3 heteroreceptors on dopaminergic neurons and, possibly, cholinergic neurons (sites of action of imetit and immepip). The findings obtained with H_3 receptor agonists and antagonists point to the involvement of H_{3A} and H_{3B} receptor subtypes in the modulation of acetylcholine release.

4. HIPPOCAMPUS STIMULATION INCREASES ACETYLCHOLINE RELEASE IN THE NUCLEUS ACCUMBENS

The nucleus accumbens receives glutamatergic innervation from the fornix/fimbria tract [21]. Electrical stimulation of the hippocampal afferents increases the outflow of glutamate and acetylcholine in the nucleus accumbens in a TTX-sensitive way. The stimulation-induced release of both acetylcholine and glutamate is enhanced on superfusion of the nucleus accumbens with histamine, and the histamine effect is abolished by triprolidine (Table 1). Moreover, the stimulation-induced release of acetylcholine is abolished by the NMDA receptor antagonists ($\pm$)-2-amino-5-phosphonopentanoic acid (AP-5) and 6,7-dinitroquinoxaline-2,3-dione (DNQX). Hence, glutamatergic neurons of the hippocampus modulate the release of acetylcholine in the nucleus accumbens in a dual way: glutamate stimulates directly acetylcholine release by activating NMDA receptors located on cholinergic neurons and indirectly by stimulating NMDA receptors located on histaminergic neurons thus releasing histamine which, in turn, enhances cholinergic and glutamatergic transmission via H_1 receptors (unpublished observations).

5. HISTAMINERGIC AND CHOLINERGIC TRANSMISSION IN COGNITION

We have used the olfactory, social memory test [22] to investigate the effects of FMH and histamine receptor ligands on short-term memory. The test is based on the time needed by an adult rat to recognize a young rat. Intracerebroventricular injection of histamine, its precursor histidine or thioperamide, that enhances histamine release, reduces recognition time thus improving short-term memory. On the contrary, inhibition of neuronal histamine synthesis by FMH prolongs recognition time. Since FMH worsens, while short-term memory is improved by thioperamide, histamine and histidine, histaminergic neurons of the brain seem to facilitate memory [23].

Table 1
Effects of electrical stimulation of the hippocampus and drugs applied to the nucleus accumbens on the release of acetylcholine and glutamate in the nucleus accumbens

	Acetylcholine	Glutamate
	Release	
ES	+	+
ES + AP-5	0	
ES + AP-5 + DNQX	0	
ES + histamine	+++	+++
ES + histamine + triprolidine	0	0

ES Electrical stimulation of the hippocampus, + increased release, +++ further increase in release, 0 elimination of ES-induced release by AP-5 and AP-5+DNQX and histamine-induced release by triprolidine

   Determination of acetylcholine revealed that, during exposure of a young rat to an adult rat, its release is increased in the nucleus accumbens of the adult rat, whereby degree of release and recognition time are reduced when exposure is repeated. Moreover, intracerebroventricular administration of thioperamide (5 µg) together with famotidine (20 µg) further diminishes recognition time and acetylcholine outflow in the nucleus accumbens. The findings suggest that the memory facilitating property of histamine may not be dependent on cholinergic transmission. On the other hand, preliminary results indicate that histaminergic neurons are implicated in the aversive stimulus-induced acetylcholine release. The involvement in these processes of other neurons like dopaminergic, GABAergic, glutamatergic neurons, which also modulate histaminergic and cholinergic transmission, is under investigation.

REFERENCES

1. C. Kamei, Y. Okumura and K. Tasaka, Psychopharmacology, 111 (1993) 376.

2. M.A. De Almeida and I. Izquierdo, Arch. Int. Pharmacodyn., 283 (1986) 193.
3. M.A. De Almeida and I. Izquierdo, Arch. Int. Pharmacodyn. Ther., 291 (1988) 202.
4. P. Blandina, M. Giorgetti, L. Bartolini, M. Cecchi, H. Timmerman, R. Leurs, G. Pepeu and M.G. Giovannini, Br. J. Pharmacol., 119 (1996) 1656.
5. H.L. Haas, O.A. Sergueeva, V.S. Vorobjev and I.N. Sharonova, Behav. Brain Res., 66 (1995) 41.
6. S. Miyazaki, M. Imaizumi and K. Onodera, Life Sci., 57 (1995) 2137.
7. P. Ghi, M. Orsetti, S.R. Gamalero and C. Ferretti, Pharmacol. Biochem. Behav., 64 (1999) 761.
8. K. Onodera, S. Miyazaki, M. Imaizumi, H. Stark and W. Schunack, Naunyn-Schmiedeberg's Arch. Pharmacol., 357 (1998) 508.
9. A. Philippu, H. Prast and N. Singewald, Sci. Pharm., 64 (1996) 609.
10. N. Singewald and A. Philippu, Prog. Neurobiol., 56 (1998) 237.
11. A. Philippu, Pharmacopsychiatry, (in press).
12. T. Mochizuki, A. Yamatodani, K. Okakura, M. Takemura, N. Inagaki and H. Wada, Naunyn-Schmiedeberg's Arch. Pharmacol., 343 (1991) 190.
13. R. Oishi, N. Adachi, K. Okada, N. Muroi and K. Saeki, J. Neurochem., 55 (1990) 1899.
14. J. Ono, A. Yamatodani, J. Kishino, S. Okada and H. Wada, Methods Find. Exp. Clin. Pharmacol., 14 (1992) 35.
15. H. Prast, H.P. Fischer, M. Prast and A. Philippu, Naunyn-Schmiedeberg's Arch. Pharmacol., 350 (1994) 599.
16. H. Prast and A. Philippu, Naunyn-Schmiedeberg's Arch. Pharmacol., 346 (1992) 1.
17. J. Kollonitsch, L.M. Perkins, A.A. Patchett, G.A. Doldouras, S. Marburg, D.E. Duggan, A.L. Maycock and S.D. Aster, Nature, 274 (1978) 906.
18. H. Prast, M.H. Tran, H. Fischer, M. Kraus, C. Lamberti, K. Grass and A. Philippu, Naunyn-Schmiedeberg's Arch. Pharmacol., 360 (1999) 558.
19. H. Prast, M.H. Tran, C. Lamberti, H. Fischer, M. Kraus, K. Grass and A. Philippu, Naunyn-Schmiedeberg's Arch. Pharmacol., 360 (1999) 552.
20. H. Prast, M.H. Tran, H. Fischer and A. Philippu, J. Neurochem., 71, (1998) 266.
21. I. Walaas and F. Fonnum, Neuroscience, 5 (1980) 1691.
22. W.J. Carr, L. Yee, D. Gable and E. Marasco, J. Comp. Physiol. Psychol., 90 (1976) 821.
23. H. Prast, A. Argyriou and A. Philippu, Brain Res., 734 (1996) 316.

Histamine Research in the New Millennium
T. Watanabe, H. Timmerman and K. Yanai (Editors)

Physiology and pharmacology of histaminergic neurons

H.L. Haas, R.E. Brown, T. Deller, K.S. Eriksson, O.A. Sergeeva and D. R. Stevens

Department of Physiology, Heinrich-Heine-University, D-40001 Düsseldorf, Germany

INTRODUCTION

Histaminergic tuberomammillary (TM) neurons project to the whole central nervous system and display regular firing related to behavioral state in a beating pacemaker pattern, which is intrinsic to individual neurons (1 – 5 Hz in the absence of extrinsic control). The broad action potentials (ca. 2 ms) are triggered by transient voltage dependent Ca^{2+}-current(s) and a noninactivating sodium current. Two transient outward currents with time constants of 150 and 600 ms inactivate slower than the classical A-current. These currents could prevent strong excitation and awakening during transitions from REM sleep. A hyperpolarisation dependent inward current (I_h) is also prominent in TM neurons, it prevents deep hyperpolarisations and may modulate TM firing. H_3-receptor activation inhibits TM firing and histamine release from TM- (and other) terminals through G-proteins and suppression of Ca^{2+}-currents.

CELLULAR PHYSIOLOGY OF TUBEROMAMMILLARY NEURONS

The properties of histaminergic neurons are in keeping with their function as a modulating pathway: they are relatively large neurones with long, arborizing, slowly conducting axons projecting to virtually the whole central nervous system[1,2,3,4]. Intracellular recording from identified histamine neurons in the tuberomammillary nucleus was achieved in slice preparations[5] (Fig 1): the neurons displayed a rather regular spontaneous activity at 1- 5 Hz as *in vivo*, time constants of ca. 20 ms, a relatively low resting potential of - 52 mV and action potentials of about 2 ms duration (at half-maximal amplitude) with a substantial Ca^{++}-component, followed by an afterhyperpolarisation of 15 - 20 mV. A number of conductances found in the histaminergic neurons give them a characteristic appearance and response to positive and negative current injection. There are two transient outward currents with differing time courses, one with a brief time constant (100ms) and sensitive to 4-aminopyridine and one with a slower decay (600 ms). These conductances markedly slow the return to the resting potential after a hyperpolarisation, prolonging the interspike interval and may serve to prevent firing of the neurons by a brief disturbance during sleep[6]. In the cat and in the rat, TM neurons fire at higher rates during waking, fire slowly during slow wave sleep and not at all during REM sleep[7,8].

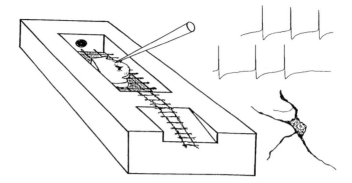

Fig. 1. Hypothalamic slice in a perfusion chamber. Microelectrode is shown recording from the TM nucleus. Most of the electrophysiological results discussed in this article were obtained from such *in vitro* recording. One TM-neurone filled with biocytin is shown and its characteristic firing pattern is illustrated.

A hyperpolarisation-activated inward current (I_h) was also found in all histaminergic neurons[5,6]. Although this current could in principle contribute to the pacemaker-like activity of TM-neurons, it does not seem to play a decisive role in the generation of the firing pattern[9] since blockers of this current do not slow firing of TM neurons. This current is known to be malleable by cyclic AMP, it is also modulated by intracellular Ca^{2+} indirectly, making it sensitive to cellular activity. If its activation range is shifted by phosphorylation, it may well adopt a role as an excitatory factor.

A low threshold Ca^{++}-current exists in TM-neurons with activation at subthreshold membrane potentials. Ca^{++}-dependent, Ni^{++}-sensitive prepotentials are observed in the absence of sodium action potentials[10]. Calcium action potentials can be recorded in tuberomammillary neurons. Under voltage-clamp, the properties of calcium currents in TM neurons have been further examined. TM neurons exhibit both low and high threshold Ca^{++} currents, conforming to the inactivating T (for transient) -type low threshold current with activation beginning near -70 mV, and high threshold currents of both inactivating and non inactivating types[10,11].

A persistent sodium current may contribute to the spontaneous firing[12], but a role in the approach to threshold has not been demonstrated[13]. Llinas and Alonso[12] have described a tetrodotoxin-sensitive plateau potential in tuberomammillary neurons, suggesting that noninactivating sodium channels underlie this potential and that such channels would provide a depolarizing influence and drive the cells to threshold. Using acutely isolated neurons from the TM we have demonstrated, under voltage clamp, a tetrodotoxin-sensitive current present in the steady state current-voltage relationship[13]. This current activates near the threshold for firing. We have also observed single channels with the expected behavior of sodium channels which exhibited a delayed inactivation. Thus two lines of evidence suggest that noninactivating sodium channels are present which provide a depolarizing influence.

In acutely isolated TM neurons we have observed the persistence of spontaneous activity. Single neurons having the morphology of TM neurons are harvested and used for whole cell recording. Before breaking of the membrane, that is, in the cell attached configuration, TM neurons exhibited capacitative transients reflective of spontaneous action potentials, indicating that spontaneous firing is an intrinsic property of individual neurons and not dependent on network properties. After recording we have harvested mRNA by suction through the patch-electrode and confirmed the identity of the cells by detecting the expression of histidine-decarboxylase (single cell RT-PCR, fig. 2).

The activity of spontaneously firing histamine neurons indicates that some intrinsic, active process brings these neurons to threshold. Spontaneous activity is not always monotonous, and misses can be observed. On the occasion of a missed action potential, one often sees a small depolarizing potential. Tetrodotoxin (TTX) blocks spontaneous action potentials, but spontaneous depolarizations persist. Similarly, with the membrane potential slightly hyperpolarized to prevent spontaneous firing, depolarizing current pulses activate a small positive potential which does not decay in a single exponential manner as would be expected of a passive membrane. Instead, the membrane often continues to depolarize before recovery. Such departures from monoexponential decay result from activation of voltage-dependent conductances. It is not blocked by TTX, suggesting that ion channels other than sodium channels are activated in the subthreshold region. The subthreshold potentials are voltage-dependent, and largely blocked by cadmium, a calcium channel blocker[10]. Nickel also reduces firing in TM neurons, and in the presence of TTX, reduces subthreshold depolarizations. Thus it appears likely that calcium as well as sodium channels contribute to the firing pattern of histaminergic neurons.

Repetitive activation of TM neurons resulting from a prolonged depolarizing current pulse results in a prolonged afterhyperpolarization (slow AHP). This event is associated with a decrease in membrane resistance, suggesting opening of ion channels[6]. The slow AHP is relatively insensitive to cadmium, but is blocked by apamin, a component of bee venom which blocks a class of calcium activated potassium channels. Apamin-sensitive calcium-activated potassium channels are a common target of metabotropic neurotransmitters such as histamine, norepinephrine and acetylcholine. Application ot tetraethylammonium (TEA), a blocker of the delayed rectifier type of potassium channel causes increased firing, spike broadening, and in the presence of TTX, enhances calcium action potentials resulting in generation of plateau potentials. The effects of TEA indicate the presence of a delayed rectifier in TM neurons.

Thus, the histaminergic neurons are enabled to fire tonically through their membrane properties, this basic behavior is modulated by a number of afferent transmitters and perhaps further factors. It should be noted in this context that most of the histaminergic neurons are located in very close proximity to the cerebrospinal fluid, the mammillary recess of the third ventricle and the subarachnoidal space near the foramina Luschkae where they may react to components of the CSF.

PHARMACOLOGY OF HISTAMINERGIC NEURONS

The firing of histaminergic neurons reflects their intrinsic properties; they are, however, also recipients of inputs from a number of brain areas including the preoptic area, and other aminergic nuclei, including the cholinergic nuclei. A notable feature of TM neurons is the presence of spontaneous synaptic activity. Spontaneous IPSPs are seen in most TM neurons pinpointing an important synaptic influence, predominantly from GABAergic neurons in the ventral-lateral preoptic area; these neurons are active at the onset of sleep and may serve to reduce histaminergic tone prior to sleep[14]. They also contain galanin[15], which inhibits TM neurons[16] and reduces N-type calcium currents in a variety of cells. Whole cell chloride

42

currents were evoked by brief exposure of isolated TM neurones to GABA and glycine. Single cell RT-PCR was used to identify these neurons as histaminergic (Fig. 2). The gabaergic input is regulated by presynaptic $GABA_B$-receptors[17].

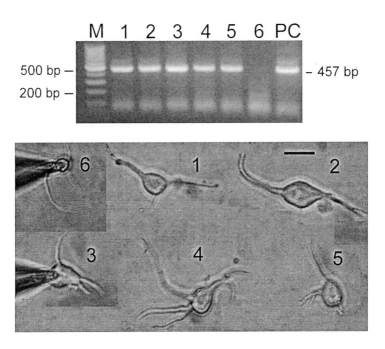

Fig. 2. Single cell RT-PCR revealed the expression of histidine decarboxylase in 5 large cells (1 – 5) but not in a small neurone (6) isolated from the tuberomammillary nucleus. PC: positive control, total mRNA isolated from TM region. M: base pair ladder.

Alpha-bungarotoxin binding is high in the posterior hypothalamus, including areas containing histamine neurons indicating the presence of nicotinic acetylcholine receptors. We have seen rapid depolarizations associated with inward membrane currents following pressure application of nicotine, ACh and DMPP (all nicotinic agonists) in TM neurons[18]. These depolarizations were blocked by α-bungarotoxin. The characteristics of these responses resemble closely those observed for alpha7 subunit-containing receptors which are not involved in synaptic transmission, but exhibit very high sensitivity to nicotine and relatively low sensitivity to ACh. ATP has also recently been identified as a fast transmitter, it depolarizes TM neurons by opening non-selective cation channels[19].

The other biogenic amine systems also project to the TM and affect the neurones as well as the afferent transmission. Serotonin is excitatory through a 5HT 2C-receptor[20] adrenergic effects are fast excitatory (α1), inhibitory (α2) or slow excitatory (β) on the neurons and inhibitory on gabaergic input[21]. Several peptides such as nociceptin[22] and the orexins exert strong actions on the tuberomammillary neurons.

CONCLUSION

The above described selected actions of histamine are in keeping with the proposed role for the tuberomammillary histamine neurons and their projections. A relatively small number of neurones send their multifold arborizing axons in all regions of the central nervous system. The TM neurons fire according to behavioral state, fast in waking, slow in sleep. They receive input from the preoptic area and maintain mutual connections with the other amine nuclei, including the basal forebrain. The location of many TM neurons at the inner or outer surface of the brain indicates their sensing of humoral signals from the cerebrospinal fluid. Their message has to be a modulatory one, the setting or switching of functional states in the brain[23].

REFERENCES

1. Watanabe T, Taguchi Y, Hayashi H, Tanaka J, Shiosaka S, Tohyama M, Kubota H, Terano Y and Wada H (1983) Neurosci. Lett. 39(3):249-54.
2. Panula P, Yang H-YT and Costa E (1984) Proc. Natl. Acad. Sci. USA 81:2572-2576.
3. Watanabe T, Taguchi Y, Shiosaka S, Tanaka J, Kubota H, Terano Y, Tohyama M and Wada H (1984) Brain Res. 295:13-25.
4. Wada H, Inagaki N, Yamatodani A and Watanabe T (1991) TINS 14:415-418.
5. Haas HL and Reiner PB (1988) J. Physiol-Lond. 399:633-646.
6. Greene RW, Haas HL and Reiner PB (1990) J. Physiol. Lond. 420:149-163.
7. Lin JS, Sakai K and Jouvet M (1988) Neuropharmacology 27:111-122.
8. Steininger T, Alam M, Gong H, Szymusiak R, McGinty D (1999) Brain Res 840:138-147
9. Kamondi A and Reiner PB (1991) J. Neurophysiol. 66:1902-11.
10. Stevens DR and Haas HL (1996) J. Physiol.-Lond 493:747-754.
11. Takeshita Y, Watanabe T, Sakata T, Munakata M, Ishibashi H, Akaike N. (1998) Neuroscience 87:797-805.
12. Llinas RR and Alonso A (1992) J. Neurophysiol. 68:1307-1320.
13. Uteshev V, Stevens DR and Haas HL (1995) Neuroscience 66:143-149.
14. Sherin JE, Shiromani PJ, McCarley RW and Saper CB (1996) Science 271:216-219.
15. Köhler C, Ericson H, Watanabe T, Polak J, Palay SL, Palay V and Chan Palay V (1986) J. Comp. Neurol. 250:58-64.
16. Schönrock B, Büsselberg D and Haas HL (1991) Agents Actions 33:135-137.
17. Stevens DR, Kuramasu A, Haas HL (1999) Europ. J. Neurosci. 11: 1148-1154
18. Uteshev V., Stevens D.R. and Haas H.L. (1996) Pflügers Archiv 432:607-613
19. Furukawa K, Ishibashi H and Akaike N (1996) J. Neurophysiol. 71(3):868-873.
20. Eriksson KS, Stevens DR, Haas HL (2000) Neuropharmacology in press
21. Kuramasu A, Haas HL and Stevens DR (2000) Neuropharmacology submitted
22. Eriksson KS, Stevens DR, Haas HL (2000) Neuropharmacology 39: 2492-2498.
23. Brown RE Stevens DR and Haas HL (2000) Progr.Neurobiol. in press

Histamine Research in the New Millennium
T. Watanabe, H. Timmerman and K. Yanai (Editors)

Histaminergic modulation of basal forebrain cholinergic neurons

M.B. Passani, L. Bacciottini, I. Cangioli, L. Giovannelli, P.F. Mannaioni and P. Blandina

Dipartimento di Farmacologia Preclinica e Clinica, Università di Firenze, V.le G. Pieraccini 6, 50139 Firenze, Italy

The aim of this review is to summarize our most recent work on the histaminergic modulation of the basal forebrain cholinergic neurons. The importance of the neuromodulatory effect that histamine exerts on acetylcholine (ACh) release is becoming poignant, since the regulation of ACh release in some brain district affects cognitive processes. The microdialysis technique is being used in association with immunohistochemistry and behavioral experiments to determine the molecular and functional relevance of the interactions between the histaminergic and cholinergic systems.

1. INTRODUCTION

One of the most intriguing and controversial roles of brain histamine is its involvement in modulating cognitive processes. Recent evidence has shown that manipulation of the histaminergic system exerts either memory enhancing or memory impairing effects, depending on what brain region and which histaminergic receptor subtypes are investigated [1, 2]. There is compelling evidence, though, that the effects of histamine on cognition, appear to involve the modulation of the cholinergic system [2-4]. The role of forebrain cholinergic neurons in the modulation of learning and memory and attentional processing is well known [5, 6]. Indeed, the procognitive effects of cholinomimetic agents and the amnesic action of muscarinic receptor antagonists have been observed in a variety of tasks, suggesting that the cholinergic transmission plays a crucial role in cognition [7]. Cholinergic and memory deficits occur both in normal aging [8, 9] and in Alzheimer's disease [10, 11]. Interestingly, another salient feature of this neurodegenerative disease is the loss of histaminergic fibers and receptors [12, 13].

The most compelling evidence that relates the cognitive effects of histamine to modifications of ACh neurotransmission, stems from studies showing that systemic administration of H3 receptor agonists impaired rat performance in cognitive tasks, that require an intact cortex, at the same doses that reduced ACh release from the cortex of freely moving rats [14, 15]. In addition, H3 receptor antagonists have shown procognitive properties in scopolamine-impaired rats [16], and senescence-accelerated mice [17], as well as in normal animals [18, 19].

The morphological features of both the histaminergic and cholinergic systems with a widespread distribution of fibers suggest that they may interact in other brain regions. These interactions may have potential relevance in cognitive processes. Cholinergic somata in the basal forebrain are clustered in the septum and diagonal band from where they mainly innervate the hippocampus. In both rats and humans projections from the nucleus basalis magnocellularis (NBM) provide the majority of cholinergic innervation to the cortex and the amygdala [20-22]. Histaminergic fibers originate exclusively from the hypothalamic tuberomammillary bodies and project to all brain regions [23, 24].

Whereas there is conclusive evidence showing histaminergic-cholinergic interactions in the cortex [25] and hippocampus [26, 27], much less is known about histaminergic modulation of cholinergic neurons in the septum, the NBM and the amygdala [3]. Bath application of histamine to guinea pig basal forebrain slices depolarized NBM cholinergic neurons mainly through H_1 receptor activation [28]. Histaminergic and cholinergic fibers are found in the amygdala [23, 24], a brain region that is involved in modulating memory consolidation of aversive events [29, 30]. In laboratory animals, aversive events such as a foot shock elicit the expression of stereotyped behaviors, the acquisition of which requires the integrity of the intra-amygdalar cholinergic system [31]. However, nothing is known about histaminergic modulation of cholinergic neurons in these brain regions. Hence, our interests to understand if and how histamine modulates the release of ACh in well defined brain areas and the behavioral relevance of such interactions. We are currently testing the hypothesis that the activation or blockade of histaminergic receptors, not only modulate ACh release, but also affects the expression of *c-fos*, an immediate-early gene linked to genomic events in response to environmental signals. This proto-oncogene provides a useful marker for tracing the effects of pharmacological, electrical and physiological stimuli in the CNS [32].

2. HISTAMINE MODULATES ACh RELEASE IN SEVERAL BRAIN REGIONS: FUNCTIONAL IMPLICATIONS

2.1 . Histamine modulates the cholinergic septum-hippocampal pathway

The hippocampal formation is a brain region primarily involved in spatial learning. Early studies showed that ACh release from the hippocampus of anesthetized rats increased after electrical stimulation of the tuberomamimllary bodies, where histaminergic cell bodies are located. The same pattern of stimulation increased histamine release in the medial septal area (MSA) [33]. The neuromodulatory action of histamine on ACh release in the hippocampus is most probably exerted through the activation of histamine receptors in the MSA, because microdialysis experiments failed to show modifications of ACh release when histamine was locally administered into the hippocampus [27]. Recently it was demonstrated in our laboratory that intraseptal administration of either thioperamide or ciproxifan increased significantly the spontaneous release of ACh from the hippocampus of freely moving rats by up to about 100%. The effect of the two H_3 receptor antagonists was fully antagonized by intraseptal co-administration of the H_2 receptor antagonist cimetidine [27, 34]. It was assumed that intraseptal administration of thioperamide, by blocking H_3 presynaptic autoreceptors, increased extracellular levels of endogenous histamine, that interacted with postsynaptic H_2 receptors. Thus far, it is not clear yet whether H_2 receptors are located on the septal cholinergic cell bodies, or on hypothetical interneurons, which in turn facilitate the release of hippocampal ACh.

Interestingly, the expression of *c-fos* immunoreactivity was detected in the medial septum 90 min after intraseptal administration of ciproxifan. This effect was fully antagonized by cimetidine [34]. Morphological features indicated that *c-fos* was expressed in neuronal cells, but the type of neuron has not been identified yet. Although increased hippocampal ACh release and *c-fos* expression might be dissociated processes, despite the identity of the stimulus, these observations may have implications for the treatment of disorders associated with impaired septum-hippocampal cholinergic functions.

2.2. Local administration of histamine in the NBM modifies cortical ACh release

We have recently demonstrated that perfusing the NBM with histaminergic drugs, the rate of cortical ACh spontaneous release is modified using the dual-probe microdialysis method [35, 36]. A vertical microdialysis probe was implanted in the NBM to deliver drugs locally, and a transverse microdialysis fiber was inserted through the fronto-parietal cortex to measure ACh extracellular levels. It was found that administration of histamine into the NBM stimulated dose-dependently ACh release from the cortex of freely moving rats. The release of cortical ACh elicited by application of histamine onto NBM neurons is attributable to activation of H_1 receptors. Indeed, methylhistaprodifen, a highly selective H_1 receptor agonist, released cortical ACh with a pattern similar to that of histamine, whereas histaminergic agonists dimaprit and R-alpha-methylhistamine, added to the NBM-perfusing medium at concentrations sufficient to fully activate H_2 and H_3 receptors, respectively, are completely inactive in modulating cortical release of ACh [36]. Furthermore, histamine-evoked release of cortical ACh is resistant to antagonism by cimetidine at concentration more than 400 times its K_d for the H_2 receptor [36]. Given the action of methylhistaprodifen and the lack of effects shown by R-alpha-methylhistamine, it appears that H_1 receptors must be responsible for the stimulation by histamine of NBM cholinergic neurons. Further support to the hypothesis of H_1 receptor involvement is added by the blockade of histamine- and methylhistaprodifen-evoked release of ACh produced by H_1 receptor antagonists, such as triprolidine and mepyramine, at concentrations consonant with their affinities at H_1 receptors [36]. The report that histamine depolarized the membrane and increased the tonic firing of guinea-pig NBM cholinergic neurons mainly through H_1 receptor activation [28] is consonant with the findings shown in this study. Analogously, H_1 receptor activation is responsible for stimulation of the cholinergic neurons of the mesopontine tegmentum [37].

The behavioral significance of the interactions between histaminergic and cholinergic systems in the NBM has yet to be tested. The observation that performance in attention-demanding tasks deteriorates after treatment with H_1 receptor antagonist at doses that fail to cause changes in subjective sleepiness [38] indicates a role in cognitive processes.

2.3. Administration of histaminergic compounds in the rat amygdala affects both ACh release and fear conditioning

A single microdialysis probe was used to perfuse histaminergic compounds in the basolateral complex of the amygdala (BLA) and collect the dialysate. The H_3 receptor antagonists clobenpropit and thioperamide locally administered to the BLA decreased ACh spontaneous release (Table 1) an effect antagonized by the simultaneous perfusion of the amygdala with the H_2 receptor antagonist cimetidine [39]. These observations suggest that endogenous histamine is released in the BLA and moderates ACh output. Indeed, the decrease of amygdalar ACh release could be most simply explained by an interaction with H3 autoreceptors. Blockade of these receptors caused an increase of extracellular levels of endogenous histamine [40]. Therefore, the present study suggests that activation of histaminergic neurons projecting to the amygdala inhibits locally the cholinergic tone. Postsynaptic H_2 receptors seem to mediate this effect, since pretreatment with cimetidine fully antagonized the effect of thioperamide and clobenpropit. Whether H_2 receptors are located on cholinergic terminals, or on hypothetical interneurons is not clear yet.

Activation of cholinergic receptors within the amygdala appears to be crucial in the memory for aversive stimuli [31]. Memory in inhibitory avoidance task and in contextual fear conditioning was enhanced after post-training injections of the muscarinic agonist oxotremorine [41, 42]. On the other hand, systemic administration of scopolamine, and intra-amygdala post-training injections of the muscarinic antagonist atropine, prevented memory enhancement produced by systemic administration of muscarinic agonists [42, 43]. The neuromodulatory effect of H3 receptor antagonists in the BLA may also conceivably influence memory consolidation indirectly. To examine the physiological relevance of histamine as a neuromodulator in the amygdala, we are currently testing the effect of intra-BLA injections of H3 receptor antagonists on fear conditioning.

Table 1
Effects of local administration of H3 receptor antagonists in the BL-amygdala. ** $p<0.001$ ***; $p<0.01$ (two way ANOVA and Scheffe's test); thio, thioperamide; clob, clobenpropit; cim, cimetidine; (n).

	Amygdala	
	Spont. rel. (pmol/20 min)	Treatment (pmol/20 min)
300 nM Thio	0.26 ± 0.05	0.11 ± 0.01 ** (4)
300 nM Clob	0.28 ± 0.05	0.10 ± 0.04 *** (4)
100 μM Cim 300 nM Thio	0.42 ± 0.05	0.42 ± 0.06 (5)
100 μM Cim 300 nM Clob	0.3 ± 0.03	0.24 ± 0.04 (6)

3. CONCLUSIONS

There is clear evidence of the important role that neuronal histamine exerts in cognition. An accredited hypothesis, that our experiments are currently testing, is that the effector (or one of the effectors) of the histaminergic cognitive action is the cholinergic system. Infact, although ACh has a central role in learning and memory, interactions with other neurotransmitters, such as dopamine, GABA, noradrenaline, are essential for the formation of memory. Novel approaches for treating cognitive dysfunctions are required since the clinical outcome of cholinomimetic strategies (ChEIs) has been far from satisfactory [44]. HA receptors might represent a target for non-cholinergic drugs that potentiate cholinergic functions. Appropriate histaminergic drugs could produce beneficial effects on disorders associated with impaired cholinergic functions, such as AD disease. However, our data, as well as electrophysiological evidence indicate that ACh/histamine interactions are complex and multifaceted. Indeed, H_3 receptor antagonists have opposite neuromodulatory effects on ACh release in, e.g., the NBM and the amygdala. Unfortunately, the potential for opposite effects in different brain regions may restrict their systemic use and produce contrasting results.

REFERENCES

1. Klapdor, K., R.U. Hasenöhrl, and J.P. Huston. Behav Brain Res, 1994. **61**: p. 113-116.
2. Bacciottini, L., et al. Beh Brain Res, in press.
3. Passani, M.B., et al. Neurosci Biobehav Rev, 2000. **24**(1): p. 107-114.
4. Passani, M. and P. Blandina. Meth Find Exp Clin Pharmacol, 1998. **20**(8): p. 725-733.
5. Sarter, M. and J.P. Bruno. Neuroscience, 2000. **95**(4): p. 933-952.
6. Everitt, B.J. and T.W. Robbins. Annu Rev Psychol, 1997. **48**: p. 649-684.
7. Woolf, N. Neurobiology of Learning and Memory, 1996. **66**: p. 258-266.
8. Decker, M.W. Brain Res Rev, 1987. **12**: p. 423-428.
9. Kubanis, P. and S.F. Zornetzer. Behav Neural Biol, 1981. **31**: p. 115-172.
10. Davies, P. and A. Maloney. Lancet, 1976. **2**: p. 1403-1405.
11. Perry, E.K., et al. Br Med J, 1978. **2**: p. 1457-1459.
12. Panula, P., et al. Neuroscience, 1997. **82**: p. 993-997.
13. Higuchi, M., et al. Neuroscience, 2000. **99**: p. 721-729.
14. Blandina, P., et al. Br J Pharmacol, 1996. **119**: p. 1656-1664.
15. Leurs, R., et al. Trends Pharmacol Sci, 1998. **19**: p. 177-183.
16. Giovannini, M.G., et al. Behav Brain Res, 1999. **104**: p. 147-155.
17. Meguro, K.-I., et al. Biogenic Amines, 1992. **8**: p. 299-307.
18. Ligneau, X., et al. J Pharmacol Exp Ther, 1998. **287**: p. 658-666.
19. Prast, H., A. Argyriou, and A. Philippu. Brain Res, 1996. **734**: p. 316-318.
20. Eckenstein, F.P., R.W. Baughman, and J. Quinn. Neuroscience, 1988. **25**: p. 457-474.
21. Mesulam, M.M., et al. Neuroscience, 1983. **10**: p. 1185-1201.
22. LoConte, G., et al. Archs Ital Biol, 1982. **120**: p. 176-188.
23. Panula, P., et al. Neuroscience, 1989. **28**: p. 585-610.
24. Inagaki, N., et al. J Comp Neurol, 1988. **273**: p. 283-300.
25. Blandina, P., et al. Inflamm Res, 1996. **45**: p. S54-S55.

26. Bacciottini, L., et al. *Abs. of XVIIth Annual Meeting of the European Histamine Research Society.* 1998. Lodz (PL), May 20-23.
27. Bacciottini, L., et al. Inflamm Res, 1999. **48**: p. S63-S64.
28. Khateb, A., et al. Neuroscience, 1995. **69**: p. 495-506.
29. McGaugh, J.L. Science, 2000. **287**: p. 248-251.
30. LeDoux, J.E. Annual Review of NEuroscience, 2000. **23**: p. 155-184.
31. McGaugh, J.L., L. Cahill, and B. Roozendaal. Proc. Natl. Acad. Sci., 1996. **93**: p. 13508-13514.
32. Sheng, M. and M.E. Greenberg. Neuron, 1990. **4**: p. 477-485.
33. Mochizuki, T., et al. J Neurochem, 1994. **62**: p. 2275-2282.
34. Bacciottini, L., et al. Inflamm Res, 2000. **49**: p. S41-S42.
35. Cecchi, M., et al. Inflamm. res, 1998. **47**: p. S32-S33.
36. Cecchi, M., et al. Eur J Neurosci, in press.
37. Lin, J.S., et al. J Neurosci, 1996. **16**: p. 1523-1537.
38. Okamura, N., et al. Br J Pharmacol, 2000. **129**: p. 115-123.
39. Passani, M.B., et al. Inlamm Res, 2000. **49**: p. S43-S44.
40. Arrang, J.M., M. Garbarg, and J.C. Schwartz. Nature, 1983. **302**: p. 832-837.
41. Vazdarjanova, A. and J.L. McGaugh. J Neurosci, 1999. **19**: p. 6615-6622.
42. Introini-Collison, I.B., C. Dalmaz, and J.L. McGaugh. Neurobiol Learn Mem, 1996. **65**: p. 57-64.
43. Dalmaz, C., I.B. Introini-Collison, and J.L. McGaugh. Behavioural Brain Research, 1993. **58**: p. 167-174.
44. Kelly, J.S. Trends Pharmacol Sci, 1999. **20**: p. 127-129.

Histamine Research in the New Millennium
T. Watanabe, H. Timmerman and K. Yanai (Editors)

The interaction between the histaminergic system and the NO-cGMP pathway: A functional neuroanatomical study in the mammillary region and cerebral cortex of the rat

Harry W.M. Steinbusch, Gary V. Allen[1], Jan de Vente and David A. Hopkins[1]

European Graduate School of Neuroscience (EURON), Maastricht University, Dept. Psychiatry & Neuropsychology, Division Neuroscience, Maastricht, The Netherlands; [1]Dept. Anatomy & Neurobiology, Dalhousie University, Halifax, N.S., Canada

The mammillary body, as one of the constituents of the limbic system, has been implicated in three general spheres of interest: 1. learning and memory, 2. autonomic function and motivation and emotion, and 3. propagation and initiation of seizures. In the present study we have investigated the possible interaction between the distribution of the histaminergic neurons and fibres in the mamillary region and the appearance of the nitric oxide synthase positive (NOS) cells and fibres and NO-mediated cGMP-fibres in that same region using the activation of the guanylyl cyclase by NO as a tool to visualize cGMP activity. Brain histamine is exclusively contained within and released from neurons whose cell bodies are clustered in the tuberomammillary nucleus (TM) of the posterior hypothalamus. The mammillary bodies contain three distinctive histaminergic cell groups of which the tuberomamillary and the ventrolateral parts are most compact and well defined. These histaminergic cell groups project to various parts of the limbic system and the cerebral cortex. Previous data have also shown that the mammillary region is highly innervated with cGMP-immunoreactive fibres and contain an elaborated NOS neuronal system. Using double immunostaining procedures with antibodies to histidine decarboxylase (HDC), the acetylcholine transporter (VChAt), neuronal NOS and cGMP, the cellular structures were visualized in which NO-mediated cGMP was increased after stimulation of histamine activity or cholinergic and NMDA-receptor blocking.

1. INTRODUCTION

Historically histamine has been ascribed a neurotransmitter role in the mammalian central nervous system (CNS) on the basis of an impressive amount of indirect - mainly neurochemical – evidence[16,17,20]. Neurochemical studies using radio-enzymatic assays carried out in the early 1970's demonstrated that histamine is distributed extensively, but unevenly throughout the brain[8]. Thus, the concentration of this monoamine appeared to be highest in the hypothalamus, intermediate throughout the telencephalon, and lowest in the brain stem and cerebellum. A similar global distribution was found for the synthesizing enzyme HDC[10,16,17,20]. Other studies have proven that histamine exerts potent effects on specific central neurons, revealing three specific receptor systems (H1,H2 and H3)[2,4,17]. It was demonstrated that in the striatum the activity of the cholinergic neurons is permanently modulated by neighbouring histaminergic nerve terminals and axons via H3 auto- and heteroreceptors. Histamine released from histaminergic nerve terminals increases the release of acetylcholine in part by inhibition of dopamine release which, in turn, decreases the GABAergic transmission.

The application of immunohistochemical and autoradiographic techniques to study the distribution of histamine has unveiled the presence of this monoamine throughout the rat and guinea-pig CNS. Histamine-producing cells contain a specific HDC that is different from the L-aromatic aminoacid decarboxylase, present in catecholaminergic as well as indolaminergic neurons[16,17]. Watanabe and coworkers[32,33] purified HDC from fetal rat liver and raised antibodies against the enzyme to localize immunohistochemically HDC-positive cell bodies and fibres in rat brain. Another immunohistochemical approach which has been applied successfully to localize other monoaminergic systems is to use antibodies directed against the monoamine neurotransmitter itself, following its coupling to a carrier protein[23]. Since then a number of studies have localized histaminergic neurons using antibodies directed against HDC[11,15,19,26,32,33] or against histamine conjugated to a carrier protein [1,7,13,22,24,34]. These studies have shown the presence of histaminergic fibres in the brain. They originate from only a modest number of perikarya located mainly in three cell clusters in the tuberomammillary region of the posterior hypothalamus. Some of the histamine-containing neurons appear to contain also other neuroactive substances, i.e. gamma-aminobutyric acid, glutamic acid decarboxylase, galanin, Met-Enk-Arg-Phe heptapeptide, adenosine deaminase and substance P[12,14,18,21,27,30,31]. Cells in the tuberomammillary region have also been reported to contain immunoreactivity for these neuroactive substances but not for HDC[12]. In order to study the anatomical connectivity of the histaminergic neurons, it is therefore a prerequisite to combine tracing techniques with immunocytochemistry for HDC or histamine to specifically identify the involved neurons as histaminergic[35].

The aim of this paper is to present a brief summary of histaminergic neurons in the rat brain and a detailed description of the localization of histaminergic fibres and fibres related to the NO-cGMP pathway. This is important since we have observed that histamine is related to memory processes, high levels of cGMP are beneficial for memory recognition and that hippocampal NO is not critically involved in place learning in rats[10].

2. MATERIALS AND METHODS

Information on the immunohistochemical staining of HDC, histamine, NOS or cGMP can be found elsewhere [23,28,29]. The antibody to HDC was a generous gift of Dr. Watanabe.

3. RESULTS and DISCUSSION

3.1. Localization of histaminergic neurons in the rat brain

Histidine decarboxylase- or histamine (HA$_i$)-immunoreactive perikarya are strictly confined to the region of the mammillary nuclei and the ventral part of the posterior hypothalamus (Figs. 1 A,C,E,F). They are arranged in three clusters. The most prominent group of HA$_i$-cell bodies was found between levels A 2800 and A 3800. It is mostly confined to the caudal magnocellular nucleus (CM). The caudal magnocellular nucleus is located immediately below the pial surface of the posterior hypothalamic area. This cluster is large and consists of a single layer of maximally four or five cells thick. Another bridge of HDC-immunoreactive neurons connects the caudal one-third of the CM and the lateral sulcus of the mammillary recess of the third ventricle. The cell bridges of both sides meet in the roof and the floor of the mammillary recess. Caudally, the CM is continuous with a second cluster of histaminergic neurons, the caudal magnocellular postmammillary nucleus (PCM), of which the main portion also lies directly beneath the pial surface, lateral and slightly dorsal to the lateral mammillary nucleus. The PCM extends to the caudalmost pole of the postmammillary nucleus. Caudally, they appear ventrolateral to the nucleus mammillaris lateralis, immediately adjacent to the basal surface of the brain. Rostrally, this cell group extends to the recessus mammillaris, to form a narrow band of HA_i-perikarya ventral to and within the nucleus mammillaris lateralis.

In the rat, the most rostral and third cluster is found immediately dorsal and lateral to the point where the mammillary recess emerges from the third ventricle. This cluster is called the tuberal magnocellular nucleus (TM). It is situated mainly between levels A 3400 and A 4400. This cell group is not as compact as the previous one. Rostrally, this group can be followed until the level of the third ventricle, where the HA_i-cell bodies are situated between the dorso- and ventromedial hypothalamic nuclei. In addition to these cell groups, scattered HA_i-cell bodies were observed throughout the posterior hypothalamus. Caudally, at level A 2800, some HA_i-cell bodies were demonstrated in the dorsal part of the nucleus mammillaris medialis and lateralis, just ventrally to the fasciculus mammillothalamicus. Rostrally, at the posterior edge of the recessus mammillaris no cells were found. At level A 3400, we observed some HA_i-perikarya throughout the nucleus premammillaris ventralis.

At that same level, a few HA_i-cells were demonstrated in the nucleus premammillaris dorsalis. Rostrally between levels A 3800 and A 4400, these cells can be found in the posterior hypothalamic nucleus and in the ventrolateral aspects of the hypothalamus, e.g. the region situated between the medial forebrain bundle (MFB) and the basal surface of the brain. Some HA_i-cells can be found within the MFB itself. A few solitary HDC-immunoreactive cells can further be seen in the supramammillary region, in areas lateral to the entrance of the fornix into the mammillary body, and immediately below the caudal surface of the mammillary body.

Apart from these HA_i-neurons, HA_i-mast cells were found at the basal surface of the hypothalamus, where they were especially prominent at the level of the median eminence, immediately beneath the meninges.

3.2. Histaminergic Neuronal Projections and Areas of Termination

Our findings indicate that HA_i-varicose fibers innervate almost all regions of the rat CNS. The HA_i-varicose fibers appeared most abundant in the di- and telencephalon. Within the diencephalon the highest density was found in the median eminence, the ventromedial hypothalamic nucleus and adjacent areas. Within the telencephalon the following areas contain HA- or HDC-immunoreactive fibers: the nucleus olfactorius anterior, the entire cerebral cortex (no laminar prevalence), the amygdaloid complex, especially the medial amygdaloid nucleus, the nucleus of the diagonal band of Broca, the lateral and medial nuclei of the septal complex, the nucleus accumbens and the caudate-putamen complex (in the latter structure only scattered fibers). On the basis of preliminary data obtained in experiments examining the immunocytochemical localization of histamine together with the anterograde transport of lectins (Phaseolus vulgaris), three pathways can be traced: two ascending (one periventricularly, and the other laterally through the medial forebrain bundle) and one descending. Both ascending pathways enter the basal telencephalon and combine in the diagonal band of Broca.

The dorsal ascending pathway arises from the HA_i-cell bodies situated in the region between levels A 3400 and A 4400, i.e., the HA_i-perikarya close to the fibers do not enter the MFB but are situated dorsolaterally to it. The main areas of termination of this pathway are the caudate-putamen complex, the globus pallidus and the nucleus accumbens.

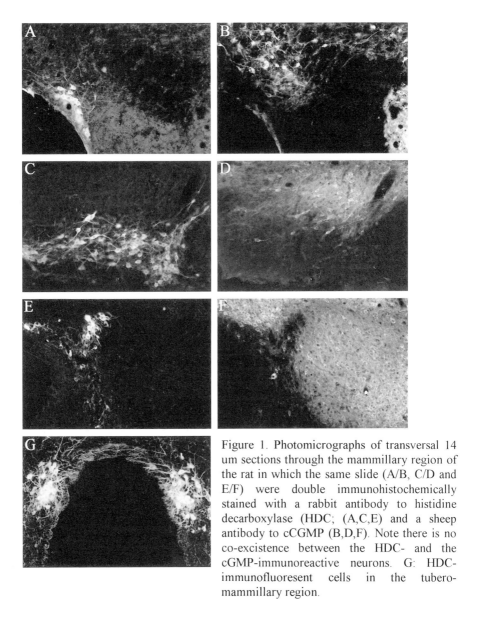

Figure 1. Photomicrographs of transversal 14 um sections through the mammillary region of the rat in which the same slide (A/B, C/D and E/F) were double immunohistochemically stained with a rabbit antibody to histidine decarboxylase (HDC; (A,C,E) and a sheep antibody to cCGMP (B,D,F). Note there is no co-excistence between the HDC- and the cGMP-immunoreactive neurons. G: HDC-immunofluoresent cells in the tubero-mammillary region.

The ventral ascending pathway arises from the HA_i-cell bodies situated more ventrolaterally in the posterior hypothalamus, between levels A 2800 and A 3800, and its fibers enter the MFB. The highest density of histaminergic fibers has been observed within the diencephalon in the ventral half of the posterior hypothalamic area, i.e. in the median eminence, the ventromedial nucleus of the hypothalamus and throughout the mammillary bodies. Histaminergic fibers are furthermore found in the suprachiasmatic and paraventricular nuclei. In the thalamus a few fibers appear to be present in the periventricular nucleus and in the lateral geniculate body. Rostrally, fibers leave the MFB to enter the fasciculus retroflexus, and distribute to the nucleus medialis habenulae and other thalamic structures. At this level some fibers enter the median eminence and run through the infundibulum to the pars nervosa of the pituitary. Further rostrally, fibers leave the MFB to enter the nucleus lateralis hypothalami, the suprachiasmatic nucleus and the amygdala complex, by means of the striae terminalis. Finally, some HA_i-fibers reached the prefrontal-, frontal-, neo-entorhinal- and hippocampal cortices via the cingulum bundle.

In serial sections it was observed that the periventricular and lateral fiber bundles and the diagonal band of Broca provide the telencephalic structures. The periventricular fiber group emanates fibers which pass dorsolaterally and enter the stria terminalis, to reach the amygdaloid complex. Fibers dissociating from the lateral group enter the capsula interna to course to the caudate-putamen complex and the cerebral cortex. Other fibers emanating from this group join the amygdalofugal pathway and terminate in the amygdalar complex and in the prepiriform cortex. The fibers in the diagonal band of Broca distribute to the nucleus of the same name, the septal nuclei, the nucleus accumbens, and to the cerebral cortex. Extensive descriptions of the distribution of the ascending histaminergic fibers in the rat brain have been published[11,22], whereas recently mappings have been published of the distribution of histaminerg ic fibers in the guinea pig brain[1,19]. In particular, limbic structures (prepiriform cortex, entorhinal area, septal area, amygdalar complex) receive a relatively dense input from the magnocellular nuclei[12]. Little is known about the differential distribution of the histaminergic fibers. At issue here is the question whether neurons in all the clusters of histaminergic neurons send fibers to all brain areas, or whether specific clusters of histaminergic neurons send their efferent fibers to specific brain areas. The only studies so far in which this question has been addressed according to a combined immunocytochemical tracing approach were conducted [5,25]. Steinbusch et al.[25] injected the retrograde fluorescent tracer Granular Blue (GB) in the caudate-putamen complex of rats and immunostained the posterior hypothalamus. Co-localization of HDC-immunofluorescence and GB-fluorescence in cell bodies of neurons in the posterior hypothalamus indicated that these histaminergic cells project to the caudate-putamen complex. The authors noted that 20-25% of the cells belonging to the histaminergic population, mainly cells in the CM and PCM, project to the caudate-putamen complex. Ericson et al.[6] injected the fluorescent tracer Fast Blue in various brain areas, and also found co-localization of the fluorescent tracer and HDC-immunofluorescence scattered in the tuberomammillary region. Thus, the scant evidence available suggests that there is no histaminergic cell cluster of which all cells project specifically to the caudate-putamen complex or, perhaps, to any brain region. Contrary, the evidence so far suggests that all clusters of histaminergic neurons contribute to the histaminergic innervation of particular brain areas.

3.3. Localization of NOS and NO-receptive elements in the Telencephalon

$cGMP_i$ was prominently present in a network of varicose fibers in the cingulate, frontal, parietal, and piriform cortices. The density of the neuronal network appeared to be slightly greater in the more superficial layers (layers I - III) of the cortex. In all cell layers, we observed occasionally glial and neuronal cell somata. In these cortical areas, NOS-IS was found in a varicose fiber network with few somata. NO activated the sGNC in a network which, like the NOS-containing network, stretches throughout the cortical areas. In the cortical areas cGMP was not observed in NOS-$_i$ structures.

The area of the corpus callosum (CC) is one of regions of the brain which is scarcely innervated with NOS-$_i$ fibers. Occasionally a NOS containing cell soma was observed. In agreement with this observation, there are relatively few fibers which show cGMP-$_i$ in this area. In addition, many astrocytes were observed in the region of the genu of the CC, whereas cGMP-$_i$ astrocytes were scarce in other parts of the CC. cGMP-$_i$ was not observed in NOS-positive structures in the CC, although some degree of colocalization might possibly be observed in the cortical layer bordering on the CC.

A dense network of NOS-$_i$ varicose fibers was observed in the caudate putamen complex. A small number of NOS-$_i$ cells bodies was observed. NO induces cGMP-accumulation in a dense varicose fiber network that appeared to be uniformly distributed throughout the caudate putamen complex. No colocalization of NOS was observed in the cGMP-$_i$ structures. In the nucleus accumbens cGMP-$_i$ and NOS-$_i$ were present in dense, overlapping but not colocalizing, fiber networks, and, in addition, NOS-IS was found in some cell bodies. In the globus pallidus, a relative absence of cGMP-$_i$ was found, i.e. cGMP-$_i$ was observed in fibers encircling the myelinated fiber bundles in a manner similar to that observed for the NOS-positive fibers, although no colocalization was observed.

In the amygdala region we found the central amygdala to be relatively devoid of NOS-i, whereas cGMP-$_i$ was strong in this region. The median preoptic nucleus showed intense cGMP-$_i$ and in this area NOS-$_i$ was prominent in a large number of cells and fibers also, both dorsal and ventral of the anterior commissure. At this level of resolution it cannot be definitely proven that there is, or is not, colocalization of cGMP and NOS in this nucleus, however, actual colocalization was not observed.

The localization of NO-receptive structures in the hippocampus has been described in detail previously. The fimbria showed cGMP-$_i$ and NOS-$_i$ in a large number of varicose fibers with the occasional cell somata. A dense cGMP-$_i$ network of varicose fibers was observed throughout the hippocampus and double immunostaining revealed an absence of colocalization between nNOS and cGMP. Pyramidal cells were often observed encircled by cGMP-$_i$ fibers, but no cGMP-$_i$ was found in these cells.

3.4. Localization of NOS and NO-receptive elements in the Diencephalon

In the medial habenula we found a number of NOS-containing cells that also stained for cGMP, however, not all NOS-IS cells were also cGMP-$_i$. In contrast, the medial aspect of the lateral habenula, showed a dense immunostaining for both cGMP and NOS in a multitude of fibers and punctate staining structures that was highly suggestive for an extensive colocalization in this area. Intense cGMP-$_i$ was observed in the fibers running along the dorsolateral side of the dorsal geniculate nucleus, whereas in the more medial part a multitude of thin varicose cGMP-$_i$ fibers were observed. In the same region we observed also intense NOS staining. In the dorsomedial and the dorsoventral thalamic nuclei we found a dense network of cGMP-$_i$ fibers whereas NOS-IS was relatively scarce in varicose fibers. In the area adjacent to the thalamic reticular nucleus, we found a group of NOS positive cells that were also cGMP-$_i$. Not all cGMP-$_i$ cells appeared to be NOS-positive. Again, the general pattern of the fiber staining was very similar for cGMP and NOS, although colocalization at the level of fibers could not be ascertained. Strong cGMP-$_i$ and NOS-$_i$ was observed in the zona incerta, both stainings showing a typical similar pattern. In the subthalamic nucleus we observed numerous NOS-positive cell bodies and a typical honeycomb-like pattern in the fiber staining. A similar pattern was found for cGMP-$_i$ with some cell somata being cGMP-positive. cGMP-positive and NOS-positive cells could be observed adjacent to each other but no colocalization was observed (Figs 1 B,D,F.).

NOS-immunostaining in the hypothalamic area was very dense in thin varicose fibers. cGMP-$_i$ was also found in varicose fibers; the density of the cGMP-$_i$ fibers varied somewhat between different areas of the hypothalamus, with the ventromedial hypothalamic areas showing relatively little cGMP-$_i$. Few cell somata were positive for cGMP. The suprachiasmatic nucleus stained intensely for cGMP in the ventral part, whereas in the dorsal part cGMP-$_i$ was very weak. No NOS-$_i$ could be found in the suprachiasmatic nucleus. In the region of the arcuate nucleus and median eminence we observed cGMP-$_i$ fibers and cell somata. In the median eminence we found a very intense, punctate-like staining for cGMP and also for NOS. An extensive colocalization between these two markers was found in this area. We also observed intensely cGMP-$_i$ somata, which in addition showed a lightly stained, NOS-positive, cytoplasm. In the mammillary region we noted a sharp delineation between the supramammillary nucleus and the medial mammillary region indicated by the NOS-IS and also by the cGMP-$_i$. A strong punctate staining was observed for both NOS and cGMP, although a colocalization could not be observed.

4. CONCLUDING REMARKS

It is worth noting the striking general agreement between the distribution of histaminergic neurons suspected on the basis of neurochemical findings and that revealed thus far in our immunohistochemical studies as well as those of others. The data obtained thus far suggest that the arrangement of the histaminergic neuronal system, viz. a compact cell group with a widespread distribution of fibers, resembles that of other monoaminergic systems, particularly the serotonergic, dopaminergic and noradrenergic systems in the nucleus raphe dorsalis, substantia nigra and locus coeruleus, respectively. The widespread distribution of histaminergic fibers suggests that histamine, like the catecholamines and serotonin, may be involved in a large variety of physiological functions ruled by the CNS. Four general comments with regard to the distribution of histaminergic fibers throughout the rat CNS can be made. 1: The histaminergic system is a very widespread system in the sense that there are hardly any brain regions which are not innervated by histaminergic fibers. 2. The strongest projections are ascending. Descending projections are much weaker developed. 3. The density of the innervation of the brain by histaminergic fibers is considerably less than we presently know to occur by other monoaminergic systems such as the dense serotonergic innervation, the relatively dense dopaminergic innervation in the forebrain, and the presence of a strong noradrenergic and adrenergic innervation of the rhombencephalon. 4. In some areas of the CNS there is a strong relationship between histaminergic fibers and intracerebral blood vessels.

In the present study we have investigated the possible interaction between the distribution of the histaminergic neurons and fibers in the mammillary region and the appearance of the nitric oxide synthase-positive (NOS) cells and fibers and NO-mediated cGMP-fibers in that same region using the activation of the guanylyl cyclase by NO as a tool to visualize cGMP activity. Previous data from our group have shown the anterograde messenger role of NO in cholinergic neurons and that NO-mediated cGMP synthesis may play a role in acetylcholine release. The mammillary bodies contain three distinctive histaminergic cell groups of which the tuberomamillary and the ventrolateral parts are most compact and well defined. These histaminergic cell groups project to various parts of the limbic system and the cerebral cortex. We have presented evidence for functional neuroanatomical interactions between the histaminergic system and the NO-cGMP cascade within the mammillary bodies, and the cholinergic system in the cerebral cortex. The system is of clinical interest because patients with Alzheimer's and/or Parkinson's disease are reported to exhibit characteristic pathology and cell loss in the regions of the hypothalamus were histaminergic neurons are localized[40,41,42,43].

5. References:

1. M. Airaksinen and P. Panula, J. Comp. Neurol. 273 (1988) 163-186.
2. H. Prast, M.H. Tran, C. Lamberti, H.P. Fischer, M. Kraus, K. Grass and A. Philippu, Naunyn-Schmiedeberg's Arch. Pharmacol. 360 (1999) 552-557.
3. M.B. Passani and P. Blandina, Methods Finf. Exp. Clin. Pharmacol. 20 (1998) 725-733.
4. H. Prast, M.H. Tran, C. Lamberti, H.P. Fischer, M. Kraus, K. Grass and A. Philippu, Naunyn-Schmiedeberg's Arch. Pharmacol. 360 (1999) 558-564.
5. H. Ericson, T. Watanabe and Ch. Köhler, J. Comp. Neurol. 263 (1987) 1-24.
6. H. Ericson, A. Blomqvist and Ch. Köhler, J. Comp. Neurol. 281 (1989) 169-192. L.B. Hough and J.P. Green, In: Lajtha A, ed. Handbook of Neurochemistry, Vol. 6, New York: Plenum Press, 1984:145-211.
7. K.A. Manning, J.R. Wilson and D.J. Uhlrich, J. Comp. Neurol. 373 (1996) 271-282.
8. A. Khateb, P. Fort, A. Pegna, B.E. Jones and M. Mühlethaler, Neuroscience 69 (1995) 495-506.
9. S. Miyazaki, K. Onodera, M. Imaizumi and H. Timmerman, Life Sci. 61 (1997) 355-361.
10. A. Blokland, J. De Vente, J. Prickaerts, W. Honig, M. Markerink-van Ittersum and H. Steinbusch, Eyr. J. Neurosci. 11 (1999) 223-232.
11. N. Inagaki, A. Yamatodani, M. Ando-Yamamoto, M. Tohyama, T. Watanabe and H. Wada, J. Comp. Neurol. 273 (1988) 283-300.
12. Ch. Köhler, L.W. Swanson, L. Haglund and J.-Y. Wu, Neuroscience 16 (1985) 85-110.
13. P. Panula, H.-YFT. Yang and E. Costa, Proc. Natl. Acad. Sci. USA 81 (1984) 2572-2576.
14. B.T. Patel, N. Tudball, H. Wada and T. Watanabe, Neurosci. Lett. 63 (1986) 185-189.
15. H. Pollard, I. Pachot and J.-C. Schwartz, Neurosci. Lett. 54 (1985) 53-58.
16. J.-C. Schwartz, Life Sci. 17 (1975) 503-518.
17. J.-C. Schwartz, H. Pollard and T.T. Quach, J. Neurochem. 35 (1980) 26-33.
18. E. Senba, P.E. Daddona, T. Watanabe, J-Y. Wu and J.I. Nagy, J. Neuroscience 5 (1985) 3393-3402.
19. R.P.J.M. Smits, H.W.M. Steinbusch and A.H. Mulder, J. Chem. Neuroanat. 3 (1990) 85-100.
20. S.H. Snyder and K.M. Taylor, In: Snyder S.H., ed. Perspective in Neuropharmacology: A tribut to Julius Axelrod. New York: Oxford University Press, 1974.
21. W.A. Staines, P.E. Daddona and J.I. Nagy, Neuroscience 23 (1987) 571-596.
22. H.W.M. Steinbusch and A.H. Mulder, In: Björklund A., Hökfelt T., and Kuhar M.J., eds., Handbook of Chemical Neuroanatomy, Vol. 3. Amsterdam: Elsevier Science Publishers, 1984:126-140.
23. H.W.M. Steinbusch and F.J.H. Tilders, In: Monoaminergic Neurons: Light Microscopy and Ultrastructure (ed. Steinbusch H.W.M.) IBRO Handbook Series: Methods in the Neurosciences Vol. 10. Wiley, Chicester, UK, 1987:125-166.

24. H.W.M. Steinbusch and A.H. Mulder, In: Gannelin J. and Schwarz J.-C., eds, Frontiers in Histamine Research. Adv. Biosciences 51. New York: Plenum Press, 1985:119-131.

25. H.W.M. Steinbusch, Y. Sauren, H. Groenewegen, T. Watanabe and A.H. Mulder , Brain Res. 368 (1986) 389-393.

26. N. Takeda, S. Inagaki, S. Taguchi, M. Tohyama, T. Watanabe and H. Wada, Brain Res. 323 (1984a) 55-63.

27. N. Takeda, S. Inagaki, S. Shiosaka, Y. Taguchi, W.H. Oertel, M. Tohyama, T. Watanabe and H. Wada, Proc. Natl. Acad. Sci. USA 81 (1984b) 7647-7650.

28. J. de Vente, D.A. Hopkins, M. Markerink-van Ittersum, P.C. Emson, H.H.H.W. Schmidt and H.W.M. Steinbusch, Neuroscience 87 (1998) 207-241.

29. J. de Vente, M. Markerink-van Ittersum, J. van Abeeleen, P.C. Emson, H. Axer and H.W.M. Steinbusch, Eur. J. Neurosci. 12 (2000) 507-519.

30. S.R. Vincent, T. Hökfelt and J-Y. Wu, Neuroendocrinology 34 (1982) 117-125.

31. S.R. Vincent and T. Hökfelt T. Science 220 (1983) 1309.

32. T. Watanabe, Y. Taguchi, H. Hayashi, H. Wada, H. Kubota, Y. Terano, J. Tanaka, S. Shiosaka and M. Tohyama, Neurosci. Lett. 39 (1983) 249-254.

33. T. Watanabe, Y. Taguchi, S. Shiosaka, J. Tanaka, H. Kubota, Y. Terano, M. Tohyama and H. Wada H., Brain Res. 295 (1984) 13-25.

34. B.J. Wilcox and V.S. Seybold, Neurosci. Lett. 29 (1982) 105-110.

35. F.G. Wouterlood, J.G.J.M. Bol and H.W.M. Steinbusch, J. Histochem. Cytochem. 35 (1987) 817-823.

36. M.B. Passani, L. Bacciottini, P.F. Mannaioni and P. Blandina, Neurosci. Biobehav. Rev. 24 (2000) 107-113.

37. P. Panula, J. Rinne, K. Kuokkanen, K.S. Eriksson, T. Sallmen, H. Kalimo and M. Relja, Neuroscience 82 (1998) 991-997.

38. E. Nakazato, T. Yamamoto, M. Ohno and S. Watanabe, Life Sci. 67 (2000) 1139-1147.

39. J.R. Wilson, K.A. Manning, D.M. Forrester, S.E. Counts and D.J. Uhlrich, Anat. Rec. 255 (1999) 295-305.

40. C.B. Saper and D.C. German, Neurosci. Lett. 74 (1987) 3364-3370.

41. M.S. Airaksinen, A. Paltau, L. Paljärvi, K. Reinikainen, P. Riekinen, R. Suomalainer and P. Panula, Neuroscience 44 (1991) 465-481.

42. H. Braak and E. Braak, Progr. Brain Res. 93 (1992) 3-14.

43. D.F. Swaab, M.A. Hofman, P.J. Lucassen, J.S. Purba, F.C. Raadsheer and J.A.P. Van de Nes, Anat. Embryol. 187 (1993) 317-330.

The Histamine H3 receptor and its legends; from gene to clininc

Histamine Research in the New Millennium
T. Watanabe, H. Timmerman and K. Yanai (Editors)

Molecular identification of the human and rat histamine H_3 receptors: New pharmacological and functional insight

Timothy W. Lovenberg, Sandy Wilson, Jayashree Pyati, Hong Chang, Barbara Roland, Changlu Liu

R.W. Johnson Pharmaceutical Research Institute, 3210 Merryfield Row, San Diego, CA 92121

Histamine regulates neurotransmitter release in the central and peripheral nervous systems through H_3 presynaptic receptors. Although the existence of the histamine H_3 receptor was pharmacologically demonstrated 15 years ago, intensive efforts have failed to reveal its molecular identity. As part of a directed effort to discover novel G-protein coupled receptors through homology searching of expressed sequence tag (EST) databases, we identified a partial cDNA clone (GPCR97) that had significant homology to biogenic amine receptors. Expression of its full-length sequence in cells conferred an ability to inhibit adenylate cyclase in response to histamine, as well as various H_3 receptor agonists. Radioligand binding analysis revealed a pharmacological profile consistent with that for the histamine H_3 receptor. The definitive assignment of GPCR97 as the human histamine H_3 receptor has opened the door to advance our understanding of the histamine H_3 receptor to a new level. This presentation highlights the identification of the human and rat histamine H_3 receptor cDNAs, their tissue distributions, and pharmacological profiles (both binding and functional). Also highlighted is the discussion of putative receptor subtypes such as alternative splice forms vs. novel molecular entities.

1. INTRODUCTION

The histamine H_3 receptor was first identified as a presynaptic autoreceptor on histamine neurons in the brain controlling the stimulated release of histamine (1). It has subsequently been shown to be a presynaptic heteroreceptor in non-histamine containing neurons in both the central and peripheral nervous systems (2). Many potent agonists and antagonists of the H_3 receptor have been described over the past 15 years, and much promise has been made about the use of such compounds as human therapeutics. Despite this promise, the actual molecular identity of the H_3 receptor has remained an enigma and thus left investigators to ponder the exact nature of the receptor or receptors for which they are developing ligands. The advent of advanced molecular sequencing techniques has led to an explosion in the amount of genetic information available in public and private databases. We, and others, have taken advantage of these databases through systematic mining in search of novel receptors. We used this approach to identify an orphan G-protein coupled receptor which we called GPCR97. We demonstrated that GPCR97 was indeed the human H_3 receptor cDNA (3) and showed that the recombinant H_3 receptor is a G-protein coupled receptor that signals through the inhibition of adenylate cyclase. Our subsequent cloning of the rat histamine H_3 receptor revealed some interesting pharmacological distinctions between the two species (4).

Additionally, we have used the recombinant receptor clones to examine some of the agonist/antagonist properties of various known H_3 receptor ligands. These findings reveal some here-to-fore unpredicted properties of certain H_3 ligands that should form the basis of future studies to determine how accurately the recombinant receptors predict the nature of these compounds *in vivo*.

1.1 Identification of the human histamine H_3 receptor

The human H_3 receptor is a 445 amino acid protein that exhibits most homology (albeit less than 25%) to the muscarinic acetylcholine receptor family. This is rather low by receptor standards and puts the H_3 receptor in a category by itself. The H_3 receptor clearly fits into the biogenic amine receptor family with the highly conserved aspartic acid residue in the putative third transmembrane domain. The human H_3 receptor mRNA is most abundantly expressed in the central nervous system, particulary in the regions of the striatum, thalamus, hypothalamus, and cortex. The human H_3 receptor displays high affinity for the known H_3 agonist radioligands [^{3}H]-R-alpha-methylhistamine (0.6 nM) and [^{3}H]-N-methylhistamine (0.8 nM), as well as modest affinity for [^{3}H]-histamine (11 nM). Binding of these radioligands is competitively displaced by known H_3 ligands, including both agonists and antagonists (Table 1). Functionally, the human H_3 receptor appears to mediate signal transduction through inhibition of adenylate cyclase. Inhibition of adenylate cyclase is achieved by histamine and the known H_3 agonists imetit, immepip, R-alpha-methylhistamine, N-methylhistamine, and S-alpha-methylhistamine. The inhibition of adenylate cyclase by any of these agonists can be competitively antagonized by thioperamide or clobenpropit. For the most part, the binding affinities and functional properties are consistent with what is expected based on literature values using guinea pig ileum or rat cerebral cortex. One notable exception is thioperamide, which has been shown to be high affinity in rodent tissue, but appears to exhibit a lower affinity at the human receptor. West and coworkers have reported in rodent tissue that thioperamide binds to both high (H3a, 5nM) and low (H3b, 68nM) affinity sites, thus possibly distinguishing between two distinct populations of receptor (5). In order to determine if the human clone that we found represented the putative H3b subtype or whether there existed a simple species difference, we cloned and characterized its rat homolog and determined the pharmacological properties.

1.2 Identification of the rat histamine H_3 receptor

The rat H_3 receptor is the same size as human (445 amino acids) and is nearly 93% identical. It is significantly more homologous to its human counterpart than are the similar rat/human pairs of H_1 or H_2 receptors at 78% and 86%, respectively. Within the putative transmembrane, the homology reaches 97% identity, corresponding to a total of only five amino acid differences, with 2 found in third transmembrane domain and a single change found in each of fourth, sixth, and seventh transmembrane domains. As with the human receptor, the rat ortholog of human H_3 receptor is robustly expressed in various regions of the rat brain, most notably the cerebral cortex, striatum, hypothalamus and thalamus. Specific expression is also detected in the tuberomammilary nuclei and locus coeruleus. The rat H_3 receptor also couples negatively to adenylate cyclase and binds the H_3 radioligands with high affinity. The rank order of potency is similar to that seen for the human recombinant receptor and rat cerebral cortex (Table 1). However, the antagonist thioperamide was more potent vs. the rat receptor than for the human receptor, showing a distinct species difference. Clobenpropit displayed high affinity for both receptors (approx. 0.5 nM). We performed a correlation analysis comparing the pK_i values for rat recombinant receptor binding vs the human recombinant receptor binding. A highly significant correlation ($r^2=0.956$) was observed when thioperamide was left out of the analysis, whereas a poor correlation ($r^2=0.711$) was observed when thioperamide was included. This analysis included both agonists and antagonists (4).

1.3 Heterogeneity of histamine H_3 receptors.

A recent report of the cloning of the guinea pig H_3 receptors described the existence of splice forms of the H_3 receptor (6). Focusing on the region between transmembrane five and six, we examined the expression of the human H_3 receptor by both PCR and RNase protection. Interestingly, we were only able to identify one isoform of the human mRNA which corresponded to the isoform originally reported (3). We were however, able to demonstrate in a parallel experiment, the existence of splice forms in rat brain, one of which corresponded to the splice form identified in guinea pig. These splice forms in rat correspond to three unannotated sequences submitted to Genbank (Itadani, AB015646, 2000). We believe that the splice forms seen in rat represent real mRNAs but are most likely artifacts of aberrant splicing events. We do not think that these splice forms have any correlates in humans (7).

1.4 Functional analysis in recombinant cells shows that ability to detect partial agonism

Tissue preparations are normally used to evaluate the agonist/antagonist potential of compounds. Obtaining fresh human tissue is problematic and thus studying ligand-receptor interactions in recombinant systems is a convenient way to evaluate the intrinsic efficacy of compounds against human receptors. Leurs et al. (8) have reported complex binding behavior of several known histamine analogs. We tested these analogs in the recombinant system and found they do indeed possess complex behavior even in response the single receptor entity expressed in the cells. These data are summarized in Table 3. Histamine, as expected, is a full agonist with a potency of approximately 6 nM. Addition of an extra methylene between the imidazole ring and the primary amine (impropamine) results in a decrease in potency, yet retains full efficacy as an agonist. An additional methylene yields imbutamine which is also a full efficacy agonist, but is more potent than histamine. A further methylene extension yields impentamine which exhibits a complex behavior. By itself, impentamine can inhibit adenylate cyclase, but only with approximately 60% of efficacy of histamine. In the presence of histamine, impentamine displays antagonist properties and thus would be considered a partial agonist. The final compound, imhexamine, which has an additional methylene, behaves as a pure, competitive antagonist. Another compound which behaves as a full agonist is chloroproxyfan. Interestingly, the classical H_2/H_3 antagonist burimamide does not act as an antagonist at the recombinant human or rat H_3 receptors. Burimamide appears to be a full agonist at the rat receptor and a partial agonist at the human receptor. The agonistic effect of burimamide can be competitively antagonized by clobenpropit (Figure 1). These findings of complex compound behavior in the simple H_3 expression system suggest that many of the complexities observed in tissue are the result of intrinsic properties of the compounds and not heterogeneity of the H_3 receptor system.

2.0 DISCUSSION

The recent cloning of the human and rat histamine H_3 receptor cDNA opens up a new area of study for function and pharmacological intervention of histamine function in the central nervous system. We have demonstrated that the recombinant H_3 receptors bind the known histamine ligands and accurately predict agonist/antagonist properties of a majority of these ligands. We have also suggested some previously unsuspected properties of certain putative H_3 antagonists such as burimamide which appears to have agonist properties in the recombinant systems. There are many caveats that may be associated with studying drug/receptor interactions in recombinant, overexpressed systems and it can easily be conceived that the overexpressed receptor may identify aspects of ligand that is not reflective of a real tissue situation. However, these recombinant systems provide an excellent opportunity for identifying the intrinsic potential of various H_3 ligands, which can then be evaluated in tissue preparations.

Table 1. K_i values of known histamine agonists and antagonists.

	Rat H_3 K_i (nM) AVG ± SD	Human H_3 K_i (nM) AVG ± SD	Rat Cortex K_i (nM) AVG ± SD
Imetit	0.2 ± 0.1	0.6 ± 0.1	0.1 ± 0.1
Immepip	1.4 ± 0.5	1.6 ± 0.1	0.5 ± 0.1
N-methylhistamine	1.5 ± 0.5	2.4 ± 0.5	1.2 ± 0.2
RAMH	1.9 ± 0.6	2.1 ± 0.9	1.5 ± 0.1
Clobenpropit	0.4 ± 0.1	0.6 ± 0.1	0.5 ± 0.1
Thioperamide	4.2 ± 1.8	58.0 ± 19.3	10.2 ± 3.4
Histamine	13.2 ± 1.0	15.2 ± 3.9	12.0 ± 4.2
Clozapine	1750 ± 350	>10000	3000

Values were determined by competition binding with [^{3}H]-N-methylhistamine to cell membranes from either rat recombinant H_3-expressing cells, human recombinant H_3-expressing cells, or rat cerebral cortex. Values represent the average plus/minus the standard deviation of at least three experiments.

Table 2. Summary of binding potency (pK_1), agonist potency (pEC$_{50}$), antagonist potency (pA$_2$), and intrinsic agonist efficacy of various histamine analogs.

Compound	n =	pK$_I$ n=3	pEC$_{50}$ n=3	pA$_2$ n=3	Agonist Efficacy
Histamine	1	8.22 ± 0.17	8.18 ± 0.27	ND	100%
Impropamine	2	7.35 ± 0.14	7.39 ± 0.26	ND	100%
Imbutamine	3	8.90 ± 0.07	9.04 ± 0.04	ND	100%
Impentamine	4	8.05 ± 0.02	7.77 ± 0.20	7.52 ± 0.24	60%
Imhexamine	5	7.56 ± 0.04	ND	7.03 ± 0.13	<10%

Agonist potency was determined by the inhibition of forskolin-stimulated cAMP accumulation in SK-N-MC cells expressing the recombinant human H$_3$ receptor. Receptor binding was determined using the same cells with [^{3}H]-N-methylhistamine as a radioligand.

Figure 1. Agonist effects of burimamide on human or rat recombinant H_3 receptors.

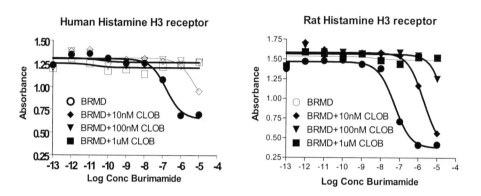

Burimamide (BRMD) was incubated with increasing concentrations of clobenpropit (CLOB) Cyclic AMP accumulation was indirectly measured by reporter gene assay measuring the absorbance of a beta-galactosidase substrate at A570.

REFERENCES
1. Arrang, J. M., M. Garbarg, and J. C. Schwartz (1983) Autoinhibition of brain histamine release mediated by a novel class (H3) of histamine receptor. *Nature (London)* **302**:832-837.
2. Hill, S. J., C. R. Ganellin, H. Timmerman, J. C. Schwartz, N. P. Shankley, J. M. Young, W. Schunack, R. Levi, and H. L. Haas (1997) International Union of Pharmacology. XIII. Classification of histamine receptors. *Pharmacol. Rev.* **49**:253-278.
3. Lovenberg, T. W., B. L. Roland, S. J. Wilson, X. Jiang, J. Pyati, A. Huvar, M. R. Jackson, and M. G. Erlander (1999) Cloning and functional expression of the human histamine H3 receptor. *Mol. Pharmacol.* **55**:1101-1107.
4. Lovenberg, T.W., Pyati, J., Chang, H., Wilson, S.J. and Erlander, M.G. (2000) Cloning of rat histamine H3 receptor reveals distinct species pharmacological profiles, *J. Pharmacol. Exp. Ther.*, **293**:771-778.
5. West, R. E., Jr., A. Zweig, N. Y. Shih, M. I. Siegel, R. W. Egan, and M. A. Clark (1990) Identification of two H3-histamine receptor subtypes. *Mol. Pharmacol.* **38**:610-613.
6. Tardivel-Lacombe, J., Rouleau, A., Heron, A., Morisset, S., Pillot, C., Cochois, V., Schwartz, J.-C., Arrang, J.-M. (2000) Cloning and cerebral expression of the guinea pig histamine H3 receptor: evidence for two isoforms, *NeuroReport*, **11**:755-759.
7. Liu, C., Ma, X.-J., Lovenberg, T.W. (2000) Alternative splicing of the histamine H3 receptor mRNA at the third cytoplasmic loop is not detectable in humans. *Molecular Brain Res.* (in press).

8. Leurs, R., Kathman, M., Vollinga, R.C., Menge, W.M.P.B., Schlicker, E., Timmerman, H. (1996) Histamine homologues discriminating between two functional H3 receptor assays. Evidence for H3 receptor heterogeneity. *J. Pharmacol. Exp. Ther.* **276:**1009 - 1015.

Histamine Research in the New Millennium
T. Watanabe, H. Timmerman and K. Yanai (Editors)

Cloning, functional characterisation and CNS expression of H3 receptor isoforms

R. Leurs[1], N. Peitsaro[2], G. Drutel[1], K. Wieland[1], K. Karlstedt[2], M. J. Smit[1†], H. Timmerman[1], and P.Panula[2, 3].

[1] LACDR, Vrije Universiteit Amsterdam, Division of Medicinal Chemistry, De Boelelaan 1083, 1081 HV Amsterdam, The Netherlands.

[2]Department of Biology Åbo Akademi University, Biocity, Artillerigaten 6 A, FIN-20520 Turku, Finland.

[3]Institute of Biomedicine, Department of Anatomy, University of Helsinki, POB 9, 00014 Helsinki, Finland.

Following the cloning of the human H_3 receptor by Lovenberg *at al*, we found the H_3 receptor gene to be localised on human chromosome 20. Since the gene contains at least 2 introns, we started a RT-PCR approach on whole rat brain cDNA to identify potential H_3 receptor isoforms. We cloned the cDNAs of three functional rat H_3 receptor isoforms (H_{3A}, H_{3B} and H_{3C}), that are generated as a result of alternative splicing. The receptor isoforms show high homology to the cloned human H_3 receptor and vary in the length of the third intracellular loop. The three subtypes show different efficacies for coupling to adenylate cyclase or p44/p42 MAPK, a newly identified signalling pathway for the H_3 receptor. The three isoforms also display distinct CNS expression, which adds a new level of complexity to our understanding of the role of histamine and the H_3 receptor in brain function.

1. INTRODUCTION

The presynaptic histamine H_3 autoreceptor is an important regulatory unit for histamine homeostasis in the CNS [1]. However, the histamine H_3 receptor not only regulates the release of histamine from histaminergic nerve terminals, but is also present in non-histaminergic nerve terminals, where it acts as a heteroreceptor modulating the release of e.g. other biogenic amines such as acetylcholine, serotonin, noradrenaline, and dopamine [2].

Important progress has recently been made in the understanding of the physiological role of the H_3 receptor. Clear indications for the therapeutic use of H_3 receptor agonists and antagonists are now available [2], and clinical trials are in progress or being planned. For H_3 receptor agonists, especially the feedback mechanism on sensory C-fibres and resulting anti-inflammatory effects suggest a potential peripheral application in the treatment of migraine and inflammatory disorders, such as arthritis and Bowel disease [2]. The CNS effects of the H_3 antagonists make them interesting candidates for the treatment of several CNS-related disorders [2]. These drugs show potential therapeutic effects in e.g. models of obesity and epilepsy. Intriguing are also the observations that H_3 receptor antagonists have beneficial

† Supported by the Royal Dutch Academy of Arts and Sciences.

effects on learning parameters in both pharmacological (e.g. scopolamine-induced amnesia) and natural (senescence-accelerated mice, ADHD models) models of memory impairment [2]. The possible relevance of these findings to diseases such as age-related memory disorders, Alzheimer's disease and ADHD is currently considered and awaits confirmation from clinical trials.

2. CLONING OF THE H₃ RECEPTOR

Whereas the H_3 receptor has been considered for many years as a potentially interesting therapeutic target, the lack of information on the actual molecular target has been a major drawback for the therapeutic development of selective ligands. Despite considerable efforts to clone the H_3 receptor gene details on the molecular structure of this therapeutically interesting receptor subtype have been lacking until June 1999 [3]. Whereas homology based approaches and expression-cloning strategies by various laboratories were unsuccessful, information from an EST-database finally led to the identification of the H_3 receptor as a G-protein coupled receptor (GPCR) [3]. Lovenberg and colleagues identified an EST sequence (GPCR97) with 35 % homology to transmembrane domain 7 of α_2 adrenergic receptors. Predominant expression of the EST sequence in the CNS prompted Lovenberg *et al.* to clone the full length sequence (Genbank AF140538) from a human thalamic cDNA library [3]. Signal transduction assays and radioligand binding studies revealed that GPCR97 was, in fact, the G_i-coupled histamine H_3 receptor [3].

3. H₃ RECEPTOR HETEROGENEITY?

Recent pharmacological studies have provided indirect evidence for the existence of H_3 receptor heterogeneity [4, 5]. This suggestion was furthermore supported by the lack of clear mRNA expression of the cloned H_3 receptor gene in peripheral tissues, despite the clear pharmacological identification of H_3 receptor effects in the periphery. Although the lack of detection of H_3 receptor expression in the periphery can be due to its low abundancy, it could also indicate the potential existence of H_3 receptor subtypes. With the cloning of the H_3 receptor gene new experimental approaches to study H_3 receptor heterogeneity became available

Submission of the human H_3 receptor cDNA sequence to the Genbank database locates the human H_3 receptor gene at human chromosome 20 (accession number: 7263900). Comparison of the reported human cDNA [3] and the genomic sequence reveals that the human H_3 receptor gene consists of at least 3 exons separated by two introns. Exon 1 encodes the first 84 amino acids of the human H_3 receptor and is interrupted by intron of 1063bp. Exon 2 encodes for the amino acids 85 to 139 and is separated by a second intron of 1564 bp from exon 3, which encodes for the rest of the human H_3 receptor (amino acids 140 to 445).

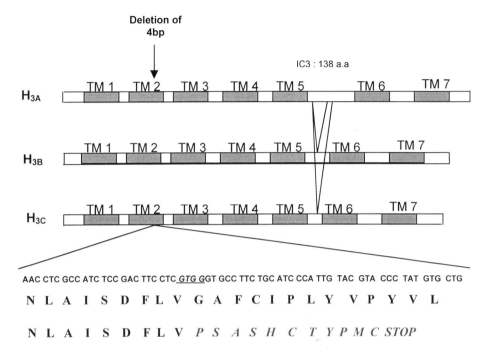

Fig. 1 Schematic representation of the identified H₃ receptor isoforms after RT-PCR on whole rat brain cDNA. The H₃A receptor is 445 amino acids long and contains an IC3 loop of 138 amino acids. The H₃B and H₃C isoform lack 32 and 48 amino acids in the intracellular IC3 loop , whereas the H₃T variant represents a truncated variant as a result of a 4 bp deletion (underlined) [6].

4. CLONING OF H₃ RECEPTOR ISOFORMS

Since the identification of at least two introns in the human H₃ receptor gene suggest the existence of potential H₃ receptor isoforms as a result of alternative splicing we started a RT-PCR approach on whole brain rat cDNA. This approach resulted in the cloning of the cDNAs of three functional rat H₃ receptor subtypes, named H₃A, H₃B and H₃C, which vary in length of their third intracellular loop (IC3) with H₃B and H₃C lacking 32 and 48 amino acids, respectively [6]. Moreover, we identified a 4 bp deletion variant, that results in a frame-shift and to a truncated receptor protein with 11 amino acid changes and a stop codon in transmembrane domain 2 (H₃T) (Fig. 1).

The rat H₃A receptor protein is 93% homologous to its human counterpart [3] and corresponds to the rat variant that was recently reported by Lovenberg *et al.* [7]. In the human gene the first intron of 1063bp is exactly located at the position of the identified 4 bp deletion, suggesting that the rat H₃T variant is likely the result of alternative splicing of intron 1. The second intron is located at the border of transmembrane 3 (DRY motif), but so far no isoforms have been found that are related to alternative splicing of this intron. The observed variations in IC3 are the result of the use of different splicing donor and acceptor sites (H₃B and H₃C) or the complete retention of the nucleotide sequence (H₃A) [6].

5. CNS EXPRESSION OF THE H₃ RECEPTOR ISOFORMS

To study the mRNA expression of the various isoforms we performed *in situ* hybridization on rat brain slices. The general distribution of the H_3 receptor mRNA as revealed with a non-selective H_3 receptor probe (H_{3X}, fig. 2) resembled that described in some brain areas by Lovenberg et al. [3]. Using isoform selective oligonucleotide probes, it was observed that the H_3 receptor isoforms display differential expression in key areas involved in regulation of the sensory, endocrine and cognitive functions in the brain (fig. 2). All isoforms were expressed in the tuberomammillary histamine neurons, but differential expression of the H_3 receptor isoforms in e.g. the dentate gyrus and hippocampal subfields was found. The relatively strong expression of the H_{3A} isoform in the hippocampus renders it a likely candidate for regulation of hippocampal functions. Strong expression of H_{3B} and H_{3C} isoforms in the locus coeruleus and dorsal raphe nucleus suggests that these isoforms may be responsible for inhibition of noradrenaline [8] and serotonin [9] release, respectively. H_{3c} receptor mRNA was also abundant in striatal cells, which may thus mediate the inhibitory effect on dopamine release from striatal dopaminergic terminals [10]. Cerebellar Purkinje cells strongly expressed the H_{3C} isoform, whereas the H_{3A} isoform was found in granule cells, suggesting that histamine regulates motor functions in cerebellum through H_{3A} and H_{3C} receptor isoforms.

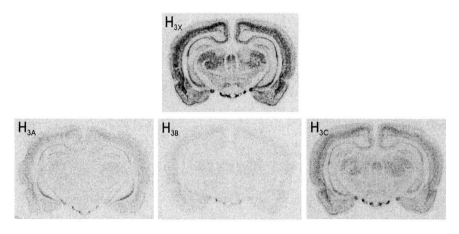

Figure 2
Histamine H_3 receptor isoform mRNA expression in rat brain. The expression pattern seen with the H_{3X} probe resembles that seen with the H_{3C} probe. The H_{3A} and H_{3B} expression pattern clearly differs from that of H_{3C} and H_{3X}. Control hybridization with a 100-fold excess of unlabelled H_{3X} probe results in a completely abolished signal.

6. FUNCTIONALITY OF THE H₃ RECEPTOR ISOFORMS

For the functional analysis the H_3 receptor isoforms were transiently expressed in COS-7 cells and analysed for H_3 agonist and antangonist radioligand binding. As expected, the H_{3T} receptor isoform did not bind any radioligand and was also unable to give rise to any signal transduction upon stimulation with H_3 agonists. The other isoforms all bound both agonist and antagonist radioligand with high affinity. No major differences were observed for the affinities of various H_3 antagonists. In contrast, all agonists bound with significant lower affinity to the full length H_{3A} isoform (fig. 3) [6].

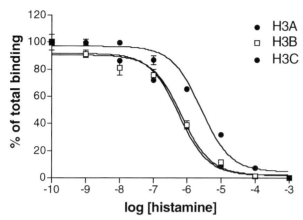

Figure 3
Agonist binding to the histamine H_3 receptor isoforms after expression in COS-7 cells. Cell membrenes were incubated with [^{3}H]-N$^\alpha$-methylhistamine and increasing concentrations of histamine. Similar results were obtained with other H_3 agonists like, (R)-α-methylhistamine, immepip and impentamine.

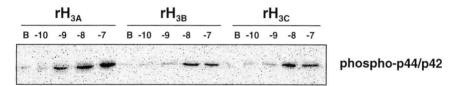

Figure 4
Activation of MAPK in COS-7 cells by the three H_3 receptor isoforms by various concentrations of immepip. MAPK activation was assessed using a phospho-p44/p42 specific antibody.

In signal transduction assays coupling of all three functional isoforms to a G_i protein mediated inhibition of adenylate cyclase was observed. In these assays the H_{3A} receptor was less effectively coupled to the inhibition of forskolin-mediated cAMP production [6]. In contrast, the H_{3A} receptor stimulated the tyrosine kinase MAP kinase at lower H_3 agonist concentrations compared to the other two isoforms, as assessed by the amount of phosphorylated p42/44 MAPK (fig. 4). The stimulation of MAPK is a new signaling pathway for the H_3 receptor. In view of the described importance of MAPK activation in hippocampal long-term potentiation [11] and the distinct H_3 receptor localization in this important brain area, the discovery of MAPK activation as a downstream signalling mechanism of the H_3 receptor is highly interesting and deserves further attention.

7. CONCLUSIONS

We cloned the cDNAs of three functional rat H_3 receptor isoforms (H_{3A}, H_{3B} and H_{3C}) and one non-functional, truncated form (H_{3T}), that are generated as a result of alternative splicing. The functional isoforms vary in the length of the third intracellular loop and show different efficacies for coupling to adenylate cyclase or p44/p42 MAPK, a newly identified signalling pathway for the H_3 receptor. The three isoforms also display distinct CNS expression, which adds a new level of complexity to our understanding of the role of histamine and the H_3 receptor in brain function [6].

8. REFERENCES

1. Arrang, J.M., M. Garbarg and J.C. Schwartz, Nature **302**: (1983) p. 832-837.
2. Leurs, R., P. Blandina, C. Tedford and H. Timmerman, Trends Pharmacol. Sci. **19**: (1998) p. 177-183.
3. Lovenberg T.W., B.L. Roland,S.J. Wilson, X. Jiang, J. Pyati, A. Huvar, M.R. Jackson and M.G. Erlander, Mol. Pharmacol. **55**: (1999) p. 1101-1107.
4. Leurs R, M. Kathmann, R.C. Vollinga, W.M.P.B. Menge, E. Schlicker and H. Timmerman, J. Pharmacol. Exp. Ther. **276**: (1996) p. 1009-1015.
5. West, R.E., A. Zweig, N. Shih, M.I. Siegel and R.W. Egan, Mol. Pharmacol. **38**: (1990) p. 610-613.
6. Drutel, G., N. Peitsaro, K. Karlstedt, K. Wieland, M. J. Smit, H. Timmerman, P. Panula and R.Leurs, Mol, Pharmacol. **59**: (2001) p. 1-8.
7. Lovenberg, T.W., J. Pyati, H. Chang, S.J. Wilson and M.G. Erlander, J. Pharmacol. Exp. Ther. **293**: (2000) p. 771-778.
8. Schlicker, E, K. Fink, M. Hinterthaner and M. Göthert, Arch. Pharmacol. **340**: (1989) p. 633-638.
9. Schlicker, E,R. Betz and M. Göthert, Arch. Pharmacol. **337**: (1988) p. 588-590.
10. Schlicker, E, K. Fink, M. Detzner and M. Gothert, J. Neural. Transm. **93**: (1993) p. 1-10.
11. Bhalla, U.S. and R. Iyengar, Science **283**: (1999) p. 381-387.

Histamine Research in the New Millennium
T. Watanabe, H. Timmerman and K. Yanai (Editors)

Partial agonists for the histamine H₃ receptor with high in vivo activity

W. Schunack[a], A. Sasse[a], H. Stark[a], S. Elz[a], X. Ligneau[b], C.R. Ganellin[c], and J.-C. Schwartz[d]

[a]Institut für Pharmazie, Freie Universität Berlin, Königin-Luise-Strasse 2+4, 14195 Berlin, Germany

[b]Laboratoire Bioprojet, 9 rue Rameau, 75002 Paris, France

[c]Department of Chemistry, Christopher Ingold Laboratories, University College London, 20 Gordon Street, London WC1H 0AJ, U.K.

[d]Unité de Neurobiologie et Pharmacologie Moléculaire (U. 109), Centre Paul Broca de l'INSERM, 2ter rue d'Alésia, 75014 Paris, France

Novel (partial) agonists are discussed which lack a second basic moiety in the side chain of the molecule. All compounds described contain a 3-(1*H*-imidazol-4-yl)propyl structural element which is connected to a bulky residue by an ether or a carbamate moiety. Some of these lipophilic compounds display partial intrinsic activity in vitro in the [³H]histamine release assay on synaptosomes of rat cerebral cortex at nanomolar concentrations and partial or even full agonist activity with low ED_{50} values in mouse cerebral cortex following oral administration. A pair of enantiomers (FUB 593 and FUB 594) are of special interest because of their differences in intrinsic activities and agonist potencies in vitro as well as in vivo.

1. INTRODUCTION

Histamine H₃-receptor agonists exert a stimulating effect on the histamine H₃ autoreceptor, thus reducing the synthesis and release of histamine [1,2]. In addition, histamine H₃ heteroreceptors inhibit the release of various neurotransmitters [3]. Possible therapeutic targets of histamine H₃-receptor agonists might be migraine and sleep disorders [4]. Classical agonists of the histamine H₃ receptor, e.g., (*R*)-α-methyl-histamine [5] and imetit [6] (cf. Chart 1), consist of an imidazole nucleus, an alkyl spacer, and a basic moiety in the side chain of the molecule. Under physiological conditions this basic group is protonated and presumably interacts with a carboxylate group of the receptor, leading to a change in conformation of the receptor protein,

Chart 1

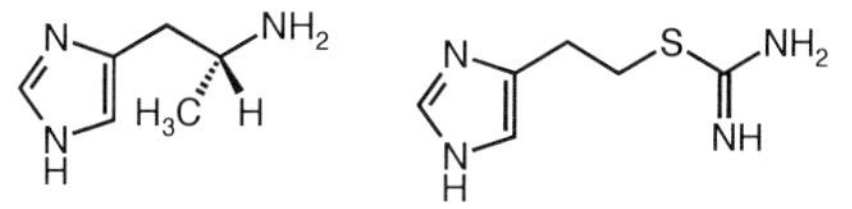

(*R*)- α-Methylhistamine   Imetit

thus inducing a cellular response. Unfortunately, these highly hydrophilic agonists penetrate the blood-brain barrier only poorly. One approach to overcome this problem was to design prodrugs of (*R*)-α-methylhistamine, e.g., BP 2.94 [7], thus increasing the amount of drug in the CNS.

Although there has been some evidence for partial agonist behaviour at the histamine H_3 receptor by lipophilic compounds devoid of a basic amino moiety in the side chain, e.g., iodoproxyfan [8,9], which is inactive under in vivo conditions in mouse brain after oral administration, this promising approach needed further exploration. Therefore, novel histamine H_3-receptor ligands lacking a basic moiety in the side chain of the molecule were investigated with special emphasis on (partial) agonist behaviour in the CNS.

2. HISTAMINE H_3-RECEPTOR AGONISTS LACKING A SECOND BASIC MOIETY

2.1. Ethers
In the series of aliphatic ethers containing a terminal bulky group, the distance of the ether moiety from the bulky aliphatic group as well as the type of the bulky group, e.g., isopropyl or *tert*-butyl, seem to be important for inducing (partial) agonism in vitro and in vivo (Table 1).

Table 1
Histamine H_3-receptor (partial) agonist/antagonist potency of aliphatic ethers

	R	$K_i^{a,b}$ (nM) $\bar{x} \pm$ sem	$EC_{50}^{a,c}$ (nM) $\bar{x} \pm$ sem	α^e	ED_{50}^d (mg/kg) $\bar{x} \pm$ sem	α^e	Ref.
FUB 396		139 ± 56		f	0.74 ± 0.12	f	10
FUB 373		14 ± 4	128 ± 86	~ 0.22	0.51 ± 0.26	1.0	10
FUB 397		9.4 ± 1.6	n.c.^{g}	~ 0.25	0.15 ± 0.08	0.6	10
FUB 407		10 ± 3	45 ± 10	0.55	0.29 ± 0.17	1.0	10
FUB 665		$24 \pm 3^{h,f}$	n.d.^{i}		0.13 ± 0.07	0.6	11
FUB 666		$44 \pm 4^{h,f}$	n.d.^{i}		1.4 ± 0.4	f	11
UCL 1470	CF$_3$	8.4 ± 2.5	98 ± 32	0.40	0.6 ± 0.3	1.0	12

^{a}K$^+$-Evoked [^{3}H]histamine release assay on synaptosomes of rat cerebral cortex [6]; ^{b}compound tested as antagonist; ^{c}compound tested as agonist; ^{d}central H_3-receptor screening assay after po administration to mice, measuring the modulation of N^τ-methylhistamine level [6]; $^e\alpha$ = intrinsic activity; ^{f}no agonism evidenced; ^{g}n.c. = not calculable; ^{h}functional H_3-receptor assay on guinea-pig ileum [13-15], K_B-value; ^{i}n.d. = not determined.

The occurrence of (partial) agonism and the intrinsic activity strongly depend on *distinct steric parameters*. The short-chained isobutyl derivative FUB 396 and on the other hand FUB 666, which contains the longest alkyl spacer with a terminal *tert*-butyl group (5,5-dimethylhexyl derivative), display purely *antagonist* behaviour in vitro as well as in vivo. The alkylaryl ether UCL 1470 which belongs to a different chemical class within the group of ethers shows partial agonist activity in vitro and full agonist action at low dosage in vivo [12].

However, the most potent (partial) agonist in the series of ethers is the 3,3-dimethylbutyl derivative FUB 407, displaying high in vitro potency on the K^+-induced [^{3}H]histamine release assay on rat synaptosomes (EC_{50} = 45 nM, $\alpha = 0.55$). In vivo screening of FUB 407 in mouse brain with oral administration showed full intrinsic activity at low dosage (ED_{50} = 0.29 mg/kg, α = 1).

2.2. Diarylmethyl carbamates

In the series of diarylmethyl carbamates, first a new lead compound was defined (FUB 316, Fig. 1, R^1, R^2 = H, Table 2), displaying partial agonist activity in vitro and full intrinsic activity in vivo. Substitution of aryl residues did not lead to increased agonist potency, although some intrinsic activity was retained in vitro by diphenylmethyl carbamates mono-substituted in 3-position (Table 2). However, due to low intrinsic activity EC_{50} values could not be calculated in each case. Substitution with methyl or chlorine in 2- or 4-position led to a dramatic drop in histamine H_3-receptor potency.

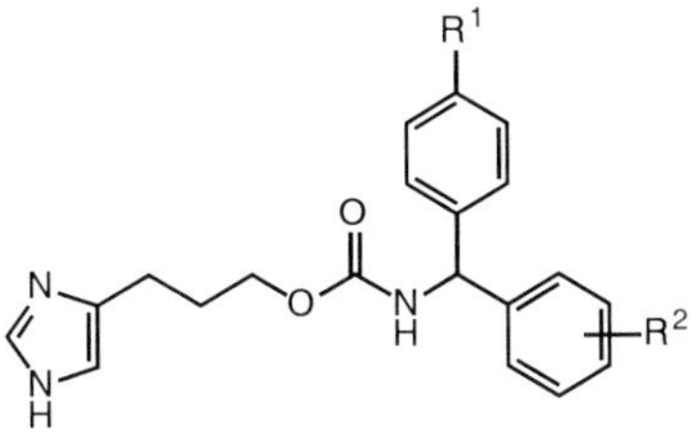

Fig. 1 Diphenylmethyl carbamates

Table 2

Histamine H_3-receptor (partial) agonist/antagonist potency of substituted diphenylmethyl carbamates[a]

	R^1	R^2	K_i (nM)[b,c] $\bar{x} \pm$ sem	EC_{50} (nM)[b,d] $\bar{x}$	α^f	ED_{50} (mg/kg)[e] $\bar{x} \pm$ sem	α^f	Ref.
FUB 316	H	H	26 ± 14	~ 100	0.2	5.3 ± 2.6	1.0	16
FUB 516	H	2-CH$_3$	≥ 1 500	> 10 000	$-^g$	> 10	-	16
FUB 517	H	3-CH$_3$	31 ± 10	n.c.^{g}	0.2	~ 30	~ 1	16
FUB 546	H	4-CH$_3$	279 ± 140		$-^h$	> 10	-	16
FUB 519	CH$_3$	4-CH$_3$	> 1 500	> 10 000	$-^g$	> 10	-	16
FUB 529	H	2-Cl	380 ± 100		$-^h$	> 10	-	16
FUB 530	H	3-Cl	21 ± 5	n.c.^{g}	0.1	> 10	-	16
FUB 531	H	4-Cl	137 ± 36		$-^h$	> 10	-	16
FUB 540	Cl	4-Cl	258 ± 61		$-^h$	> 10	-	16
FUB 547	H	3-CF$_3$	41 ± 15	~ 20 000	~ 0.4	> 10	-	11
FUB 518	F	4-F	54 ± 22		$-^h$	~ 10	-	16

[a]For general structure of compounds refer to Fig. 1; [b]K^+-evoked [^{3}H]histamine release assay on synaptosomes of rat cerebral cortex [6]; [c]compound tested as antagonist; [d]compound tested as agonist; [e]central H_3-receptor screening assay after po administration to mice, measuring the modulation of N^τ-methylhistamine level [6]; [f]α = intrinsic activity; [g]n.c. = not calculable; [h]no agonism evidenced.

This effect was not observed for the 4-fluoro derivative FUB 518, suggesting that steric demand of the lipophilic pocket of the receptor protein is responsible for this observation rather than electronic properties of the substituent.

On exchange of a phenyl ring by a cyclopropyl or cyclohexyl residue, agonist activity was lost as well, but in vitro antagonist affinity for the histamine H_3 receptor was retained (Fig. 2; Table 3, e.g., FUB 559, FUB 560). Introduction of a heterocyclic aromatic ring system such as thiophene led to partial agonist activity in vitro and full intrinsic activity in vivo after oral application to mice (FUB 557, ED_{50} = 3.4 mg/kg, α = 1). In vivo partial agonist activity was observed for the dithienyl derivative FUB 591.

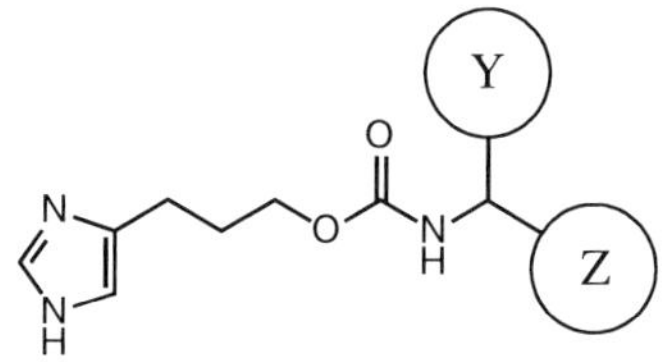

Fig. 2 (Hetero)aryl (heteroaryl/cycloalkyl) methyl carbamates

Table 3
Histamine H_3-receptor (partial) agonist/antagonist potency of aryl heteroaryl/cycloalkyl methyl carbamates[a]

	Y	Z	K_i (nM)[b,c] $\bar{x} \pm$ sem	EC_{50} (nM)[b,d] $\bar{x} \pm$ sem	α^f	ED_{50} (mg/kg)[e] $\bar{x} \pm$ sem	α^f	Ref.
FUB 560	phenyl	cyclopropyl	44 ± 9		-^{g}	~ 10	-	11
FUB 559	phenyl	cyclohexyl	54 ± 14		-^{g}	15 ± 2	-	11
FUB 532	phenyl	3-pyridyl	96 ± 35		-^{g}	> 10	-	16
FUB 557	phenyl	2-thienyl	14 ± 4	557 ± 196	0.27	3.4 ± 1.4	1.0	16
FUB 591	2-thienyl	2-thienyl	11 ± 4^{g,h}	n.d.^{i}		3.0 ± 1.9	0.8	16

[a]For general structure of compounds refer to Fig. 2; [b]K^+-evoked [^{3}H]histamine release assay on synaptosomes of rat cerebral cortex [6]; [c]compound tested as antagonist; [d]compound tested as agonist; [e]central H_3-receptor screening assay after po administration to mice, measuring the modulation of N^τ-methylhistamine level [6]; [f]α = intrinsic activity; [g]no agonism evidenced; [h]functional H_3-receptor assay on guinea-pig ileum [13-15], K_B-value; [i]n.d. = not determined.

Although these compounds possess structural similarities to histamine H_1-receptor antagonists, e.g., a diarylalkyl moiety, selectivity towards the H_3 receptor was high. The compounds of this series show (non-)competitive antagonist behaviour on H_1 and H_2 receptors in functional assays with pA_2 or $pD'_2 \leq 5.4$ [16].

2.3. Alkyl carbamates

Investigation of branched alkyl carbamates, structurally similar to aliphatic ethers mentioned in section 2.1, led to highly interesting results (Table 4). Compounds containing one methyl-branch in the α- or β-position to the carbamate nitrogen displayed H_3-receptor antagonist potency in vitro as well as in vivo. However, by introduction of a second methyl branching group, (partial) agonist activity was obtained (e.g., FUB 415→379, FUB 378→FUB 592, FUB 378→FUB 475).

Racemate FUB 562 is of special interest, as it displays full intrinsic activity and high agonist potency in vivo after oral application to mice. On screening of FUB 562 on other neurotransmitter receptors (e.g. H_1, H_2, M_3, α_{1D}, $\beta_{1/2}$, 5-HT$_{2A}$, 5-HT$_3$, 5-HT$_4$ receptor) high selectivity for the histamine H_3 receptor was observed (≥ 250).

Table 4
Histamine H_3-receptor (partial) agonist/antagonist potency of alkyl carbamates

	R	$K_i^{a,b}$ (nM)	$EC_{50}^{a,c}$		ED_{50}^{d} (mg/kg)		Ref.
		$\bar{x} \pm$ sem	$\bar{x} \pm$ sem	α^e	$\bar{x} \pm$ sem	α^e	
FUB 415		82 ± 16		$-^f$	15 ± 5	$-^f$	17
FUB 378		30 ± 10		$-^f$	≥ 10	$-^f$	17
FUB 592		$22 \pm 3^{g,f}$	n.d.^{h}		0.51 ± 0.38	0.6	18
FUB 379		$60 \pm 10^{g,f}$	n.d.^{h}		0.9 ± 0.1	0.7	10
FUB 475		23 ± 4	n.c.^{i}	~ 0.15	0.48 ± 0.15	0.7	10
FUB 562		13 ± 3	n.c.^{i}	~ 0.2	0.31 ± 0.06	1.0	18
FUB 593		10 ± 2	46 ± 35	0.45	0.27 ± 0.10	1.0	18
FUB 594		13 ± 1	n.c.^{i}	~ 0.1	0.75 ± 0.34	0.45	18

^{a}K$^+$-Evoked [^{3}H]histamine release assay on synaptosomes of rat cerebral cortex [6]; ^{b}compound tested as antagonist; ^{c}compound tested as agonist; ^{d}central H$_3$-receptor screening assay after po administration to mice, measuring the modulation of N^τ-methylhistamine level [6]; $^e\alpha$ = intrinsic activity; ^{f}no agonism evidenced; ^{g}functional H$_3$-receptor assay on guinea-pig ileum [13-15], K_B-value; ^{h}n.d. = not determined; ^{i}n.c. = not calculable.

Due to these exciting observations the pure enantiomers of FUB 562 were prepared and investigated pharmacologically (Table 4) [11,18]. FUB 593, the S-enantiomer of FUB 562, shows higher agonist potency in vitro as well as in vivo (EC_{50} = 46 nM, α = 0.45; ED_{50} = 0.27 mg/kg, α = 1). FUB 594, the distomer, displays only low partial intrinsic activity in vitro and in vivo as well as lower potency. Thus, the ligand-receptor interaction leading to a change in receptor conformation seems to depend strongly on the stereochemistry of the bulky group attached to the carbamate nitrogen.

3. SUMMARY

The described novel histamine H_3-receptor (partial) agonists are structurally diverse from classical agonists as they are lacking a second basic moiety in the side chain of the molecule. These novel compounds belong to the class of aliphatic ethers and carbamates with a bulky terminal group. Of special interest is an *enantiomeric pair* of chiral aliphatic carbamates showing different intrinsic activity and agonist potency in vitro as well as in vivo.

REFERENCES

1. J.-M. Arrang, M. Garbarg, and J.-C. Schwartz, Nature (London), 302 (1983) 832.
2. J.-M. Arrang, M. Garbarg, and J.-C. Schwartz, Neuroscience, 23 (1987) 149.
3. S.J. Hill, C.R. Ganellin, H. Timmerman, J.-C. Schwartz, N.P. Shankley, J.M. Young, W. Schunack, R. Levi, and H.L. Haas, Pharmacol. Rev., 49 (1997) 253.
4. R. Leurs, P. Blandina, C. Tedford, and H. Timmerman, Trends Pharmacol. Sci., 19 (1998) 177.
5. J.-M. Arrang, M. Garbarg, J.-C. Lancelot, J.-M. Lecomte, H. Pollard, M. Robba, W. Schunack, and J.-C. Schwartz, Nature (London), 327 (1987) 117.
6. M. Garbarg, J.-M. Arrang, A. Rouleau, X. Ligneau, M.D. Trung Tuong, J.-C. Schwartz, and C.R. Ganellin, J. Pharmacol. Exp. Ther., 263 (1992) 304.
7. A. Rouleau, M. Garbarg, X. Ligneau, C. Mantion, P. Lavie, C. Advenier, J.-M. Lecomte, M. Krause, H. Stark, W. Schunack, and J.-C. Schwartz, J. Pharmacol. Exp. Ther., 281 (1997) 1085.
8. E. Schlicker, M. Kathmann, H. Bitschnau, I. Marr, S. Reidemeister, H. Stark, and W. Schunack, Naunyn-Schmiedeberg's Arch. Pharmacol., 353 (1996) 482.
9. G.F. Watt, D.A. Sykes, S.P. Roberts, N.P. Shankley, and J.W. Black, Proceedings of the British Pharmacological Society, P153, September 2-4, Edinburgh, U.K. (1997).
10. A. Sasse, H. Stark, S. Reidemeister, A. Hüls, S. Elz, X. Ligneau, C.R. Ganellin, J.-C. Schwartz, and W. Schunack, J. Med. Chem., 42 (1999) 4269.
11. A. Sasse, PhD thesis, Berlin, Germany (1999).
12. N. Pelloux-Léon, A. Fkyerat, W. Tertiuk, W. Schunack, H. Stark, M. Garbarg, X. Ligneau, J.-C. Schwartz, and C.R. Ganellin, 29th Meeting of the European Histamine Research Society (EHRS), Abstract 31, 17-21 May, Nemi (Rome), Italy (2000).
13. R.C. Vollinga, O.P. Zuiderveld, H. Scheerens, A. Bast, and T. Timmerman, Meth. Find. Exp. Clin. Pharmacol., 14 (1992) 747.
14. E. Schlicker, M. Kathmann, S. Reidemeister, H. Stark, and W. Schunack, Br. J. Pharmacol., 112 (1994) 1043. Erratum, 113 (1994) 657.
15. X. Ligneau, M. Garbarg, M.L.Vizuette, J. Diaz, K. Purand, H. Stark, W. Schunack, and J.-C. Schwartz, J. Pharmacol. Exp. Ther., 271 (1994) 452.
16. A. Sasse, H. Stark, X. Ligneau, S. Elz, S. Reidemeister, C.R. Ganellin, J.-C. Schwartz, and W. Schunack, Bioorg. Med. Chem., 8 (2000) 1139.
17. A. Sasse, K. Kiec-Kononowicz, H. Stark, M. Motyl, S. Reidemeister, C.R. Ganellin, X. Ligneau, J.-C. Schwartz, and W. Schunack, J. Med. Chem., 42 (1999) 593.
18. A. Sasse, H. Stark, S. Elz, X. Ligneau, C.R. Ganellin, A. Rouleau, J.-M. Arrang, J.-C. Schwartz, and W. Schunack, Arch. Pharm. Pharm. Med. Chem., 333 (Suppl. 2) (2000) 9.

Histamine Research in the New Millennium
T. Watanabe, H. Timmerman and K. Yanai (Editors)

Structure-activity relationship of histamine H$_3$-ligands: Organic synthesis of imidazole *C*-nucleoside derivatives

Shinya Harusawa,[a] Tomonari Imazu,[a] Seiichiroh Takashima,[a] Lisa Araki,[a] Hirofumi Ohishi,[a] Takushi Kurihara,[a] Yasuhiko Sakamoto,[b] Yumiko Yamamoto,[c] Takeshi Hashimoto,[c] and Atsushi Yamatodani[c]

Osaka University of Pharmaceutical Sciences,[a] R&D Division, AZWELL Inc.,[b] and School of Allied Health Sciences, Faculty of Medicine, Osaka University[c]

The four possible stereoisomers of two novel imidazole *C*-nucleoside derivatives were synthesized by a new synthetic method using a phenylseleneyl group. Among them, (+)-4(5)-[(2*R*,5*R*)-5-(aminomethyl)tetrahydrofuran-2-yl]imidazole (imifuramine) exhibited clear agonistic activity for the H$_3$ receptor by a brain microdialysis method, but its activity was weak for the *in vitro* test using guinea pig ileum.

1. Introduction

The histamine H$_3$(H$_3$) receptors exist on the histaminergic fibers in the brain and modulate the synthesis and release of histamine as an autoreceptor. H$_3$-antagonists are now expected to be potential drugs for memory degenerative disorders such as Alzheimer's disease. This type of receptor can be also found in many peripheral tissues. (*R*)-α-Methylhistamine, imetit and immepip, which are potent and selective H$_3$-agonists, have been well used as pharmacological tools. H$_3$-agonists are regarded as a target for development of new therapeutics for bronchial asthma. On the other hand, theoretical calculations of histamine or some H$_3$-agonists have predicted the importance of an intramolecular hydrogen-bonding between the cationic primary amine and the N atom of the imidazole. We recently reported the β-stereoselective synthesis of C-4 linked imidazole nucleosides[1]. On the basis of these studies, we envisioned that, while the *cis*-isomer (**1**) could adopt a folded conformation through intramolecular hydrogen-bonding, the *trans*-isomer (**2**) would form the extended one (Fig.1). In this presentation, we report the synthesis of the respective four stereoisomers (**1** - **4**, *ent* **1 – 4**) of two novel imidazole *C*-nucleoside derivatives using a synthetic method characterized by use of a PhSe group for the formation of the tetrahydrofuran ring. It is of particular interest to find from the preliminary results using an *in vivo* brain microdialysis that, among them, only (+)-**2** (imifuramine) exhibited histamine H_3-agonistic activity .

2. Synthesis [2,3]

Phenylselenation of γ-butyrolactone **5** provided α-and β-selenolactones **6** and **7**, both of which were used as substrates to prepare key intermediates **11** and **12** (Fig. 2). Reduction of the major isomer **6** with DIBAL-H followed by an addition of 5-lithioimidazole **8** gave a diol **9** (73%) with a C1' *S* configuration. The 1',

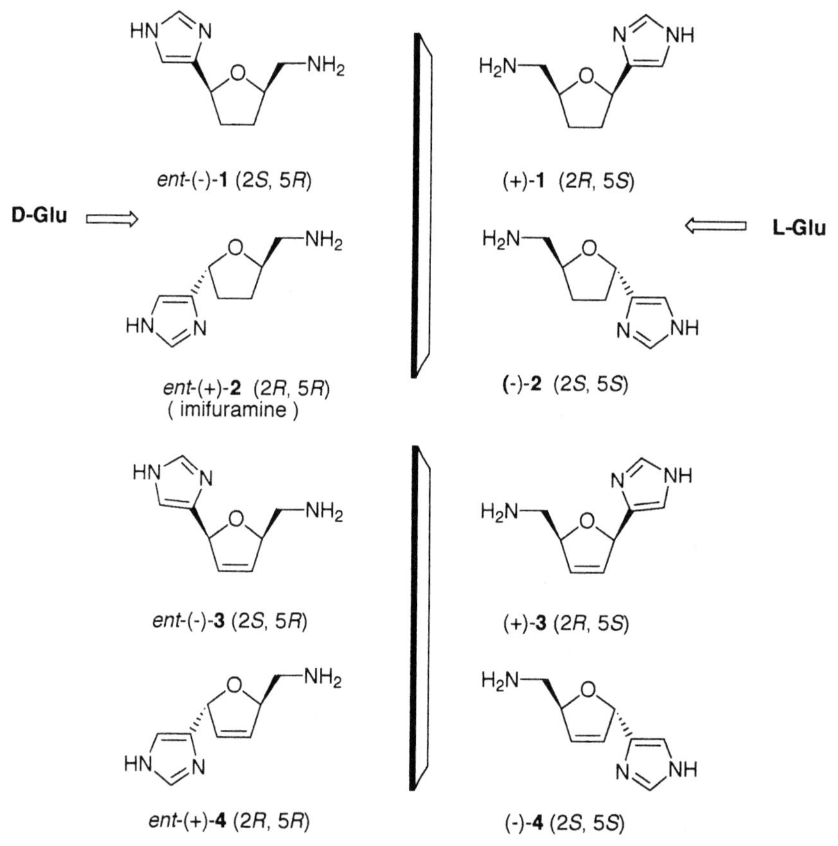

ent-(-)-**1** (2*S*, 5*R*)

(+)-**1** (2*R*, 5*S*)

D-Glu ⟹

⟸ **L-Glu**

ent-(+)-**2** (2*R*, 5*R*)
(imifuramine)

(-)-**2** (2*S*, 5*S*)

ent-(-)-**3** (2*S*, 5*R*)

(+)-**3** (2*R*, 5*S*)

ent-(+)-**4** (2*R*, 5*R*)

(-)-**4** (2*S*, 5*S*)

Fig. 1

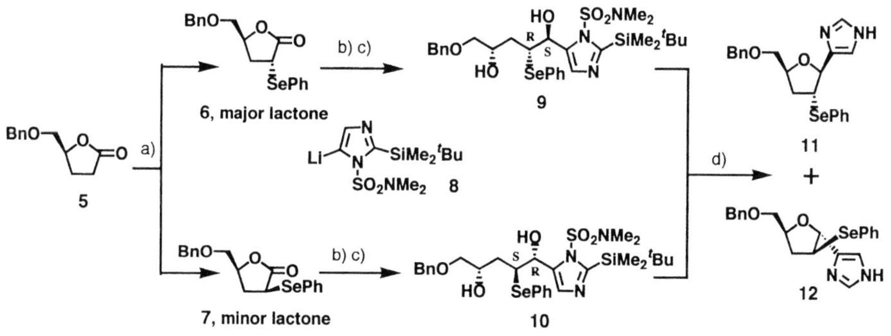

Reagents : a) (i) LHMDS , TMSCl; (ii) PhSeBr; b) DIBAL; C) **8**; d) (i) aqueous 1.5N HCl-THF; (ii) benzene, reflux, Dean - Stark water separator; Yields **11** (42%), **12** (56%) from **9**; **11** (35%), **12** (53%) from **10**

Fig. 2

2'-*anti*-selectivity for **9** may be accounted for by a chelation-cyclic model as shown in Fig. 3. Deprotection of **9** under reflux in HCl-THF followed by dehydration in the reaction mixture afforded easily separable β- and α-nucleosides **11** (42%) and **12** (56%). The formation of **11** and **12** can be reasonably rationalized as shown in Fig. 4. To date, this synthetic approach for the preparation of C-nucleosides using a combination of the elimination of PhSeCl and selenocyclization has not been reported. The minor lactone **7** also effectively supplied **11** and **12** by a parallel sequence of reactions.

Ethoxycarbonylation of the β-anomer **11** followed by free radical deselenylation gave benzyl ether **14** (Fig. 5). Debenzylation of **14** and subsequent phthaloylimination afforded 5'-substituted phthalimide **15**. Double deprotection of **15** with hydrazine hydrate yielded (+)-**1**. Alternatively, synthesis of *trans* isomer (-)-**2** was attained in 87.5% overall yield from α-anomer **12** by the synthetic procedures previously described. Their configuration counterparts (-)-**1** and (+)-**2** (imifuramine) were also synthesized starting from D-glutamic acid by the same methodology.

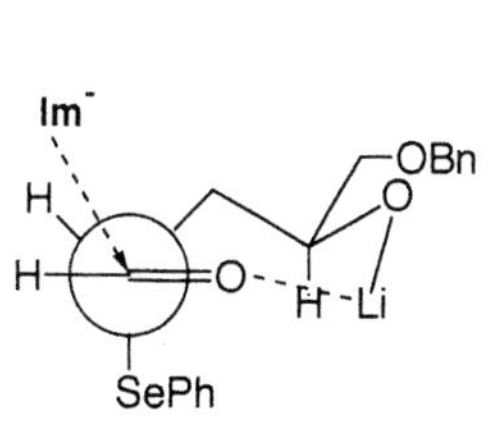

Fig. 3 The *anti*-selectivity for **9** by a chelation-cyclic model

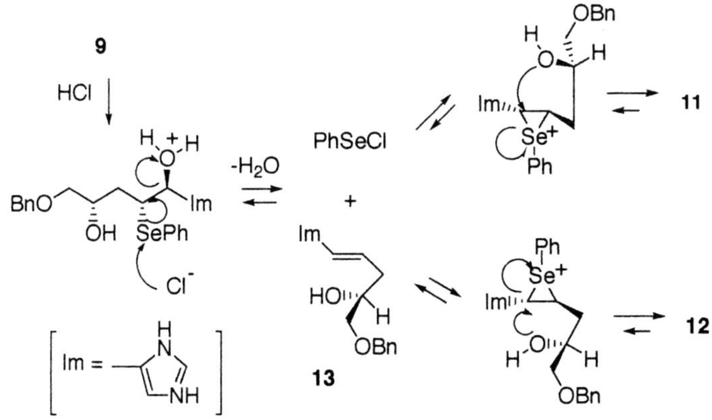

Fig. 4

It is well known that the oxidation of a phenylselenenyl group gives the formation of a double bond, so we next tried to synthesize the C2'-C3' unsaturated compounds from the key intermediates (Fig. 5). Oxidation of the β-selenonucleosides **11** with hydrogen peroxide resulted in the formation of the double bond at the C2'-C3' position of a benzyl ether **16**. In the following debenzylation, we encountered some difficulties but fortunately found the use of sodium naphthalenide was effective. Treatment of the benzyl ether with sodium naphthalenide gave a primary alcohol in 93 % yield. Then, protection of the imidazole moiety, the conversion of the primary alcohol into a phthalimide, and finally deprotection with methylamine gave the *cis*-dihydrofuranylimidazole (+)-**3** in 84% overall yield from the alcohol **17**. The *trans* isomer (-)-**4** and two

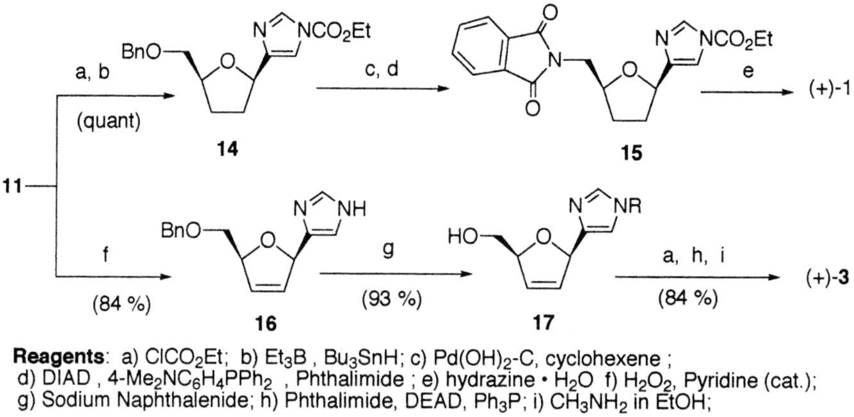

Reagents: a) ClCO₂Et; b) Et₃B , Bu₃SnH; c) Pd(OH)₂-C, cyclohexene ;
d) DIAD , 4-Me₂NC₆H₄PPh₂ , Phthalimide ; e) hydrazine • H₂O f) H₂O₂, Pyridine (cat.);
g) Sodium Naphthalenide; h) Phthalimide, DEAD, Ph₃P; i) CH₃NH₂ in EtOH;

Fig. 5

Fig. 6 Effect of Imifuramine and Clobenpropit on the *in vivo* release of Histamine

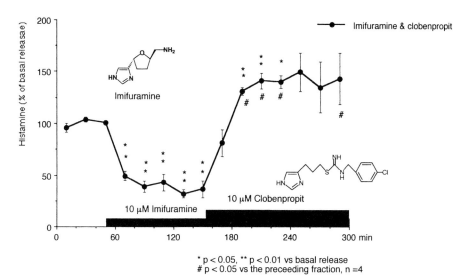

* p < 0.05, ** p < 0.01 vs basal release
# p < 0.05 vs the preceeding fraction, n =4

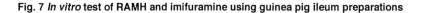

Fig. 7 *In vitro* test of RAMH and imifuramine using guinea pig ileum preparations

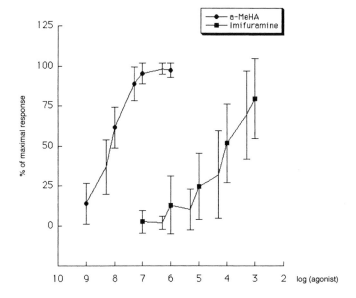

enantiomers (*ent*-3, 4) could be synthesized from the corresponding selenonucleosides.

3. Pharmacology

Using an *in vivo* microdialysis method, we first examined whether the eight synthesized stereoisomers had any effect on the release of histamine in the brain of rats. Among them, only imifuramine exhibited H_3- agonistic activity (Fig. 6). The administration of 10 μM of imifuramine to the perfusion fluid decreased histamine release to about 30% of the basal release. Further, the co-perfusion with an H_3- antagonist, clobenpropit (10 μM), fully antagonized this effect and increased histamine release to about 160% of the basal levels. The activity of imifuramine measured by the microdialysis was approximately equal to that of immepip. These facts support the H_3-agonistic activity of imifuramine. The other isomers had no effect on the histamine release at 10 μM concentration.

We next carried out *in vitro* assay of imifurmine using guinea pig ileum preparation (Fig. 7). The dose-response curve obtained for imifuramine (pD_2 = 4) appears to be shifted the right, compared to the curve of R-α-methylhistamine (pD_2 = 8). These results indicated imifuramine is a relatively weak H_3-agonist in the *in vitro* test system.

The synthesis and biological evaluation of related imidazol *C*-nucleoside derivatives are in progress in our laboratories.

REFERENCES

1. S. Harusawa , Y.Murai, H. Moriyama, T. Imazu, H. Ohishi, R. Yoneda, and T. Kurihara, J. Org. Chem., 61 (1996) 4405.

2. S. Harusawa , T. Imazu, S. Takashima, L. Araki, H. Ohishi, T. Kurihara, Y. Yamamoto and A. Yamatodani, Tetrahedron Lett., 40 (1999) 2561.

3. S. Harusawa , T. Imazu, S. Takashima, L. Araki, H. Ohishi, T. Kurihara, Y. Sakamoto, Y. Yamamoto and A. Yamatodani, J. Org. Chem., 64 (1999) 8608.

Histamine H1 antagonists

© 2001 Elsevier Science B.V. All rights reserved.
Histamine Research in the New Millennium
T. Watanabe, H. Timmerman and K. Yanai (Editors)

Role of protein kinase C-α in signalling from the histamine H_1-receptor to the c-fos promoter

S.J. Hill, A.C. Megson and E. M. Walker

Institute of Cell Signalling, Medical School, Queen's Medical Centre, Nottingham, NG7 2UH, United Kingdom

The histamine H_1-receptor produces its intracellular effects via the activation of the heterotrimeric $G_{q/11}$ family of G-proteins. Stimulation of H_1-receptors has been shown to stimulate cellular proliferation and to induce the expression of the proto-oncogene c-fos in a number of cell types. In the present study we have investigated whether specific isoforms of PKC mediate the effect of H_1-receptor stimulation on signalling to the c-fos promoter.

1. INTRODUCTION.

The histamine H_1-receptor produces its intracellular effects via the activation of the heterotrimeric $G_{q/11}$ family of G-proteins [1-3]. Activation of this receptor leads to stimulation of phospholipase Cβ which catalyzes the hydrolysis of phosphatidylinositol 4,5-bisphosphate to form inositol-1,4,5-trisphosphate (IP_3) and diacylglycerol. IP_3 released into the cytoplasm causes the mobilization of calcium from intracellular stores, whilst diacylglycerol activates protein kinase C [1-3]. Stimulation of histamine H_1-receptors has also been shown to stimulate cellular proliferation and to induce the expression of the proto-oncogene c-fos in human smooth muscle cells [4,5]. In addition, H_1-receptor stimulation has been shown to induce c-fos expression in hypothalamic neurones [6].

The c-fos promoter contains several regulatory sequences in its 5'-untranslated region, which include the serum response element (SRE) and a cyclic AMP response element (CRE) [7,8]. At the SRE, a ternary complex forms between serum response factor (SRF) and a ternary complex factor (TCF) to mediate responses to growth factors and mitogens via the activation of mitogen-activated protein kinases (MAPKs) [8, 9].

Recent studies have begun to provide evidence for the role of specific protein kinase C isoforms in the activation of MAPKs in different cell types, and in response to particular growth factors [10-12]. In the present study, we address the question of whether specific isoforms of protein kinase C mediate the effect of histamine H_1-receptor stimulation on signalling to the c-fos promoter.

2. METHODS.

2.1 C-fos luciferase activity.

CHO-K1 cells expressing recombinant bovine histamine H_1-receptors at a level of 3 pmol/mg protein (CHO-H1; [13]) were grown at 37°C in a humidified air/CO_2 atmosphere (95:5) in 75 cm² flasks. For measurement of c-fos promoter activity, CHO-H1 cells were secondarily transfected with a reporter vector encoding firefly luciferase under the control of the full c-fos promoter. Confluent CHO-H1 cell monolayers, in 24 well cluster dishes, were incubated at 37°C in a humidified air/CO_2 atmosphere (95:5) for 24h in 1ml serum-free DMEM/F12 media. Agonists (10μl) or foetal calf serum (100μl; total volume 1ml) were then added and the incubation continued for 6h. Luciferase activity in cell lysates was then monitored using the Promega luciferase assay system.

2.2 Down-regulation of PKC isoforms.

CHO-H1 cells, grown to 80% confluency, were treated for a further 24 h with the active phorbol ester phorbol 12,13-dibutyrate (PDBu, 1 μM), its inactive analogue 4α-phorbol (1 μM) or vehicle control, in DMEM/F12 media (1:1) supplemented with 2 mM L-glutamine, 1% foetal calf serum, 100 U/ml penicillin, 100 μg/ml streptomycin, and 250 ng/ml amphoterocin B. After this period, the now confluent cell monolayers were washed twice with ice-cold phosphate buffered saline and then harvested from the culture flasks using either a cell scraper or by incubation with 1 mM EDTA in PBS. The detached cells were collected by centrifugation at 700 g for 5 min. For determination of the expression of the PKC isoforms detergent extracts were prepared from the collected cells by homogenizing them in 100 μl ice-cold extract buffer (20 mM Tris-HCl, 1% (v/v) Triton X-100, 10 mM EGTA, 1 mM EDTA, 1 mM dithiothreitol, 0.1 mM leupeptin, 1 μg/ml soybean trypsin inhibitor, 1 mM benzamidine, 0.1 mM phenylmethylsulphonylfluoride, pH 7.4, followed by centrifugation for 15 min at 36,000g, 4 °C. The protein content of the supernatant, containing cytosolic and membrane proteins, was determined by the method of Bradford [14], using bovine serum albumin as a standard. Samples (15-40 μg protein) were heated to 95 °C in SDS/PAGE sample buffer (0.5 M Tris-HCl, 10% (v/v glycerol), 2% (w/v) sodium dodecyl sulphate, 5% 2-mercaptoethanol, 0.05% (v/v) bromophenol blue, pH 6.8), and then subjected to Western blot analysis.

2.3 Western blot analysis.

Protein samples were separated by SDS/PAGE (7.5% acrylamide gel) using the Bio-Rad Mini-Protean II system. Following transfer of proteins to nitrocellulose membranes, the membranes were blocked overnight in blocking buffer (5% (w/v) low fat dried milk in PBS/0.1% (v/v) Tween 20), at 4 °C. The blots were then incubated with primary anti-PKC antibodies (Transduction Laboratories, distributed by Affiniti Research Products Ltd, Exeter, UK) for 2 h at room temperature in blocking buffer. The blots were washed briefly in washing buffer (PBS/0.1% (v/v) Tween 20), then for 15 min and a further two times for 5 min with fresh changes of the washing buffer. The blots were then incubated with secondary antibody (horseradish-peroxidase conjugated goat anti-mouse IgG, Fc specific, affinity isolated antibody, Sigma), in blocking buffer, for 1 h at room temperature. The secondary antibody was removed, the blots washed twice briefly with washing buffer, then for 15 min and a further four times for 5 min, before developing the blots using the Enhanced Chemiluminescence detection system (Amersham). For the studies looking at the prolonged effect of PDBu treatment on PKC-α expression, an alternative primary anti-PKC antibody was used (Gibco-Life Technologies). The washing buffer used was PBS/1% (v/v) Tween 20, the blocking buffer additionally contained 1% BSA (w/v), and the secondary antibody was horseradish-peroxidase conjugated swine anti-rabbit IgG supplied by DAKO, Denmark. Otherwise, all the other conditions of Western blot analysis were identical.

3. RESULTS

CHO-H1 cells, expressing a luciferase reporter gene (pGL3 basic) under the transcriptional control of the human c-fos promoter, responded to a variety of different stimuli, including 10% foetal calf serum, histamine, thrombin, the adenylyl cyclase activator forskolin and the phorbol ester PDBu, but not ATP and Cholecystokinin (CCK) (Figure 1). The response to histamine (EC_{50} 9.8 ± 0.9 nM; n=14) was antagonised by the H_1-receptor selective antagonist mepyramine (100nM; apparent K_D = 0.65 ± 0.19 nM; n=3), although there was a small reduction in the maximal response to histamine.

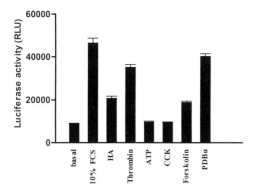

Figure 1. Effect of FCS, histamine (HA; 100μM), thrombin (1U/ml), ATP (100μM), CCK (1μM), forskolin (3μM) and PDBu (1μM) on c-fos luciferase activity in CHO-H1 cells. Values represent mean ± S.E.M. of triplicate determinations in a single experiment, representative of two others.

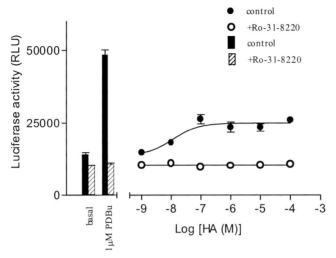

Figure 2. Effect of the protein kinase C inhibitor
Ro-31-8220 (10µM) on histamine-stimulated c-fos luciferase activity.
Values represent mean ± S.E.M. of triplicate determinations in a
single experiment. Similar data were obtained in two other
experiments.

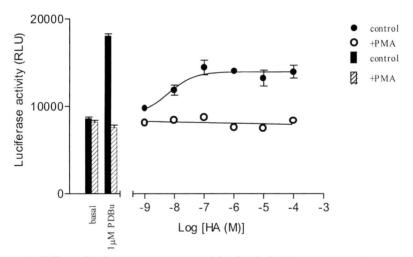

Figure 3. Effect of 24h pre-treatment with phorbol-12-myristate-13-
acetate (PMA; 3µM) on histamine-stimulated c-fos-luciferase expression.
Values represent mean ± S.E.M. of triplicate determinations in a single
experiment. Similar results were obtained in 3 further experiments.

Table 1.
Effect of 24h treatment with 4-α-phorbol (1μM) and PDBu (1μM) on PKC isoform expression.

PKC Isoform	4-α-Phorbol treatment (% of control)	PDBu treatment (% of control)	n
PKC-α	103.7 ± 3.6	5.7 ± 3.8	3
PKC-δ	94.5 ± 3.9	2.1 ± 0.6	3
PKC-ι	110.3 ± 8.7	102.5 ± 14.5	3
PKC-μ	101.6 ± 5.3	106.9 ± 13.3	3
PKC-ζ	96.2 ± 7.0	98.1 ± 2.3	3

Values represent mean ± S.E.M. of n determinations. Bands from Western blots were subjected to laser densitometry and compared to control, protein-matched, lanes.

The bisindolylmaleimide PKC inhibitor, Ro-31-8220 (10μM; Figure 2) and the indolocarbazole PKC inhibitor Go6976 (1μM), markedly inhibited the c-fos promoter-mediated activation of luciferase expression induced by histamine. The response to histamine was also completely attenuated following pre-treatment of CHO-H1 cells with the protein kinase C activator phorbol-12-myristate-13-acetate (PMA; 3μM) for 24h (Figure 3).

Several forms of protein kinase C (PKC-α, PKC-δ, PKC-μ, PKC-ι, PKC-ζ) could be detected in cell extracts from CHO-H1 cells by Western blot analysis (Table 1). The expression of the phorbol ester sensitive isoforms PKC-α and PKC-δ, but not the atypical isoforms PKC-μ, PKC-ι and PKC-ζ, were down-regulated by 24h treatment with PDBu, but not by 4-α-phorbol, the negative control (Table 1). Of the two isoforms that were down-regulated, only protein kinase C-α was translocated to CHO-H1 cell membranes following stimulation with histamine (100μM; 5 min stimulation).

4. DISCUSSION.

Previous studies have shown that distinct pathways can mediate the effect of G_i - and G_Q -coupled receptors on MAP kinase activation [15]. Thus, while G_i-coupled receptors stimulate the MAP kinase pathway via $G\beta\gamma$ subunits and Ras, G_Q-coupled receptors stimulate MAP kinase activation and cell proliferation via PKC and c-Raf [15]. However, in certain cells (e.g. PC12 cells) activation of protein kinase C is not required for activation of MAP kinase pathways via G_Q-coupled receptors such as the alpha-1A-adrenoceptor [16]. In the present study we provide evidence that activation of the human c-fos promoter via histamine H_1-receptor activation requires activation of protein kinase C-α. Thus, the c-fos response to histamine is completely attenuated by down-regulation of PKC-α and PKC-δ, and the non-selective protein kinase C inhibitor Ro-318220. Furthermore, histamine was able to stimulate the translocation of protein kinase C-α to the plasma membrane. Finally, the indolocarbazole PKC inhibitor Go 6976, which inhibits cPKC isoforms and PKC-μ but not nPKCs [17] was able to markedly attenuate the activation of the c-fos promoter by histamine.

REFERENCES.

[1] Hill, S.J. (1990) Pharmacol. Rev. **42**: 45-93.
[2] Leurs, R., Smit, M.J. and Timmerman, H. (1995) Pharmacol. Ther. **66**: 413-   463.
[3] Hill, S.J, Ganellin, C.R., Timmerman, H., Schwartz, J.C., Shankley, N.P., Young, J.M., Schunack, W., Levi, R. and Haas, H.L (1997) Pharmacol. Rev. **49**: 253-278.
[4] Satoh, T., Sugama, K., Matsuo, A., Kato, S., Ito, S., Hatanaka, M. and Sasaguri, Y. (1994) Atherosclerosis **110**: 53-61
[5] Panettieri, R.J., Yadvish, P.A., Kelly, A.M., Rubinstein, N.A.and Kotlikoff, M.I. (1990) American J. Physiol. **259**: L365-L371
[6] Kjaer.,A. Larsen, P.J., Knigge, U., Moller, M. and Warberg, J. (1994) Endocrinology. **134**: 82-491
[7] Yalkinoglu, A.O., Spreyer, P., Bechem, M., Apeler, H.and Wohlfeil, S. (1995) J. Receptor and Signal Transduction Research **15**: 117-130
[8] Hill, C.S. and Treisman, R. (1995) EMBO J. **14**:.5037-5047
[9] Price, M.A., Hill, C.S. and Treisman R (1996) Phil. Trans. Royal Society series B: Biological Sciences **351**: 551-559.
[10]Ueda, Y., Hirai, S, Osada, S and Suzuki, A (1996) J. Biol. Chem. **271**: 23512-23519.
[11]Mackenzie, S., Fleming, I., Houslay, M.D., Anderson, N.G. and Kilgour, E. (1997) Biochem. J. **324**: 159-165.
[12]Kim, J.Y., Yang, M.S., Oh, C.D., Kim, K.T., Ha, M.J., Kang, S.S. and Chun, J.S. (1999) Biochem. J. **337**: 275-280.
[13]Iredale, P.A., Fukui, H. and Hill, S.J. (1993) Biochem. Biophys. Res. Commun. **195**: 1294-1300.
[14]Bradford MM (1976). Anal Biochem. **72**: 248-254.
[15]Hawes, B.E., Van Biesen, T., Koch, W.J., Luttrell, L.M. and Lefkowitz, R.J. (1995). J. Biol. Chem. **270**: 17148-17153.
[16]Berts, A., Zhong, H. and Minneman, K.P.(1999) Molec. Pharmacol. **55**: 296-303.
[17]Way, K.J., Chou, E. and King, G.L. (2000) Trends Pharmacol. Sci. **21**: 181-187.

We thank the MRC and Wellcome Trust for financial support and Prof P E Shaw and Prof H Fukui for the cDNA for the human c-fos promoter and the bovine H$_1$-receptor respectively.

© 2001 Elsevier Science B.V. All rights reserved.
Histamine Research in the New Millennium
T. Watanabe, H. Timmerman and K. Yanai (Editors)

Molecular basis for the cardiovascular adverse effects of first- and second-generation antihistamines

Maurizio Taglialatela, Pasqualina Castaldo, Anna Pannaccione, Francesca Boscia, Adriana Canitano, and Lucio Annunziato

Section of Pharmacology, Department of Neuroscience, School of Medicine, University of Naples Federico II; Naples - Italy

Over the last decade, cardiac safety has been a major concern in the therapeutic selection among antihistamines to treat allergic diseases. In fact, congeners belonging to this therapeutic class like terfenadine or astemizole are provided of the ability to cause rare but potentially fatal adverse effects such as QT interval prolongation, "torsade de pointes" polymorphic ventricular arrhythmias, syncope and cardiac arrests. Blockade of cardiac K^+ channels, and in particular of the I_{Kr} component of the cardiac repolarizing K^+ current underlined by the Human Ether-à-Gogo Related Gene-1 (HERG1), has been demonstrated as the mechanism responsible for the cardiac toxicity of these compounds. In the present work we have studied and compared the inhibitory effects of several second-generation H_1 receptor antagonists (terfenadine, astemizole, cetirizine, loratadine, and mizolastine) at the level of HERG1 K^+ channels, using three complementary experimental models: 1. Xenopus oocytes heterologously expressing HERG1 K^+ channels; 2. Human neuroblastoma cells (SH-SY5Y cells) constitutively expressing I_{HERG}; and 3. Human Embryonic Kidney cells (HEK-293 cells) stably transfected with HERG1 cDNA. Collectively, the results obtained from these models suggested that second-generation H_1 receptor antagonists display marked heterogeneity in their blocking ability of HERG1 K^+ channels. In particular, while loratadine and cetirizine lack of significant HERG1-blocking ability, terfenadine and astemizole potently inhibit HERG1 K^+ channels. Mizolastine, a novel second-generation H_1 receptor antagonist recently available in Europe, displays a certain degree of HERG1 inhibitory action, although the concentrations required to exert such effect are 10-100 times higher than those of astemizole or terfenadine. The recognition of severe cardiac adverse effects by second-generation antihistamines has also raised the issue of the potential cardiotoxicity of older antihistamines. Recently, it has been found that micromolar concentrations of both diphenhydramine and hydroxyzine inhibited HERG1 K^+ channels; these concentrations are similar to those able to block I_{Kr} in guinea-pig ventricular myocytes and are within the plasma concentration range found in poisoned patients.

The present results might be of some clinical significance for those patients at risk of developing cardiac arrhythmias undergoing therapy with first- and second-generation antihistamines. In addition, the observation that antihistamines greatly differ in their ability to interfere with HERG1 K^+ channels and, consequently, to determine cardiotoxic effects, emphasizes the importance of an evaluation of the possible blockade of HERG1 K^+ channels during the early developmental phases of novel compounds belonging to this therapeutical class.

Finally, direct comparison of HERG1-blocking properties by different H_1 receptor blockers, together with recent site-directed mutagenesis experiments, has allowed to provide further insights into the structure-activity relationships for these molecules and on the molecular determinants for drug binding in HERG1 K^+ channels.

1. ANTIHISTAMINES AND CARDIAC TOXICITY

1.1 First- and second-generation antihistamines

Compounds able to block histamine responses at the level of H_1 receptors (antihistamines) have represented a major improvement in the therapy of allergic diseases, such as allergic rhinitis, chronic urticaria, and atopic dermatitis. For these indications, older first-generation molecules, such as hydroxyzine and diphenhydramine, have been progressively replaced by more recently-introduced less lipophylic drugs, in order to overcome the blood-brain barrier crossing ability and central sedating action of older congeners, which was responsible for decreased verbal learning, decision-making ability, and psychomotor speed (1). These newer second-generation antihistamines, such as astemizole, cetirizine, ebastine, fexofenadine, loratadine, mizolastine, and terfenadine, are characterized by an improved selectivity for histamine receptors over serotoninergic-, muscarinic- and α_2-adrenergic-receptors, and, possibly, by antiallergic properties distinct from their antihistaminic activity (2). Although the pharmacodynamic and pharmacokinetic profile of second-generation compounds bears an obvious clinical advantage in the therapy of allergic diseases, adverse cardiovascular effects associated with the use of some congeners belonging to this therapeutical class have been recently reported. The concern over the potentially severe arrhythmogenic properties of second-generation antihistamines is regarded nowadays as one of the major criteria in the therapeutic selection of antihistamines (3).

1.2 QT prolongation and"torsade de pointes" by second-generation antihistamines

In the last fifteen years, an increasing number of reports have appeared in the literature showing an association between astemizole and terfenadine assumption and the occurrence of prolongation of the QT interval, leading to the appearance of a rare form of polymorphic ventricular arrhythmia called "torsade de pointes", syncope, and cardiac arrests. "Torsade de pointes", as first described by Dessertenne (4), consists of a progressive modification of the amplitude and polarity of the QRS complexes on the surface ECG, which appear to be twisting around an imaginary isoelectric baseline (5). This cardiotoxic manifestation occurred either in patients taking the recommended doses of terfenadine or astemizole, or in patients with intentional or accidental overdoses of these two second-generation antihistamines (6-13). Despite the low number of cases in the literature, a careful evaluation of the conditions under which the toxic effects arose has led to the clarification of the predisposing factors to second-generation antihistamines-induced cardiotoxicity. In particular, the case of a 39-year old woman who experienced several syncopes and "torsade de pointes" ventricular arrhythmias during assumption of the standard therapeutic dose of terfenadine (120 mg per day for 12 days) only after she started self-medication with the antimycotic ketoconazole, pointed toward an impaired liver metabolism as one of the main predisposing factor (7). In fact, ketoconazole is a well-known inhibitor of the CYP3A4 P450 enzyme, a primary metabolizing pathway for several drugs including terfenadine (14). Therefore, while in most normal subjects terfenadine levels in the plasma are below the detection limits, the impaired metabolism of terfenadine induced by ketoconazole in that woman likely caused an abrupt increase in terfenadine plasma levels, thus unmasking the cardiac adverse effect of the antihistaminic molecule.

As a matter of fact, most of the cases describing cardiotoxic effects of second-generation antihistamines involved the concomitant use of inhibitors of the CYP3A4 P450 enzyme, such as ketoconazole, itraconazole, or macrolide antibiotics. Also patients with an impaired liver function (cirrhosis, ethanol abuse) were at risk of developing arrhythmias. Fexofenadine, the main metabolic product generated by the hepatic metabolism of terfenadine, retains the histamine H_1 receptor antagonist and non-sedative properties of the parent compound, but does not seem to affect the cardiac QT interval in pre-clinical and clinical studies (15) and does not undergo further hepatic metabolism (16). However, the cardiac safety of fexofenadine has recently been questioned (17). On the other hand, astemizole also undergoes extensive first-pass liver metabolism, with one of its main metabolites being desmethylastemizole. Preliminary studies suggest that also this metabolite is provided of significant cardiotoxic potential (18).

Other clinical conditions of pre-existing cardiac dysfunctions, such as congenital QT prolongation (see below), ischemic heart diseases, and congestive heart failure, or electrolyte imbalance, such as hypokalemia and hypomagnesemia, may also precipitate the arrhythmic episodes by second-generation antihistamines (2). Finally, an additional risk factor which might precipitate adverse cardiac events upon exposure to H_1 receptor antagonists is the simultaneous assumption of QT-prolonging antiarrhythmic drugs such as quinidine.

1.3. Cardiac potassium channels and long QT syndrome (LQTS).

The coordinated contraction of the cardiac muscle is due to the sequential opening of several classes of ion channels. The duration of the cardiac action potential is controlled by a fine equilibrium between inward and outward currents (19).

Most of the arrhythmic episodes occurring in predisposed patients upon assumption of terfenadine and astemizole were polymorphic ventricular tachycardias with "torsade de pointes" ventricular fibrillation. "Torsade de pointes" generally occur in the setting of a marked bradycardia with prolongation of the QT interval (generally >440 ms).

Drug-induced prolongation of the cardiac action potential is generally consequent to the blockade of the repolarizing currents mainly carried by K^+ channels. Under physiological conditions, several classes of K^+ currents shape the action potential in cardiac cells (20): the transient outward current (I_{to}), the delayed rectifier repolarizing current made up of both rapid (I_{Kr}) and slow (I_{Ks}) components (21), and the inward rectifier I_{K1} current, which participates in the final phases of repolarization. Other K^+ channels are also active during the action potential plateau in selective heart regions, such as the acetylcholine-activated K^+ channel ($I_{K(Ach)}$) in the atria and the Purkinje fibers; or under specific pathological conditions, such as the ATP-dependent K^+ channel ($I_{K(ATP)}$), the Na^+-dependent K^+ current ($I_{K(Na)}$), and the fatty-acid activated K^+ current ($I_{K(FA)}$) (19). Such functional diversity of cardiac K^+ currents is matched by an extraordinary degree of structural heterogeneity, as revealed by the recent cloning of most of the genes encoding for cardiac K^+ channels. In general, K^+ channels can be classified on the basis of several criteria, including putative transmembrane arrangement, pharmacological selectivity, permeation and rectification properties, as well as gating mechanisms (22).

A major contribution to the identification of the molecular basis for most of the currents involved in cardiac repolarization has been given by the study of the molecular genetics of the Long QT syndrome (LQTS).

This life-threatening genetically-transmitted human disease is characterized by a marked prolongation of the QT interval on the ECG and by frequent episodes of syncope or cardiac arrest usually occurring during conditions of psychological or physical stress (23). Similarly to the acquired LQTS induced by cardiotoxic second-generation antihistamines, these syncopal episodes are due to "torsade de pointes" ventricular arrhythmias that often degenerate into ventricular fibrillation and eventually result in the sudden death of the affected patient (24). In the last five years several genetic defects have been recognized as responsible for LQTS. In particular, mutations in five genes have been associated to LQTS (25-29). Two of these genes (HERG1 and K_vLQT1) encode for the main subunits of cardiac K^+ channels, one (SCN5A) for a Na^+ channel subunit, and the last two (MinK and MiRP1) for accessory subunits regulating K^+ channel function. Due to these achievements, the genes underlying each of the cardiac K^+ currents are now known. In particular, HERG1 (an acronym for Human Ether-a-Gogo-Related Gene-1, attributed to this gene as it was cloned by homology to another K^+ channel-encoding gene named Ether-a-Gogo) (30) was soon recognized to encode for the main subunit of the rapid component of the ventricular repolarizing current I_{Kr} (31). More recently, it has been proposed that the association between HERG1 and other accessory subunits encoded by MinK or MiRP1 reproduces the biophysical and pharmacological properties of native I_{Kr} (29,32). The predicted protein encoded by HERG1 shares considerable sequence similarity with other K^+ channels, displaying a putative topological arrangement with six α-helical transmembrane domains, the N- and C-termini located in the cytoplasm, a cyclic nucleotide-binding domain in the C-terminus, and a pore-forming region between the transmembrane segments S_5 and S_6. Mutations in HERG1 have been proposed to impair the rapid component of the ventricular repolarizing current I_{Kr}, thus causing delayed repolarization, which represents a triggering mechanism for "torsade de pointes". The analogies existing between drug-induced acquired LQTS and genetically-determined LQTS, also revealed by the recent identification of a MiRP1 mutation in a patient experiencing arrhythmias upon treatment with chlaritromycin (29), suggest that acquired arrhythmias can result from inheritance of a mutant K^+ channel subunits that reduces cardiac repolarization capacity. Thus, the study of the molecular basis of congenital LQTS, beside clarifying the role played by specific ion channel subunits in cardiac repolarization, have also shed light onto the physiopathological mechanisms involved in drug-induced arrhythmias.

1.4. HERG1 K^+ channels as molecular targets for the cardiotoxic effects of second-generation antihistamines.

The crucial role played by HERG1 K^+ channels in the control of cardiac repolarization has prompted several studies attempting to correlate the in vivo propensity of a drug to cause delayed repolarization and "torsade de pointes" with its inhibitory action at the level of HERG1 K^+ channels in vitro. Given the complexity of isolating I_{Kr} in cardiac tissue, where several K^+ currents are simultaneously expressed in the same cell type, these studies have often utilized several cellular models where HERG1 K^+ currents could be properly resolved. These models include either cells in which HERG1 K^+ channels are constitutively expressed (33-35), or cells in which the heterologous expression of the channel can be achieved either by cDNA or cRNA microinjection techniques (such as the Xenopus oocytes) (36) or by transient or permanent transfection techniques (such as the Human Embryonic Kidney-293 or HEK-293 cells) (37). Although each of these cellular models has specific advantages and drawbacks, a complete picture of the effect of a drug on a particular class of ionic channels generally emerges upon comparison and careful evaluation of the results obtained in each of these different cellular models.

Soon after the description of HERG1 K^+ channels as the main constituents of the cardiac repolarizing current I_{Kr}, the observation that both terfenadine (38) and astemizole (39) effectively blocked HERG1 K^+ channels suggested a novel mechanism for cardiotoxic H_1 receptor antagonists to delay action potential repolarization, and cause the occurrence of the arrhythmic episode. The concentrations of terfenadine and astemizole required to produce HERG1 K^+ channels blockade were clearly within the range found in those clinical situations (hepatic diseases; co-administration of itraconazole, ketoconazole, or macrolide antibiotics, see above) in which patients experienced a cardiotoxic manifestation by these two second-generation antihistamines (40,41).

The important cardiotoxic effects exerted by two of the most widely-used second-generation antihistamines have prompted speculations on whether other molecules belonging to this therapeutic class might also be provided with similar pharmacological effects (2,42,43). To address such a question, comparative studies among several second-generation antihistamines (terfenadine, astemizole, loratadine, and cetirizine) have been recently performed (44), showing that second generation antihistamines display marked differences in their ability to block HERG1 K^+ channels. In fact, while terfenadine and astemizole were provided with such pharmacological action at nanomolar concentrations, the piperazine derivative cetirizine was shown to be devoid of HERG1-blocking ability both upon the heterologous expression of this channel in Xenopus oocytes or in HEK-293 cells, as well as in cells constitutively expressing HERG K^+ channels. This lack of effect was observed for concentrations of cetirizine (1-30 µM) comparable to those achieved in the plasma of normal subjects (1-5 µM) after the administration of doses 2-6 times higher than the commonly recommended daily therapeutical dose (45). Although caution should be exercised when establishing a direct correlation between the pharmacological actions of a drug in vitro and their possible clinical implications in vivo, the observation that cetirizine was completely devoid of any interference with endogenously or heterologously expressed HERG1 K^+ channels seems to suggest that "torsade de pointes" are not likely to occur during conventional therapy with this drug (2,46). As a matter of fact, cetirizine did not display significant prolongation of the QT interval in experimental animals (47) or humans (45). Furthermore, both I_{Kr} and I_{Ks} in guinea-pig ventricular myocytes have been shown to be quite insensitive to cetirizine (48).

Using the same expression systems, the piperidinic second-generation antihistamine loratadine was shown to be unable to block HERG1 K^+ channels at concentrations up to 10 µM (44). These results are in agreement with the results obtained in guinea pig ventricular myocytes (up to 3 µM) (49); however, higher concentrations (3-30 µM, depending on the expression system) of loratadine blocked both heterologously and constitutively-expressed HERG1 K^+ channels (44,50). Given that the concentrations of loratadine required to block HERG1 K^+ channels were at least 30 times higher than those achieved in the plasma during conventional therapy (51), these results might also explain the lack of cardiac side effects associated with its use in humans (52,53) and experimental animals (54). In fact, it should be considered that in a recent pharmacosurveillance study in which the risk profile for heart rhythm disorders and cardiac deaths has been determined for some of the most common non-sedating antihistamines, cetirizine and loratadine displayed the lowest adverse drug reaction report rate per million of defined daily doses sold (55).

However, it should be underlined that recent experiments performed in HERG1-transfected HEK-293 cells showed that, when more physiological recording conditions (low extracellular K^+ concentration, 37°C temperature, and low pacing rates), loratadine was equipotent to terfenadine in blocking HERG1 K^+ channels (56); thus, the reasons for the described differences in the incidence of severe, life-threatening arrhythmias between loratadine and terfenadine are still matter of debate.

Ebastine is another second-generation antihistamine which bears considerable structural similarities with terfenadine. In vivo studies in laboratory animals have revealed that this compound might exert a QT-prolonging effects (47), although the effects are smaller than with terfenadine and only evident upon concomitant administration of ketoconazole which, by itself, is known to cause an increase in the QT interval when administered alone in the same experimental paradigm (57); nevertheless, in vitro studies revealed that ebastine was able to block both HERG1 K^+ channels heterologously expressed in Xenopus oocytes and native I_{Kr} in ventricular guinea-pig myocytes (49). Interestingly, in both in vivo and in vitro models, the liver metabolic product of ebastine, carebastine, failed to show any cardiotoxic effect. Although the structural similarities between terfenadine and ebastine should not be overlooked (58), the possible clinical relevance of these studies is still under investigation.

Mizolastine is a new potent and selective second-generation H_1 receptor blocker available in Europe, which is effective in relieving the symptoms of allergic rhinitis (59,60) and urticaria (61). This compound, structurally related to astemizole, is devoid of sedative (62,63) and antimuscarinic (64) properties, and displays a more hydrophilic profile which confers to the molecule a lower distribution volume, good bioavailability, and limited metabolic conversion by the hepatic CYPs 3A4 and 2A6 (65). When the effects of mizolastine on HERG1 K^+ channels were investigated, it was found that this benzimidazole compound blocked HERG1 K^+ channels either heterologously expressed in amphibian (Xenopus oocytes) (Fig. 1) or in mammalian (HEK-293) cells (Fig. 2), as well as constitutively present in SH-SY5Y human neuroblastoma cells (66). The potency of mizolastine in inhibiting HERG1 K^+ channels appears to be at least 10 times lower than that of astemizole (37,39); this lower potency could be at least in part ascribed to the faster dissociation rate of mizolastine from its receptor site on the channel when compared to astemizole. The potential clinical relevance of a certain inhibitory action by mizolastine on HERG1 K^+ channels is worth considering since the drug reached a C_{MAX} of 0.3-1 µM during standard therapy (10-20 mg/die) (67,68), a concentration range which clearly showed significant HERG1 inhibitory action. However, it should be noted that the steady-state levels achieved by the drug in standard therapeutic settings are much lower than the C_{MAX}, and that the potency for HERG1 K^+ channels blockade by mizolastine is much lower than that exerted by the same drug at the level of H_1 receptors in vitro (69). In vitro studies performed on guinea pig ventricular myocytes have suggested that mizolastine is unable to lengthen cardiac action potential duration, even at concentrations 10-30 times above the standard therapeutic range (70). Furthermore, clinical studies in both healthy volunteers (68) and in allergic patients (65) have shown that mizolastine showed no significant effect on cardiac repolarization. Therefore, the results of both animal and clinical studies argue against the possible occurrence of cardiotoxic events during standard therapy with this novel H_1 receptor blocker. However, it should be underlined that the recognition of the potential for cardiotoxicity exerted by terfenadine and astemizole has required more than 10 years of extensive world-wide clinical use of these drugs (40). Despite the relatively high concentrations of mizolastine required to inhibit HERG1 K^+ channels, which appear to be above the steady-state plasma levels required to exert its therapeutical action, the present results might be of some clinical significance for those patients at risk of developing cardiac arrhythmias undergoing therapy with mizolastine.

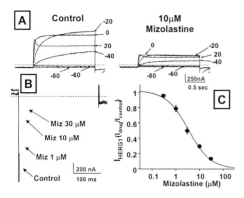

Figure 1. <u>Effect of mizolastine on the K$^+$ currents carried by hERG1 K$^+$ channels expressed in Xenopus oocytes.</u> *Panel A.* Representative outward current traces recorded with the two-microelectrode voltage-clamp technique from a Xenopus oocyte expressing HERG1 K$^+$ channels recorded in control condition and after 5 minutes perfusion with 10 μM mizolastine. Holding potential : -90 mV; test potentials from -80 mV to +20 mV in 20 mV steps; return potential : -100 mV. The dashed lines in the panel indicate the zero current level. *Panel B..* Representative current traces recorded with the two-microelectrode voltage-clamp technique from a single HERG1-expressing oocyte exposed to control condition, and after perfusion with 1, 10, and 30 μM mizolastine (5 minutes for each concentration).

Holding potential: -90 mV; test potential: 0 mV; return potential: -100 mV. Only the tail currents recorded upon return to –100 mV are shown. The dashed line in the panel indicate the zero current level. *Panel C.* Dose-dependence of HERG1 K$^+$ currents inhibition by mizolastine. The inhibitory effect of the different concentration of the H$_1$ receptor antagonist on the peak of the inward HERG1 K$^+$ currents recorded at -100 mV was calculated for several cells and plotted against drug concentrations. The solid line represents the fit of the experimental data to the following binding isotherm: $y=max/(1+X/IC_{50})^n$, where X is the drug concentration and n the Hill coefficient. The fitted value for n was between 0.72 and 0.96. Each point is the mean±S.E.M. of 3-6 determinations. Data reprinted from Ref. 66.

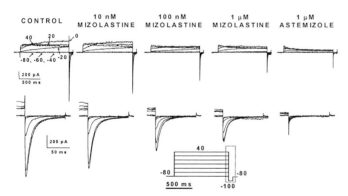

Figure 2. <u>Effect of mizolastine on I$_{HERG1}$ heterologously expressed in HEK-293 cells stably transfected with HERG1 cDNA.</u> Representative current traces recorded in the whole-cell configuration of the patch-clamp technique from a single HERG1-transfected HEK-293 cell.

Records were obtained in control conditions, after 5 minutes perfusion with increasing concentrations of extracellular mizolastine (10 nM, 100 nM, and 1 μM), and after 5 minutes exposure to 1 μM extracellular astemizole. The pulse protocol (shown at the bottom of the Figure) was the following: holding potential: -80 mV; test potentials from -80 mV to +40 mV in 20 mV steps (1 sec duration); return potential: -100 mV. The bottom panels of the figure (corresponding to the time region indicated by the boxed area in the voltage pulse protocol) show the inward tail currents recorded upon repolarization to –100 mV on an expanded time and current scale. Data reprinted from Ref. 66.

1.5. Potential cardiotoxicity of first-generation antihistamines.

The large number of studies demonstrating the cardiotoxicity of some second-generation antihistamines, as well as the similarities in the chemical structures between older and newer H_1 receptor blockers, has prompted a re-examination of the possible cardiac adverse effects of older first-generation molecules. These drugs are generally considered to be free from cardiac toxicity and are widely sold in most western countries as "over the counter" (OTC) or prescribed medications. Since these drugs are rather easily available to the public and are frequently implicated in accidental or intentional poisoning, this reassessment seems of particular pharmacological relevance. The issue of the potential cardiotoxicity of older antihistamines has also been raised by some recent studies. Khalifa et al. (71) reported that diphenhydramine blocked the repolarizing K^+ currents in guinea-pig ventricular myocytes, an effect also shared by chlorpheniramine and pyrilamine (72); furthermore, the same study also showed the ability of therapeutical dosages of diphenhydramine to lengthen cardiac repolarization in vivo in normal volunteers and in patients undergoing angioplasthy (71). The ability of diphenhydramine, as well as of other "conventional" antihistamines, to interfere with cardiac repolarization has also been confirmed in vitro by another study performed in feline hearts (73). In this model, the EC_{50s} for the ability of these older molecules to delay cardiac repolarization did not differ significantly from those of the two well-known cardiotoxic second-generation antihistamines astemizole or terfenadine. A review of the available literature on clinical cases describing possible association between the administration of older antihistamines and cardiac adverse effects shows that both diphenhydramine (74-76) and the cetirizine metabolic precursor hydroxyzine (Fig. 3C) (77,78), when taken in larger than therapeutic doses, display the ability of inducing QT prolongation, in some cases leading to the occurrence of cardiac arrhythmias of the "torsade de pointes" type. The concentration of diphenhydramine and hydroxyzine found in the blood of intoxicated individuals (ranging 20 to 200 μM) were much higher than those considered to be within the standard therapeutic range (≈ 0.2-2 μM). The rare cardiovascular adverse effects observed with older antihistamines have often been interpreted as a consequence of their antimuscarinic properties; however, the antimuscarinic actions of older antihistamines seem to not always be directly related to their cardiac toxicity (74,77).

Prompted by these observations, the in vitro blockade of HERG1 K^+ channels by hydroxyzine and diphenhydramine has been recently investigated (79). The results obtained suggest that micromolar concentrations of both compounds (Fig. 3A and 3B) exerted an inhibitory action on this class of K^+ channels; these concentrations of the two older antihistamines are similar to those found to block I_{Kr} in guinea-pig ventricular myocytes (71), and, more importantly, are within the plasma concentration range found in patients undergoing poisoning with these first-generation congeners. These experimental, clinical, and pharmaco-epidemiological data support the notion that older H_1 receptor antagonists provided with HERG1-blocking ability could also exert cardiotoxic manifestations under specific clinical settings, as it can occur with some of the second-generation antihistamines. This conclusion seems to find support in the results of a recent study showing that the incidence of life-threatening ventricular arrhythmic events and cardiac arrests was higher in patients receiving OTC antihistamines (mainly diphenhydramine), than in those receiving terfenadine or a reference drug (ibuprofen) (80). However, the identification of the predisposing factors to such adverse reactions are yet unknown, largely due to the little knowledge available on the pharmaco-metabolic profile of such compounds (81,82).

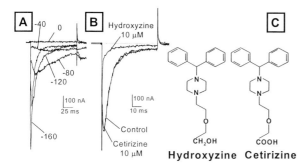

Figure 3. Effect of the extracellular perfusion with cetirizine or hydroxyzine on I_{HERG} constitutively expressed in SHSY-5Y human neuroblastoma cells. *Panel A.* Representative I_{HERG} current traces recorded in the whole-cell configuration of the patch-clamp technique from a single SHSY-5Y human neuroblastoma cell. The pulse protocol was the following: holding potential: -70 mV; depolarizing test potential: 0 mV for 10 sec; hyperpolarizing return potentials: from 0 to -160 mV in -40 mV steps for 125 ms; return potential: -70 mV. Only approximately the last 150 ms of each pulses are shown. *Panel B.* Effect of the sequential perfusion of the same cell as in panel A with cetirizine (10µM, 3 min perfusion) or with hydroxyzine (10µM, 3 min perfusion). Extracellular [K$^+$]: 100 mM. Holding potential: -60 mV; test potential 0 mV for 10 sec; return potential -160 mV. Only the last 150 ms of each pulse are shown. *Panel C.* Molecular structure of hydroxyzine and cetirizine.

1.6. Structure-activity relationships for HERG1 K$^+$ channel blockade by second-generation antihistamines.

A direct comparison of HERG1-blocking properties by different H$_1$ receptor blockers also allows to provide further insight into the structure-activity relationships for these molecules. In fact, it has been suggested that the HERG1 K$^+$ channel-blocking properties of terfenadine and its structural analogue ebastine are at least in part related to the tertiary amine substituent of the molecule rather than to the presence of the piperidine ring, or to the aromatic ring structures conferring H$_1$ receptor blocking activity (83); no correlation has been recently found between the ability to prolong the cardiac action potential duration, an effect possibly related to HERG1 K$^+$ channels blockade, and the H$_1$ antagonistic activity by several antihistamines (79,83). Lipophilicity and bulkiness appear to be the two crucial parameters in the tertiary amine group substituents conferring HERG1 K$^+$ channel-blocking capacity to the antihistaminic molecule. In fact, the second-generation antihistamine cetirizine, which appears to lack of significant HERG1-inhibitory properties (44), has polar and smaller substitutions at the nitrogen atom (amido and carboxyl groups, respectively); on the other hand, terfenadine, astemizole, and ebastine, the H$_1$ receptor antagonists most effective in inhibiting HERG1 K$^+$ channels, have less polar and bulkier phenyl rings in the substituting side chains. Mizolastine, on the other hand, is characterized by a lower lipophylicity and thus by a low tissular penetration and distribution volume (65). The lower lipophilicity of mizolastine could explain the lower potency of this novel congener in inhibiting HERG1 K$^+$ channels when compared to astemizole or terfenadine.

HERG1 K$^+$ channels blockade by terfenadine (38) and astemizole (39,44), as well as by the antiarrhythmic methanesulfonanilides such as dofetilide and MK-499 (84), seems to occur at a site located on the cytoplasmic side of the channel. Recent structure-function studies performed by site-directed mutagenesis in HERG1 K$^+$ channels have addressed the issue of the high degree of selectivity for HERG1 K$^+$ channels over other cardiac ion channels displayed by second-generation antihistamines as well as by other potent compounds such as methanesulfonanilides (85) and cisapride (86). The results of these studies have revealed that the pore helix located between the S_5-S_6 linker region and the S_6 transmembrane domain participate in the formation of the cavity where terfenadine binds (87,88) (Fig. 4). In particular, electrostatic interactions between hydrogen atoms of the aromatic residues at positions 652 and 656 and the π electrons of the phenyl ring of the drug molecule are crucial for high affinity drug binding to HERG1 channels. The presence of such aromatic residues is highly characteristic for HERG1 K^+ channel sequence, and might at least in part explain the molecular basis for the preferential binding of these drugs to this subclass of cardiac K^+ channels.

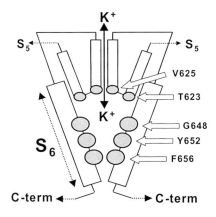

Figure 4. Schematic drawing of the pore region and of the S_6 transmembrane segment of hERG1. Only two of the four channel-forming subunits of hERG1 channels are drawn. According to the reported alanine-scanning mutagenesis data (88) and to the model of the KscA channel structure (92), the residues T623 and V625 (in the P-region) and G648, Y652, and F656 (in S_6), which appear to be crucial for drug binding to hERG1 channels, are shown.

CONCLUSIONS

The description of potentially-fatal cardiac arrhythmias induced by H_1 receptor antagonists in predisposed patients or in intoxicated individuals, has introduced important safety considerations in the therapeutical strategy for selecting drugs to treat allergic diseases. The achievements in molecular genetics, electrophysiology, and pharmacology here briefly reviewed, have improved our basic knowledge of the molecular mechanisms controlling cardiac action potential repolarization and have allowed an understanding of the molecular mechanisms underlying drug-induced cardiac adverse effects; pre-clinical tests (both in vivo and in vitro) displaying a certain degree of predictive efficacy for cardiotoxic effects are now available. In view of these considerations, the use of safer drugs to treat often non-life threatening diseases appears mandatory. It seems possible to foresee that the impact of such expanding knowledge will transcend the field of antihistamines, to also affect other therapeutical classes, such as antipsychotics and antidepressants, which are known to possess the potential to induce similar cardiovascular side-effects (89). In fact, it should be remembered that the issue of the potential proarrhythmic effects of non-cardiac drugs is becoming increasingly important from both clinical and regulatory standpoints (90), and the list of drugs able to induce cardiotoxic arrhythmic effects is rapidly expanding (91).

References
1. K. Yanai, N. Okamura, M. Tagawa, et al. Clin. Exp. Allergy 1999; 29 (Suppl. 3): 29.
2. R.L. Woosley. Ann. Rev. Pharmacol. Toxicol. 1996; 36: 233.
3. J.W. Slater, A.D. Zechnich, and D.G. Haxby. Drugs 1999; 57: 31.

4. F. Dessertenne. Arch. Mal. Coeur 1966; 95: 263.
5. A. Genovese, and G. Spadaro. Allergy 1997; 52 (Suppl. 34): 67.
6. A.J. Davies, V. Harindra, A. McEwan, and R.R. Ghose. Br. Med. J. 1989; 298: 325.
7. B.P. Monahan, C.L. Ferguson, E.S. Killeavy, et al. J. Am. Med. Ass. 1990; 264: 2788.
8. T.M. Craft. Br. Med. J. 1986; 292: 660.
9. J. Snook, D. Boothman-Burrell, J. Watkins, and D. Colin-Jones. Br. J. Clin. Pract. 1988; 42: 257.
10. F.E. Simons, M.S. Kesselman, N.G. Giddins, et al. Lancet 1988; 2: 624.
11. R.O. Bishop, and P.L. Gaudry. Arch. Emerg. Med. 1989; 6: 63.
12. J. Leor, M. Harman, B. Rabinowitz, and B. Mozes. Am. J. Med. 1991; 91: 94.
13. K. Hoppu, T. Tikanoja, P. Tapanainen, et al. Lancet 1991; 338: 538.
14. D.A. Garteiz, R.H. Hook, B.J. Walker, and R.A. Okerholm. Arzneimittelforschung 1982; 32: 1185.
15. C. Pratt, A.M. Brown, D. Rampe, et al. Clin. Exp. Allergy 1999; 29 (Suppl. 3): 212.
16. A. Markham, and A.J. Wagstaff. Drugs 1998; 55: 269.
17. Y.M. Pinto, et al. Lancet 1999; 353: 980.
18. V.R. Vorperian, Z. Zhou, S. Mohammad, et al. J. Am. Coll. Cardiol. 1996; 28: 1556.
19. E. Carmeliet. Eur. Heart J. 1993; 14: 3.
20. D.M. Barry, and J.M. Nerbonne. Annu. Rev. Physiol. 1996; 58: 363.
21. M.C. Sanguinetti, and N.K. Jurkiewicz. J. Gen. Physiol. 1990; 96: 195.
22. L.Y. Jan, and Y.N. Jan. Annu. Rev. Neurosci. 1997; 20: 91.
23. P.J. Schwartz, E.H. Locati, C. Napolitano, and S.G. Priori. In : Zipes DP and Jalife J, eds. Cardiac electrophysiology. From cell to bedside. 2nd Ed. Philadelphia, PA: WB Saunders, Co; 1995: 788-811.
24. C. Napolitano, S.G. Priori, and P.J. Schwartz. Drugs 1994; 47: 51.
25. Q. Wang, M.E. Curran, I. Splawski, et al. Nature Genet. 1996; 12: 17.
26. M.E. Curran, I. Splawski, K.W. Timothy, et al. Cell 1995; 80: 795.
27. Q. Wang, J. Shen, I. Splawski, et al. Cell 1995; 80: 805.
28. I. Splawski, M. Tristani-Firouzi, M.H. Lehmann, et al. Nature Genet. 1997; 17: 338.
29. G.W. Abbott, F. Sesti, I. Splawski, et al. Cell 1999; 97: 175.
30. J. Warmke, R. Drysdale, and B. Ganetzky. Science 1991; 252: 1560.
31. M.C. Sanguinetti, C. Jiang, M.E. Curran, and M.T. Keating. Cell 1995; 81: 299.
32. T.V. McDonald, Z. Yu, Z. Ming, et al. Nature 1997; 388: 289.
33. L. Bianchi, B. Wible, A. Arcangeli, et al. Cancer Res. 1998; 58; 815.
34. R. Schafer, I. Wulfsen, S. Behrens, et al. J. Physiol. (Lond) 1999; 518: 401.
35. T. Yang, D.J. Snyders, and D.M. Roden. Circulation 1995; 91: 1799.
36. M. Taglialatela, P. Castaldo, S. Iossa, et al. Proc. Natl. Acad. Sci. U S A 1997; 94: 11698.
37. Z. Zhou, Q. Gong, B. Ye, et al. Biophys. J. 1998; 74: 230.
38. M-L. Roy, R. Dumaine, and A.M. Brown. Circulation 1996; 94: 817.
39. H. Suessbrich, S. Waldegger, F. Lang, and A.E. Busch. FEBS Lett. 1996; 385: 77.
40. P. Honig, and J.N. Baranjuk. In: F. Estelle R. Simons, ed. Histamine and H_1-receptor antagonists in allergic diseases. New York: Marcel Dekker Inc. 1996: 383-412.
41. E.M. Sorkin, and R.C. Heel. Drugs 1985; 29: 34.
42. A.P. Good, R. Rockwood, and P. Schad. Am. J. Cardiol. 1994; 74: 1240.
43. L.M. DuBuske. Clin. Therapeutics 1999; 21: 281.
44. M. Taglialatela, A. Pannaccione, P. Castaldo, et al. Mol. Pharmacol. 1998; 54: 113.
45. M.E. Sale, J.T. Barbery, R.L. Woosley, et al. Clin. Pharmacol. Ther. 1994; 56: 295.

46. J.A. Hey, M. del Prado, J. Sherwood, et al. Arznemittel-Forschung Drug Res. 1996; 46: 153.
47. P. Coulie, A. Delaere, C. De Vos, et al. Lancet 1998; 351: 451.
48. E. Carmeliet. Br. J. Pharmacol. 1998;124: 663.
49. C.M. Ko, I. Ducic, J. Fan, et al. J. Pharmacol. Exp. Ther. 1997; 281: 233.
50. A.E. Lacerda, M-L. Roy, E.W. Lewis, and D. Rampe. Mol. Pharmacol. 1997; 52: 314.
51. M. Haria, A. Fitton, and D.H. Peters. Drugs 1994; 48: 617.
52. M. Brannan, P. Reidenberg, E. Radwanski, et al. Clin. Pharmacol. Ther. 1995; 58: 269.
53. R.L. Woosley, and W.P. Darrow. Am. J. Cardiol. 1994; 74: 208.
54. J.A. Hey, M. del Prado, R.W. Egan, et al. Int. Arch. Allergy Immunol. 1995; 107: 418.
55. M. Lindquist, and I.R. Edwards. Lancet 1997; 349: 1322.
56. W.J. Jr. Crumb. J. Pharmacol. Exp. Ther. 2000; 292: 261.
57. J. Gras, J. Llenas, J.M. Palacios, and D.J. Roberts. Br. J. Pharmacol. 1996; 119: 187.
58. D.J. Roberts. Inflamm. Res. 1998; 74: S36.
59. F. Leynadier, J. Bousquet, M. Murrieta, and P. Attali. Ann. Allergy Asthma Immunol. 1996; 76: 163.
60. A.J. Tasman, and P. Weber. Allergy 1995; 50: 79.
61. J. Brostoff, P. Fitzharris, C. Dunmore, et al. Allergy 1996; 51: 320.
62. A. Patat, M.C. Perault, B. Vandel, et al. Br. J. Clin. Pharmacol 1995; 39: 31.
63. E.F. Vuurman, M.M. Uiterwijk, P. Rosenzweig, and J.F. O'Hanlon. Eur. J. Clin. Pharmacol. 1994; 47: 253.
64. P. Danjou, P. Molinier, I. Berlin, et al. Br. J. Clin. Pharmacol 1992; 34: 328.
65. M.C. Delauche-Cavallier, S. Chaufour, E. Gueralt, et al. Clin. Exp. Allergy, 1999; 29: 206.
66. M. Taglialatela, A. Pannaccione, P. Castaldo, et al. Br. J. Pharmacol. 2000; 131:1081.
67. O. Chosidow, C. Dubruc, P. Danjou P, et al. Eur. J. Clin. Pharmacol. 1996; 50: 327.
68. S. Chaufour, H. Caplain, N. Lilienthal, et al. Br. J. Clin. Pharmacol., 1999; 47: 515.
69. J. Benavides, H. Schoemaker, C. Dana, et al. Arzneimittelforschung 1995; 45: 551.
70. B. Biton, S. Maitre, D. Godet, et al. Allergy, 1998; 43 (suppl.): 160.
71. M. Khalifa, B. Drolet, P. Daleau, et al. J. Pharmacol. Exp. Ther. 1999; 288: 858.
72. J.J. Salata, N.K. Jurkiewicz, A.A. Wallace, et al. Circ. Res. 1995; 76: 110.
73. W.X. Wang, S.N. Ebert, X.K. Liu, et al. J. Cardiovasc. Pharmacol. 1998; 32: 123.
74. R.F. Clark, and M.V. Vance. Ann. Emerg. Med. 1992; 21: 318.
75. H.E. Hestand, and D.W. Teske. J. Pediatr. 1977; 90: 1017.
76. W. Zareba, A.J. Moss, S.Z. Rosero, et al. Am. J. Cardiol. 1997; 80: 1168.
77. B.E. Magera, C.J. Betlach, A.P. Sweatt, and C.W. Derrick. Pediatrics 1981; 67: 280.
78. L.E. Hollister. Psychopharmacol. Commun. 1975; 1: 61.
79. M. Taglialatela, H. Timmermann, and L. Annunziato. Trends Pharmacol. Sci. 2000; 21:52.
80. C.M. Pratt, R.P. Hertz, B.E. Ellis, et al. Am. J. Cardiol. 1994: 73: 346.
81. B.A. Hamelin, A. Bouayad, B. Drolet, et al. Drug Metab. Dispos. 1998: 26: 536.
82. M.S. Lennard. Drug Saf. 1993; 9: 60.
83. M-Q. Zhang. Curr. Med. Chem., 1997; 4: 187.
84. J. Kiehn, A. Lacerda, B. Wible, and A.M. Brown. Circulation 1996; 94: 2575.
85. J.J. Lynch, A.A. Wallace, R.F. Stupienski, et al. J. Pharmacol. Exp. Ther. 1994; 269: 541.
86. S. Mohammad, Z. Zhou, Q. Gong, and C.T. January. Am. J. Physiol. 1997; 42: H253.
87. J.P. Lees-Miller, Y. Duan, G.Q. Teng, and H.J. Duff. Mol. Pharmacol. 2000; 57: 367.

88. J.S. Mitcheson, J. Chen, M. Lin, et al. Proc. Natl. Acad. Sci. USA 2000; 97: 12329.
89. Y.G. Yap, and J. Camm. Br. Med. J. 2000; 320:1158.
90. European Agency for the Evaluation of Medicinal Products: Committee for Proprietary Medicinal Products. 1997; CPMP/986/96.
91. Among others available on the Internet, an updated database on QT-prolonging drugs is kept at the Georgetown Center for Education and Research on Therapeutics (www.qtdrugs.org;)
92. D.A. Doyle, J. Morais Cabral, R.A. Pfuetzner, et al. Science 2000; 280: 69.

Histamine Research in the New Millennium
T. Watanabe, H. Timmerman and K. Yanai (Editors)

THE SKIN REACTIVITY TO HISTAMINE:
THE TRAPS OF THE INVESTIGATION

J.-P. Rihoux, FFPM and A. Campbell, PHD
UCB SA, chemin du Foriest, 1420 Braine-l'Alleud, Belgium

INTRODUCTION

Since the description by Lewis of the histamine-induced triple skin reaction, the histamine skin test has been widely used for investigating the pharmacodynamic aspects of new H_1-antagonists and more especially for performing comparative studies. This skin test might appear very simple and very easy to perform, at least at first glance, but several publications show that it is not really the case. The aim of the present paper is to discuss some of the most frequent difficulties encountered and or errors that may be linked to this very classical investigation of skin reactivity to histamine.

RESPECTIVE POTENCIES OF DIFFERENT DRUGS

In 1995, Rosenzweig *et al* compared the respective anti H_1 potencies of cetirizine 10 mg, loratadine 10 mg, mizolastine 10 mg and terfenadine 120 mg using the histamine-induced skin wheal and flare reaction.(1). They showed that the % change from baseline of wheal area reached a maximum of 67 % four hours after loratadine intake while the three other drugs resulted in a change of greater than 100 %.

They concluded that the antihistamine activity of mizolastine 10 mg is very close to those of cetirizine 10 mg and terfenadine 120 mg.

The fact that a mean inhibition of more than 100 % was observed for 3 drugs indicates that there is a problem involving the methodology of this study.

Using exactly the same method, ie 2 µg histamine injected I.D. in the skin in a volume of 0.1 ml saline, Hüther et al showed in 1977 that the maximum mean percent change in histamine wheal area after p.o administration of terfenadine 60 and 200 mg was close to 100 %, with no significant difference between these 2 doses. (2)

In contrast, Shall et al compared the respective potencies of terfenadine 60,120 and 240 mg using the same skin test but a higher histamine concentration (20 µg in 0.1 ml saline) and showed a dose-effect relationship as far as the wheal was concerned together with a correlation between the inhibiting effect of the drug and the plasma concentration of its major metabolite (3). In addition, Rafferty and Holgate demonstrated a very clear dose-effect response for terfenadine 60, 120 and 180 mg using skin prick tests and increasing concentrations of histamine (4 to 128 mg/ml). (4)

These data clearly demonstrate that some studies allow one to demonstrate significant differences between drugs or between different doses of the same drugs whilst others do not, depending on the methods used.

THE PLATEAU EFFECT: AN ARTIFACT?

Some results obtained during pharmacodynamic studies carried out with cetirizine 10 mg po in healthy subjects and atopics tend to demonstrate that the antihistaminic effect of the drug at skin level is almost maximum 3 hours after p.o. intake and remains close to the maximum until 9 to 12 hours post-dosage (5). Such a characteristic is often interpreted as a plateau effect (see graph I).

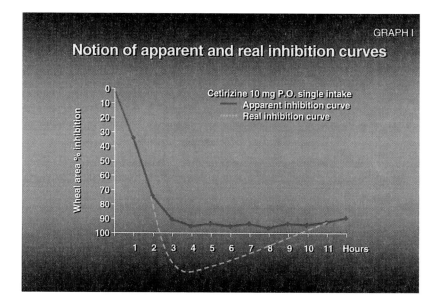

In fact, this particular shape of the curve is probably due to the use of a too low histamine concentration when investigating a very potent antagonist. This leads to an apparent inhibition curve as shown on graph I, whilst the true inhibition curve (dotted line) can not be demonstrated. This artifact is the main reason why some comparative studies do not allow discrimination between different drugs or different doses of the same drug as already mentioned.

SELECTION OF THE ADEQUATE HISTAMINE CONCENTRATION

Several comparative studies have been performed using just a single concentration of histamine and in these cases it is difficult to know if this concentration is the ideal one for each compound under test? This is the reason why some investigators prefer to use a range of concentrations in order to obtain histamine-wheal concentration response curves (4) (6) (7). It goes without saying that the higher the histamine concentration, the less the inhibition by a given antagonist. Nevertheless, several years ago we carried out a clinical pharmacology study in healthy subjects who took cetirizine 20 and 40 mg as single intake and were skin tested with histamine I.D (0.1, 1 and 10 µg in 10 µL saline). Under these experimental conditions, the % inhibition of wheal surface area was significantly higher for the highest histamine concentration than for the lowest one (graph II).

This apparently paradoxical result is easy to explain. On one hand, the wheal surface area was larger after ID injection of the high histamine concentration, as expected. On the other hand, after an ID injection of histamine, there is usually after H_1-blockade a significant residual wheal which is not H_1-dependent. After H_1-blockade by 2 high doses of cetirizine, the mean areas of the H_1-independent residual wheals were similar, while the histamine-induced skin reactions were proportional to the injected concentrations. As a consequence, the inhibition of skin reactions, when expressed in Δ %, was higher when the wheal area before drug intake was larger, ie when induced by the highest histamine concentration.

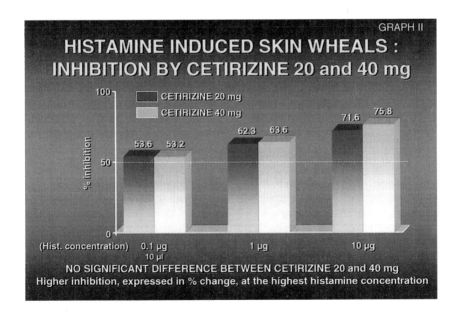

This story deserves 2 comments:

- the ID injection of the agonist histamine seems inappropriate since it induces the appearance of a non specific-wheal,
- if a drug is very potent, it will be difficult, if not impossible, to select the adequate histamine concentration for skin test. We once tested a solution of histamine at 500 mg/ml for Prick tests (8) and despite this concentration, the inhibition of the skin reaction by cetirizine 10 mg reached 100 % in several volunteers. Moreover, it is difficult to prepare a stable solution of histamine at a concentration higher than 500 mg/ml, and even at 500 mg, some volunteers develop very large satellite wheals which render difficult the objective quantification of the reactions very difficult.

THE USE OF THE ED_{50} IN SKIN REACTIONS

Taking into account all the above-mentioned difficulties and objections, Ramboer et al performed a nice pharmacodynamic comparative experiment in 14 healthy subjects taking cetirizine and loratadine (9). Depending on the relative potencies of both drugs, they gave the volunteers increasing doses of loratadine, ie 10, 20 and 40 mg single p.o administration, and decreasing doses of cetirizine, ie 10, 5 and 2.5 mg. They performed prick tests in order to avoid non specific skin reactions due to the volume injected, and they used a range of histamine concentrations: 10, 100 and 500 mg/ml. The experiment was double-blind, cross-over, randomized and placebo-controlled. Using such a protocol, they could calculate the dose of each drug required to inhibit histamine-induced skin reactions by 50 % at each experimental time. Calculation of the ED_{50} demonstrated that, on an average, cetirizine is seven to nine times more potent than loratadine.

CONCLUSION

The correct use of histamine-induced skin reaction for comparative pharmacodynamic studies in humans is neither difficult nor complicated. Nevertheless, this kind of investigation is not always as simple as it might first appear. Not only are the skills of the investigators of importance in order to ensure reproducible results, but also a number of other factors must be taken into account. The development of very potent antagonists such as cetirizine, epinastine and levocetirizine will probably necessitate the systematic use of the ED50 approach for accurate pharmacodynamic comparisons. This will not simplify the life of the investigators since such experiments require a high number of consecutive sessions for the volunteers. The solution for the future could be to perform fewer studies, but studies of higher quality.

REFERENCES

1. P. Rosenweig, H. Caplain, S. Chaufour, N. Ulliac, M.J. Cabanis, J.J. Thebault. Comparative wheal and flare study of mizolastine vs terfenadine, cetirizine, loratadine and placebo in healthy volunteers. Br J Clin Pharmacol 1995;40:459-465

2. K.J. Hüther, G. Renftle, Barraud N, J.T. Burke, and J. Koch Weser. Inhibitory activity of terfenadine on histamine-induced skin wheals in man. Eur J Clin Pharmacol 1977;12:195-199

3. L. Shall, R.G., M. Lush, R. Marks. Dose-response relationship between objective measures of histamine-induced weals and dose of terfenadine. Acta-Derm. Venereol. 1991,71,3:199-204

4. P. Rafferty and ST. Holgate.Terfenadine (Seldane) is a potent and selective histamine H_1 receptor antagonist in asthmatic airways. Am Rev Respir Dis 1987;135:181-184

5. FER Simons, JL McMillan, KJ Simons. A double-blind, single-dose, crossover comparison of cetirizine, terfenadine, loratadine, astemizole, and chlorpheniramine versus placebo: suppressive effects on histamine-induced wheals and flares during 24 hours in normal subjects. J Allergy Clin Immunol 1990;86:540-547

6. J-P Rihoux, L.Ghys, and P. Coulie. Compared peripheral H_1 inhibiting effects of cetirizine 2 HCl and loratadine. Annals of Allergy 1990;65(2):139-142

7. N. Frossard, M. Melac, O. Benabdesselam, G. Pauli. Consistency of the efficacy of cetirizine and ebastine on skin reactivity. Annals of Allergy, Asthma and Immunology 1998,80,1:61-65

8. PJ Coulie, L Ghys and J-P Rihoux. Cetirizine, oxatomide, ketotifen and placebo. Pharmacological evaluation of their respective anti-H_1-histamine, antipruritic and sedating effects. Drug Invest 1991;3(5):324-327

9. I. Ramboer, R. Bumbacea, D. Lazarescu, JR. Radu. Cetirizine and Loratadine: a comparison using the ED_{50} in skin reactions. The Journal of International Medical Research 2000;28:69-77

Safety and efficiency of histamine H1 antagonists

© 2001 Elsevier Science B.V. All rights reserved.
Histamine Research in the New Millennium
T. Watanabe, H. Timmerman and K. Yanai (Editors)

Efficacy and safety of H_1-receptor antagonists in the treatment of allergic disorders: an overview

F. Estelle R. Simons, M.D., FRCPC

Bruce Chown Professor and Head, Section of Allergy & Clinical Immunology, Department of Pediatrics & Child Health, University of Manitoba, Winnipeg, Manitoba, Canada[1]

1   INTRODUCTION

Allergic disorders such as rhinitis, urticaria, atopic dermatitis, and asthma are among the commonest chronic afflictions of the human race[1]. H_1-receptor antagonists are the most frequently used medications for the treatment of these disorders. Based on chemical structure, H_1-antagonists are classified as ethylenediamines, ethanolamines, alkylamines, phenothiazines, piperazines, and piperidines. They are also classified in a clinically useful way, as either "first-generation", potentially sedating H_1-antagonists, for example, chlorpheniramine, diphenhydramine, hydroxyzine, promethazine, and triprolidine, or "second-generation" relatively non-sedating H_1-antagonists, for example, cetirizine, ebastine, fexofenadine, loratadine, and mizolastine.

Since 1990, there have been attempts to introduce the term "third-generation" H_1-antagonist, however, this has not yet been adopted as there is no consensus as to how it should be defined. Initially, it was applied to H_1-antagonists with anti-allergic effects. More recently, it has been applied to H_1-antagonists which are metabolites, H_1-antagonists with unique pharmacologic or pharmaco-kinetic properties, H_1-antagonists which are free from cardiac toxicity, and H_1-antagonists which are non-sedating even at supratherapeutic doses.

H_1-antagonists with excellent clinical pharmacology, efficacy and safety profiles are now available for use[2,3]. Here we present a brief, state-of-the-art

1   Dr. F.E.R. Simons
Children's Hospital of Winnipeg, 820 Sherbrook Street, Winnipeg, Manitoba, Canada
R3A 1R9   Phone: (204) 787-2440   FAX: (204) 787-5040   e-mail: lmcniven@hsc.mb.ca

review of their efficacy and safety, with emphasis on the second-generation medications.

2 EFFICACY

2.1 Clinical Pharmacology

H_1-antagonists act at histamine H_1-receptors on post-capillary venules and sensory nerves, and also have dose-dependent anti-allergic and anti-inflammatory activities, most of which do not involve the H_1-receptor.

The second-generation H_1-antagonists are well-absorbed after oral administration. Terminal elimination half-life values range from 2-24 hours[3]. Some, such as ebastine, loratadine, and mizolastine are transformed into active metabolites by the hepatic cytochrome P450 system. Others such as acrivastine, cetirizine and fexofenadine are less extensively metabolized (50%, 40%, and <1% respectively in adults), and may have a reduced likelihood of drug-drug interactions and of requiring special dosage regimens in patients with impaired hepatic or renal function.

All H_1-antagonists suppress the histamine- or allergen-induced wheal and flare (erythema) in the skin. This bioassay is used in dose-response studies, and in pharmacodynamic studies in which the relationship between the plasma concentration and the intensity of the pharmacological effects is defined using frequent tests during a 24-hour dosing interval. Another, less commonly used bioassay involves H_1-antagonist-induced suppression of $\alpha2$-macroglobulin concentrations in nasal lavage fluid after histamine challenge on the nasal mucosa.

Most H_1-antagonists have clinically relevant activity within 1-2 hours after a single dose and a duration of action of 12-24 hours, facilitating once- or twice-daily dosing. They play an important role in the treatment of allergic rhinitis and urticaria. During months of regular daily administration, tachyphylaxis to their effects does not develop.

2.2 Allergic Rhinitis

In some countries, up to 40% of individuals currently suffer from this disorder. The evidence base for effectiveness of H_1-antagonists in intermittent or perennial allergic rhinitis consists of hundreds of large, prospective, randomized, double-blind, clinical trials, most of which are placebo-controlled, and last for 1-4 weeks. H_1-antagonists provide excellent relief of nasal itching, sneezing and rhinorrhea and of associated ocular itching, erythema, and tearing, but incomplete relief of nasal congestion. They are effective in reducing the morbidity of allergic rhinitis, as reflected in significant improvement in quality of life assessments. Topical intranasal or conjunctival application of H_1-antagonists such as azelastine or levocabastine provide an additional treatment option.

Although one or more allergic rhinitis clinical trials can usually be found to support the superiority of any H_1-antagonist over its commercial competitors, where statistically significant differences in efficacy among these medications have been identified, their magnitude has seldom been clinically important. All H_1-antagonists have similar effectiveness when used in a clinical setting. Higher doses than those recommended by the manufacturer are unlikely to result in significant additional relief of allergic rhinitis symptoms and non-responders to H_1-antagonists require intranasal glucocorticosteroid treatment[2,4].

2.3   Chronic Urticaria

H_1-antagonists are the most important medications available for the symptomatic treatment of chronic urticaria, defined as persistent or recurrent hives of at least six weeks duration. Their beneficial effects have been well-documented for reducing the frequency urticarial episodes and for reducing the number, size, itching, and duration of individual urticarial lesions. In prospective, randomized, placebo-controlled, double-blind studies, second-generation, non-sedating H_1-antagonists such as cetirizine have been found to be as effective as first-generation, sedating ones such as hydroxyzine. For optimal effectiveness in chronic urticaria treatment, H_1-antagonists should be given on a regular basis rather than on an "as needed" basis.

If an unsatisfactory response to H_1-antagonists occurs, the treatment options for an individual with chronic urticaria are somewhat limited. An H_1-/H_2- antagonist such as doxepin can be given, or an H_2-antagonist such as cimetidine or ranitidine can be administered concurrently with an H_1-antagonist for a 4-week trial. A course of prednisone, or an even more potent immunomodulator such as cyclosporin, may be needed[2,5].

2.4   Other Allergic Disorders

In atopic dermatitis, oral H_1-antagonists are used in conjunction with topical glucocorticoids to reduce itching. In this disorder, while H_1-antagonists have some glucocorticoid-sparing effect, they are less effective than they are in urticaria[2].

In patients with mild seasonal asthma associated with allergic rhinitis, H_1-antagonists decrease both asthma and rhinitis symptoms significantly and improve pulmonary function. In placebo-controlled, double-blind studies of 1-3 years duration in high risk infants with atopic dermatitis and/or elevated serum IgE and a family history of atopy, cetirizine or ketotifen appear to delay the onset of asthma[6].

In systemic anaphylactic or anaphylactoid reactions, H_1-antagonists play a subordinate role to the prompt injection of epinephrine, but they are useful for relief of the acute urticaria and intense pruritus associated with these reactions[2]. Indeed, this is one of the few remaining indications for a first-generation H_1-

antagonist such as diphenhydramine, which unlike the second-generation H_1-antagonists, is available in solution for injection; the sedative effects of diphenhydramine are not a major concern during emergency treatment.

3   SAFETY

The greatest advance in H_1-antagonist treatment during the past sixty years has been the development of medications in this class which are free from adverse central nervous system and cardiac effects[2,7].

3.1   Central Nervous System (CNS) Effects
The first-generation H_1-antagonists cause daytime somnolence in 40-80% of users. Some of them, eg. diphenhydramine and doxylamine are among the most commonly used non-prescription sedatives in the world. In contrast, second-generation H_1-antagonists are relatively free from CNS adverse effects, primarily because they do not cross the blood-brain barrier to the same degree that their predecessors did. Although the second-generation medications (cetirizine, ebastine, fexofenadine, loratadine, and mizolastine) differ from each other in their ability to cause adverse CNS effects, they are all associated with fewer CNS effects than the first-generation H_1-antagonists such as chlorpheniramine, diphenhydramine, hydroxyzine, promethazine, or triprolidine. Furthermore, in contrast to the older H_1-antagonists, they do not potentiate the adverse effects produced by other CNS-active medications or by ethanol[2,7-9].

The second generation H_1-antagonists are also free from minor, but annoying adverse effects such as anticholinergic effects (dry mouth, dysfunctional urine voiding), anti-serotonin effects (inappropriate weight gain), or dysgeusia (bitter taste).

3.2   Cardiac Toxicity
The H_1-antagonists astemizole and terfenadine are no longer approved by regulatory agencies because of their well-documented ability to prolong the QT interval on the electrocardiogram, cause torsade de pointes, syncope at rest or with exertion, loss of consciousness, palpitations and, rarely, death. The mechanism of the cardiac toxicity involves blockade of the IKr rapidly activating delayed rectifier potassium current in the ventricular myocardium. While IKr is the major time-dependent outward current determining the duration of the action potential, IKi, IKs and other ion currents may also be involved.

Susceptibility to cardiac toxicity from H_1-antagonists is increased in females, elderly individuals, those with pre-existing cardiac or hepatic disorders or electrolyte imbalance, and those who are concomitantly taking other CYP450 inhibitors or medications which themselves prolong the QT interval. Most of the second generation H_1-antagonists which remain approved by regulatory agencies are unlikely to cause cardiac toxicity[2,10].

3.3 Long-Term Safety

With the exception of the 18-month duration Early Treatment of the Atopic Child (ETAC) study in 800 toddlers, which confirmed the safety of cetirizine in this age group[11], there are no prospective, randomized, double-blind, placebo-controlled, long-term safety studies of H_1-antagonists. In particular, studies in infants and in the elderly are long overdue.

Although no H_1-antagonist can be declared to be absolutely safe for use during pregnancy, two second-generation medications, cetirizine and loratadine, are considered to be relatively safe (US Food and Drug Administration Category B)[12].

There is no evidence that H_1-antagonists which have been approved by regulatory agencies have carcinogenic or tumor-promoting effects in humans[13].

4 SUMMARY

New H_1-antagonists such as carebastine, desloratadine, emedastine, epinastine, levocetirizine, norastemizole, and rupatidine are being developed and introduced for use. Some of them are H_1-antagonist metabolites (carebastine, desloratadine, norastemizole), or enantiomers (levocetirizine), which have an improved therapeutic index compared to their predecessors.

A novel polymorphism has been discovered in the gene encoding the H_1-receptor: a single amine substitution on codon 356 within the third intracellular loop, which is a critical area for receptor phosphorylation[14]. At this time, the clinical significance of this polymorphism is unknown, however, in the future using genotyping and phenotyping of the pharmacodynamic response, it may be possible to identify H_1-antagonist responders and non-responders and direct therapy accordingly.

REFERENCES:

1.   The International Study of Asthma and Allergies in Childhood (ISAAC) Steering Committee. Worldwide variation in prevalence of symptoms of asthma, allergic rhinoconjunctivitis, and atopic eczema: ISAAC. Lancet 1998;351:1225-32.
2.   Simons FER, Simons KJ. The pharmacology and use of H_1-receptor antagonist drugs. N Engl J Med 1994;330:1663-70.

3. Simons FER, Simons KJ. Clinical pharmacology of new histamine H_1-receptor antagonists. Clin Pharmacokinet 1999;36:329-52.
4. Dykewicz MS, Fineman S. Diagnosis and Management of Rhinitis: Parameter Documents of the Joint Task Force on Practice Parameters in Allergy, Asthma, and Immunology. Ann Allergy Asthma Immunol 1998;81:463-518.
5. Greaves MW. Chronic urticaria. N Engl J Med 1995;332:1767-72.
6. Wahn U, for the ETAC Study Group. Allergic factors associated with the development of asthma and the influence of cetirizine in a double-blind, randomised, placebo-controlled trial: first results of ETAC. Pediatr Allergy Immunol 1998;9:116-24.
7. Simons FER. Non-cardiac adverse effects of antihistamines (H_1-receptor antagonists). Clin Exp Allergy 1999;29 (Suppl. 2):125-32.
8. Hindmarch I, Shamsi Z. Antihistamines: models to assess sedative properties, assessment of sedation, safety and other side-effects. Clin Exp Allergy 1999;29 (Suppl. 3):133-42.
9. Simons FER, Fraser TG, Reggin JD, Simons KJ. Comparison of the central nervous system effects produced by six H_1-receptor antagonists. Clin Exp Allergy 1996;26:1092-7.
10. Yap YG, Camm AJ. Arrhythmogenic mechanism of non-sedating antihistamines. Clin Exp Allergy 1999;29 (Suppl. 3):174-81.
11. Simons FER, on behalf of the ETAC Study Group. Prospective, long-term safety evaluation of the H_1-receptor antagonist cetirizine in very young children with atopic dermatitis. J Allergy Clin Immunol 1999;104:433-40.
12. Schatz M, Petitti D. Antihistamines and pregnancy. Ann Allergy Asthma Immunol 1997;78:157-9.
13. Weiss SR, McFarland BH, Burkhart GA, Ho PTC. Cancer recurrences and second primary cancers after use of antihistamines or antidepressants. Clin Pharmacol Ther 1998;63:594-9.
14. Dewar JC, Hall IP. A novel degenerate polymorphism in the human histamine H_1-receptor gene. Am J Respir Crit Care Med 1998;157:A773.

© 2001 Elsevier Science B.V. All rights reserved.
Histamine Research in the New Millennium
T. Watanabe, H. Timmerman and K. Yanai (Editors)

Histaminergic Neurons and Sleep-Wake Regulation

J.S. Lin, G. Vanni-Mercier and R. Parmentier

INSERM U480, Department of Experimental Medicine, Faculty of Medicine, Claude Bernard University, 8 avenue Rockefeller 69373 Lyon, France

The history for the functional importance of histamine (HA) in waking can be traced back as far as the 1930's when the classic antihistaminic drugs were discovered in France. This class of drugs, now designated as H1-receptor antagonists, has notoriously been known to cause sedation and drowsiness in man when they are used in the treatment of allergic diseases, as Douglas described: "*In therapeutic doses, all H1 brokers elicit side effects, the side effect with the highest incidence, and the one common to all drugs in this group, is sedation*" (1). However, the cause of this so called "side effect" has, until recently, not been studied by neuroscientists. Only after the recent discovery that HA is also a neurotransmitter in the brain, was it hypothesized that a blockade of HA transmission could be responsible for the sedation caused by antihistaminics. Here, experimental data are provided supporting our hypothesis that histaminergic (HArgic) neurons play an important role in cortical activation and wakefulness (W).

1. Histaminergic neurons and their fiber projections

In the mammalian brain, HA is synthesized from L-histidine by histidine decarboxylase (HDC) and is predominantly inactivated by histamine-N-methyltransferase. The central actions of HA are mediated by postsynaptic H1- and H2-receptors and by H3-receptors possessing characteristics of auto- and hetero-receptors (2). In addition to a large body of neuroanatomical data obtained in rats and other species by other groups (e.g., 3-5), we have demonstrated, in the cat (6), that HArgic neurons are located exclusively in the tuberomammillary nucleus (TM) and adjacent areas of the posterior hypothalamus, a brain area known for its importance in waking (see review in Refs. 6,7). These neurons send widespread ascending and descending inputs to various brain areas, especially those involved in controlling the sleep-wake states, such as the cortex, thalamus, preoptic/anterior hypothalamus, posterior hypothalamus (including the dorsolateral and perifornical areas) and periaqueductal gray, and to brainstem and forebrain cholinergic and monoaminergic neurons(6). In addition, HA is also present in mast cells and the endothelium of microvessels, whereas HA H1- and H2-receptors have been identified not only on neurons, but also on glial cells (2), suggesting that non-neuronal HA may also regulate brain functions. Consistent with the widespread outputs of HArgic cells, we have recently used *in situ* hybridization (6) to demonstrate strong expression of H1-receptor mRNA in neuronal populations of large brain areas in guinea-pigs, e.g. in the cortex, intralaminar nuclei of the thalamus and mesencephalic reticular formation. H2-receptor mRNA also has been identified in large cell populations in the cortex, thalamus and basal forebrain in guinea-pigs (8). The anatomical organization of HArgic neurons suggests that this system may influence the neuronal excitability and activity of large brain areas. Electrophysiological data support this idea.

126

2. Discharge pattern of histaminergic neurons and postsynaptic actions of histamine

In the rat brain slice *in vitro*, HA neurons are spontaneously active with a discharge rate of 2.1 ± 0.6 Hz (9,10). In the freely-moving cat, presumed HArgic neurons present a waking-state specific (W-on) activity, discharging tonically and specifically during W, with their activity decreasing significantly as soon as cortical spindles appear (drowsiness) and becoming totally silent during deep slow wave sleep (SWS) and paradoxical sleep (PS). In the cat hypothalamus, this kind of activity is exclusively recorded in the TM and adjacent ventrolateral posterior hypothalamus (7,11). Similar W-on discharge pattern has been recently recorded in the TM and adjacent areas in freely-moving rats (12). In order to bring new insights into the histological nature of these W-on cells, we have recently carried out unitary recordings in the same region of freely-moving cat, combined with systemic or *in situ* injection of highly potent and selective ligands of H3-receptors (13) which control the activity of HA neurons through mechanisms of autoinhibition (2). We have found that intramuscular injection of ciproxifan (H3-receptor antagonist, 1 mg/kg), induces a significant increase in the discharge rate of W-on cells during active and quiet waking (Fig. 1). Conversely,

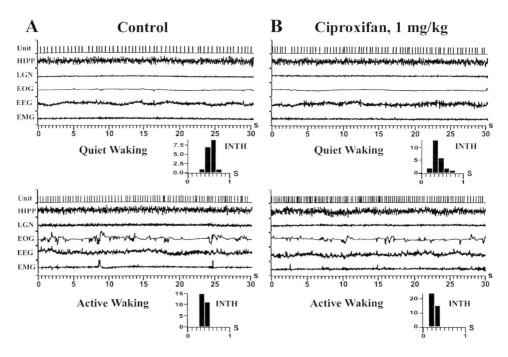

Figure 1: Representative example of the effect of ciproxifan (1 mg/kg, im) on the discharge of a W-on cell recorded from the cat ventrolateral posterior hypothalamus. Samples of polygraphic and unitary recordings before (A) and within one hour after injection (B), as well as the interval histograms (INTH) of spikes, showing a significant enhancement of the neuronal discharge after ciproxifan injection during both quiet and active waking. The mean discharge rates (Hz) of 16 tested W-on cells ±SEM before and after the ciproxifan injection were: 1.64 ±0.05 vs 2.46 ±0.06 for quiet waking and 2.30 ±0.07 vs 3.15 ±0.12 for active waking (p<0.001, ANOVA).

intramuscular injection of imetit (H3-receptor agonist, 1 mg/kg) or microinjection of α-methylhistamine (α-MHA, another H3-receptor agonist, 0.05 μg/0.2μl) in the vicinity of recorded cells, results in a significant decrease in their discharge rate. The effect of ciproxifan on the neuronal discharge of W-on cells is reversed by either intramuscular injection of imetit or microinjection of α-MHA, suggesting that the changes in neuronal discharge rate seen with the used ligands is, indeed, due to a modulation on H3-receptors. Moreover, administrations of the same ligands have no effect on other types of neuronal discharges recorded in the posterior hypothalamus (13). Our data thus provide further experimental evidence for the HAergic nature of the W-on cells recorded in the cat posterior hypothalamus.

Consistent with the high discharge rate of presumed HArgic neurons during W, it has also been demonstrated in rodents that the release and turnover of HA is high during darkness, the period in which the animals are active and spend a large part of their time in W (14). In monkeys, increased HA release in the posterior hypothalamus occurs on awakening and is maintained during each waking episode (15).

At the postsynaptic level, recent *in vitro* intracellular recording studies have revealed that activation of H1-receptors on thalamic relay neurons results in slow depolarization by suppression of leakage potassium current. Activation of H2-receptors, on the other hand, induces a small depolarization, associated with an increase in hyperpolarization current. As a result, this combined action of HA can cause a switch of neuronal discharge from rhythmic bursts to tonic activity, and therefore might promote the switch from SWS to W (16). Similar results have been obtained in human cortical neurons (17) and guinea-pig mesopontine and basal forebrain cholinergic neurons (18). Activation of H2-receptors also causes shortening of afterhyperpolarization and may facilitate cortical and hippocampal activity (9,10). Moreover, in rat cortical or hippocampal cultures or isolated neurons, HA has been shown to enhance NMDA receptor-mediated synaptic transmission by as yet undefined receptors and mechanisms (19).

All these electrophysiological data suggest that HArgic cells increase their activity during wake state and activate or facilitate the neuronal activity of large brain areas, such as the cortex, thalamus, and basal forebrain, thus contributing to generalized cortical activation. In order to evaluate this assumption, we have carried out a series of systemic and *in situ* pharmacological studies in the cat, data summarized below.

3. Histaminergic transmission and the sleep-wake cycle

In cats (6) as in rats (20,21), intraperitoneal injection of α-fluoromethylhistidine (α-FMH), a specific inhibitor of the HA synthesis enzyme, induces a slowly-developed and significant decrease in W and an increase in SWS without modifying PS, the time-course of the effects paralleling the reduction in brain HA content. In the posterior hypothalamus where HA neurons are located, blockade of HA synthesis by microinjection of α-FMH also causes a significant increase in deep SWS. In contrast, blockade of HA catabolism at the same site by microinjection of SKF-91488 (an inhibitor of histamine-*N*-methyltransferase) results in long-lasting W (6). Concerning data about the functional role of HA receptors, we have shown that:

Firstly, intraperitoneal injection of mepyramine, a H1-receptor antagonist, causes an increase in cortical slow waves, as revealed by power spectral analysis, this slow activity being indistinguishable from that seen during SWS in the control recording. This effect is seen on EEG scoring as a decrease in latency to SWS and an increase in the time spent in

128

SWS, at the expense of an decrease in both W and PS (6). In man, H1-receptor antagonists have been shown to impair vigilance during W and to reduce performance (22). These data obtained using H1-receptor antagonists are consistent with the sedation and drowsiness caused in man by classical antihistaminics, now designated as H1-receptor antagonists (1,2) and provide experimental confirmation to this well-known clinical observation.

Secondly, intraventricular injection of ranitidine, a H2-receptor antagonist, also increases SWS in the cat, the effect being slow and progressive (6). Whereas the exact role of H2-receptors on sleep-wake cycle remains to be established by using potent and specific brain-penetrating agonists and antagonists, the effect seen with ranitidine seems to be consistent with antagonism of central H2-receptors processing a mode of action of facilitation (2,,9,10,16).

Thirdly, HA controls its own release and synthesis by autoinhibition mediated by H3-receptors. Potent and selective agonists and antagonists of H3-receptors have been identified and shown to be able to alter the release and synthesis of HA and the turnover of HArgic neurons (2). We have previously shown in cats that sleep can be increased or decreased via systemic administration of agonists or antagonists of H3-receptors (6). Indeed, oral application of BP2-94, a H3-receptor agonist (kindly provided by Bioprojet, Paris) induces in the cat a dramatic increase in the power spectral density of cortical slow activity, accompanied by an significant increase in SWS (6), while, in contrast, intraperitoneal injection of ciproxifan, a H_3-receptor antagonist (also provided by Bioprojet, Paris), induces cortical EEG desynchronization and waking in mice. This waking effect seems to depend on the endogenous HA and postsynaptic H1-receptors, because the same dose of ciproxifan has no effect on HDC or H1-receptors knock-out mice (23). In the cat, oral application of a small dose of ciproxifan causes a total suppression of cortical slow activity and spindles and marked enhancement of fast rhythms, and consequently induces W (6). Because the occurrence of cortical fast rhythms is closely associated with the so-called high mental activities, such as attention, alertness, and leaning, these results thus suggest that the HArgic system plays a role not only in waking, the basis for all other high brain functions, but also in some cognitive processes.

All these data indicate that various administrations impairing brain HArgic transmission, such as the blocking of HA synthesis or postsynaptic receptors, all increase cortical slow activity and SWS. In contrast, enhancement of HArgic transmission, e.g. by blocking its autoinhibition, promotes W. These results, taking together with the recent in vitro electrophysiological data, have let to a general hypothesis concerning cellular mechanisms involved in HArgic arousal (6), summarized as follows. Activation of H1-receptors, by suppressing the leakage potassium current and by slow depolarization, would trigger the tonic neuronal discharge of large brain target cells and other physiological responses, such as glycogenolysis, required for high energy output, leading consequently to general brain arousal and increased vigilance. Activation of H2-receptors, on the other hand, by increasing neuronal excitability and discharge rate via hyperpolarization and afterhyperpolarization currents might facilitate cortical activation and W. H1- and H2-receptors might therefore act in a synergic manner, through, respectively, direct neuronal depolarization or facilitation. Finally, H3-receptors are involved in the sleep-wake cycle by a negative control over HA release and synthesis. The significance of the HA-mediated enhancement of NMDA transmission (19) in sleep-wake regulation remains to be investigated.

4. Induction of sleep in different experimental conditions by inactivation of the posterior hypothalamic containing histaminergic cell-bodies

The role of the posterior hypothalamus containing HA neurons in W is also supported by the fact that sleep can be induced in different experimental conditions by inactivation of the posterior hypothalamus (6). For this, we used microinjection of muscimol, a potent GABA agonist, because HA neurons have been shown to be contacted by GABA synapses (24). Furthermore, Haas et al. have shown by *in vitro* elecrophysiological studies that functional GABA inputs and GABAa receptors are present in HA cell membranes and that GABA induces hyperpolarization of HA neurons (9,10). Like GABA, muscimol is able to suppress neuronal activity of virtually all the neurons in the CNS and its microinjection may therefore mimic a localized and reversible lesion. We found that muscimol microinjection into the preoptic/anterior hypothalamus or the hypothalamo-mesencephalic junction provokes increased W and hyperactivity. In sharp contrast, the same injection in the rostral and middle parts of the posterior hypothalamus (including the TM and adjacent areas) induces pronounced and long-lasting increase in deep SWS, accompanied by a reduction in, or suppression of, PS. When the injection is performed in the caudal part, the increase in deep SWS is followed by an increase either in W or PS, depending upon the exact injection site. In the latter case, PS can even directly follow waking. In both the rostral and caudal parts, induction of deep SWS is seen with a shorter latency when injection is made ventrally, rather than dorsally. We have, therefore, defined a hypothalamic "waking territory" which covers TM and adjacent areas and which is, up to present, the sole brain region where such a pronounced hypersomnia in SWS following the use of muscimol has been reported (6).

The importance of the posterior hypothalamus in waking, as well as that of its inactivation in sleep onset and maintenance is further supported by the fact that, in different experimental insomniac models in the cat, sleep can be induced by neuronal inactivation of the posterior hypothalamus using muscimol microinjection (6). For example, it is well known that para-chlorophenylalanine, an inhibitor of the serotonin synthesizing enzyme, produces total insomnia 24-48h after injection and we have previously reported that muscimol microinjection into the tuberal and mammillary regions of the lateral posterior hypothalamus restores both SWS and PS with a short latency, insomnia reappearing once the effect of muscimol has worn off. Similarly, lesioning of the preoptic and anterior hypothalamus results in long-lasting insomnia and hyperthermia as shown by Sallanon et al. (25), both effects being reversed by muscimol microinjection into the ventrolateral posterior hypothalamus with restoration of both SWS and PS (25). In addition, amphetamine, a well-known psychostimulant and dopaminergic transmission-enhancing drug, is known to cause behavioral excitation and EEG activation. We recently found that, following 2h activation with amphetamine, microinjection of muscimol into the TM area suppresses, with a short latency, the effects of amphetamine by restoring both cortical slow activity and spindles and inducing deep SWS, these effects being accompanied by all behavioral signs of sleep; PS is, however, not restored (6). Finally, modafinil is a newly-discovered wake-promoting drug now being used in the treatment of hypersomnia and narcolepsy. Unlike amphetamine, modafinil induces long-lasting quiet W in the cat without causing marked behavioral excitation and subsequent sleep rebound. To assess if inactivation of the posterior hypothalamus is able to reverse its waking effect, apparently by mechanisms distinct from those of amphetamine and other psychostimulants, we have also carried out muscimol microinjection in this structure at the right moment of modafinil's effect and found that the induced W is also blocked by muscimol microinjection into the TM area, inducing the reappearance of SWS with short latency, accompanied by both cortical slow activity and spindles (6). From these results, it therefore seems clear that inactivation of the posterior hypothalamus containing HA cell bodies induces hypersomnia in normal cats and restores sleep in various models of insomnia provoked by different experimental means, suggesting the key role of this region in the mechanisms and maintenance of cortical activation and waking state.

So far, these results are obtained by reversible neuronal inactivation of the posterior hypothalamus, which contains both HArgic and non-HArgic neurons. Our understanding on the functions of HA neurons will be far from complete if we are unable to determine the effects of long-term suppression of HA or its receptors on the sleep-wake cycle. For this reason, we have studied the sleep-wake cycle in mice devoid of HDC or H1-recptors (23).

5. Role of histamine in sleep-wake regulation in rodents, as demonstrated by using knock-out mice

Using inbred HDC knock-out mice established from 129/Ola strain by Drs. H. Ohtsu and T. Watanabe (Tohoku University, School of Medicine), we have found that the wild type animals, like other rodents, respond to the beginning of the lights-off period with a significant increase in W whereas the mutant mice show a marked deficit of waking just before and after lights-off. In spite of this, there is no major difference in term of daily amount of spontaneous W between the wild type and mutant mice, suggesting that some physiological mechanisms must have compensated for the loss of HA. However, a clear difference in waking between the wild type and mutant mice is seen when we provoke a behavioral challenge, such as housing them in a new environment by changing their habitual round cage to a rectangular one. As shown in Fig. 2, after changing the cage, HDC+/+ mice maintain W for several hours, perhaps interested in the new environment. In contrast, HDC-/- mice seem to be indifferent to the new environment because they fall asleep soon after the cage change (Fig. 2)(23).

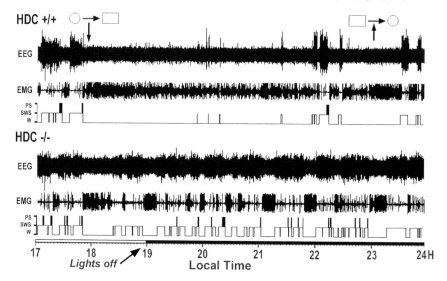

Figure 2   Effects of environmental change on cortical EEG and sleep-wake cycle in wild type and HDC knock out mice. The moments of the cage change are indicated by an arrow. See text for details.

Using H1-receptor knock-out (H1R-/-) mice (established from C57BL/6J strain by Dr. T. Watanabe, Kyushu University) and homozigoute H1R+/+ mice as experimental control, we have found that H1R-/- mice share the main characteristics of HDC-/- mice in both sleep-wake and behavioral aspects, i.e. 1) a decrease in W during the periods before and after lights-off. This deficit is, however, smaller in amplitude (per unit time) but longer in the duration (>8h), compared with that seen using HDC-/- mice (~ 4h); and 2) a similar inability to maintain W in response to behavioral challenges such as environmental change (23).

These data suggest that, by a compensatory mechanism which remains to be determined, mice lacking HA synthesis or H1-receptors can reach a daily amount of waking near to the normal level that is indispensable for their survival. However, at moments when a high level of vigilance is required, such as a lights-off period or environmental change, they are unable to maintain awake, a condition necessary for responding to behavioral and cognitive challenges. From these results, we suggest that, in addition to their importance in arousal demonstrated in the cat, HA neurons could also play an important role in maintaining the brain awake in the presence of behavioral challenges and this role is ensured, at least in part, by H1-receptors. The involvement of H2-receptors in this function and behavioral regulation remains to be determined.

6. Ability of histaminergic neurons to induce cortical activation demonstrated in brain transectioned cats

In order to further evaluate the ability of HArgic neurons and their ascending projections to induce cortical activation and W, we have performed rostral mesencephalic transection in the cat (the *cerveau isolé* preparation, in which HArgic cell-bodies and their ascending fibers, situated rostrally to the section, are intact, while their descending axons and ascending projections from the brainstem to the rotral brain are cut), and examined the effects of the H3-receptor antagonist ciproxifan on cortical EEG and expression of the immediate early gene, *c-fos* (6). H3-receptor antagonists currently constitute the only experimental means of selectively stimulating HA neurons (2).

As previously described by in the cat (7), during the first 2-3 days, these transections result in a continuous high voltage and slow activity of the cortical EEG, the β and γ rhythms being weak. Subsequently, the cortical EEG displays alternating highly synchronized and less synchronized or desynchronized activities. Moreover, under the present experimental conditions, most animals exhibit a clear circadian rhythm of cortical slow waves, i.e. a diurnal occurrence of cortical slow activity in abundance ("synchrony period", characterized by successive and long lasting episodes of deep SWS) and a nocturnal appearance in much less amount ("low synchrony period"). During the entire survival period, PS occurs regularly and frequently. PS episodes are accompanied by either cortical synchronization or desynchronization in a completely random fashion. This preparation, as well as the circadian pattern of cortical slow waves have allowed us to observe any desynchronizing effect during the acute phase and chronic "synchrony period" and any synchronizing effect during the chronic "low synchrony period".

During either the acute phase or chronic "synchrony period", intramuscular injection of small doses (0.3-2 mg/kg) of ciproxifan induces cortical desynchronization, the intensity and duration of which being dependent on the dose used and the number of days post-surgery. This desynchronizing effect is seen as early as the first day after brain transection, when spontaneous cortical activation is totally absent. Starting at day 3-4, ciproxifan causes total and long-lasting suppression of cortical slow activity and spindles, accompanied by continuous hippocampal θ waves, suggesting that the induced cortical arousal is similar to that seen in normal cats during periods of vigilance or attention. In addition, PS decreases, but one or two episodes with full desynchronization can appear. These effects of ciproxifan on the cortical and hippocampal EEG are abolished by subsequent injection of small doses of mepyramine, a H1-receptor antagonist, which restored both the cortical and hippocampal EEG to the state prior to ciproxifan injection, suggesting that the ciproxifan-induced arousal results from enhanced HA transmission. In contrast, during the chronic "low synchrony period", intramuscular injection of imetit (0.25-3 mg/kg, a H3-receptor agonist) or mepyramine (0.25-1 mg/kg) elicits a marked and continuous cortical and hippocampal high-voltage and slow activity.

To determine if the EEG arousal induced by ciproxifan is, indeed, due to activation of HA neurons, we used *c-fos* as an experimental marker to examine cellular activation after 1h activation by ciproxifan or after control saline injection. Cats were perfused under deep anesthesia with fixatives and the brains subjected to double-immunohistochemical labeling for *c-fos* and HA. Following ciproxifan injection, the great majority of HArgic TM neurons display dense *c-fos* labeling. In contrast, after saline injection very little *c-fos* labeling is seen in the TM nucleus and adjacent areas and elsewhere in the brain (6).

It should be emphasized that, in the cat, expression of *c-fos* in HArgic neurons has only been seen, up to the present, using ciproxifan and not using other waking substances, such as modafinil, or psychostimulants, like amphetamine and methylphenidate, suggesting that only stimuli specific to the HArgic system can induce *c-fos* expression within its cell bodies. Since in this preparation the descending projections of HA neurons and the ascending projections from the lower brainstem are largely, if not totally, interrupted, these data therefore support the importance of HArgic ascending projections in cortical arousal by demonstrating their ability to ensure cortical activation in the case of a deficit of more caudal brainstem ascending activating systems. In a medical point of view, the clear arousing effect of ciproxifan demonstrated in both acute and chronic phases of transectioned cats also suggests that H3-receptor antagonists might constitute a novel approach for the restoration of cortical activation in comatose or brain-traumatized patients. Finally, the fact that systemic administration of ciproxifan is able to enhance the release and turnover of HArgic neurons and to cause their activation seen in the present study using *c-fos* might constitute an helpful experimental mean for their pharmacological identification when their unitary activity is recorded *in vivo*, method that has been used in our current studies (13).

7. Hypothalamo-preoptic histaminergic projections and their interaction with neurons in the preoptic area

Among the different ascending pathways of HArgic neurons involved in arousal, mention should be made of those projecting to the preoptic/anterior hypothalamus. This region is considered to play an important role in sleep generation, mainly because its lesion, probably by destruction of neurons discharging in high rate during SWS, causes insomnia. The preoptic area is probably the brain structure with the greatest density of HArgic fibers, terminals, and receptors. We have previously shown that the action of HA in this region is to enhance W, probably by H2-receptors, and suggested that HA cells can exert control over the preoptic sleep-generating mechanisms (6). Taking together with the fact that the insomnia induced by preoptic lesion is reversed by inactivation of the ventrolateral posterior hypothalamus (25), these data indicate the importance of an intrahypothalamic interaction in the alternation of the sleep-wake cycle, an idea that is consistent with the long-standing hypothesis of Nauta (26), and suggest that this interaction in the caudo-rostral sense might be, at least in part, HArgic. As regards interaction in the rosto-caudal sense, recent studies have indicated that GABA neurons in the preoptic area send heavy projections to the posterior hypothalamus and TM neurons (e.g. Ref. 27), and functional GABA innervation of HArgic cells has been demonstrated (9). Furthermore, electrical stimulation of the ventrolateral preoptic area, in which neurons exhibit increased discharge during SWS and PS, induces hyperpolarization of TM neurons in brain slices (28). Finally, as indicated in the above section, muscimol microinjection into the posterior hypothalamus containing HA cells, induces hypersomnia. Taking together, all these results tend to suggest that the interactions between HA and GABA neurons might constitute one of the important hypothalamic mechanisms underlying the alternation of sleep and W. Other sources of GABA in the posterior hypothalamus, such as that in the afferents from the mesopontine tegmentum and adjacent regions (29) and that from local interneurons, are also present, but their role in the inactivation of HA cells during sleep and in sleep induction remains to be determined. Furthermore, the determination of the functional significance of the presence of GABA within HA neurons, currently reported only in the rodent (25,30), constitute a challenge for our understanding of HArgic transmission and neuronal functions.

8. Histaminergic ascending and descending projections and their interaction with cholinergic neurons

Among the HArgic ascending pathways, those projecting to the basal forebrain and to the cholinergic neurons present in this region should also be noted. Our double immunohistochemical studies have shown that, in the substantia innominata, a dense network of HArgic fibers and terminal-like structures is found in close proximity to a great number of cholinergic cells, with which they appear to make contact (6). Furthermore, our studies in the guinea-pig, using *in situ* hybridization, together with choline acetyltransferase immunocytochemistry, have demonstrated strong expression of H1-receptor mRNA in a great number of cholinergic neurons in the substantia innominata and adjacent basal forebrain, suggesting HArgic innervation of these neurons (6). With regard to the descending projections of HA neurons, we have found that these neurons also send out substantial inputs to the brainstem. In particular, numerous axons are seen to reach the mesopontine tegmentum, (6), which contains cholinergic neurons playing a key role in tonic cortical activation, by their diencephalic projections (7). In this structure, HArgic axons form dense networks of very fine varicose fibers and terminal-like dots in close proximity to a large number of cholinergic neurons, with which they seem to make contact (6). Moreover, we have found that, in the guinea-pig, almost all mesopontine cholinergic neurons strongly express H1-receptor mRNA (6). All these anatomical data clearly indicate that both basal forebrain and mesopontine cholinergic neurons constitute particularly important targets for the HArgic system, and that the activity of these neurons may be under ascending and descending control by HA neurons. In support of this and from a functional point of view, Katheb et al. have shown in guinea-pig brain slices that HA induces direct depolarization of cholinergic neurons and significantly increases their discharge rate; these effects are observed not only in the mesopontine tegmentum, but also in the basal forebrain, and are mediated by H1-receptors (18).

To explore the functional role on cortical activation of the HArgic descending inputs to the mesopontine tegmentum, we have performed *in situ* pharmacological studies coupled with polygraphic recordings and spectral analysis of the cortical EEG in the cat (6). In the cholinergic mesopontine tegmentum, application of HA by microdialysis or microinjection of a H1-receptor agonist results in disruption of cortical spindles and slow waves and enhances cortical fast rhythms, resulting in a long-lasting quiet waking state. The effects of HA are attenuated by systemic or *in situ* pretreatment with mepyramine, which, when injected alone, produces an increase in SWS. In contrast, microinjection of H2-receptor agonists into the same area has no effect on either the cortical EEG or the waking state. Since, in the mesopontine tegmentum, presumed cholinergic ascending neurons discharge tonically during cortical activation of W (7), and since HA causes excitation of mesopontine cholinergic neurons via H1-receptors (18), we suggest that the HArgic descending afferents in the mesopontine tegmentum could promote cortical activation and W, at least partially via activation of H1-receptors situated on cholinergic neurons (6).

In a reciprocal manner to that for the HArgic inputs, mesopontine cholinergic cells send ascending projections to the TM nucleus and adjacent areas and to the thalamic intralaminar nuclei (7), and micro-administration of carbachol, a cholinergic-receptor agonist, into these two structures suppresses cortical slow activity and increases W. (7 & our unpublished data), suggesting that cholinergic ascending inputs to the posterior hypothalamus and intralaminar nuclei constitute, in turn, important excitatory afferents for the thalamo- and hypothalamo-cortical systems and thus for ascending cortical activation. The anatomical and functional links demonstrated here between HArgic and cholinergic systems have led to our hypothesis (6), according to which HA neurons could activate the cortex, either directly by their widespread cortical projections or indirectly via the thalamocortical system. In addition, they could promote cortical activation via the cholinergic system by dual activation of the corticopetal system, originating from the basal forebrain, and the pontothalamic and ponto-hypothalamic systems, arising from the mesopontine group. The reciprocal and excitatory interactions between HArgic and cholinergic neurons in the mesopontine tegmentum, posterior hypothalamus, and basal forebrain, therefore, constitute a crucial circuit within the whole ascending network responsible for the maintenance of cortical activation and W.

9. Conclusions

Wakefulness is a brain functional state that allows the performance of several "high brain functions", such as diverse behavioral, cognitive, and emotional activities. Present knowledge at the whole animal or cellular level suggests that the maintenance of the cerebral cortex in this highly complex state necessitates the convergent and divergent activity of an ascending network within a large reticular zone, extending from the medulla to the forebrain and involving four major subcortical structures (the thalamus, basal forebrain, posterior hypothalamus, and brainstem monoaminergic nuclei), their integral interconnections, and several neurotransmitters, such as glutamate, acetylcholine, histamine and noradrenaline. Classical and recent experimental data have been provided here supporting the hypothesis that 1) as one of the major excitatory sources for cortical activation during waking, histaminergic neurons play an important role in arousal and in maintaining the brain awake in the presence of behavioral challenges; 2) the mechanisms involved include both their ascending and descending projections and implicate their interactions with other brain activating systems, such as, cholinergic neurons; 3) the close interactions between histaminergic and cholinergic systems and the increase in cortical fast rhythms seen with activating histaminergic system also suggest a cognitive function for histaminergic neurons.

Acknowledgments: The authors wish to thank Profs. M. Jouvet and J.C. Schwartz for constant support and Dr. K. Sakai for advice and the performance of brain transections. We also would like to thank Bioprojet (Paris, France) for kind gift of BP2-94 and ciproxifan. This work was supported by INSERM U52 & U480, Department of Experimental Medicine, Faculty of Medicine, Claude Bernard University, Lyon, France.

References

1. Douglas WW. In: Gilman, Goodman, Rall & Murad (eds), *The Pharmacological Basis of Therapeutics*, New York, Macmillan 1985; 605-638.
2. Schwartz JC, Arrang JM, Garbarg M, Pollard H, Ruat M. *Physiol Rev* 1991; 71: 1-51.
3. Panula P, Yang HYT & Costa E. *Proc. Natl. Acad. Sci. USA.*, 1984, 81: 2572-2576.
4. Steinbusch HWM & Mulder AH. In Björklund, Hökfelt & Kuhar (eds): *Handbook of Chemical Neuroanatomy.* Amsterdam: Elsevier, 1984; 3:126-140.
5. Watanabe T, Taguchi Y, Shiosaka S, Tanaka J, Kubota H, Terao Y, Tohyama M, Wada H. *Brain Res*, 1984; 295: 13-25.
6. Lin JS, Sleep Medicine Reviews, 4(5)(2000)471-503
7. Sakai K, El Mansari M, Lin JS, Zhang JG, Vanni-Mercier G. In: Mancia & Marini (eds), *The Diphencephalon and Sleep,* New York: Raven Press, Ltd. 1990; 171-198.
8. Vizuete ML, Traiffort E, Bouthenet ML, Ruat M, Souil E, Tardivel-Lacombe J, Schwartz JC. *Neurosci.*1997; 80: 321-343.
9. Haas HL Reiner PB, Greene RW. In: Watanabe & Wada (eds), *Histaminergic neurons: morphology and function,* Boca Raton: CRC Press 1991; 195-208.
10. Haas HL. In: Schwartz & Haas (eds), *The histamine receptors*, New York Wiley-Liss 1992, 161-178.
11. Vanni-Mercier G, Sakai K, Salvert D, Jouvet M. *C R Acad Sci* 1984; 298:195-200.
12. Steininger TL, Alam MN, Gong H, Szymusiak R, McGinty D. *Brain Res* 1999; 840: 138-147.
13. Vanni-Mercier G, Gigout S and Lin JS. In preparation
14. Orr E, Quay WB. *Endocrinology* 1975; 96: 941-945.
15. Onoé H, Yamatodani A, Watanabe Y, Mochizuki T, Wada H, Hayashi O. *J Sleep Res* 1992; 1(Suppl. 1): 166.
16. McCormick DA. *Prog Neurobiol* 1992; 39 337-388.
17. Reiner PB, Kamondi A. *Neurosci.*1994; 59: 579-588.
18. Khateb A, Fort P, Pegna A, Jones BE, Mühlethaler M. *Neurosci.*1995; 69: 495-506.
19. Vorobjev VS, Sharonova IN, Walsh IB, Haas HL. 1993; 11: 837-844.
20. Kiyono S, Seo M, Shibagaki M, Watanabe T, Maeyama K, Wada H. *Physiol. Behav.* 1984; 34: 615-617.
21. Monti JM, D'Angeto L, Jantos H, Pazos S. *J Neural Transm* 1988; 72: 141-145.
22. Nicholson AN, Stone BM. *Eur J Clin Pharmacol* 1986; 30: 27-32.
23. Parmentier R, Ohtsu H, Djebbara Z, Valatx JL, Watanabe T, Watanabe T and Lin JS. In preparation.
24. Ericson H, Köhler C, Blomqvist A. *J Comp Neurol* 1991; 305: 1-8.
25. Sallanon M, Denoyer M, Kitahama K, Aubert C, Gay N, Jouvet M. *Neurosci.*1989; 32: 669-683.
26. Nauta WJH. *J Neurophysiol* 1946; 9: 285-316.
27. Sherin JE, Elmquist JK, Torrealba F, Saper CB. *J Neurosci* 1998; 18: 4705-4721.
28. Steininger TL, Stevens DR, Haas HL, McGinty D, Szymusiak R. *Sleep Res* 1997; 26: 45.
29. Ford B, Holmes CJ, Mainville L, Jones BE. *J Comp Neurol* 1995; 363: 177-196.
30. Airaksinen MS, Alanen S, Szabat E, Visser T, Panula P. *J Comp Neurol* 1992; **323**: 103-116.

2001 Elsevier Science B.V.
Histamine Research in the New Millennium
T. Watanabe, H. Timmerman and K. Yanai (Editors)

Brain penetration of ebastine evaluated in human by positron emission tomography (PET)

M. Tagawa[a], K. Yanai[a], M. Kano[a], N. Okamura[b], M. Higuchi[b], M. Matsuda[d], Y. Mizuki[d], R. Iwata[c], H. Arai[b], T. Fujii[d], T. Ido[c], M. Itoh[c], H. Sasaki[b], and T. Watanabe[a]

Departments of [a]Pharmacology and [b]Geriatric Medicine, Tohoku University School of Medicine, Seiryo-cho 2-1, Aoba-ku, Sendai 980-8575, Japan. [c]Cyclotron Radioisotope Center, Tohoku University, Aramaki Aza-aoba, Aoba-ku, Sendai 980-8578, Japan. [d]Developmental Research Laboratories, Dainippon Pharmaceutical Co.,Ltd., Enoki-cho 33-94, Suita 564-0053, Japan

Antihistamines (AHs) have been often applied to peripheral allergic diseases such as urticaria and rhinitis, however, a sedation induced by these agents were well-known to be as a serious adverse effect. We have examined the mechanism of sedation induced by AHs in humans using positron emission tomography (PET) and cognitive tasks. In this report, we showed the non-sedative properties of second-generation AHs using ebastine as compared with *d*-chlorpheniramine (CP), a classical one, which were demonstrated by measuring their brain histamine H_1-receptor (H_1R) occupancies using PET, and the cognitive performance using reaction time tasks. In the PET study with [^{11}C] doxepin (a potent H_1 antagonist), the H_1R occupancies after the ebastine 10mg treatment in the H_1R-rich regions such as cortices, cingulate gyrus, and thalamus were significantly lower than those after the CP 2mg treatment. The values of H_1R occupancies in the cortices were calculated to be about 10% by ebastine and about 50% by oral CP 2mg dosing. In the cognitive study, ebastine 10mg did not affect the cognitive performance (reaction time and accuracy) and the subjective sleepiness. In contrast, CP 2 and 6mg significantly deteriorated the performance and increased the sleepiness. These results demonstrated that ebastine does not induce a sedation because of its low occupancy of brain H_1Rs, which is comparable to those of terfenadine 60mg (*ca.* 12%) and epinastine 20mg (*ca.* 8%) well-known as a non-sedating AH. Moreover, it was revealed that CP induces a sedation at even a low dose of 2mg (OTC medication dose) due to about 50% occupation of brain H_1Rs, and that both sedation and H_1R occupancy increase along with the plasma CP concentration.

Keywords: H_1-receptor occupancy, cognition, ebastine, *d*-chlorpheniramine, PET (positron emission tomography)

Abbreviations: AH (antihistamine), H_1R (histamine H_1-receptor), PET (positron emission tomography), BP (binding potential), CP (*d*-chlorpheniramine), RT (reaction time), AC (accuracy)

138

1. *Introduction*

Antihistamines (AHs) are widely used for treatments of peripheral allergic diseases. The sedative issues of AHs are well-known to be of central importance, because of their wide-spread uses in current clinical medications including the OTC medications. Practically, sedative properties of classical antihistamines were reported to cause accidents while driving and working and to contribute to a decline in productivity and learning efficiency [1,2,3,4]

We have visualized the brain distribution of histamine H_1-receptors (H_1Rs) and have quantified the available brain H_1Rs using human by the development of a positron emission tomography (PET) technique, which is an non-invasive and non-surgical method, with [^{11}C]doxepin and [^{11}C]pyrilamine (potent H_1 antagonists) [5,6,7]. The PET technologies have contributed to our investigation of the mechanism of AH-induced sedation. We previously reported that the impaired cognitive functions induced by intravenously injection of *d*-chlorpheniramine (CP) were caused by the occupation of brain H_1Rs [8]. In this report, we used ebastine, one of second-generation AHs, and CP, one of classical ones, and compared the influences of these drugs on cognitive performance and brain H_1R bindings using cognitive tasks and PET, in order to better understand the sedative or non-sedative effects of AHs. Furthermore, we compared the H_1R occupancies of a variety of AHs including sedating- and non-sedating agents, and examined the receptor occupancies in relation to plasma concentrations of AHs.

2. *Methods*

2.1. *Cognitive tasks*

Visual discrimination tasks adopted as an attention-demanding cognitive task were used in order to objectively evaluate cognitive functions [8]. In brief, due to keeping a highly attention-demanding condition, the visual stimuli used in these tasks were presented with near-visual threshold presentation time of 3, 5, 7 or 20 msec. Subjects viewed single visual stimulus displayed on an AV tachistoscope, subtending 2°×2° of visual angle. The task was to distinguish target stimuli (10 kinds of digits) from non-target stimuli (46 kinds of Japanese phonogram called "hiragana") and to push a reaction button promptly with the right index finger when the target stimulus was presented. Target stimuli were presented with a probability of 20% of total stimuli. In total, one-hundred and twenty single digits or letters were serially presented during each 3 min-session. Task performance was evaluated by measuring 2 kinds of parameters, the reaction time (RT) and the accuracy (AC), and then the ratios (after/before drug administration) of them were used for the data evaluations.

2.2. *PET studies*

(*E*)-Doxepin labeled with carbon-11 was prepared by N-alkylation of the desmethylated (*E*)-doxepin with [^{11}C]iodomethane as described previously [9]. Young male volunteers between 20 and 27 years of age received a variety of AHs and thereafter dynamic PET scans were conducted for 90 min after an injection of [^{11}C]doxepin with a SET2400W and a ECAT PT931 scanners. Binding potential (BP) of doxepin (Bmax/Kd), which was used for the parameter of density and affinity of an available receptor population, was determined by a graphical analysis [10]. Parametric neuroimages of BPs were statistically analyzed on a voxel-by-voxel bases by the statistical parametric mapping (SPM96) software [11,12], in order to compare the H_1R bindings by ebastine 10mg and CP 2mg treatments. Moreover, the H_1R occupancies in the interested regions such as cortices, cingulate gyrus and thalamus were calculated by the following equation: 100 - (BP in each treated subject) / (mean value of BPs in non-drug- or placebo-treated subjects) × 100 (%).

3. *Results*

3.1. *Cognitive effects of antihistamines; a comparative study of ebastine and d-chlorpheniramine*

Drugs used in this crossover study were ebastine 10mg, CP 2 and 6mg, and placebo. The tasks were given healthy male volunteers twice, first before drug administrations and secondly near respective T_{max} of drugs (ebastine: *ca.* 5hrs, and CP: *ca.* 2hrs) [13,14]. The changes of the task performance (RT and AC) by ebastine were almost the same level as those by placebo. On the other hand, the performance were significantly deteriorated after oral treatments of two CP doses. The RTs were prolonged and the AC were decreased as compared with the placebo treatment. (only the 5 and 7 msec-task data shown in Fig. 1a, b)

The relationships between the task performance and plasma drug concentration were examined. The ratios of the RT and AC were not depended on the plasma concentration of carebastine, an active metabolite of ebastine (Fig. 2a), however, those were significantly correlated with the plasma CP concentration (Fig. 2b).

In addition, during the task performance study, the subjective sleepiness was also monitored. The subjective sleepiness was estimated with Stanford Sleepiness Scale composing a 7-level self-report measure for assessment [15]. It was revealed that the results for the sleepiness were comparable to the task performance study. The sleepiness was not changed by ebastine as well as by placebo, but those by both CP doses were significantly increased against that by placebo (Fig. 1c).

These results obviously suggested that ebastine, a second-generation AH, did not affected to cognitive functions, differently from CP, a classical one.

3.2. *Brain H_1-receptor bindings of antihistamines; a comparative study of ebastine and d-chlorpheniramine*

PET scans were started at around respective T_{max} after oral ebastine 10mg and CP 2mg treatments in the crossover study. The distribution patterns of [^{11}C]doxepin after ebastine treatment were similar to those of the non-drug treated group (Fig. 3a, b). In both groups, high radioactivity was detected in the frontal, temporal and occipital cortices, cingulate gyrus, striatum and thalamus, where the density of H_1R was high. On the other hand, in the above areas, the radioactivity was observed to be relatively low after the CP treatment (Fig. 3c). Comparing the parametric neuroimages of BPs between the ebastine and CP treatments, the BPs in the above areas after the ebastine treatment were significantly higher than those after the CP treatment (Fig. 4a), but, in contrast, it was not detected any areas where the BPs after the CP treatment were significantly higher than those after the ebastine treatment (Fig. 4b). It was suggested that the H_1R occupancy of CP was higher than that of ebastine in these areas. Furthermore, focusing on the cortices, cingulate gyrus and thalamus, the H_1R occupancies were calculated, when the occupancies in the non-drug treated group were regarded as 0%.

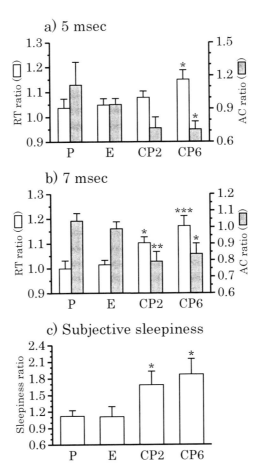

Figure 1 Effects of four drugs, placebo (P), ebastine (E) and *d*-chlorpheniramine 2mg (CP2) and 6mg (CP6) on the reaction time (RT), accuracy (AC) of the visual discrimination task with 5 msec- (a) and 7 msec- (b) presentation time and the subjective sleepiness (c). Data are represented as mean ± se of 12 subjects. Y-axes show ratios of RT, AC or sleepiness of post-dose to those of pre-dose. : * $p<0.05$, ** $p<0.01$ and *** $p<0.001$ vs. placebo, statistically analyzed by Dunnett's multiple comparison test.

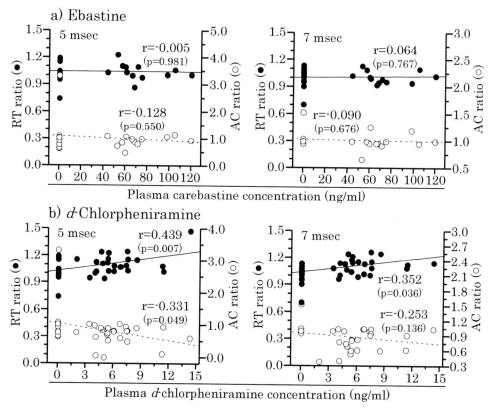

Figure 2 Relationships between plasma drug concentrations and ratios of RT and AC of the visual discrimination task with 5 and 7 msec-presentation time after the a) ebastine and b) d-chlorpheniramine treatments. The X-axis for ebastine shows carebastine concentration. A slope of a regression line was statistically analyzed by Pearson's correlation.

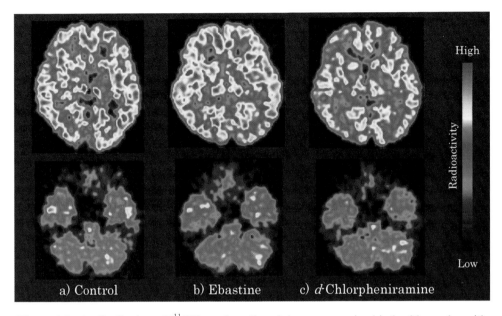

a) Control   b) Ebastine   c) *d*-Chlorpheniramine

Figure 3 Brain distribution of [^{11}C]doxepin radioactivity was examined in healthy males with or without the oral treatments of antihistamines, a) non-drug treatment, b) ebastine 10mg, and c) *d*-chlorpheniramine 2mg. The representatives of PET images are shown at the striatal and cerebellar levels.

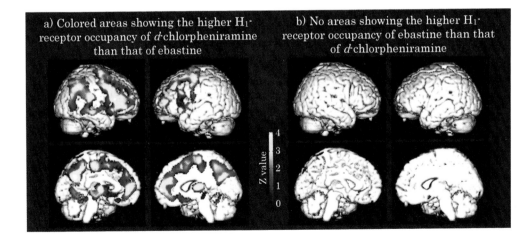

a) Colored areas showing the higher H$_1$-receptor occupancy of *d*-chlorpheniramine than that of ebastine

b) No areas showing the higher H$_1$-receptor occupancy of ebastine than that of *d*-chlorpheniramine

Figure 4 Comparison of the binding potentials of doxepin after the oral treatments of ebastine 10mg and *d*-chlorpheniramine 2mg. The colored areas show that the binding potentials after the a) ebastine or b) *d*-chlorpheniramine treatment was statistically higher than those after the a) *d*-chlorpheniramine or b) ebastine treatment ($p < 0.05$, uncorrected).

The respective occupancies were about 9.9%, 3.2% and 14.4% in the ebastine 10mg treatment, and were about 50.3%, 49.2% and 49.7% in the CP 2mg treatment, showing that the H_1R occupancy of CP 2mg was significantly higher than that of ebastine (Table).

3.3. Brain H_1-receptor occupancy of a variety of antihistamines

Figure 5 shows the H_1R occupancies of a variety of AHs including sedating- and non-sedating-drugs. PET scans were also conducted using healthy male volunteers. The drugs which were high potent of sedation occupied a large amount of H_1Rs, showing about 85% (CP 5mg IV), 75% (ketotifen 1mg), 60% (CP 2mg IV) and 50% (oxatomide 30mg and CP 2mg PO) occupation.

Table. H_1-receptor occupancies in cortex, anterior cingulate cortex and thalamus by antihistamines

Brain region	Ebastine (10mg)	d-Chlorpheniramine (2mg)
	(%)	
Cortex	9.9 ± 3.3	50.3 ± 5.0*
Anterior cingulate cortex	3.2 ± 7.9	49.2 ± 6.4*
Thalamus	14.4 ± 5.3	49.7 ± 6.3*

Values are mean ± se of 6 subjects. *p<0.005: Statistically analyzed by Wilcoxon-test (Ebastine vs. d-Chlorpheniramine).

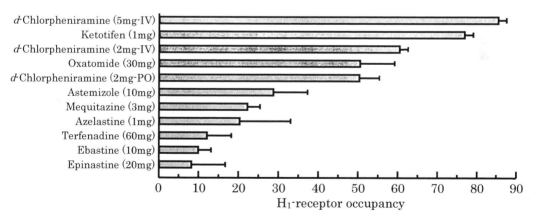

Figure 5 Brain H_1-receptor occupancies of a variety of antihistamines in healthy male subjects. These values are obtained from the regions of front-temporal cortices. Data are represented as mean ± se.

In contrast, the non-sedating drugs, generally called second-generation agents, occupied a small amount of the H₁Rs in the range from about 10 to 30% occupation. Especially, the occupancies of epinastine, ebastine and terfenadine, which have been recognized as non-sedating agents in clinical practices, were very low with the values of about 8, 10 and 12%, respectively.

3.4. Brain H₁-receptor occupancies in relation to plasma drug concentrations

During the PET scans of the CP-, ebastine- and epinastine-treated subjects, the respective drugs in plasma were analyzed for a correlation to the receptor occupancy. In the CP treatment, BP was relatively low in low plasma concentration range against other two drugs. Then, as the plasma concentration of CP increased, the BP was significantly decreased, suggesting that the H₁R occupancy of CP was increased (Fig. 6a). In contrast, the BPs after ebastine and epinastine treatments were relatively high in the respective low plasma concentration ranges, and the BP was not depended on the plasma concentration of carebastine, an active metabolite of ebastine, practically (Fig. 6b). However, as for epinastine, the BP were tended to decrease along with the increase of plasma concentration (Fig. 6c). This fact obtained from the epinastine study suggested that a kind of non-sedating AHs could occupy the serious amount of brain H₁Rs along with plasma concentration.

4. Discussion

We investigated the sedation induced by AHs using cognitive tasks as an objective method, and the H₁R bindings of AHs using PET with [¹¹C]doxepin, and then clearly demonstrated that the differential sedative properties of sedating- and non-sedating AHs were caused by the difference of brain H₁R occupancies of the agents, namely, the differences of brain penetration through blood-brain-barrier (BBB). Practically, ebastine with about 10% occupation of brain H₁Rs hardly induced a sedation, in contrast, CP with about 50% occupation of the receptors at even a low dose of 2mg, significantly induced a sedation.

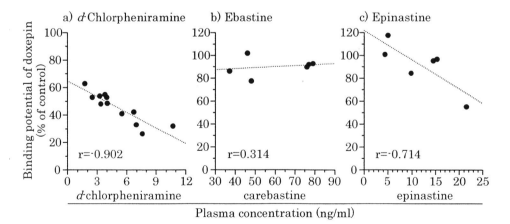

Figure 6 Relationships between plasma drug concentrations and the binding potentials of doxepin after the a) *d*-chlorpheniramine, b) ebastine and c) epinastine treatments. The X-axis of the ebastine is plasma concentration of carebastine, and the Y-axes show the binding potential of doxepin as a percentage of the mean control values. Relationship between the occupancy and the plasma concentration was analyzed by Spearman's rank test.

The differences of the penetration into brain between these-agents were thought to be caused by the differences of the physical, chemical and biological properties such as the lipophilicity, the ionization and the binding affinity to serum proteins [16]. Moreover, there is recently thought to be a possible factor that a few AHs are the substrates of the active transport protein expressed on the plasma membranes in BBB such as P-glycoprotein and organic anion transport proteins (OATP), and these facts were known in some reports that carebastine and fexofenadine, which are respective carboxylic metabolites of ebastine and terfenadine, would be possible substrates of these transport proteins [17,18,19]. It is suggested that the brain penetration of these agents are more difficult than other non-sedating AHs.

Contrarily considering the brain penetrations, non-sedating agents could seriously penetrate into brain under some conditions such as over-dosing, co-existence of inhibitors for the transporters mentioned above or the drug-metabolizing enzymes, and then could induce sedation. We do emphasize, however, that possibilities of sedation induced by non-sedating AHs differ in degree, but are generally low.

References

1) Cimbura G, Lucas DM, Bennett RC, Warren RA, Simpson HM. Incidence and toxicological aspects of drugs detected in 484 fatally injured drivers and pedestrians in Ontario. *J Forensic Sci* 1982; 27: 855-867
2) Fireman P. Treatment of allergic rhinitis: effect on occupation productivity and work force costs. *Allergy Asthma Proc* 1997; 18: 63-67
3) Gilmore TM, Alexander BH, Mueller BA, Rivara FP. Occupational injuries and medication use. *Am J Ind Med* 1996; 30: 234-239
4) Vuurman EF, van Veggel LLM, Uiterwijk MM, Leutner D, O'Hanlon JF. Seasonal allergic rhinitis and antihistamine effects on children's learning. *Ann Allergy* 1993; 71: 121-126
5) Yanai K, Watanabe T, Hatazawa J, *et al.* Visualization of histamine H_1 receptors in dog brain by positron emission tomography. *Neurosci Lett* 1990; 118: 41-44
6) Villemagne VL, Dannals RF, Sanchez-Roa PM, *et al.* Imaging histamine H_1 receptors in the living human brain with carbon-11-pyrilamine. *J Nucl Med* 1991; 32: 308-311
7) Yanai K, Watanabe T, Yokoyama H, *et al.* Histamine H_1 receptors in human brain visualized in vivo by [^{11}C]doxepin and positron emission tomography. *Neurosci Lett* 1992; 137: 145-148
8) Okamura N, Yanai K, Higuchi M, *et al.* Functional neuroimaging of cognition impaired by a classical antihistamine, *d*-chlorpheniramine. *Br J Pharmacol* 2000; 129: 115-123.
9) Yanai K, Watanabe T, Yokoyama H, *et al.* Histamine H_1 receptors in human brain visualized *in vivo* by [^{11}C]doxepin and positron emission tomography. *Neurosci Lett* 1992; 137: 145-148

10) Logan J, Fowler JS, Volkow ND, *et al.* Graphical analysis of reversible radioligand binding form time-activity measurements applied to [N-^{11}C-methyl]-(-)-cocaine PET studies in human subjects. *J Cereb Blood Flow Metab* 1990; 10: 740-747.

11) Friston KJ, Holmes AP, Worsley KJ, *et al.* Statistical parametric maps in functional imaging: A general linear approach. *Human Brain Mapping* 1995; 2: 189-210

12) Higuchi M, Yanai K, Okamura N, *et al.* Histamine H$_1$ receptors in patients with Alzheimer's disease assessed by positron emission tomography (PET). *Neuroscience* 2000; 99: 721-729

13) Yamaguchi T, Hashizume T, Matsuda M, *et al.* Pharmacokinetics of the H$_1$-receptor antagonist ebastine and its active metabolite carebastine in healthy subjects. *Arzneimittelforschung Drug Res* 1994; 44: 59-64

14) Peets EA, Jackson M, Symchowicz S. Metabolism of chlorpheniramine maleate in man. *J Pharmacol Exp Ther* 1972; 180: 464-474

15) Hoddes E, Zarcone V, Smythe H, Phillips R, Dement WC. Quantification of sleepiness: a new approach. *Psychophysiology* 1973; 10: 431-436

16) Timmerman H.: Why are non-sedating anti-histamines non-sedating? *Clin Exp Allergy* 1999; 29 (Suppl 3): 13-18

17) Tamai I. *et al.*: Blood-brain barrier transport of H$_1$-antagonist ebastine and its metabolite carebastine. *J Drug Target* (accepted)

18) Hait WN. *et al.*: Terfenadine (Seldane): a new drug for restoring sensitivity to multidrug resistant cancer cells. *Biochem Pharmacol* 1993; 45: 401-406.

19) Cvetkovic M. *et al.*: OATP and P-glycoprotein transporters mediate the cellular uptake and excretion of fexofenadine. *Drug Metab Dispos* 1999; 27: 866-871.

Single transduction

© 2001 Elsevier Science B.V. All rights reserved.
Histamine Research in the New Millennium
T. Watanabe, H. Timmerman and K. Yanai (Editors)

Pathways of histamine H_1 receptor-induced Ca^{2+} entry in human astrocytoma cells

M.M.-P. Wong and J.M. Young

Department of Pharmacology, University of Cambridge, Tennis Court Road, Cambridge CB2 1QJ, U.K.

Abstract. Histamine causes an inhibition of forskolin and isoprenaline-stimulated cyclic AMP accumulation in U373 MG cells which is dependent on Ca^{2+} entry. The differential effect of a low concentration of La^{3+} in preventing the inhibitory actions of histamine and thapsigargin provides evidence that at least two, and possible three, Ca^{2+} entry pathways are involved.

1. HISTAMINE H_1 RECEPTOR-MEDIATED RESPONSES IN ASTROCYTES

The functional role of histamine H_1 receptors in the CNS is not well understood, but they may well have an important role in astrocytes, particularly the type-2 astrocytes identified in primary cultures. These cells express H_1 receptors and are involved in the propagation of inflammatory-like responses in the CNS. H_1 receptors on type-2 astrocytes have been characterised in terms of coupling to phospholipase C (PLC) and the mobilisation of intracellular Ca^{2+} (Kondou *et al.*, 1991; Peakman & Hill, 1995). However, much less is known about the pathways by which histamine induces influx of extracellular Ca^{2+}. The work of Schwartz and his collaborators demonstrated that histamine-induced glycogenolysis in slices of mouse cerebral cortex, mediated exclusively by H_1 receptors and almost certainly an astrocyte response, was dependent on extracellular Ca^{2+} (Quach *et al.*, 1980). A similar Ca^{2+}-dependence was observed for the H_1-receptor component of glycogenolysis in primary cultures of rat astrocytes (Arbonés *et al.*, 1990) and in the human UC11 MG astrocytoma cell line (Medrano *et al.*, 1992). However none of these studies yielded information on the nature of the pathways of Ca^{2+} entry involved. There is evidence for a close association between Ca^{2+} entry sites in the plasma membrane and the effectors that they modulate, as is the case for the Ca^{2+}-sensitive isozymes of adenylyl cyclase, which are selectively regulated by Ca^{2+} entry through the so-called capacitative pathway linked to the refilling of 1,4,5-IP_3-sensitive intracellular stores (Cooper *et al.*, 1995). This means that changes in bulk intracellular Ca^{2+} ($[Ca^{2+}]_i$) in the cell may not reflect the extent of changes immediately below the plasma membrane in the vicinity of the Ca^{2+}-sensitive effector. Indeed if the assembly also includes Ca^{2+} extrusion sites, then changes in bulk cytoplasmic Ca^{2+} might be very small. We therefore set out to investigate routes of histamine-induced Ca^{2+} entry by monitoring the effect on a Ca^{2+}-sensitive effector. We have used human astrocytoma cells as a model system, particularly the U373 MG cell line, which has been widely used for studies on astrocyte activation by pro-inflammatory cytokines (see e.g. Lieb *et al.*, 1996). We have previously investigated the Ca^{2+}-dependence of histamine-induced PLC activation in these cells, but although inositol phosphate formation does show some dependence on extracellular Ca^{2+} in the millimolar concentration range (Arias-Montaño et al., 1994), the effect was too small for a detailed study of the pathways involved. We therefore looked for other Ca^{2+}-dependent responses to histamine to use as a reporter system.

2. GLYCOGENOLYSIS IN UC11 MG AND U373 MG CELLS

Human UC11 MG and human U373 MG astrocytoma cells share a number of characteristics, including histamine H_1 receptor-mediated stimulation of PLC (Johnson & Johnson, 1992; Arias-Montaño et al., 1994) and Ca^{2+} mobilisation (Lucherini & Gruenstein, 1992; Young et al., 1998a). Histamine-induced glycogenolysis has been described in UC11 MG cells and this therefore appeared to be a promising starting point. Both UC11 MG and U373 MG cells incorporated [^{3}H]-glucose into glycogen (as confirmed by the action of the enzyme amyloglucosidase) with a similar time-course and in UC11 MG cells histamine caused a statistically significant decrease in the level of [^{3}H]-glycogen (20 ± 2% decrease, n=8), which was prevented in the presence of the H_1-antagonist mepyramine (2 μM), but not by the H_2-antagonist tiotidine (10 μM), as reported by Medrano et al. (1992). However, in U373 MG cells 100 μM histamine had no consistent or statistically significant effect on the level of [^{3}H]-glycogen, mean 103 ± 6% of control (n=3).

Thapsigargin (5 μM), which activates Ca^{2+} entry through store-refilling-activated channels (capacitative Ca^{2+} entry), secondary to inhibition of Ca^{2+} uptake into intracellular stores and the emptying of the store by Ca^{2+} leakage, stimulated glycogenolysis in UC11 MG cells (15 ± 2% decrease, n=5) to an extent that did not differ significantly to that induced by 100 μM histamine measured concurrently. This indicates that Ca^{2+} entry through capacitative Ca^{2+} entry channels alone is sufficient to cause the same degree of activation of glycogenolysis as that produced by histamine. However, the rather small (and often erratic) response discouraged us from undertaking a more detailed investigation to establish whether this is the only pathway of Ca^{2+} entry operated by histamine. The failure to detect any histamine-induced glycogenolysis in U373 MG cells underlines the problems in attempting to relate responses in different astrocytoma cell lines and their limitations as model systems.

3. Ca^{2+}-DEPENDENT INHIBITION OF CYCLIC AMP ACCUMULATION

We have previously reported that in U373 MG cells histamine alone has no effect on the level of cyclic AMP (Young et al., 1998a). However, in the presence of a stimulator of adenylyl cyclase cyclic AMP accumulation was strongly inhibited. The action of histamine was completely dependent on the presence of extracellular Ca^{2+}, but was independent of whether isoprenaline or forskolin was used to stimulate cyclic AMP accumulation (Wong et al., 2000). The effect of histamine was duplicated by the NK-1 selective agonist [Sar^9,Met(O$_2$)^{11}]-substance P (Fig. 1) (IC$_{50}$ 0.84 ± 0.07 nM), although in UC11 MG cells substance P has been reported to produce a small stimulation of agonist-induced cyclic AMP accumulation (Fowler & Brännström, 1994), illustrating again that no assumptions can be made that the same effectors are expressed in different astrocytoma cell lines.

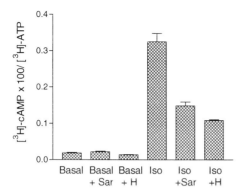

Figure 1. Inhibition of isoprenaline-stimulated cyclic AMP accumulation by histamine and [Sar^9,Met(O$_2$)^{11}]-substance P. [^{3}H]-Cyclic AMP accumulation in the presence of 0.5 mM 3-isobutyl-1-methylxanthine (IBMX), after labelling cells with [^{3}H]-adenine, was measured by the two column method of Salomon *et al.* as described in detail elsewhere (Wong *et al.*, 2000). [^{3}H]-Cyclic AMP was expressed as a percentage of the [^{3}H]-ATP formed. Incubations with 1 μM isoprenaline (Iso), with or without 10 μM histamine (H) or 1 μM [Sar^9,Met(O$_2$)^{11}]-substance P (Sar) were for 1 min.

Ca^{2+} influx induced by thapsigargin in U373 MG cells is very sensitive to inhibition by low concentrations of La^{3+} (Wong *et al.*, 2000). Similarly the inhibition of cyclic AMP accumulation by 5 μM thapsigargin measured over a 4 min incubation period was blocked in the presence of 1 μM La^{3+}. However, when the time of incubation with the cyclase stimulant was reduced to 1 min the extent of the inhibition was significantly reduced (Table 1).

The differential effect of 1 μM La^{3+} is unlikely to be a consequence of incomplete equilibration, since (a) La^{3+} was added 10 min before the isoprenaline or forskolin and (b) it acts rapidly to inhibit thapsigargin-induced Ca^{2+} entry through capacitative channels in U373 MG cells (Wong *et al.*, 2000). Further, the accumulation of stimulated cyclic AMP is approximately linear up to 4 min. One explanation is that two capacitative entry pathway are

Table 1 Time-dependence of the reversal by La^{3+} of the inhibition of drug-induced cyclic AMP accumulation

	% Reversal of the inhibition of the response to	
Incubation time	10 μM Forskolin	1 μM Isoprenaline
1 min	31 ± 11 (3)	55 ± 6 (4)
4 min	112 ± 2 (5)	108 ± 2 (4)

La^{3+} (1 μM) was added 10 min before the addition of agonist and further incubated for the time indicated. The values are means ± approximate s.e. mean, with the number of determinations in parentheses.

activated: one is relatively insensitive to block by 1 μM La^{3+}, but inactivates within 1 min, whereas the other is sensitive to low concentrations of La^{3+} and does not inactivate over the period of the experiment. What makes this explanation attractive is that there is an obvious analogy with the *trp* and *trpl* channels involved in phototransduction in *Drosophila* (Hardie & Minke, 1993; Niemeyer *et al.*, 1996), which show the same differential sensitivity to La^{3+} and which may be closely linked in the plasma membrane (Fanning & Anderson, 1999).

A notable feature of the Ca^{2+}-dependent inhibition of types V and VI adenylyl cyclase is that inhibition is mediated specifically by Ca^{2+} entry via the capacitative pathway (Cooper *et al.* 1995; Shuttleworth & Thompson, 1999). This same selectivity for the route of Ca^{2+} entry is not observed with glycogenolysis in UC11 MG cells, since ionomycin also causes a decrease in glycogen levels (Medrano *et al.*, 1992). All measurements of cyclic AMP accumulation in U373 MG cells were made in the presence of a non-selective inhibitor of phosphodiesterase, 0.5 mM IBMX, and a higher concentration, 1 mM, had no greater effect and it would thus seem likely that it is a cyclase which is the target for the Ca^{2+}-dependent inhibition. However, at present we have no direct evidence for this and it is notable that in the 1321N1 astrocytoma cell line histamine inhibition of cyclic AMP accumulation is via stimulation of a Ca^{2+}-dependent phosphodiesterase, although the inhibition in 1321N1 cells was prevented by 0.1 mM IBMX (Nakahata *et al.*, 1986). We have looked for evidence of any selectivity for capacitative Ca^{2+} entry in inhibition of cyclic AMP accumulation in U373 MG cells by examining the effect of ionomycin.

Ionomycin produced a concentration-dependent inhibition of cyclic AMP accumulation (IC$_{50}$ 0.12 ± 0.01 μM) (Fig. 2). There are reports that at concentrations of 1 μM and below ionomycin acts selectively to release Ca^{2+} from intracellular stores (Morgan & Jacob, 1994), but this appears not to be true in U373 MG cells, since 1 μM La^{3+} had only a small effect in inhibiting Ca^{2+} influx following 1 μM ionomycin, whereas 1 μM La^{3+} reduced the

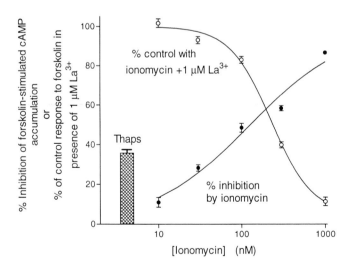

Figure 2.   Inhibition of forskolin-stimulated cyclic AMP accumulation by ionomycin and its reversal by La^{3+}. Each point is the weighted mean ± s.e. mean from 3 independent experiments. The bar shows the extent of the inhibition by 5 μM thapsigargin (Thaps) measured in the same experiments. Incubations with 10 μM forskolin were for 4 min.

thapsigargin-stimulated increase in $[Ca^{2+}]_i$ to basal levels. Consistent with 1 μM ionomycin causing a generalised influx of Ca^{2+} across the plasma membrane, the inhibition of cyclic AMP accumulation by 1 μM ionomycin was practically unaffected by 1 μM La^{3+} (Fig. 2), whereas at concentrations of ionomycin up to approximately 100 nM, which produced the same level of inhibition as 5 μM thapsigargin in these experiments, 1 μM La^{3+} prevented the inhibitory action (Fig. 2).

Caution must be exercised in interpreting experiments with ionomycin, since it could produce a very high concentration of Ca^{2+} in the vicinity of the plasma membrane not evident in measurements of bulk cytoplasmic Ca^{2+}. However, the evidence that Ca^{2+} entry pathways other than those coupled to store-refilling can lead to inhibition of cyclic AMP accumulation was strengthened by the weak effect of 1 μM La^{3+} on the inhibition produced by histamine. Whereas the action of thapsigargin on isoprenaline-stimulated cyclic AMP accumulation over a 4 min incubation is completely reversed by 1 μM La^{3+}, the inhibition produced by histamine, measured concurrently, was only reversed to a modest extent (Fig. 3A), mean reversal 29 ± 3% (n=7). Similar observations were made with forskolin as the cyclase stimulant, 35 ± 3% reversal (n=4). There was no indication that histamine and thapsigargin are acting at different sites to inhibit cyclic AMP accumulation, since the effect of the two inhibitors acting together was not significantly different from that of either acting alone (Fig. 3B). The apparent implication is that histamine activates a pathway of Ca^{2+} entry that is separate from the store refilling pathway(s) activated by thapsigargin.

Histamine will presumably also activate the store-refilling channels in U373 MG cells, since there is evidence that the increase in intracellular Ca^{2+} induced by histamine is via 1,4,5-IP₃-sensitive Ca^{2+} stores (Young et al., 1998b). This would imply that histamine can open at least two, possibly three, separate Ca^{2+} entry pathways in U373 MG cells. A number of human TRP channels have now been characterised (Harteneck et al., 2000), certain of which are non-selective cation channels with a relatively low sensitivity to La^{3+}, and there is evidence from transfected CHO-K1 cells that H_1 receptors can mediate opening of both store-refilling and non-store-refilling-activated TRP channels (Hofmann et al., 1999). The

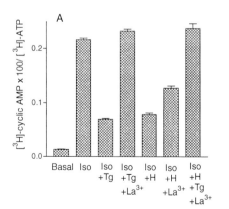
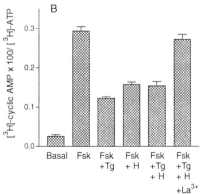

Figure 3.   A. Effect of 1 μM La^{3+} of the inhibition of isoprenaline-induced cyclic AMP accumulation by 10 μM histamine (H) and 5 μM thapsigargin (Tg). (Reproduced with permission from Wong et al., 2000). B. Lack of additivity between 10 μM histamine (H) and 5 μM thapsigargin (Tg). In A & B incubation with 1 μM isoprenaline was for 4 min.

detailed mechanisms by which TRP channels are activated, in particular the role of IP_3 receptors and lipid mediators, remain unclear (Harteneck *et al.*, 2000). There is evidence in DDT_1 MF-2 cells that histamine can stimulate Ca^{2+} entry via the formation of arachidonic acid (van der Zee *et al.*, 1995), but how that might relate to TRP channel activation is unknown.

There is one surprising observation that might ultimately help shed some light on the mechanism by which histamine stimulates Ca^{2+} entry, namely that in the presence of histamine *and* thapsigargin the inhibition can be reversed by 1 μM La^{3+} (Figs 3A & B). The explanation of this effect is at present not clear. There is no evidence of any marked direct inhibition by thapsigargin at the level of H_1 receptor activation of PLC (Wong *et al.*, 2000), but it is known to have inhibitory actions on channels (Treiman *et al.*, 1998). It is possible that thapsigargin might inhibit a histamine-operated TRP channel. The elucidation of exactly how many Ca^{2+} entry pathways are stimulated by histamine in U373 MG cells may well have to await the availability of inhibitors that are more channel-selective than La^{3+}.

REFERENCES

Arbonés L., Picatoste F. and Garcia A. (1990) Mol. Pharmacol., 37, 921-927.
Arias-Montaño J.-A., Berger V. and Young J.M. (1994) *Br. J. Pharmacol.*, 111, 598-608.
Cooper D.M.F., Mons N. and Karpen J.W. (1995) *Nature*, 374, 421-424.
Fanning A.S and Anderson J.M. (1999) *Current Opinion Cell Biol.*, 11, 432-439.
Fowler C.J. and Brännström G. (1994) *Meth. Find. Exp. Clin. Pharmacol.*, 16, 21-28.
Hardie R.C. and Minke B. (1993) *Trends Neurosci.*, 16, 371-376.
Harteneck C., Plant T.D. and Schultz G. (2000) *Trend Neurosci.*, 23, 159-166.
Hofmann T., Obukhov A.G., Schaefer M., Harteneck C., Gudermann T. and Schultz G. (1999) *Nature*, 397, 259-263.
Johnson C.L. and Johnson C.G. (1992) *J. Neurochem.*, 58, 471-477.
Kondou H., Inagaki N., Fukui H., Koyama Y., Kanamura A. and Wada H. (1991) *Biochem. Biophys. Res. Commun.*, 177, 734-738.
Lieb K., Kaltschmidt C., Kaltschmidt B., Baeuerle P.A, Berger M., Bauer J. and Fiebich B.L. (1996) *J. Neurochem.*, 66, 1496-1503.
Lucherini M.J. and Gruenstein E. (1992) *Brain Res.*, 592, 193-201.
Medrano S., Gruenstein E. and Dimlich R.V.W. (1992) *Brain Res.*, 592, 202-207.
Morgan A.J. and Jacob R. (1994) *Biochem. J.*, 300, 665-672.
Nakahata N., Martin M.W., Hughes A.R., Hepler J.R. and Harden T.K. (1986) *Mol. Pharmacol.*, 29, 188-195.
Niemeyer B.A., Suzuli E., Scott K., Jalink K. and Zuker S. (1996) *Cell*, 85, 651-659.
Peakman M.-C. and Hill S.J. (1995) *Br. J. Pharmacol.*, 115, 801-810.
Quach T.T., Duchemin A.-M., Rose C. and Schwartz J.-C. (1980) *Mol. Pharmacol.*, 17, 301-308.
Shuttleworth T.J. and Thompson J.L. (1999) *J. Biol. Chem.*, 274, 31174-31178.
Treiman M., Caspersen C. and Christensen S.C. (1998) *Trends Pharmacol. Sci.*, 19, 131-135.
Van der Zee L., Nelemans A. and Den Hertog A. (1995) *Biochem. J.*, 305, 859-864.
Wong M.-P.M., Cooper D.M.F., Young K.W. and Young J.M. (2000) *Br. J. Pharmacol.*, 130, 1021-1030.
Young K.W., Pinnock R.D., Gibson W.J. and Young J.M. (1998a) *Br. J. Pharmacol.*, 123, 545-557.
Young K.W., Pinnock R.D. and Nahorski S.R. (1998b) *Cell Calcium*, 24, 59-70.

Histamine Research in the New Millennium
T. Watanabe, H. Timmerman and K. Yanai (Editors)

Qualitative Structure Activity Relationships for inverse agonism at the histamine H_2 receptor

A.E. Alewijnse, A. Jongejan, D. Dijkstra, W.M.P.B. Menge, T. Ter Laak, H. Timmerman and R. Leurs

Leiden/Amsterdam Center for Drug Research, Division of Medicinal Chemistry, Faculty of Sciences, Vrije Universiteit, De Boelelaan 1083, 1081 HV Amsterdam, The Netherlands

Previous studies by our group (1) showed that some H_2 antagonists behave as inverse agonists at the constitutively active H_2 receptor whereas e.g. burimamide is devoid of negative intrinsic activity. In the present study some structural elements important for the negative intrinsic activity of H_2 ligands are determined.

1. INTRODUCTION

Previous studies showed that the wild-type histamine H_2 receptor, expressed in various cell lines, is constitutively active (1, 2, 3). Most classical H_2 antagonists act as inverse agonists at the constitutively active H_2 receptor (1, 3). However, the first developed H_2 antagonist, burimamide (4) does not inhibit the constitutive H_2 receptor signalling but acts either as a neutral antagonist (1) or a weak partial agonist (3).

At this moment it is not known why some H_2 antagonists as e.g. cimetidine and ranitidine posses negative intrinsic activity and others like e.g. burimamide not. Interestingly, metiamide, a compound which is structurally very closely related to burimamide behaves as a partial inverse agonist at the constitutively active H_2 receptor (unpublished observations). Therefore, in the present study burimamide and metiamide were taken as lead compounds to investigate the structural requirements for inverse agonism. To enable the detection of differences in the negative intrinsic activity of compounds and to increase the sample throughpout, the highly sensitive luciferase assay was used. The structural basis for inverse agonism of histamine H_2 antagonists was further investigated using series of structurally related H_2 antagonists.

2. RESULTS

COS-7 cells transiently expressing the rat histamine H_2 receptor (B_{max} = 5.6 ± 2.7, mean ± S.E.M, n=4) and a reporter gene plasmid with the luciferase gene under control of 21 cAMP response elements (CREs) were incubated with the test ligands directly after transfection. The luciferase reporter gene assay is an easy to perform and highly sensitive assay to determine constitutive H_2 receptor activity and to detect inverse agonism.

2.1. Negative intrinsic activity of structurally related H_2 ligands

Introduction of a methyl substituent at the 4 position in the imidazole ring of burimamide, giving methylburimamide, does not significantly change the pharmacological properties of the compound (Figure 1). Methylburimamide has, like burimamide, partial agonistic properties in the luciferase assay. Introduction of the methyl substituent does also not significantly affect the affinity of burimamide (Table 1).

In contrast, introduction of a sulphur atom in the side chain of burimamide, giving thiaburimamide, changed the intrinsic activity from a partial agonist to a partial inverse agonist (α=-0.35 ± 0.04, mean ± S.E.M, n=3).

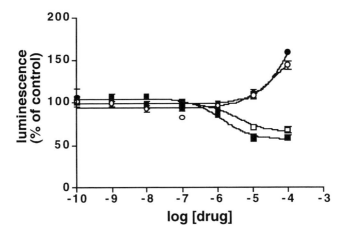

Figure 1. Effect of increasing concentrations of methylburimamide (open circles), burimamide (closed circles), metiamide (closed squares) and thiaburimamide (open squares) on the basal luciferase activity in COS-7 cells transiently expressing the H_2 receptor and the 21-CRE luciferase construct. The luciferase activity is expressed as a percentage of the basal luminescence measured for each construct (basal luminescence is 100%). Data presented are from one typical experiment out of at least three independent experiments performed in triplicate.

The negative intrinsic activity of thiaburimamide is comparable to the negative intrinsic activity of metiamide (Figure 1, Table 1). Introduction of the sulphur atom also significantly affects the H_2 receptor affinity of burimamide. The affinity of thiaburimamide is increased compared to burimamide but still significantly lower than that of metiamide (Table 1).

For the partial inverse agonist metiamide the sulphur atom in the side chain is important for its negative intrinsic activity (Table 1). The effect of removal of the side chain sulphur atom was also investigated for other H_2 ligands. The ligands tested differ in their heterocyclic ring system.

Table 1 Effect of the sulphur atom in side chain on negative intrinsic activity, potency and affinity of H_2 antagonists

structure	ligand	pIC_{50}	α_{inv}	pK_i
	burimamide X = S	-	p.a.	5.09 ± 0.17
	thiaburimamide X = CH_2	5.60 ± 0.11	0.35 ± 0.04	5.48 ± 0.05
	methylburimamide X = S	-	p.a.	5.21 ± 0.02
	metiamide X = CH_2	5.95 ± 0.06	0.41 ± 0.02	6.17 ± 0.05
	cimetidine X = S	5.77 ± 0.07	0.68 ± 0.05	5.98 ± 0.12
	VUF5651 X = CH_2	-	0	5.13 ± 0.12
	SK&F92.857 X = S	6.08 ± 0.09	1.00 ± 0.01	6.76 ± 0.11
	SK&F93.162C X = CH_2	5.62 ± 0.08	0.93 ± 0.01	6.32 ± 0.04

The negative intrinsic activity (α_{inv}) and the potency of inhibition (pIC_{50}) were determined from the dose-dependent inhibition curve of the different drugs in a luciferase assay. The negative intrinsic activity of ranitidine is defined as 1. The affinity (pK_i) is determined from competition experiments with 0.3 nM [^{125}I]-APT. Data shown are mean ± S.E.M from at least three independent experiments. p.a. means partial agonist. 0 means neutral antagonist.

Removal of the sulphur atom in the side chain of cimetidine, resulting in VUF5651, dramatically affects the intrinsic activity of the ligand. VUF5651 has no negative intrinsic activity but behaves as a neutral antagonist (Table 1). Removal of the side chain sulphur atom also significantly decreases the affinity of the compound. Interestingly, removal of the sulphur atom in SK&F92.857 does not drastically affect the negative intrinsic activity (Table 1). The affinity and the potency are however slightly decreased upon removal of the sulphur atom in SK&F92.857 (Table 1).

2.2. Ligand Modelling studies

Energy profile plots for rotation of the imidazole ring around the marked bond in the presence or absence of a sulphur atom in the side chain were made for the depicted molecules (Figure 2).

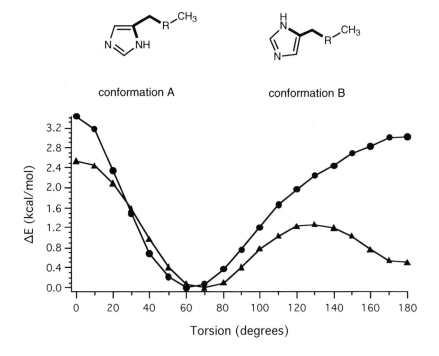

Figure 2. Energy profile for the rotation of the imidazole ring in the presence of either a -CH$_2$- (black triangles) or -S- (black circles) in the β position. The ring is protonated at the π-position. The geometry of the initial structure was optimized at the 6-31G(d,p) level using GAMESS-US. The torsion angle, N-C-C-X, was incremented in steps of 10 degrees to generate the structures with a torsion angle between 0 and 180 degrees. The energy of the resulting structures was calculated at the 6-31G(d.p)level of theory.

It is found that in the presence of a sulphur atom, as in thiaburimamide and metiamide, conformation A (torsion angle N-C-C-S is approximately 60 degrees), a folded conformation is highly preferred (Figure 2). In the absence of a sulphur atom, as in burimamimide and methylburimamide, both a folded conforamtion (conformation A) and an extended conformation (torsion angle N-C-C-CH$_2$ is approximately 120 degrees, conformation B) are low energy conformations (Figure 2).

3. DISCUSSION

In previous studies we showed that burimamide behaves, dependent upon the system, either as a neutral antagonist (1) or a weak partial agonist (3). Interestingly, the structurally closely related compound metiamide is a partial inverse agonist at the constitutively active H$_2$ receptor (unpublished observations).

The introduction of a methyl substituent at the 4 position of the imidazole ring of burimamide does not induce negative intrinsic activity, as methylburimamide is still a partial agonist in this test system. Moreover, the negative intrinsic activity of metiamide was not affected by removal of the 4-methyl substituent. The 4-methylsubstituent, however, slightly increases the affinity of the compounds. The effect found on affinity is probably due to the enhanced ability of the N$^\tau$ atom to accept a proton (ring pK$_a$ increase). As demonstrated by Nederkoorn et al. (1994) H$_2$ agonist potency of imidazole derivatives is dependent on the proton acceptor capacity of the tele nitrogen (N$^\tau$) atom which might consequently also affect affinity of antagonistic ligands (5).

In contrast to the 4-methyl substituent the presence of a sulphur atom in the side chain is a prerequisite for negative intrinsic activity of imidazole containing H$_2$ ligands. Thiaburimamide was found to be a partial inverse agonist with a negative intrinsic activity comparable to that of metiamide. Investigation of the conformational differences between burimamide, methylburimamide, thiaburimamide and metiamide revealed that both burimamide and methylburimamide prefer a conformation in which the proton of the imidazole ring points away from the methylene group in the side chain (conformation B, Figure 2). In contrast, in thiaburimamide and metiamide the proton of the imidazole ring seems to prefer a position in which it points towards the side chain sulphur atom (conformation A, Figure 2).

Our findings are in agreement with earlier crystallography findings. The crystal structures of metiamide and thiaburimamide (6) differ significantly from that of burimamide; the molecules are not extended (as in burimamide) but folded; an intramolecular hydrogen bond is formed between the thiourea -NH and the imidazole N^π-atom, leading to the formation of an eight or ten-membered ring. In burimamide such thiourea-imidazole contacts have not been identified (7). The difference in conformational flexibility between burimamide and metiamide might thus be a possible explanation for the obtained difference in the intrinsic activity of these compounds.

Interestingly the presence of a sulphur atom in the side chain is not important for H_2 ligands containing other heterocyclic ring systems (Table 1). Probably these ligands, which generally have higher basicity, may bind in a different way to the receptor than the imidazole-containing ligands. No data supporting the hypothesis that non-imidazole containing ligands bind differently to the H_2 receptor are, however, available currently and further investigations are therefore needed.

In summary, the present study shows that for imidazole-containing antagonistic ligands the presence of a sulphur atom in the side chain is required for negative intrinsic activity. However, the presence of a sulphur atom in the side chain is not required for negative intrinsic activity of H_2 antagonistic ligands containing other heterocyclic ringsystems.

REFERENCES

1. M.J. Smit, R. Leurs, A.E. Alewijnse, J. Blauw, G.P. van Nieuw Amerongen, Y. van de Vrede, E. Roovers and H. Timmerman, Proc. Natl. Acad. Sci. USA, 93 (1996) 6802.
2. A.E. Alewijnse, M.J. Smit, M.S. Rodriguez Pena, D. Verzijl, H. Timmerman and R. Leurs, FEBS Lett., 419 (1997) 171.
3. A.E. Alewijnse, M.J. Smit, M. Hoffmann, D. Verzijl, H. Timmerman and R. Leurs, R, J. Neurochem., 71 (1998) 799.
4. J.W. Black, W.A.M. Duncan, C.J. Durant, C.R. Ganellin and E.M. Parsons, Nature, 236 (1972) 385.
5. P.H.J. Nederkoorn, P. Vernooijs, G.M. Donné-Op den Kelder, E.J. Baerends and H. Timmerman, J. Mol. Graphics, 12 (1994) 242.
6. K. Prout, S.R. Critchley, C.R. Ganellin et al., J. Chem. Soc., Perkin II (1977) 68.
7. B. Kamenar, K. Prout and C.R. Ganellin, J. Chem. Soc., Perkin II (1973) 1734.

Histamine Research in the New Millennium
T. Watanabe, H. Timmerman and K. Yanai (Editors)

Constitutive signalling of the human histamine H₁ receptor[*]

R. A. Bakker, M. J. Smit[†], H. Timmerman, and R. Leurs.

LACDR, Dept. Medicinal Chemistry, Vrije Universiteit Amsterdam, De Boelelaan 1083, 1081 HV Amsterdam, The Netherlands.

Both the histamine H_1 receptor and the transcription factor nuclear factor kappa B (NF-κB) are important factors in inflammatory conditions. In this study we show that the histamine H_1 receptor activates NF-κB in both a constitutive and agonist-dependent manner. Moreover, the observed constitutive NF-κB activation is inhibited by various H_1-receptor antagonists, suggesting that inverse agonism may account, at least in part, for their ascribed anti-allergic properties.

1. INTRODUCTION

NF-κB is a ubiquitous transcription factor that is considered to play an important role in inflammatory processes [1] and can be activated by many stimuli. Inactive NF-κB is sequestered in the cytoplasm by inhibitory proteins (inhibitor kappa B, IκB) [2]. Phosphorylation of the NF-κB/IκB complex by IκB kinase (IKK) and subsequent ubiquination and degradation of IκB releases the active NF-κB, which then translocates to the nucleus to stimulate transcription of a wide variety of genes. The physiological roles, including lymphocyte activation and protection from apoptosis, for the heterogeneous family of NF-κB proteins, and activators thereof, have recently gained much interest because of their potential therapeutic use (see [3]). Elevated levels of activated NF-κB are found in asthmatic individuals [4], and NF-κB is thought to have a pivotal role in asthma [5].

The $G\alpha_{q/11}$-coupled histamine H_1 receptor [6] is expressed in a variety of cells and is believed to mediate diverse cellular actions of histamine, including many of the histamine-induced symptoms of allergic reactions. Consequently, during the past 20 years H_1-receptor antagonists have become one of the most prescribed drug families in Western countries [7] to relieve the symptoms of allergic reactions. In a previous study we have shown constitutive activation of phospholipase C by the human histamine H_1 receptor [8]. Moreover, the agonist-independent accumulation of inositol phosphates was selectively inhibited by several therapeutics formerly known as H_1 antagonists, which has led to the reclassification of various H_1 antagonists as inverse H_1 agonists [8].

[*] The presented work has been supported by UCB Pharma, Belgium.
[†] Supported by the Royal Dutch Academy of Arts and Sciences.

In this report we show that H_1 agonists induce NF-κB and SRE activation via the H_1 receptor. All tested H_1 antagonists, including those that are clinically used to relieve symptoms of allergy, inhibited the constitutive activation of NF-κB, indicating that these drugs act as inverse H_1 agonists which may represent a potential new mechanism of action of these important class of anti-allergic drugs.

2. MATRERIALS AND METHODS

Materials. pNF-κB-Luc was obtained from Stratagene (La Jolla, USA). Mepyramine (pyrilamine maleate) was obtained from RBI (USA). ATP disodium salt, bovine serum albumin, chloroquine diphosphate, cholera toxin, DEAE-dextran (chloride form), histamine dihydrochloride, and polyethyleneiminewere purchased from Sigma Chemical Company (USA). D-luciferin was obtained from Duchefa Biochemie B.V. (Haarlem, The Netherlands), glycerol was obtained from Riedel-de-Haën (Germany), and Triton X-100 was obtained from Fluka (Switzerland). Cell culture media, penicillin, and streptomycin were obtained from Life Technologies (Merelbeke, Belgium). Foetal calf serum (FCS) was obtained from Integro B.V. (Dieren, The Netherlands), dialysed foetal calf serum was obtained from HyClone® Laboratories Inc. (USA). [³H]mepyramine (30 Ci/mmol), and *myo*-[2-³H]inositol (17 Ci/mmol) were obtained from Amersham International (United Kingdom).
Gifts of acrivastine (The Wellcome Foundation Ltd, United Kingdom), (R)- and (S)-cetirizine hydrochloride (UCB Pharma, Belgium), epinastine hydrochloride (Boehringer Mannheim, Germany), mianserine hydrochloride (Organon NV, the Netherlands), pTLNTRE4-Luc and pTLNSRE3-Luc [9] (Dr. W. Born), pAP-1-fos-Luc (Dr. Gershenforn [10]), pcDEF₃ (Dr. J. Langer [11]), and of the cDNA encoding the human histamine H_1 receptor (Dr. Fukui [12]) are greatly acknowledged.

Cell culture and transfection. COS-7 African green monkey kidney cells were maintained at 37°C in a humidified 5% CO_2/95% air atmosphere in either DMEM containing 2mM L-glutamine, 50 IU/mL penicillin, 50μg/mL streptomycin and 5% (v/v) FCS. COS-7 cells were transiently transfected using the DEAE-dextran method [13]. The total amount of DNA transfected was maintained constant by addition of the empty vector (pcDEF₃ or pcDNA₃).

[³H]Inositol phosphate formation. Cells were seeded in 24-well plates and 24 hr after transfection labelled overnight in inositol-free culture medium supplemented with 1μCi/mL *myo*-[2-³H]inositol. Subsequently, the medium was aspirated and cells were incubated with drugs for 1 hr at 37°C in DMEM containing 25mM Hepes (pH 7.4) and 20mM LiCl. Aspiration of the culture medium and the addition of cold 10mM formic acid. After 90 min incubation at 4°C, [³H]inositol phosphates were isolated by anion exchange chromatography [14], and determined by liquid scintillation counting.

Reporter-gene assay. Cells transiently co-transfected with pNFκB-Luc (125 μg/1·10⁷ cells, Stratagene) and either pcDEF₃ or pcDEF₃hH₁ (25 μg/1·10⁷ cells) were seeded in 96 well blackplates (Costar) in serum free culture medium and incubated with drugs. After 48hrs, cells were assayed for luminescence by aspiration of the medium and the addition of

25µL/well luciferase assay reagent (0.83mM ATP, 0.83mM d-luciferin, 18.7mM MgCl$_2$, 0.78µM Na$_2$H$_2$P$_2$O$_7$, 38.9mM Tris (pH 7.8), 0.39% (v/v) glycerol, 0.03% (v/v) Triton X-100 and 2.6µM DTT). After 30min luminescence was measured for 3sec/well in a TopCount (Packard) or a Victor^2 (Wallac).

Histamine H$_1$ receptor binding studies. The transfected COS-7 cells that were used for radioligand binding studies were harvested after 48h and homogenised in ice-cold H$_1$-binding buffer. The COS-7 cell homogenates were incubated for 30 min at 25°C in 50mM Na$_2$/K-phosphate buffer (pH = 7.4) in 400µL with 1nM [^{3}H]mepyramine. The non-specific binding was determined in the presence of 1µM mianserin. The incubations were stopped by rapid dilution with 3mL ice-cold 50mM Na$_2$/K-phosphate buffer (pH = 7.4). The bound radioactivity was separated by filtration through Whatman GF/C filters that had been treated with 0.3% polyethyleneimine. Filters were washed twice with 3mL buffer and radioactivity retained on the filters was measured by liquid scintillation counting. Binding data were evaluated by a non-linear, least squares curve-fitting procedure using Graphpad Prism$^®$ (GraphPad Software, Inc., San Diego, CA). Proteins concentrations were determined according to Bradford [15], using BSA as a standard.

3. RESULTS

Previously, we have shown that the G$_{q/11}$-coupled H$_1$ receptor activates phospholipase C (PLC) in the absense of an agonist, resulting in spontaneous formation of inositol-1,4,5-triphosphate (InsP$_3$) in transiently transfected COS-7 cells [8]. The constitutive H$_1$-receptor activity could be inhibited by various H$_1$-antagonists [8]. We correlated the inverse agonist potencies with their H$_1$ receptor affinities obtained by [^{3}H]mepyramine displacement studies using whole cell homogenates of transfected COS-7 cells expressing the human H$_1$ receptor (Fig 1B). The inverse H$_1$ agonists display a pharmacological profile that is expected for the H$_1$ receptor, including the known stereospecificity for the stereoisomers of cetirizine [16], and the potencies as inverse agonists determined in the [^{3}H]InsP$_3$ assay correlate well with their respective pK$_i$-values (Fig 1B, slope = 0.98, r^2 = 0.97, N = 6).

As the measurement of the accumulation of [^{3}H]InsP$_3$ does not allow a semi-high-throughput screening for inverse agonism, we developed a suitable reporter-gene assay which deploys multiple integrating signalling pathways to initiate gene-transcription as an end point of receptor activity. As constitutive activity of the Gα$_{q/11}$-coupled TRH receptor has previously been described via a highly sensitive, protein kinase C (PKC)-dependent (AP-1) luciferase reporter-gene assay [10], we tested several reporter-gene assays as suitable readouts for constitutive H$_1$-receptor activity. To this end, we transiently co-transfected COS-7 cells with the pcDEF$_3$humH$_1$ plasmid together with a reporter-plasmid containing a firefly luciferase gene under the transcriptional control of either four TRE (pTLNTRE4-Luc [9]), three SRE (pTLNSRE3-Luc [9], see Fig 2), one AP-1 (pAP-1-fos-Luc [10]) or five NF-κB (pNF-κB-Luc, see Fig 2) enhancer elements. In fact, all these reporter-gene assays may be used to measure both agonism and inverse agonism of the H$_1$ receptor in COS-7 cells (data not shown). We selected the pNFκB-Luc reporter for further experiments for its dynamic range for the measurement of both agonism and inverse agonism.

In COS-7 cells, expressing the H_1 receptor at a density of 3.2 ± 0.4 pmol/mg protein (n = 6), histamine stimulated NF-κB activation 3.6 ± 0.3-fold over basal with a pEC_{50} value of 6.8 ± 0.1 (n = 37; Fig 2B), whereas histamine did not increase NF-κB activation in mock-transfected COS-7 cells (n = 3). As found for the accumulation of $[^3H]InsP_3$ [8], the basal NF-κB activation was increased upon expression of the human H_1 receptor (see Fig 3A). This constitutive H_1 receptor activity was inhibited by the H_1 antagonist mepyramine (Fig 2 and 3), whereas mepyramine had no effect on NF-κB activation in transfected COS-7 cells that did not express the human H_1 receptor (n = 5, Fig 3A). Mepyramine inhibited the constitutive NF-κB activation by 78 ± 1 % with a pIC_{50} value of 7.9 ± 0.1 (n = 55). Whereas increased H_1-receptor expression led to a further rise in the basal response, the pIC_{50} value of mepyramine was unaffected by varying the H_1-receptor density from one to four pmol/mg protein (data not shown). Also, the inhibition of constitutive NF-κB activation by the enantiomers of cetirizine was found to be stereospecific (Fig. 3B); (R)-cetirizine inhibits the constitutive H_1 receptor activity for 59 ± 3 % with a pIC_{50} value of 8.2 ± 0.1 (n = 13), whereas (S)-cetirizine shows an inhibition of 62 ± 3 % with a pIC_{50} value of 6.6 ± 0.1 (n = 13).

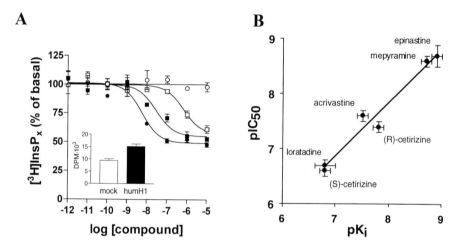

Figure 1. A, effects of mepyramine on the basal $[^3H]$inositol phosphates accumulation activity in mock transfected COS-7 cells (O) ant the effects of mepyramine (●), R- (■) and S-cetirizine (□) on the basal $[^3H]$inositol phosphates accumulation in COS-7 cells transiently expressing the H_1 receptor (3 pmol/mg protein). Inset of A, Effect of expression of the human H_1 receptor (humH1) on the basal $[^3H]$inositol phosphates accumulation in transfected COS-7 cells. B, correlation graph of the pIC_{50} values obtained for the inverse agonists in the $[^3H]InsP_3$ assay versus the pK_i values obtained by $[^3H]$mepyramine displacement in COS-7 cells expressing the human H_1 receptor. Representative experiments performed in triplicate are shown, each experiment was repeated at least three times. Data reproduced from [8] with permission of Elsevier Science B.V.

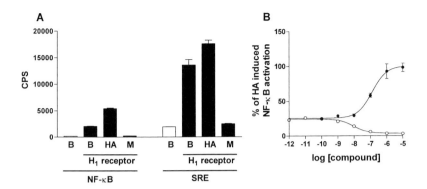

Figure 2. Histamine H₁-receptor mediated activation of SRE and NF-κB. A, COS-7 cells were transiently co-transfected with either cDNA encoding the human H₁ receptor (filled bars) or pcDEF₃ (empty bars) together with a reporter-plasmid containing a firefly luciferase gene under the transcriptional control of either five NF-κB (pNF-κB-Luc) or three SRE (pTLNSRE3-Luc [9]) enhancer elements and incubated in the absence (basal, B) or presence of either 10 μM histamine (HA) or 10 μM mepyramine (M) for 48 hr after which luminescence was measured. B, effects of histamine (●) and mepyramine (O) on the constitutive NF-κB activation in human H₁-receptor expressing COS-7 cells.

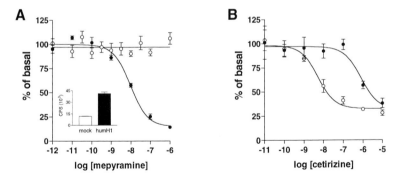

Figure 3. A, effects of mepyramine on the basal luciferase activity in mock transfected COS-7 cells (O) or in COS-7 cells transiently expressing the human histamine H₁ receptor (3 pmol/mg protein, ●). Inset of A, Effect on the basal NF-κB activation in mock or humane H₁ receptor expressing COS-7 cells (humH1). B, inhibition of constitutive H₁-receptor-mediated NF-κB activation by R- (O) and S-cetirizine (●). Representative experiments performed in triplicate are shown, each experiment was repeated at least three times.

166

4. DISCUSSION

The actual therapeutic importance of constitutive GPCR activity has so far not been fully clarified. However, for a proper evaluation of drug action this new aspect in GPCR pharmacology cannot be ignored. In view of the widespread therapeutic use of H_1 antagonists in allergic conditions [7, 17, 18], we investigated the constitutive H_1-receptor activity and inverse agonistic activity of several H_1 antagonists. In this study, we show that the H_1 receptor activates the important pro-inflammatory transcription factor NF-κB in both a constitutive and agonist-dependent manner. Moreover, the NF-κB reporter-gene assay proved to be a very sensitive discriminator between positive and negative ligand efficacy for the H_1 receptor. Although the developed NF-κB reporter-gene assay will be a useful tool to identify neutral H_1 antagonists, at this moment we can not speculate about a potential therapeutic preference for a neutral antagonist or inverse agonist for the H_1 receptor, as all of the tested H_1 antagonists are inverse H_1 agonists.

REFERENCES

1. Barnes, P.J., K.F. Chung, and C.P. Page, Pharmacol Rev, **50**: (1998). p. 515-596.
2. Baldwin, A.S., Jr., Annu Rev Immunol, **14**: (1996). p. 649-683.
3. Newton, R.C. and C.P. Decicco, J Med Chem, **42**: (1999). p. 2295-2314.
4. Hart, L.A., V.L. Krishnan, I.M. Adcock, P.J. Barnes, and K.F. Chung, Am J Respir Crit Care Med, **158**: (1998). p. 1585-1592.
5. Barnes, P.J. and I.M. Adcock, Trends Pharmacol Sci, **18**: (1997). p. 46-50.
6. Leurs, R., E. Traiffort, J.M. Arrang, J. Tardivel-Lacombe, M. Ruat, and J.C. Schwartz, J Neurochem, **62**: (1994). p. 519-527.
7. Woosley, R.L., Annu Rev Pharmacol Toxicol, **36**: (1996). p. 233-252.
8. Bakker, R.A., K. Wieland, H. Timmerman, and R. Leurs, Eur J Pharmacol, **387**: (2000). p. R5-R7.
9. Flühmann, B., U. Zimmermann, R. Muff, G. Bilbe, J.A. Fischer, and W. Born, Mol Cell Endocrinol, **139**: (1998). p. 89-98.
10. Jinsi-Parimoo, A. and M.C. Gershengorn, Endocrinology, **138**: (1997). p. 1471-1475.
11. Goldman, L.A., E.C. Cutrone, S.V. Kotenko, C.D. Krause, and J.A. Langer, Biotechniques, **21**: (1996). p. 1013-1015.
12. Fukui, H., K. Fujimoto, H. Mizuguchi, K. Sakamoto, Y. Horio, S. Takai, K. Yamada, and S. Ito, Biochem Biophys Res Commun, **201**: (1994). p. 894-901.
13. Brakenhoff, R.H., E.M. Knippels, and G.A. van Dongen, Anal Biochem, **218**: (1994). p. 460-463.
14. Godfrey, P., ed. *Inositol lipids and phosphatases.* Signal transduction. A practical approach., ed. G. Milligan. 1992, IRL Press: Oxford. 105-121.
15. Bradford, M.M., Anal Biochem, **72**: (1976). p. 248-254.
16. Moguilevsky, N., F. Varsalona, J.P. Guillaume, M. Noyer, M. Gillard, J. Daliers, J.P. Hénichart, and A. Bollen, J Recept Signal Transduct Res, **15**: (1995). p. 91-102.
17. Handley, D.A., A. Magnetti, and A.J. Higgins, Exp. Opion. Invest, Drugs, **7**: (1998). p. 1045-1054.
18. Zhang, M.-Q., R. Leurs, and H. Timmerman, *Histamine H₁-receptor antagonists*, in *Burger's Medical Chemistry and Drug Discovery,*, M.E. Wolff, Editor. 1997, John Wiley & Sons, Inc. p. 495-559.

© 2001 Elsevier Science B.V. All rights reserved.
Histamine Research in the New Millennium
T. Watanabe, H. Timmerman and K. Yanai (Editors)

H_1-Histamine receptor communicates to G_{14} with a relatively higher affinity than to G_{11}

N. Nakahata[a], Y. Sato[a], S. Ohkubo[a] and T. Nukada[b]

[a]Department of Cellular Signaling, Graduate School of Pharmaceutical Sciences, Tohoku University, Aoba, Aramaki, Sendai 980-8578, Japan.

[b]Department of Neurochemistry, Tokyo Institute of Psychiatry, Kamikitazawa 2-1-8, Setagaya-ku, Tokyo 156-8585, Japan.

H_1-Histamine receptor has been shown to couple to G_q family G proteins, and the stimulation results in Ca^{2+} mobilization mediated through phospholipase C-β and an accumulation of inositol 1,4,5-trisphosphate (IP_3). There are several G proteins in G_q family, such as G_q, G_{11}, G_{14}, G_{15} and G_{16}. It is unknown whether H_1-histamine receptor preferentially communicates to a specific G protein of G_q family, so far. In the present study, we examined whether H_1-histamine receptor specifically communicates to G_{11} or G_{14} in 1321N1 cells transfected with $G\alpha_{11}$ or $G\alpha_{14}$ cDNA. Northern blot analysis indicated that $G\alpha_{11}$ and $G\alpha_{14}$ mRNAs were detected in the cells transfected with $G\alpha_{11}$ and $G\alpha_{14}$ cDNAs, respectively. When intracellular Ca^{2+} concentration ($[Ca^{2+}]_i$) was determined, histamine, carbachol and U46619, a thromboxane A_2 agonist, increased $[Ca^{2+}]_i$ in a concentration-dependent manner in control (vector-transfected) cells. Maximum response to each agonist was augmented in $G\alpha_{11}$- and $G\alpha_{14}$-expressed cells. While carbachol caused $[Ca^{2+}]_i$ elevation to a similar extent in both $G\alpha_{11}$- and $G\alpha_{14}$- expressed cells, histamine did $[Ca^{2+}]_i$ elevation to a greater extent in $G\alpha_{14}$-expressed cells than in $G\alpha_{11}$-expressed cells. Histamine also stimulated [^{3}H]inositol phosphate production in $G\alpha_{14}$-expressed cells with a greater potency than in $G\alpha_{11}$-expressed cells, although carbachol and U46619 did the production to a similar extent in $G\alpha_{11}$- and $G\alpha_{14}$-expressed cells. These results indicate that H_1-histamine receptor, but not muscarinic or thromboxane A_2 receptor, preferentially communicates to G_{14} than G_{11} for activation of phospholipase C.

1. INTRODUCTION

It has been shown that the stimulation of H_1-histamine receptor results in an activation of G_q family G proteins, causing intracellular Ca^{2+} mobilization mediated through phospholipase C-β activation and an accumulation of inositol 1,4,5-trisphosphate (IP_3). Among trimeric G proteins, G_q family G proteins are divided into G_q, G_{11}, G_{14}, G_{15} and G_{16}. It has been shown that $G\alpha_{14}$ coexpressed with metabotropic glutamate receptors inhibits phospholipase C in *Xenopus* oocytes [1]. It is unknown whether H_1-histamine receptor preferentially communicates to a specific G protein of G_q family, so far.

We have previously demonstrated that 1321N1 human astrocytoma cells express H_1-histamine receptor, the stimulation of which results in phosphoinositide hydrolysis [2-5] mediated through G_q class of G protein and phospholipase C. In the present study, we examined whether H_1-histamine receptor specifically communicates to G_{11} or G_{14} in 1321N1 cells transfected with $G\alpha_{11}$ or $G\alpha_{14}$ cDNA.

2. METHODS

2.1 Cell culture and expression of exogenous $G\alpha_{11}$ and $G\alpha_{14}$

Human astrocytoma cells (1321N1) were grown in DMEM supplemented with 5% FCS, 50 unit/ml of penicillin and 50 μg/ml of streptomycin [6]. Cells were maintained in a humidified incubator in an atmosphere of 95% air and 5% CO_2. $G\alpha_{11}$ and $G\alpha_{14}$ cDNA clones were prepared as described previously [7]. By using a *Hind*III linker, the $G\alpha$ cDNA fragment containing the entire protein coding segment was inserted into the *Hind*III site of pKGSαN [8] to yield expression vector. Human astrocytoma cells (1321N1) in culture were transfected with above plasmids by a lipofectamine method. Among G418-resistant transformants, $G\alpha$-transformed 1321N1 cells were selected out by blot hybridization analysis.

2.2. Northern blot analysis

Total RNA in 1321N1 cells transfected with vector, $G\alpha_{11}$ or $G\alpha_{14}$ cDNA was extracted [9], and then, Northern blot analysis was performed as previously described [8] using the cDNA probes ($G\alpha_{11}$ or $G\alpha_{14}$) uniformly labeled with [^{32}P]dCTP.

2.3. Measurement of intracellular free Ca^{2+} concentration

The change in $[Ca^{2+}]_i$ was measured by monitoring the intensity of fura 2 fluorescence as described previously [10]. In brief, the cells were incubated with 1 μM fura 2-AM for 15 min, and washed with Tyrode solution. $[Ca^{2+}]_i$ in fura 2-loaded cells was determined by spectrofluorometer (Hitachi F-2000).

2.4. Assay of inositol phosphates

Phosphoinositide breakdown was monitored by measuring [^{3}H]inositol phosphates as previously described [11]. Phosphoinositides of the cells were labeled with DMEM containing [^{3}H]inositol (2 μCi/ml) for 18 to 24 h. The cells were incubated in EMEM buffered with 20 mM HEPES (EMEM/HEPES) (pH 7.4) containing 10 mM LiCl at 37°C for 10 min with or without drugs. The reaction was terminated by the addition of 1 ml of 5% trichloroacetic acid (TCA) after aspiration of the medium. Total [^{3}H]inositol phosphates in the ether-washed TCA extract were separated by anion exchange column (AG 1X-8, formate form). The TCA precipitate was dissolved in 0.5 ml of 1 N NaOH, and the [^{3}H] radioactivity was measured after neutralization for determining [^{3}H]-labeled phosphoinositides.

3. RESULTS

Northern blot analysis indicated that Gα_{11} and Gα_{14} mRNAs were detected in the cells transfected with Gα_{11} and Gα_{14} cDNA, respectively (Figure. 1). When Gα_{11} cDNA was used as a probe, endogenous Gα_{11} and Gα_{11}-like mRNA were detected in the cells transfected by vector, Gα_{11} and Gα_{14} cDNA.

When intracellular Ca^{2+} concentration ([Ca^{2+}]$_i$) was determined, histamine, carbachol, a muscrinic receptor agonist, and U46619, a thromboxane A$_2$ agonist, increased [Ca^{2+}]$_i$ in a concentration-dependent manner in control (vector-transfected) cells mediated through H$_1$-histamine, M$_3$-muscarinic and thromboxane A$_2$ receptors (Figure 2). The response to each agonist was augmented in Gα_{11}- and Gα_{14}-expressed cells. Carbachol and U46619 caused [Ca^{2+}]$_i$ elevation to a similar extent in both Gα_{11}- and Gα_{14}-expressed cells. However, histamine caused [Ca^{2+}]$_i$ elevation to a greater extent in Gα_{14}-expressed cells than in Gα_{11}-expressed cells.

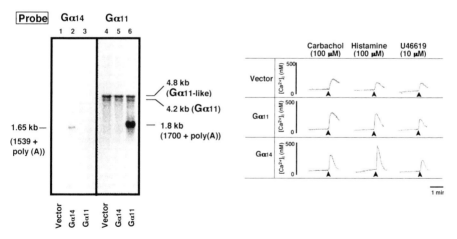

Figure 1. Northern blot analysis of Gα_{11} and Gα_{14} in Gα-expressed 1321N1 human astrocytoma cells. Vector, Gα_{11} and Gα_{14} were transfected into human astrocytoma cells, and total RNA of each cell was extracted (see "METHODS"). The cDNA probe (Gα_{11} or Gα_{14}) was uniformly labeled with [^{32}P]dCTP. Lane 1, 4; Vector-transfected cells. Lane 2,5; Gα_{14}-transfected cells. Lane 3,6; Gα_{11}-transfected cells. Lane 1-3; hybridyzed with [^{32}P]-labeled Gα_{14}. Lane 4-6; hybridyzed with [^{32}P]-labeled Gα_{11}.

Figure 2. Effects of carbachol, histamine and U46619 on [Ca^{2+}]$_i$ level in 1321N1 cells transfected with vector, Gα_{11} and Gα_{14} cDNAs. The transfected cells were loaded with fura 2-AM, and [Ca^{2+}]$_i$ was measured by spectrofluorometer. Typical responses of vector- (upper), Gα_{11}- (middle) and Gα_{14}-expressed cells (bottom) to 100 µM carbachol (left), 100 µM histamine (middle) and 10 µM U46619 (right) were indicated.

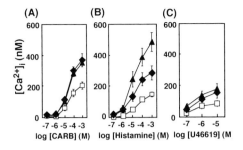

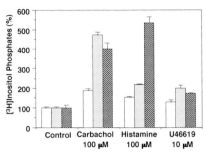

Figure 3. Concentration-dependent increases in [Ca^{2+}]$_i$ by carbachol, histamine and U46619 in 1321N1 cells transfected with vector, Gα_{11} and Gα_{14} cDNAs. The responses of the cells transfected with vector (□), Gα_{11} (◆) and Gα_{14} (▲) cDNAs to carbachol (A), histamine (B) or U46619 (C). Each point represents the mean ± SEM from 4-6 determinations.

Figure 4. Phosphoinositide hydrolysis induced by carbachol, histamine and U46619 in 1321N1 cells transfected with vector (open column), Gα_{11} (dotted column) and Gα_{14} (hatched column) cDNAs. [^{3}H]Inositol phosphates were determined in the cells labeled with [^{3}H]inositol. Each column represents the mean ± SEM from 3 determinations.

Carbachol increased [Ca^{2+}]$_i$ in a concentration-dependent manner with the EC$_{50}$ values of approximately 30 μM in control (vector-transfected), Gα_{11}- and Gα_{14}-expressed cells (Figure 3). The maximum responses to carbachol in Gα_{11}- and Gα_{14}- expressed cells were about 2-fold greater than that in control (vector-transfected) cells. U46619 concentration-dependently increased [Ca^{2+}]$_i$ in control (vector-transfected), Gα_{11}- and Gα_{14}-expressed cells with the EC$_{50}$ values of approximately 0.8 μM. The maximum responses to U46619 in Gα_{11}- and Gα_{14}-expressed cells were about 2-fold greater than that in control (vector-transfected) cells. On the other hand, histamine also increased [Ca^{2+}]$_i$ in control (vector-transfected), Gα_{11}- and Gα_{14}-expressed cells with the EC$_{50}$ values of approximately 30 μM. In contrast to carbachol or U46619, histamine increased [Ca^{2+}]$_i$ to a great extent (about 6-fold) in Gα_{14}-expressed cells, but it caused only about 2-fold increase in [Ca^{2+}]$_i$ in Gα_{11}-expressed cells. Histamine-induced [Ca^{2+}]$_i$ elevation in Gα_{14}-expressed cells was decreased by pretreatment of the cells with a Ca^{2+} chelator EGTA, indicating that Ca^{2+} was released from intracellular store sites. These results suggest that histamine increased [Ca^{2+}]$_i$ efficiently in Gα_{14}-expressed cells.

Carbachol, histamine and U46619 also accumulated [^{3}H]inositol phosphates in control (vector-transfected) cells. Although carbachol and U46619 accumulated [^{3}H]inositol phosphates to a similar extent in Gα_{11}- and Gα_{14}-expressed cells, histamine stimulated [^{3}H]inositol phosphate production in Gα_{14}-expressed cells with a greater potency than in Gα_{11}-expressed cells.

4. DISCUSSION

The present study demonstrated that the stimulation of H$_1$-histamine receptor caused phosphoinositide hydrolysis and $[Ca^{2+}]_i$ elevation to a great extent in $G\alpha_{14}$-expressed cells. Since 1) histamine only slightly stimulated $[Ca^{2+}]_i$ elevation in $G\alpha_{11}$-expressed cells, and 2) carbachol and U46619 similarly stimulated $[Ca^{2+}]_i$ elevation in both $G\alpha_{14}$- and $G\alpha_{11}$-expressed cells, the coupling of H_1-histamine receptor with $G\alpha_{14}$ might be specific. Nakamura et al. [12] demonstrated that purified G_{14} activates phospholipse β resulting in IP_3 production with a similar potency to G_{11}. Thus, G_{14} and G_{11} can stimulate phospholipse C in a similar manner. They also showed that the stimulation of muscarinic receptor resulted in an increase of $GTP\gamma S$ binding to G_{14} and G_{11} with a similar potency, consisting of the present results, which muscarinic receptor did not discriminate G_{14} and G_{11}. In spite of histamine-induced potent increase in maximum $[Ca^{2+}]_i$ elevation in $G\alpha_{14}$-expressed cells, however, histamine showed the similar EC_{50} values in control, $G\alpha_{11}$- and $G\alpha_{14}$-expressed cells. Thus, it is suggested that the affinity of H_1-histamine receptor to agonist is not changed among control, $G\alpha_{11}$- and $G\alpha_{14}$-expressed cells, and H_1-histamine receptor may preferentially couple with G_{14} to activate phospholipase C and $[Ca^{2+}]_i$ elevation. Since further study is necessary, it is a first demonstrattion that H_1-histamine receptor preferentially communicates to a G_q family G protein G_{14}.

In conclusion, the present results indicate that H_1-histamine, but not muscarinic or thromboxane A_2 receptors, preferentially communicates to G_{14} than G_{11} for activation of phospholipase C.

REFERENCES

1. K. Nakamura, T. Nukada, T. Haga and H. Sugiyama, J. Physiol. (Lond.) **474** (1994) 35.
2. N. Nakahata, M.W. Martin, A.R. Hughes, J.R. Hepler and T.K. Harden, Mol. Pharmacol. **29** (1986) 188.
3. N. Nakahata and T.K. Harden, *Biochem. J.* **241** (1987) 337.
4. N. Nakahata, M.T. Abe, I. Matsuoka, T. Ono and H. Nakanishi, J. Neurochem. **57** (1991) 963.
5. N. Nakahata, H. Ishimoto, A. Takahashi, K. Ohmori and M. Kurita, Eur. J. Pharmacol. Mol. Pharmacol. Sec. **208** (1991) 265.
6. K. Sakai, N. Nakahata, H. Ono, T. Yamamoto and Y. Ohizumi, J. Pharmacol. Exp. Ther., **276** (1996) 829.
7. F. Nakamura, K. Ogata, K. Shinozaki, K. Kameyama, T. Haga and T. Nukada, J. Biol. Chem. **266** (1991) 12676.
8. T. Nukada, M. Mishina and S.Numa, FEBS Lett. **211** (1987) 5.
9. H.C. Birnboim, Nucleic Acids Res. **16** (1988) 1487.
10. N. Nakahata, H. Ishimoto, K. Mizuno, Y. Ohizumi and H. Nakanishi, Brit. J. Pharmacol., **112** (1994) 299.
11. N. Nakahata, I. Matsuoka, T. Ono and H. Nakanishi, *Eur. J. Pharmacol.*, **162** (1989) 407.
12. F. Nakamura, M. Kato, K. Kameyama, T. Nukada, T. Haga, H. Kato, T. Takenawa and U. Kikkawa, J. Biol. Chem. **270** (1995) 6246.

Histamine Research in the New Millennium
T. Watanabe, H. Timmerman and K. Yanai (Editors)

Pathological significance of over-production of histamine and altered transcriptional regulation of H_1- and H_2-receptors during septic shock

Naoyuki Matsuda[a, b], Yuichi Hattori[a], Osamu Kemmotsu[b] and Satoshi Gando[b]

Departments of Pharmacology[a] and Anesthesiology & Critical Care Medicine[b]
Hokkaido University School of Medicine, Sapporo 060-8638, Japan

Rabbits injected with lipopolysaccharide (LPS; 100 µg/kg, i.v.) exhibited a marked elevation of plasma histamine level. Following LPS injection, there were biphasic decreases in mean arterial blood pressure (MBP). Heart rate decreased initially and then showed a lasting increase. The pharmacological analysis using the H_1-receptor antagonist diphenhydramine and the H_2-receptor antagonist ranitidine indicated that endogenous histamine contribute, at least in part, to the initial decrease in MBP through H_1-receptor activation and to the lasting tachycardia through H_2-receptor activation. Myocardial mRNA expression levels of both H_1- and H_2-receptors were significantly increased with time following LPS injection. However, there was a significant difference in the positive chronotropic effect of histamine, with the right atria isolated from LPS-treated rabbits having less sensitivity than their controls. This appeared to be associated with a decreased level of cardiac $G_{s\alpha}$ in sepsis. We thus suggest that endogenous histamine may be responsible for a part of the hemodynamic changes caused by sepsis due entirely to its excessive circulating level but not to changes in histamine receptors at the level of gene expression.

1. INTRODUCTION

Endotoxin-induced septic shock is characterized by progressive hypotension and multiple organ failure associated with extremely high mortality. This is considered to be related to excessive nitric oxide (NO) generated by inducible NO synthase (1), but sepsis may cause induction of certain autacoids that could potentially contribute to hemodynamic changes during this pathological state. Plasma histamine levels are known to be elevated during septic shock (2). In addition to serving as a mediator of inflammation, histamine exerts marked effects on cardiovascular system (3). It is thus possible that endogenous histamine may be partly involved in the cardiovascular profile of sepsis. This study was undertaken to examine a possible role of endogenous histamine in the hemodynamic changes in the rabbit which was rendered endotoxemic with *Escherichia coli* lipopolysaccharide (LPS).

2. MATERIALS AND METHODS

2.1 Hemodynamic measurements and induction of sepsis

Male New Zealand white rabbits (2 - 2.5 kg) were anesthetized with diethyl ether. Normal saline containing 2 U/ml heparin was continuously infused *via* the ear arterial catheter to maintain patency of the blood pressure cannula line. Following recovery of anesthesia, the arterial blood pressure and heart rate (HR) were continuously monitored as previously described (4). Rabbits received a slow bolus injection of 100 μg/kg LPS (*E. coli* 055:B5; List Biological Laboratories) *via* the ear vein. In untreated (control) rabbits, the same amount of normal saline was given intravenously instead of LPS.

2.2 Plasma histamine and catecholamine measurements

Blood samples were obtained at a predetermined time after LPS injection. Levels of histamine and catecholamines (norepinephrine and epinephrine) in plasma were determined using a sensitive radioimmunoassay and high-pressure liquid chromatography, respectively.

2.3. Northern blots for H_1- and H_2-receptors

Total RNA was extracted from myocardial samples using a guanidinium thiocyanate-phenol-chloroform method. RNA (30 μg/lane) was subjected to electrophoresis on agarose/formaldehyde gels and then transferred to a Hybond-N^+ nylon membrane. The membranes were incubated for 60 min at 65°C in a prehybridization buffer. The cDNA probes for H_1- and H_2-receptors were labeled by random priming methodology using [^{32}P]dCTP. The probes were hybridized at 65°C for 120 min. Following high stringency washing, the mRNA of interest (H_1- and H_2-receptors) was quantified by counting the radioactivity. In order to normalize the amount of RNA bound to membranes, all blots were also hybridized against the constitutively expressed enzyme GAPDH (5).

2.4. Western blot analysis for $G_{s\alpha}$ protein

Immunoblotting was performed as demonstrated in our previous report (5). Samples of atrial tissue homogenate were subjected to electrophoresis on polyacrylamide gels, and proteins were transferred to polyvinylidine difluoride filter membranes. After blocking with Tris-buffered saline containing 1% bovine serum albumin, membranes were incubated with primary $G_{s\alpha}$ antisera (Gramsch Laboratories). Immunolabeled $G_{s\alpha}$ was visualized by identifying the products of a reaction catalyzed by horseradish peroxidase-conjugated anti-rabbit antibody.

2.5. Organ bath experiments

Experiments were performed as described previously (6). Briefly, right atria were isolated from the hearts. The bathing solution contained (in mM): NaCl 119, KCl 4.8, $CaCl_2$ 2.5, $MgSO_4$ 1.2, KH_2PO_4 1.2, $NaHCO_3$ 24.9 and glucose 10.0, continuously gassed with 95% O_2

and 5% CO_2, and was kept at a temperature of 37°C. The spontaneous rate of contraction was counted on a chart recording its developed tension.

2.6. Statistics

The data are expressed as means ± S.E.M. Statistical analysis was performed using Student's t-test for unpaired observations. Differences were considered to be statistically significant when $P<0.05$.

3. RESULTS AND DISCUSSION

As demonstrated in our recent report (4), administration of LPS (100 µg/kg, i.v.) to the rabbit caused biphasic decreases in mean arterial blood pressure (MBP). The initial reduction in MBP appeared immediately after the addition, reaching a maximum level within 5 min. The progressive and sustained fall in MBP required a time delay of 2.5 h following administration of LPS. HR was initially reduced within 5 min after LPS injection and gradually returned to the base line by 2 h, followed by a persistent elevation over a 7-h period.

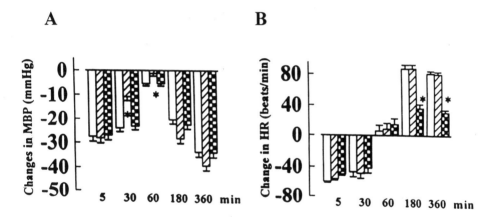

Figure 1. Effects of diphenhydramine (5 mg/kg, i.v.; hatched bars) and ranitidine (40 mg/kg, i.v.; dotted bars) on the changes in MBP (**A**) and HR (**B**) following administration of LPS (100mg/kg, i.v.) to rabbits. *$P<0.05$ compared with the corresponding values obtained from the animals without histamine antagonists (open bars).

The basal plasma concentration of histamine in the rabbit was 0.68±0.06 µM ($n = 5$). Administration of LPS elevated the histamine concentration in plasma within a few minutes. A maximum was reached at 30 min (14.57±0.93 µM) and the concentration declined thereafter, although it remained much higher than the concentration before administration (8.79±0.49 µM at 6 h).

The dramatic increase in plasma histamine concentrarion may be partly responsible for the hemodynamic alterations observed in the LPS-treated rabbit. We thus examined the effects of the H_1-receptor antagonist diphenhydramine and H_2-receptor antagonist ranitidine on the hemodynamic alterations of endotoxemia. The addition of diphenhydramine (5 mg/kg, i.v.) or ranitidine (40 mg/kg, i.v.) alone caused no significant changes in MBP and HR. Pretreatment with diphenhydramine did not affect the persistent reduction in MBP that occurred late or the HR changes following administration of LPS, but significantly accelerated the reversal of the initial hypotension (Fig. 1A). It is known that H_1-receptors are present on endothelial cells and activates the constitutively expressed endothelial isoform of NO synthase (7). Thus, the initial hypotensive phase may be due partly to activation of endothelial H_1-receptors with increased circulating histamine, resulting in increased activity of endothelial NO synthase. However, histamine does not appear to be a major determinant of MBP early after LPS treatment. The hypotension that occurred early after injection of LPS may be explained by the release of kinins or cytokines such as tumor necrosis factor-α. The previous study showing the relationship between plasma NOx (nitrite, nitrate and NO) and hemodynamic changes after LPS injection has suggested that the early hypotension is not associated with induction of inducible NO synthase, whereas the late and sustained hypotension is closely related to an increase in NO production (8).

Pretreatment with ranitidine had no effect on the changes in MBP but markedly suppressed the tachycardia that occurred late following injection of LPS (Fig.1B). Since histamine directly produces a positive chronotropic action mediated through H_2-receptors (6, 9), this finding suggests that the excessive increase in circulating histamine plays an important role in the tachycardia seen in sepsis. Thus, the increase in HR cannot be soley attributed to a reflex response to the reduced MBP. The elevated circulating concentrations of catecholamines have been reported in some animal models of endotoxemia (10, 11), and may have partially contributed to the LPS-induced increase in HR. This is most unlikely because we found in our septic model that the changes in plasma catecholamines were insignificant, at least within 6 h after LPS treatment.

In addition to the marked increase in plasma histamine concentration, sepsis may modify the expression of H_1- and H_2-receptors. We thus assessed sepsis-induced alterations in H_1- and H_2-receptors by evaluating their gene expression levels in atrial and ventricular myocardium. As shown in Fig. 2A, Northern blot analysis using the H_1-receptor probe detected two major mRNA species of approximately 3.3 and 3.9 kb in both atrial and ventricular myocardium. It has been demonstrated that the cerebrum and cerebellum express only 3.3 kb mRNA of H_1-receptors, but an additional 3.9 kb mRNA can be detected in peripheral organs including the heart (12). When GAPDH mRNA was used as an internal standard, the relative mRNA levels of H_1-receptors were increased progressively following induction of sepsis. Thus, the increases were about 13- and 23-fold in atria and about 3.6- and 4.7-fold in ventricles at 3 and 6 h after LPS injection, respectively. As presented in Fig. 2B, the identity of mRNA corresponding to H_2-receptors in myocardium was considered as a major species of approximately 3.2 kb. The levels of H_2-receptor mRNA in atrial and ventricular myocardium increased by about 2- and 5-fold at 3 h after LPS injection, respectively, and the increases remained constant in 6-h sepsis. These results suggest significant transcriptional regulation of H_1- and H_2-receptor gene products during septic shock.

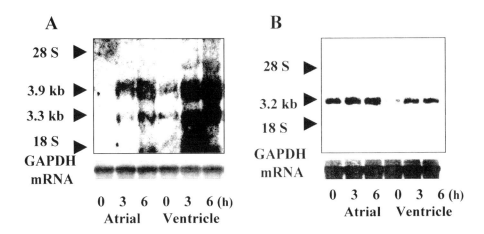

Figure 2. Representative autographs of Northern blot analysis of mRNA expression of H_1-receptors (**A**) and H_2-receptors (**B**) in atrial and ventricular myocardium from control and septic (3 and 6 h after LPS injection) rabbits. The blots were sequentially hybridized using probes for H_1- or H_2-receptors and GAPDH. The location of the 28-S and 18-S ribosomal RNA is indicated.

Despite the increased level of H_2-receptor mRNA, the positive chronotropic effect of histamine was significantly impaired in right atria from LPS-treated rabbits. Thus, an overall shift in both sensitivity and maximum response was evident at 6 h of sepsis. The reason for this apparent discrepancy may be explained by that changes in H_2-receptor protein levels do not always correspond to changes in its mRNA levels. However, we favor an alternative explanation, namely, that the impaired chronotropic responsiveness of atria to histamine is associated with a marked reduction in expression of G_s, which couples the H_2-receptor to its effector, in sepsis. We have recently provided evidence that the levels of $G_{s\alpha}$ protein and mRNA are greatly reduced in ventricular myocardium from LPS-treated rabbits (4). In the current study, determination of expression of $G_{s\alpha}$ protein in atrial myocardium by Western blotting showed a reduction of $57 \pm 3\%$ ($n = 4$) at 6 h of sepsis.

In conclusion, we found that H_1- and H_2-receptor antagonists significantly modified the hemodynaminc alterations in the rabbit model of septic shock. The data suggest that the hemodynamic alterations during sepsis is mediated in part by the overall 10- to 20-fold increase in circulating levels of histamine acting on H_1- and H_2-receptors. Our present results also indicated that cardiac H_1- and H_2-receptors and their signal transduction systems may be diversely modulated at the transcriptional levels during sepsis. However, it is unlikely that the contribution of endogenous histamine to the hemodynamic alterations of endotoxemia involves increased histamine receptors occurring at the level of gene expression.

REFERENCES

1. C.E. Wright, D.D. Rees and S. Moncada, Cardiovasc. Res., 26 (1992) 48.
2. D.J. Brackett, S.A. Hamburger, M.R. Lerner, S.B. Jones, C.F. Schaefer, D.P. Henry and M.F. Wilson, Agents Actions, 31 (1990) 263.
3. S.J. Hill, Pharmacol. Rev., 42 (1990) 45.
4. N. Matsuda, Y. Hattori, Y. Akaishi, Y. Suzuki, O. Kemmotsu and S. Gando, Anesthesiology, 93 (2000) (in press).
5. N. Matsuda, Y. Hattori, S. Gando, S. Watanuki, O. Kemmotsu and M. Kanno, Naynun-Schmiedeberg's Arch. Pharmacol., 361 (2000) 53.
6. Y. Hattori, I. Sakuma and M. Kanno, Eur. J. Pharmacol., 153 (1988) 221.
7. J. Van de Voorde and I. Leusen, Eur. J. Pharmacol., 87 (1983) 113.
8. P.R. Forfia, X. Zhang, F. Ochoa, M. Ochoa, X. Xu, R. Bernstein, P.B. Sehgal, N.R. Ferreri and T.H. Hinze, Am. J. Physiol., 274 (1998) H193.
9. Y. Hattori, Methods Find. Exp. Clin. Pharmacol., 21 (1999) 123.
10. S.B. Jones and F.D. Romano, Circ. Shock, 28 (1989) 59.
11. R.E. Shepherd, C.H. Lang and K.H. McDonough, Am. J. Physiol., 252 (1987) H410.
12. Y. Horio, Y. Mori, I. Higuchi, K. Fujimoto, S. Ito and H. Fukui, J. Biochem., 114 (1993) 408.

Histamine Research in the New Millennium
T. Watanabe, H. Timmerman and K. Yanai (Editors)

Histamine receptors in the chick cerebral cortex: effects on cyclic AMP formation and characterization by radioreceptor binding

J.B. Zawilska[a,b], A. Woldan-Tambor[a,b] and J.Z. Nowak[a]

[a]Department of Biogenic Amines, Polish Academy of Sciences, P.O.Box-225 Lodz-1, 90-950 Poland

[b]Department of Pharmacodynamics, Medical University of Lodz, 1 Muszynskiego St., Lodz, 90-151 Poland

Histamine (HA) is an established neurotransmitter/neuromodulator in the central nervous system (CNS) of vertebrate and invertebrate species [1-3]. Among various activities ascribed to HA, its ability to stimulate cyclic AMP (cAMP) formation was repeatedly demonstrated in different tissues and species, including the CNS of guinea pig and rabbit. The HA-evoked rise in cAMP formation usually results from activation of the H_2-type HA receptor. However, in some species, a H_2-receptor-mediated effect can be enhanced by a concomitant stimulation of H_1 receptors [1,3]. We have previously demonstrated that HA is a powerful stimulator of cAMP production in the pineal gland of domestic fowls, i.e., chick, duck and goose [4-7]. The action of HA was mediated by a H_2-like receptor, whose pharmacological profile is different from that described for its mammalian counterpart. In this study we characterized HA receptors in the cerebral cortex of chick using two approaches: (1) analysis of effects of selected HA-ergic drugs on cAMP synthesis, and (2) receptor binding of [^{3}H]tiotidine and [^{125}I]iodoaminopotenditine, selective H_2-antagonists.

1. MATERIALS AND METHODS
1.1. Animals
Male chicks were purchased locally on the day of hatching, and kept in warmed brooders with *ad libitum* standard food and water. Chicks were killed by decapitation; their brains were quickly removed, cerebral cortex without white matter was isolated and processed for biochemical measurements. The experiments were performed in strict accordance with the Polish governmental regulations concerning experiments on animals.

1.2 Assay of cyclic AMP formation
The formation of [^{3}H]cAMP in [^{3}H]adenine-prelabeled cortical slices (2,8-[^{3}H]adenine, 26.9 Ci/mmol, DuPont-NEN) was assayed as described by us earlier [4]. The formed [^{3}H]cAMP was isolated by a sequential Dowex-alumina chromatography, and the results were individually corrected for a percentage of recovery with the aid of [^{14}C]cAMP ([8-^{14}C]cAMP, 52.3 mCi/mmol, Du-Pont-NEN) added to each column system prior to the nucleotide extraction. The accumulation of cAMP during a 10-min stimulation period was assessed as percent conversion ([^{3}H]cAMP x 100/total ^{3}H).

1.3. Binding of [³H]tiotidine and [¹²⁵I]iodoaminopotentidine to cerebral cortical membranes

Binding assays were performed on crude membranes of chick cerebral cortex. Membranes (approximately 250 µg and 100 µg protein for [³H]tiotidine and [¹²⁵I]iodoaminopotentidine binding, respectively) were incubated in 50 mM Na_2HPO_4/KH_2PO_4 buffer, pH 7.4, for 90 min at 4°C in a total volume of 500 µl with the indicated concentrations of [³H]tiotidine (sp. act. 89.7 Ci/mmol; DuPont-NEN) or for 90 min at 30°C in a total volume of 100 µl with 0.15 nM [¹²⁵I]iodoaminopotentidine (sp. act. 2000 Ci/mmol; Amersham). The reaction was terminated by the addition of ice-cold phosphate buffer and immediate vacuum filtration through glass fiber filters GF/B. The filters were washed twice with phosphate buffer and the radioactivity trapped on the filters was measured. Specific binding of [³H]tiotidine and [¹²⁵I]iodoaminopotentidine was defined as that inhibited by 30 µM ranitidine and tiotidine, respectively. Data were analyzed using the GraphPAD InPlot program (GraphPad, San Diego, CA, USA).

1.4. Chemicals

The following chemicals were used: HA (Serva, Heidelberg, Germany); dimaprit, 2-methylHA, 4-methylHA, $N\alpha,N\alpha$-dimethylHA, *tele*-methylHA and 2-tiazolylethylamine (2-TEA) (kindly donated by Profs. R.C. Ganellin and M.E. Parsons, SmithKline & Beecham, Herts, UK); $R\alpha$-methylHA (RBI, Natick, MA, USA); aminopotentidine, and thioperamid (kindly donated by Prof. H. Timmerman, Vrije University, Amsterdam, the Netherlands), ranitidine, tiotidine and zolantidine (Tocris Cookson, Bristol, UK); mepyramine and triprolidine (Sigma Chemical Co., St. Louis, MO, USA).

2. RESULTS AND DISCUSSION

In agreement with earlier findings [8,9], in cerebral cortex of chick HA (0.1-1000 µM) stimulated cAMP production in a concentration-dependent manner, reaching maximal effect (three- to five-fold increase) at a concentration of 0.1 mM, and displaying an EC_{50} value of $\approx$ 2.5 µM (Fig. 1). Several HA-ergic compounds were tested for their ability to stimulate cAMP production in the chick cerebral cortical slices. The effect of HA was mimicked by agonists of HA receptors with the following rank order of potency: HA ($H_1 = H_2 = H_3$) $\geq$ 4-methylHA (H_2) > $N\alpha,N\alpha$-dimethylHA ($H_3 \gg H_2 = H_1$) > 2-methylHA (H_1) > $R\alpha$-methylHA (H_3) > 2-TEA (H_1) $\gg$ dimaprit (H_2) (inactive). The HA-like (imidazole-containing) compounds, known to be devoid of biological activity, such as *tele*-methylHA (Fig. 1), N-acetylHA, L-histidine, and imidazole (not shown), used at concentrations of 0.1 and 1 mM showed either no or very weak stimulatory action on cAMP accumulation.

The stimulatory effect of 100 µM HA was antagonized by selective HA H_2-receptor blockers: aminopotentidine, tiotidine, and ranitidine, of which the latter appeared to be approximately one to two orders of magnitude weaker than the two former drugs. Another selective H_2-antagonist, zolantidine, at the highest tested concentration 0.1 mM reduced the HA action only by 29%. Mepyramine and thioperamide, selective blockers of H_1- and H_3-HA-receptors, respectively, did not significantly affect the HA-evoked increase in cAMP synthesis (Fig. 2).

The results presented here extend our earlier observations made on pineal glands of chick, duck and goose [4-7] and on chick hypothalamus (unpublished data), where HA potently stimulated cAMP production, reaching maximal effect (five to ten fold increase, depending on

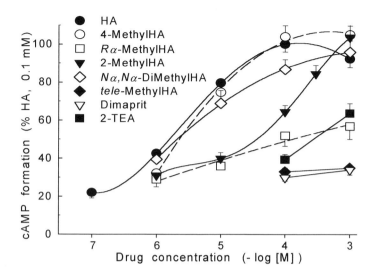

Figure 1. Effects of HA and agonists of H_1-, H_2- and H_3-HA receptors on cAMP formation in [^{3}H]adenine-prelabeled slices of chick cerebral cortex. The results are expressed as percentages of the HA response at 0.1 mM [3.88 ± 0.32% (n = 14) conversion, defined as 100%]. Data are mean ± SEM values (n = 4-12).

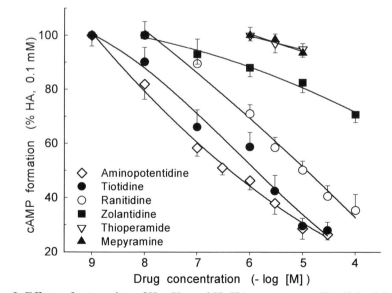

Figure 2. Effects of antagonists of H_1-, H_2- and H_3-HA receptors on HA (0.1 mM)-stimulated cAMP production in [^{3}H]adenine-prelabeled slices of chick cerebral cortex. The results are expressed as percentages of the HA response at 0.1 mM [4.01 ± 0.38% (n = 12) conversion, defined as 100%]. Data are mean ± SEM values (n = 5-12).

the tissue) also at 0.1 mM. The potency of various HA-ergic drugs to mimic or antagonize the action of HA on cAMP formation in chick cerebral cortex resembled that described for the avian pineal gland. Thus, methylated derivatives of HA, i.e., 4-methylHA, $N\alpha,N\alpha$-dimethylHA, and 2-methylHA appeared to be the most active drugs ($R\alpha$-methylHA displayed evidently poor activity), whereas compounds lacking an imidazole moiety (such as dimaprit and 2-TEA) were clearly less active or not active at all. Among tested blockers of H_2-HA receptors, zolantidine and cimetidine, displayed very weak antagonising activity towards the HA action. Taken together, the pharmacological profile of HA receptor in the chicken brain (whose activation leads to cAMP production) is different from that described for mammalian H_1-, H_2- and H_3-HA receptors.

The specific binding of [^{3}H]tiotidine to crude membranes of chick cerebral cortex was stable, saturable, reversible, and of high affinity. Concentration-dependent binding of [^{3}H]tiotidine (0.69-31.75 nM) to membranes of chick cerebral cortex resulted in a linear Scatchard plot suggesting binding to a single class of binding sites (Fig. 3). Scatchard analysis of the binding data revealed the apparent affinity constant $K_d = 4.36 \pm 0.8$ nM (n = 4) and the maximal number of binding sites $B_{max} = 369 \pm 32$ fmol/mg protein (n = 4).

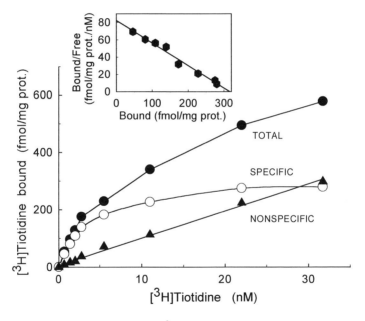

Figure 3. Concentration dependence of [^{3}H]tiotidine binding to membranes of chick cerebral cortex. Nonspecific binding was measured in the presence of 30 µM ranitidine. Specific binding was defined as total binding minus nonspecific binding. Values shown are means of a representative experiment performed in triplicate. Insert: transformation of the saturation data by the method of Scatchard.

The apparent affinity of [^{3}H]tiotidine binding sites in chick cerebral cortex is similar to that found in guinea-pig cerebral cortex ($K_d = 14.6$ nM). On the other hand, the maximum number of binding sites in chick cerebral cortex is significantly higher than the number obtained for guinea pig cerebral cortex (B_{max} = 102 fmol/mg protein)[10], a phenomenon most likely related to interspecies differences. It should be noted that using [³H]tiotidine as a radioligand, a portion of total binding accounting for so called specific binding was decisively larger in the case of the chick cortical tissue than that in guinea pig cortical membranes.

The pharmacological profile of the [³H]tiotidine and [¹²⁵I]iodoaminopotentidine binding sites in membranes of chick cerebral cortex was determined in competition experiments using selected HA-ergic compounds. The relative order of potency of the tested drugs to inhibit [³H]tiotidine binding to chick cerebral cortical membranes was: for antagonists - tiotidine >> ranitidine > zolantidine > thioperamide > triprolidine (Fig. 4A); and for agonists - HA > 4-methylHA > 2-methylHA > $R\alpha$-methylHA > dimaprit (Fig. 5). The relative order of potency of blockers of HA receptors to inhibit [¹²⁵I]iodoaminopotentidine binding to chick cerebral cortex was: aminopotentidine > zolantidine > ranitidine > tiotidine > thioperamide > triprolidine (Fig. 4B). The calculated K_i values for tiotidine (0.005 μM) and ranitidine (0.13 μM) for the inhibition of [³H]tiotidine binding to the chick cerebral cortex are similar to those obtained for the guinea-pig cerebrum [10]. However, in contrast to mammalian tissues [10,11], thioperamide and triprolidine (H₃- and H₁-receptor antagonist, respectively) inhibited [³H]tiotidine binding to the chick cerebrum, showing one- to two-orders of magnitude weaker activity than ranitidine. Thioperamide and triprolidine also inhibited the binding of [¹²⁵I]iodoaminopotentidine to chick cortical membranes (Fig. 4B).

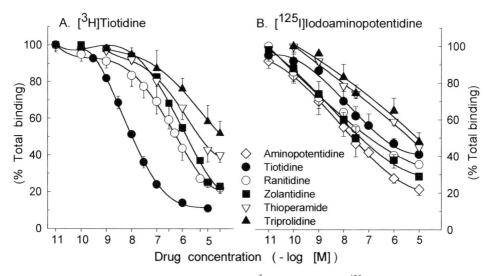

Figure 4. Competition curves for inhibition of [³H]tiotidine and [¹²⁵I]iodoaminopotentidine binding to membranes of chick cerebral cortex by antagonists of H₁-, H₂-, and H₃-HA receptors. Membranes were incubated with 1.65 nM [³H]tiotidine (**A**) or 0.15 nM [¹²⁵I]iodoaminopotentidine (**B**) and various concentrations of competing drugs. Values are means ± SEM from three to five independent experiments (each performed in triplicate).

In summary, the present data combined with our earlier results [4,5,7] indicate that chick brain contains H₂-like HA receptors. These receptors are linked to cAMP generating system

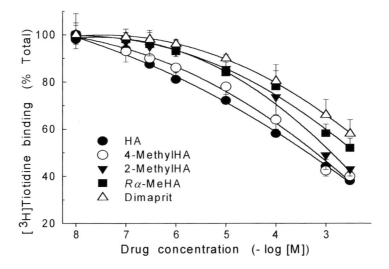

Figure 5. Competition curves for inhibition of [³H]tiotidine binding to membranes of chick cerebral cortex by agonists of H₁-, H₂-, and H₃-HA receptors. Membranes were incubated with 1.65 nM [³H]tiotidine and various concentrations of competing drugs (in the absence of GTP analogues). Values are means ± SEM from three to five independent experiments (each performed in triplicate).

and are specifically labelled by [³H]tiotidine and [¹²⁵I]iodoaminopotentidine. The pharmacological profile of the H₂-like receptor in the chick brain is different from that described for its mammalian counterpart, suggesting that it represents an avian-specific H₂-like HA receptor, or a novel HA receptor subtype.

Supported by the State Committee for Scientific Research in Poland (KBN; grant No 4 PO5A 104 16). The technical help of Mrs. T. Kwapisz and K. Konopka is highly appreciated.

REFERENCES
1. J.-C. Schwartz, J.M. Arrang, M. Garbarg, H. Pollard and M. Raut. Physiol. Rev., 71 (1991) 1.
2. D.L. Gruol and D. Weinreich. Brain Res., 162 (1979) 281.
3. S.J. Hill, C.R. Ganellin, H. Timmerman, J.-C. Schwartz, N.P. Shankley, J.M. Young, W. Schunack, R. Levi and H.L. Haas. Pharmacol. Rev., 49 (1997) 253.
4. J.Z. Nowak and B. Sek, J. Neurochem., 63 (1994) 1338.
5. J.Z. Nowak, B. Sek, T. D'Souza and S.E. Dryer. Neurochem. Int., 6 (1995), 519.
6. J.Z. Nowak, B. Sek and J.B. Zawilska. Neurosci. Lett., 202 (1995) 65.
7. J.Z. Nowak, A. Woldan-Tambor and J.B. Zawilska. Pol. J. Pharmacol., 50 (1998) 55.
8. S.R. Nahorski, K.J. Rogers, and M. Smith. Brain Res., 126 (1976) 126.
9. J.B. Zawilska, M. Kolodziejczyk and J.Z. Nowak . Pol. J. Pharmacol., 48 (1996) 589.
10. I.R. Smith, B.K. Leigh and M.E. Mylek. Agents Actions, 19 (1986) 169.
11. G.J. Sterk M.W.G. Van der Schaar, B. Rademaker, H. Van der Goot and H. Timmerman. Agents Action, 19 (1986) 131.

© 2001 Elsevier Science B.V. All rights reserved.
Histamine Research in the New Millennium
T. Watanabe, H. Timmerman and K. Yanai (Editors)

Histaminergic effect on apoptosis of small intestinal mucosa after ischemia-reperfusion in the rat

Kazuma Fujimoto, Ryuichi Iwakiri, Toshifumi Yoshida, Takahiro Noda, Masataka Kojima, Hiroyoshi Utsumi, Bin Wu, Keichiro Okada, Yasuhisa Sakata and Akifumi Ootani

Department of Internal Medicine, Saga Medical School, Nabeshima, Saga 849-8501, Japan

This study aimed to examine the relationship between a harmful effect of histamine and apoptosis following ischemia-reperfusion (I/R) in the small intestine. The superior mesenteric artery was occluded for 60 min followed by reperfusion for 60 min. Rats were infused with H_1-receptor antagonist (chlorpheniramine maleate) or H_2-receptor antagonist (cimetidine). Additional rats were pretreated with aminoguanidine. Percent fragmented DNA in the intestinal mucosa increased after reperfusion, but neither histamine antagonists had any effect on increased apoptosis. Aminoguanidine inhibited activity of diamine oxidase, increased the plasma histamine level, and attenuated the increase in apoptosis after I/R. Intestinal apoptosis induced by I/R was not related to an undesirable effect of histamine. Attenuation of increased apoptosis might be due to increased plasma histamine level and/or other pharmacological action of aminoguanidine including inhibition of inducible nitric oxide synthase.
Keywords: fragmented DNA, histamine antagonists, diamine oxidase, aminoguanidine

1. INTRODUCTION

Previous studies showed that circulating histamine, released from mucosal mast cells after prolonged ischemia-reperfusion (I/R) in the small intestine, had a systemic harmful effect on the mortality of animals [1,2]. In addition to the systemic harmful effect, histamine directly exacerbated intestinal mucosal injury after I/R and ethanol perfusion [1,3]. We have demonstrated that I/R with occlusion of the superior mesenteric artery induced apoptosis in the rat small intestinal mucosa [4], indicating that apoptosis might be related to mucosal injury after I/R in the small intestine. The aim of the present study was to examine the effect of histamine on apoptosis in order to determine whether an undesirable effect of histamine after I/R occurs through enhancement of apoptosis in the rat intestinal mucosa.

2. METHODS

2.1. Preparation of animals

Male SD rats were used in this study. Under halothane anesthesia, a laparotomy was performed. The superior mesenteric artery was occluded for 15 or 60 min with a micro-bulldog clamp, followed by reperfusion. In the rats, infused with histamine antagonists, a silicon infusion tube was introduced about 2 cm down the duodenum through the stomach [5].

2.2. Evaluation of apoptosis in the intestinal mucosa by % fragmented DNA

After euthanized, the entire small intestine was removed and placed on ice. The jejunum and ileum were removed, rinsed thoroughly with normal saline solution, and opened longitudinally to expose the intestinal epithelium. The mucosal layer was harvested by scraping of the epithelium using a glass slide. The mucosal scrapings were processed immediately after collection to minimize non specific DNA fragmentation. The amount of fragmented DNA was determined as previously described [4]. The results are expressed as percent fragmented DNA (fragmented DNA/ total DNA).

2.3. Effect of histamine antagonists and aminoguanidine on apoptosis after I/R

The animals were infused intraduodenally at 3 ml/h with saline solution (vehicle) throughout the experimental period starting just before I/R. Chlorpheniramine maleate (H_1-receptor antagonist) dissolved in vehicle at a dose of 2 μmol/h, or cimetidine (H_2-receptor antagonist) in vehicle at a dose of 10 μmol/h was infused. The additional animals were injected intraperitoneally with aminoguanidine dissolved in saline (100 mg/kg) 30 min before I/R. One h after 60 min ischemia, the animals were euthanized under anesthesia for collection of intestinal mucosa after blood sampling from the abdominal aorta.

To assay diamine oxidase activity, $[1,4-^{14}C]$putrescine was used as the substrate [1]. Homogenized intestinal mucosal scrapings were used for assay, as described elsewhere [1]. The plasma sample was treated with the perchloric acid mixture, and the clear supernatant after centrifugation (10,000 g for 30 min at 4°C) was used for histamine determination by performance liquid chromatography method [5].

3. RESULTS

3.1. Mortality rate of rats after I/R (from ref.[1])

Mortality rates of rats 24 h after 15 min or 60 min of ischemia are shown in Table 1. No rats pretreated with vehicle or aminoguanidine were dead at 24 h after sham operation or 15 min ischemia. The mortality rate of vehicle-pretreated rats following 60 min ischemia was 5/20 (25%), which was significantly increased compared to sham operation. This mortality rate after 60 min ischemia increased in rats pretreated with aminoguanidine, in which mucosal diamine oxidase activity decreased and consequently histamine content in plasma increased. The mortality rate in 60 min ischemic rats pretreated with aminoguanidine was attenuated by H_1-antagonist (chlorpheniramine maleate), but not by H_2-antagonist.

Table 1

Mortality rate of rats 24 h after ischemia induced by occlusion of superior mesenteric artery (from ref. [1])

	Duration of ischemia		
	sham	15 min	60 min
Pretreated with vehicle	0/14	0/14	5/20 *
Pretreated with aminoguanidine	0/14	0/14	12/20 **
Pretreated with aminoguanidine + H_1-receptor antagonist	—	—	2/10

Number of rats that died within 24 h after I/R of rats tested.

*=$P<0.05$, compared to sham. **=$P<0.05$, compared to vehicle pretreatment.

3.2 Effect of I/R on apoptosis in the small intestine (from ref.[4])

Results on % fragmented DNA in the jejunal mucosa before and after I/R are shown in Figure 1. In the 15 and 60 min ischemia groups, the percentage of fragmented DNA increased just after ischemia as compared to the values before ischemia ($P<0.05$ in each group), indicating that % fragmented DNA increased during ischemia. In the 60 min ischemia group, % fragmented DNA peaked at 1 h during reperfusion, and by 6 h post reperfusion, % fragmented DNA returned to baseline levels. In comparison, 15 min ischemia also resulted in enhanced

188

DNA fragmentation which peaked at 1 h during reperfusion, however, the magnitude of DNA damage at these times was less than that in the 60 min ischemia group (P<0.05).

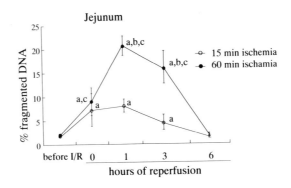

Figure 1. Percentage of fragmented DNA in the jejunal mucosa after I/R (from ref. [4])

Superior mesenteric artery was occluded for either 15 min (○) or 60 min (●) and then reperfused. a=P<0.05, compared to control value. b= P<0.05, compared to value at the end of ischemia. c=P<0.05, compared to 15-min ischemic group.

3.3 Effect of histamine antagonists and aminoguanidine on apoptosis (from ref. [7])

Table 2 shows the ratio of fragmented DNA to total DNA 60 min after 60 min ischemia in the rat intestinal mucosa. In sham treated controls, chlorpheniramine maleate, cimetidine, and aminoguanidine had no influence on % fragmented DNA, indicating that these agents themselves did not change apoptosis. Percentage of fragmented DNA increased significantly in the three I/R groups compared to the corresponding sham-treated control groups (P<0.05 in each). Both H_1-receptor antagonist and H_2-receptor antagonist had no effect on the increase of % fragmented DNA after I/R. Percent fragmented DNA increased after I/R in both the control and aminoguanidine groups (P<0.05 in each), but the increase was significantly attenuated by aminoguanidine pretreatment (P<0.05). Resolving agarose gel electrophoresis was performed for evaluation of the nature of the fragmented DNA in the jejunal and ileal mucosa after I/R. Agarose gel electrophoresis of the fragmented DNA obtained from the jejunal and ileal mucosa after I/R revealed distinct DNA ladders of characteristic of apoptosis [4,6].

Diamine oxidase activity in the intestinal mucosa was completely suppressed by aminoguanidine, an inhibitor of diamine oxidase. Concomitant with the decrease in diamine oxidase activity in the intestinal mucosa, histamine content in the plasma increased significantly (I/R rats pretreated with saline: 311 ± 55 pmol/ml, I/R rats pretreated with aminoguanidine, 2012 ± 166 pmol/ml; P<0.05).

Table 2

Effect of histamine antagonists and aminoguanidine on % fragmented DNA in the mucosa 60 min after reperfusion following 60 min ischemia induced by occlusion of superior mesenteric artery (from ref.[7])

	Ileum	Jejunum
Ischemia-reperfusion (I/R)		
Chlorpheniramine maleate (2 μmol/h)	30.4±1.1 *	31.3±4.4 *
Cimetidine (10 μmol/h)	32.0±5.1 *	36.2±5.3 *
Aminoguanidine (100mg/kg)	21.1±1.1 *,**	22.8±1.5 *,**
Vehicle	29.7±1.5 *	32.3±4.4 *
Sham		
Chlorpheniramine maleate (2 μmol/h)	4.4±1.2	5.5±2.4
Cimetidine (10 μmol/h)	3.6±2.5	4.3±3.1
Aminoguanidine (100 mg/kg)	4.4±1.2	5.5±2.4
Vehicle	4.2±2.1	6.5±1.4

*=P<0.05, compared to the corresponding sham-treated rats. **=P<0,05, compared to the corresponding rats pretreated with vehicle before I/R.

4. DISCUSSION

Histamine released from the intestinal mucosa after I/R had both an undesirable systemic effect and direct local mucosal damage of the intestine. I/R in the intestinal mucosa enhanced mucosal apoptosis [4], which might be an important factor leading to mucosal damage after I/R. Although H_1-antagonist diminished the undesirable effect of histamine after I/R, neither H_1- nor H_2- receptor antagonists had an effect on apoptosis in the intestinal mucosa after I/R with 60 min occlusion of the superior mesenteric artery. This data suggested that apoptosis in the intestinal mucosa was not related to the undesirable local effect of histamine after I/R.

Pretreatment with aminoguanidine increased histamine in the plasma concomitant with suppression of diamine oxidase activity, leading to attenuation of apoptosis in the intestinal mucosa after I/R. This result might be partly supported by previous reports that histamine, working as a growth factor, accelerated repair of damaged mucosa in the rat small intestine and that most of growth factors had an inhibitory effect on apoptosis [5,8]. Hansson et al. [9] demonstrated that monocyte-induced apoptosis in human natural killer cells was prevented by histamine, however, the histaminergic effect on apoptosis is inconsistent [10].

Aminoguanidine has other biological actions. Aminoguanidine pretreatment promoted uptake of putrescine from rat small intestine, though histamine itself competed with putrescine incorporation into rat enterocytes. Aminoguanidine, working as an inhibitor of inducible nitric oxide synthase, might attenuate apoptosis following I/R. In our preliminary study, other inhibitors of inducible nitric oxide synthase could inhibit apoptosis after I/R (data not shown).

In conclusion, the increase in apoptosis after I/R in the rat intestinal mucosa was not related to an undesirable effect of histamine. Increased histamine level pretreated with aminoguanidine attenuated intestinal mucosal apoptosis induced by I/R, which warrants further exploration regarding the effect of histamine and/or other factors including nitric oxide on apoptosis.

REFERENCES

1. J. Fujisaki, K. Fujimoto, R. Iwakiri, and Y.Yamaguchi, Dig. Dis. Sci., 38 (1993) 1195.
2. J. Kusche, W. Lorenz, C.D. Stahknecht, H. Richete, R. Hesterberg, A.Schmal, E. Hinterlang, D. Weber, and C. Ohmann, Gastroenterology, 80 (1981) 780.
3. S. Kanwar, and P. Kubes, Am. J. Physiol., 267 (1994) G316.
4. T. Noda, R. Iwakiri, K. Fujimoto, and T.Y. Aw, Am. J. Physiol., 274 (1998) G270.
5. K. Fujimoto K, I. Imamura, D.N. Granger, and P. Tso, J. Clin. Invest., 89 (1992) 126.
6. T.Y. Aw, P. Nicotera, and S. Orrenius, Arch. Biochem. Biophys., 283 (1990) 46.
7. T. Yoshida, R. Iwakiri, T. Noda, K., and K. Fujimoto, Dig. Dis. Sci., 45 (2000) 1138.
8. C.B.Thompson, Science 267 (1995) 1456.
9. M. Hansson, S. Hermodsson, and K. Hellstrand, Scand. J. Immunol., 44 (1996) 193.
10. P. Kubes and J.L.Wallace, Mediat. Inflamm., 4 (1995) 397.

Hypothalamus and histamine neurons

© 2001 Elsevier Science B.V. All rights reserved.
Histamine Research in the New Millennium
T. Watanabe, H. Timmerman and K. Yanai (Editors)

Changes in circadian rhythmicity and melatonin balance in rats with portacaval anastomosis (PCA) - relation with histamine

L. Tuomisto[1], A. Lecklin[1], V. Lozeva[1,4], M. Hippeläinen[2], M. Valtonen[3]

[1]Department of Pharmacology and Toxicology, University of Kuopio, P.O.Box 1627, FIN-70211, Kuopio, Finland

[2]Department of Surgery, Kuopio University Hospital, P.O.Box. 1777, FIN-70211, Kuopio, Finland

[3]Institute of Applied Biotechnology, University of Kuopio, P.O.Box 1627, FIN-70211, Kuopio, Finland

[4] Neuroscience Research Unit, Centre Hospitalier de l'Université de Montreal, Campus St-Luc, Montreal , Quebec, Canada

1. ABSTRACT

Patients with chronic hepatic encephalopathy (HE) have altered circadian rhythms, best demonstrated as disturbances in their sleep patterns. Similarly, the EEG recordings from rats with portacaval anastomosis (PCA), an animal model of HE, reveal less signs of drowsiness and sleepiness during the light hours, when the rats normally sleep. These rats also have flattened amplitudes of their circadian rhythms of locomotion and feeding. We have previously shown that increased brain histaminergic activity in rats with long-term PCA may have contributed to the development of these circadian changes. One potential mechanism could be a disturbance of melatonin balance. The 24 hour secretion of melatonin in the urine was highly significantly increased in rats with PCA. They also had higher daytime serum concentrations of melatonin, while the contents of melatonin and histamine in the pineal gland did not differ significantly between sham and PCA operated rats. Whether the elevation is transmitted by histaminergic system remains to be confirmed but it remains an attractive possibility.

2. BACKGROUND

Chronic hepatic encephalopathy (HE), a syndrome with a variety of CNS symptoms and signs, is a common complication of liver cirrhosis. In mild forms there may be no signs in routine clinical examination, but neuropsychological and neurophysiological tests may reveal mild personality changes, psychomotor deficits, cognitive disorders, and altered emotional behaviour and there may be EEG changes [1,2]. The quality of life of these patients may be impaired also by altered circadian rhythms, best demonstrated as disturbances in their sleep patterns [3]. Though there have been a number of studies over the years, neurochemical mechanisms of HE, also called portal systemic encephalopathy

(PSE), are still poorly understood.

Adequate animal models are helpful in establishing the mechanisms of HE. Portacaval anastomosis (PCA) technique in rats is used to bypass the liver so that the portal vein is surgically connected directly to vena cava [4,5]. This results in reduction of liver weight, reduction of growth of the animal associated with reduced food intake [6], and a number of behavioural changes related to those in clinical HE. These include disturbances in sleep patterns and diurnal rhythms [7] and a number of changes in brain neurotransmitters including GABA, glutamate and serotonin [cf. 8]. Some early findings also suggested changes in histaminergic systems [9,10].

3. NEUROCHEMICAL AND BEHAVIOURAL CHANGES IN PCA

3.1. Changes of histamine and its consequences in PCA rats

We have previously analysed histaminergic activity in the brain of rats with long-term PCA, and found that in addition to severalfold increase of histamine concentrations in the brain [11] also methylhistamine concentrations, more closely related to histamine turnover, are increased [12]. Moreover, brain dialysis studies revealed that both K^+ stimulation and administration of the H_3 antagonist thioperamide caused a larger histamine release from the hypothalamus of PCA than control rats [13] suggesting a functional increase in histaminergic systems and not simply an increase in storage (Fig.1).

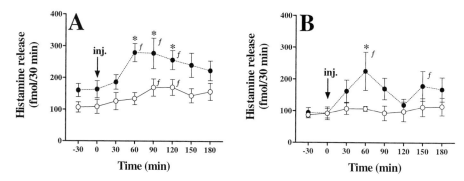

Figure 1. *Effects of systemic administration of thioperamide (3 mg/kg, i.p., indicated by an arrow), on the extracellular levels of histamine in anterior hypothalamus (**A**) and cortex (**B**) of sham-operated sham (O) or PCA operated (●) rats. Values are group means ± SEM; both n=6-7; f p<0.05 compared to basal release (repeated measures ANOVA, followed by Dunnett's test); * p<0.05 compared to sham-operated rats (ANOVA, followed by Scheffé's test).*

Histamine is involved in several rhythmic physiological functions, such as rhythms of ACTH release, locomotor activity, food intake, and sleep-wakefulness [14-16]. The release of histamine is higher during the active period [17,18], and histaminergic activity is connected with cellular mechanisms of arousal [19]. It has also been shown that histamine has a role in light entrainment of rhythms [20]. Therefore we studied possible connections between disturbed rhythms in PCA and changes in histaminergic systems

[21]. Computer-generated motility maps were produced and total activity was computed over a 72-hour period. The PCA-operation led to decreased movement time and velocity, and flattened the amplitude of the circadian rhythms of locomotion (Fig.2).

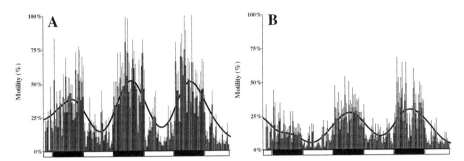

Figure 2. *Histograms of the spontaneous locomotor activity of sham-operated, saline-treated rats (A), and PCA-operated, saline-treated rats (B) with fluctuation curves of the 24-hr activity pattern. Each bar represents the mean value ± SEM of the percentage of time spent in movement in coincident 30-minute intervals of the 72-hour period of study for the 5 animals per group (100% = 30 min). Black sections in the horizontal bar indicate the dark phase. To improve the appearance of the fluctuation curves of the 24-hr activity pattern, the data were smoothed by replacing each point in the curve by the weighted average of its 13 nearest neighbours.*

Long term infusion of pyrilamine (mepyramine), an H_1 receptor blocker, by osmotic minipump increased the movement time and velocity in PCA rats, particularly in the dark phase, and improved the precision of circadian rhythms (Fig.3). This implies that a histaminergic imbalance contributes to the generation and maintenance of the decreased spontaneous locomotor activity and altered circadian rhythmicity in PCA rats.

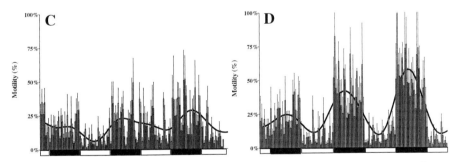

Figure 3. *Histograms of the spontaneous locomotor activity of sham-operated, pyrilamine-treated rats (C) and PCA-operated, pyrilamine-treated rats (D). Conditions as in Fig 2.*

3.2. Changes in EEG in PCA

The EEG recordings from rats with portacaval anastomosis, reveal less signs of drowsiness and sleepiness during the light hours, when the rats normally sleep [22,23]. These signs, the power density of the low frequency range, as well as the occurrence of

196

spindles, are inversely correlated with the histamine concentration in frontal cortex (Fig.4) while the power density decrease induced by H$_3$ receptor antagonist thioperamide correlates with the t-methylhistamine concentrations.

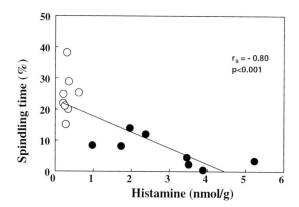

Figure 4. *Scatter plot and correlation between spindling time and frontal cortex histamine concentration in the combined group of sham- (○) and PCA-operated (●) rats 6 months after surgery. For each rat, the spindling time is expressed as percentage of the total recording time (100% = 3 hr); histamine concentrations are in nmol per gram of wet tissue weight. Statistics: Spearman rank coefficient (r$_s$).*

4. INVOLVEMENT OF MELATONIN

There are many reports linking histamine to the fundamental mechanisms of body rhythms [cf.14-16]. The suprachiasmatic nucleus, an important circadian pacemaker, receives a dense histaminergic innervation [24]. Histaminergic projections also reach the pineal gland [25] and pineal histamine concentrations exhibit a circadian rhythm 26]. The presence of histidine decarboxylase and histamine methyltransferase and the stimulation of cAMP synthesis by histamine in the chick pineal gland have been suggested to point to a regulatory function of histamine in the avian pineal gland [27]. The importance of histamine in the entrainment mechanisms of mammalian circadian rhythms has been recently emphasized [20].

Therefore one obvious question is, whether increased brain histaminergic activity in rats with long-term PCA may have contributed to the development of the observed circadian changes, and whether one potential mechanism could be an effect on melatonin balance, an important regulator of circadian rhythmicity.

The present experiments were carried out eight months after portacaval anastomosis or sham operations of the rats. The rats were housed under 12/12 hour light/dark conditions. Urine was collected for 24 hours and the rats were decapitated about 5 hours after switching on the lights. Serum was separated from the blood and the pineals were dissected. Melatonin was measured by radioimmunoassay [28] in the pineal gland, serum and urine of PCA and control rats. Pineal content of histamine was measured using HPLC [29]. Student's t-test was used to compare the means between groups.

The 24 hour secretion of melatonin in the urine was highly significantly ($p<0.001$) increased in rats with PCA as compared with the control animals (Fig 5). PCA rats also had higher daytime serum concentrations of melatonin ($p<0.01$)(Fig 5). The contents of melatonin in the pineal gland were 153.0 ± 18.5 and 122.9 ± 14.6 pg/gland and those of histamine 9 ± 3 and 20 ± 9 ng/gland in control and PCA rats respectively. These values did not differ significantly between sham and PCA operated rats.

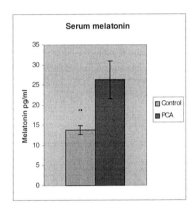 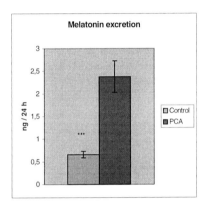

Figure 5. *Plasma concentration of melatonin (pg/ml) in control rats (n=15) and PCA operated rats (n=14) during the light hours is shown in the left figure.. Excretion of melatonin into urine during 24 hours is shown in the right figure. The values represent mean ± SEM.*

The results indicate that both the circulating melatonin levels during light hours and the excretion of melatonin are higher in PCA rats than in control rats. It is plausible that this can contribute to circadian abnormalities both in PCA and HE [30,31]. However, the mechanism of increased melatonin values cannot be resolved from these results. Melatonin is rapidly released from the gland after its synthesis, and no specific storage and release functions are known. The turnover of melatonin is fast and its half-life in the body is short. Therefore the dominating regulatory step of melatonin release is considered to be its synthesis. Whether in PCA rats the synthesis of melatonin is increased, secondary to increased histaminergic tone or by other factors related to PCA, or if its metabolism is decreased due to liver failure, remains to be examined.

REFERENCES

1. Bernuau J, Rueff B, Benhamou JP. Semin Liver Dis 1986;6:97.
2. Quero JC, Hartmann IJ, Meulstee J, Hop WC, Schalm SW. Hepatology 1996;24:556.
3. Cordoba J, Cabrera J, Lataif L, Penev P, Zee P, Blei A. Hepatology 1998;27:339.
4. Mullen KD, Roessle M, Jones DB, Grun M, Jones EA. Eur J Gastroenterol Hepatol

198

1997;9:293.

5. Lee SH, Fischer B. Surgery 1961;50:668.

6. Martin JR. Physiol Behav 1983;30:749.

7. Coy DL, Mehta R, Zee P, Salchli F, Turek FW, Blei AT. Gastroenterology 1992;103:222.

8. Butterworth RF. Adv Exp Med Biol 1994;368:79.

9. Imura K, Kamata S, Hata S, Okada A, Watanabe T, Wada H. Pharmacol Biochem Behav 1986;24:1323.

10. Fogel WA, Andrzejewski W, Maslinski C. J Neurochem 1991;56:38.

11. Fogel WA, Tuomisto L, Sasiak K, Rokicki W, Rokicki M, MacDonald E, Maslinski C. J Neurochem 1994;62:615.

12. Lozeva V, MacDonald E, Belcheva A, Hippeläinen M, Kosunen H, Tuomisto L. J Neurochem 1998a;71:1450.

13. Lozeva V, Attila M, Anttila E, Laitinen K, Hippeläinen M, Tuomisto L. Naunyn Schm Arch Pharmacol 1998b; 358:574.

14. Tuomisto L. :Involvement of histamine in circadian and other rhythms. In: Watanabe T, Wada H, editors. Histaminergic neurons: morphology and function. Boca Raton: CRC Press, 1991:283-295.

15. Schwartz JC, Arrang M, Garbarg M, Pollard H, Ruat M. Physiol Rev 1991;71:1.

16. Tuomisto L, Lozeva V, Valjakka A, Lecklin A. Behavioural Brain Res, in press.

17. Mochizuki T, Yamatodani A, Okakura K, Takemura M, Inagaki N, Wada H. Naunyn Schmiedebergs Arch Pharmacol 1991;343:190.

18. Prast H, Dietl H, Philippu A. J Auton Nerv Syst 1992;39:105.

19. McCormick DA, Williamson A. J Neurosci 1991;11:3188.

20. Jakobs EH, Yamatodani A, Timmerman H. Trens Pharmacol Sci 2000 21 293.

21. Lozeva V, Valjakka A, Lecklin A, Olkkonen H, Hippeläinen M, Itkonen M, Plumed C, Tuomisto L. Hepatology 2000;31:336.

22. Valjakka A, Vartiainen J, Kosunen H, Hippeläinen M, Pesola P, Olkkonen H, Airaksinen MM, Tuomisto L. J Neural Transm 1996;103:1265.

23. Lozeva V, Valjakka A, Anttila E, MacDonald E, Hippeläinen M, Tuomisto L. Hepatology 29 (1999) 340.

24. Panula P, Pirvola U, Auvinen S, Airaksinen MS. Neuroscience 1989;28:585.

25. Mikkelsen JD, Panula P, Moller M. Brain Res 1992;597:200.

26. Garbarg M, Julien C, Schwartz JC. Life Sci 1974;14:539.

27. Nowak JZ, Zawilska JB, Woldan-Tambor A, Sek B, Voisin P, Lintunen M, Panula P. J Pineal Res 1997;22:26.

28. Valtonen M, Laitinen JT, Eriksson L. J Endocrinol 1993;138:445.

29. Yamatodani A, Fukuda H, Wada H, Iwaeda T, Watanabe T. J Chromatogr 1985;344:115.

30. Zee PC, Mehta R, Turek FW, Blei AT. Brain Res 1991;560:17.

31. Zteindl PE, Finn B, Bendok B, Rothke S, Zee PC, Blei AT. Wien Klin Wochenschr 1997;109:741.

Histamine Research in the New Millennium
T. Watanabe, H. Timmerman and K. Yanai (Editors)

Histamine is a transmitter to maintain tonic firing of mesopontine tegmental cholinergic neurons during wakefulness

Y. Koyama, K. Takahashi and Y. Kayama

Department of Physiology, Fukushima Medical University School of Medicine, Fukushima, 960-1295, Japan

Abstract

In unanesthetized, head-restrained rats and cats, single neuronal activity was recorded from cholinergic neurons in the mesopontine tegmentum, and effects of iontophoretically-applied histamine on them were examined. The cholinergic neurons were classified into subgroups which showed different firing pattern across sleep-wakefulness conditions. Action of histamine was excitatory on virtually all cholinergic neurons active during both wakefulness and paradoxical sleep (activity during wakefulness was tonic, while that during paradoxical sleep was either tonic or bursting). Tonic activity during wakefulness, but not that during paradoxical sleep, was suppressed by application of an H_1 receptor antagonist. Cholinergic neurons of another subgroup, specifically active during paradoxical sleep and silent during wakefulness, were not affected by histamine. The results suggest that histamine is a major excitatory input to cholinergic neurons to maintain tonic firing during wakefulness.

Key words: laterodorsal tegmental nucleus, histamine, sleep, wakefulness, iontophoresis

Introduction

The cholinergic neurons in the mesopontine tegmentum, laterodorsal tegmental nucleus (LDT) and pedunculopontine tegmental nucleus (PPT), play an important role in the regulation of wakefulness (W) as well as paradoxical sleep (PS) [1-3]. A major subgroup of them in cats and rats is characterized by their tonic firing specifically during PS (PS-on neurons), while another by firing during both W and PS (WP neurons). Still another in cats is consisted of neurons showing, in addition to tonic firing during W, sporadic burst firing synchronously with PGO waves

(PGO-on neurons).

It has been hypothesized that PS is regulated by interaction of such cholinergic neurons and monoaminergic neurons which are active during W and silent during PS (PS-off neurons) [1, 2]. Histaminergic systems in the posterior hypothalamus, as well as other monoaminergic systems, have crucial roles in inducing and maintaining wakefulness [4]. The present study was done to examine the effect of histamine on the cholinergic neurons in the mesopontine tegmentum.

Materials and Methods

Male rats (Sprague-Dawley) and cats were prepared for recording single neuronal activity in unanesthetized, head-restrained condition. Under pentobarbital anesthesia (50mg/kg ip.), several stainless steel bolts were screwed to the skull to record electroencephalogram (EEG). A pair of stainless wires was inserted to the neck muscle for the recording of electromyogram (EMG). A plastic plate was mounted on the skull of the animals with dental cement; the plate was used for painless fixation of the head to a stereotaxic frame. In rats, sleep was deprived for 12 to 16 hours prior to recording session by placing them in a slowly rotating wheel while food and water were given *ad libitum*.

Neuronal activity was recorded through a glass pipette electrode filled with a 0.5 % sodium acetate solution containing 2 % Pontain Sky Blue in rats, and through a 32µm Formvar-coated stainless steel wire in cats. Drugs used were histamine dihydrochloride, noradrenaline hydrochloride, serotonin hydrochloride, diphenhydramine hydrochloride (H_1 antagonist) and sodium glutamate (All were 0.1-0.2 M). They were put in a multibarreled glass pipette which was glued to the recording electrode and were ejected iontophoretically. The cholinergic neurons in the brainstem were discriminated from the non-cholinergic ones by longer duration of action potentials [5].

Results

Histamine, when applied by current of less than 40 nA, increased firing in virtually all WP neurons in rats and cats. The excitation appeared reproducibly about 10 seconds after the current onset and continued about 20 seconds after the termination of it (Fig. 1A). Spontaneous firing of WP neurons during W was suppressed by application of H_1 antagonist (diphenhydramine), although the activity during PS was not affected by it.

Compared with the remarkable and consistent action of histamine on WP neurons, action of noradrenaline was inhibitory in rats (Fig. 1B), while excitatory in cats [6]. Action of serotonin was inhibitory in rats (Fig. 1C), though the inhibition was not so clear in cats [6].

Both in rats and cats, histamine had no effect on PS-on neurons in any sleep-wakefulness conditions. It was not due to bad condition of electrodes as checked by clear excitation by glutamate [7].

As in WP neurons, histamine exerted excitatory action in PGO-on neurons in cats; by application of histamine tonic firing increased during W or SWS. When

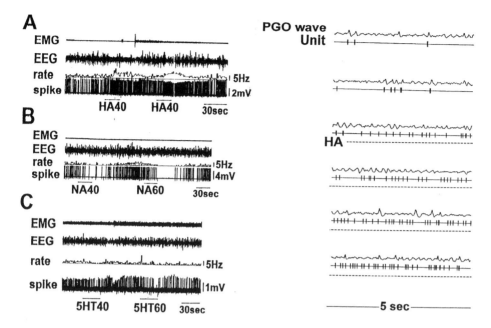

Figure 1. Effect of iontophoretically applied histamine (A), Noradrenaline (B) and serotonin (C) on cholinergic WP neuons.

Fifure 2. Change of firing pattern in a PGO-on neuron after application of histamine (dotted lines). Time proceeds from top to bottom.

histamine was applied during PS, the burst firing in synchronous with PGO waves was suppressed and replaced with tonic firing (Fig.2). Similar excitatory effect on PGO-on neurons was observed by application of glutamate or noradrenaline [6].

Discussion

In vitro studies using slice preparations have demonstrated that, a population of cholinergic neurons exhibit a burst firing which rides on a low threshold calcium spike when the neurons were hyperpolalized, while when depolarized, they show tonic firing [8, 9]. This suggest that the histamine-induced tonic firing of PGO-on neurons during PS is probably due to membrane depolalization. Thus, action of histamine was invariably excitatory, regardless of sleep-wakefulness conditions, in both WP and PGO-on cholinergic neurons.

The electrophysiological studies, showing that waking active (PS-off) neurons were recorded from the tuberomammillary region, where the histaminergic neurons were abundantly located [4, 10], strongly suggest that the histaminergic neurons in the posterior hypothalamus are waking active (PS-off) neurons similar to other monoaminergic (noradrenergic or serotonergic) neurons. It has been reported that histaminergic neurons project to wide areas in the brain including the cholinergic neurons in the LDT, and histamine infusion through microdialysis in this nucleus induces W [11]. These studies, together with the present result, suggest that histamine is a major factor for activating tonically, through H_1 receptor, the waking active mesopontine cholinergic (WP and PGO-on) neurons, and the cholinergic neurons may transmit the action to induce and/or maintain wakefulness.

Acknowledgenebts

This study was supported by a grant from the Ministry of Education, Science and Culture of Japan.

REFERENCES

1.K. Sakai, Exp. Brain Res. Suppl., 8 (1984) 3.
2.R.W. McCarley, R.W. Greene, D. Rainnie and C.M. Portas, Seminars in the Neurosc. 7 (1995) 341.
3.Y. Koyama, Y. Kayama and K. Sakai, In: B.N. Mallick, S. Inoue(eds.), Rapid Eye Movement Sleep, Narosa Publishing House, New Delhi, (1999) 221.
4.K. Sakai, M. El Mansari, J.S. Lin, J.G. Zhang and G. Vanni-Mercier, In: M. Mancia, C. Marini(eds.), The Diencephalon and Sleep, Raven Press, New York, (1990) 171.
5.Y. Koyama, T. Honda, M. Kusakabe, Y. Kayama and Y. Sugiura, Neuroscience, 83 (1998) 1105.
6.Y. Koyama and K. Sakai, Neuroscience, 96 (2000) 723.
7.K. Sakai and Y. Koyama, Neuroreport 7 (1996) 2449.
8.C.S. Leonard and R.R. Llinas, In: M. Steriade, D. Biesold(eds.), Brain Cholinergic Systems, Oxford University Press, Oxford (1990) 205.
9.A. Kamondi, J.A. Williams, B. Hutcheon and P.B. Reiner, J. Neurophysiol., 68 (1992) 1359.
10.T.L. Steininger, M.N. Alam, H. Gong, R. Szymusiak and D. McGinty, Brain Res., 840 (1999) 138.
11.J.S. Lin, Y. Hou, K. Sakai and M. Jouvet, J. Neurosci., 16 (1996) 1523.

© 2001 Elsevier Science B.V. All rights reserved.
Histamine Research in the New Millennium
T. Watanabe, H. Timmerman and K. Yanai (Editors)

Effect of leptin on feeding in histamine H_1-receptor knockout mice

Takayuki Masaki[a], Hironobu Yoshimatsu[a], Seiichi Chiba[a], Daisuke Tajima[a], Takeshi Watanabe[b] and Toshiie Sakata[a]

[a]Department of Internal Medicine, School of Medicine, Oita Medical University, Oita, Japan

[b]Department of Molecular Immunology, Medical Institute of Bioregulation, Kyushu University, Fukuoka, Japan.

Functional roles of histamine neurons in leptin signaling pathways that regulate energy intake was investigated using H_1-receptor (H_1-R) knockout (H1KO) mice. A bolus administration of leptin decreased feeding both in wild-type (WT) and H1KO mice. Leptin-induced daily feeding suppression was attenuated in H1KO mice. The result implicate that H_1-R contributes to regulation of feeding as a down-stream of leptin signals and that H1KO mice may be a useful animal model with leptin resistance.

1. INTRODUCTION

Histamine neurons originating from the tuberomamillary nucleus (TMN) project diffusely in the brain to regulate energy homeostasis and have been shown to suppress food intake through histamine H_1-receptors (H_1-R) (1, 2). Energy deficiency in the brain activates histamine neurons (3) and augments glycogenolysis in the brain (4). Leptin, an *ob* gene product, reflects energy stores in adipose tissue (5) and is capable of inhibiting food intake through action on the hypothalamus (6). Leptin has been recently demonstrated to promote histamine turnover by affecting the histamine release (7). The aim of the present study was to examine essential roles of histamine H_1-R in leptin signaling pathways using histamine H1KO mice.

2. MATERIALS AND METHODS

2.1. Implantation with a cannula into the lateral ventricle.
Mature male C57Bl/6J wild type (WT) (Seac Yoshitomi Ltd, Fukuoka, Japan) and H1KO mice (Kyushu University, Fukuoka, Japan).

2.2. Procedures of leptin treatment.
Murine recombinant leptin (Amgen Inc, Thousand Oaks, CA, USA) was injected *ip* at doses of 50μg/mouse. The procedures of PBS infusion in the control group were the same with those in the leptin group, as applicable.

204

2.3. Statistical analysis.

All the data were expressed as the mean±standard error of the mean (SEM). The statistical analysis of difference was assessed the unpaired *t* test for multiple comparison was used where appropriate control.

3. RESULTS AND DISCUSSION

Leptin infusion ip at the dose of 50 μg/mice decreased daily food intake both in H1KO and WT mice ($p<0.01$ for each). Leptin-induced feeding suppression was attenuated in H1KO mice compared with that in the corresponding WT controls ($p<0.05$). Together with the foregoing finding (6), infusion of leptin decreased food intake in WT mice. In contrast to the WT mice, the percent change in feeding induced by leptin was attenuated in H1KO mice compared with those in WT controls. It is indicated that the signaling pathways of leptin interact with those of histamine H-R in regulation of feeding.

However, the suppressive effects of leptin on feeding behavior were partially attenuated in H1KO mice, but not completely abolished. In this regard, brain mechanisms other than the H-R may contribute to feeding during leptin treatment. Our recent study demonstrated that histamine H-R regulates not only feeding but also adiposity and uncoupling protein family expression during chronic central leptin treatment (8). Taken together, H1KO mice provide an insight that H_1-R regulates energy balance as a down-stream signal of leptin's actions in the brain.

REFERENCES

1. Sakata T, Ookuma K, Fukagawa K, Fujimoto K, Yoshimatsu H, Shiraishi H, and Wada H Brain Res 441 (1988) 403-407
2. Fukagawa K, Sakata T, Shiraishi T, Yoshimatsu H, Fujimoto K, Ookuma K and Wada H Am J Physiol 256 (1989) R605-611
3. Sakata T, Kurokawa M, Oohara A, and Yoshimatsu H: A physiological role of brain histamine during energy deficiency. Brain Res Bull 35 (1994) 135-139
4. Oohara A, Yoshimatsu H, Kurokawa M, Oishi R, Saeki K, and Sakata T J Neurochem 63 (1994) 677-682
5. Zhang Y, Proenca R, Maffei M, Barone M, Leopold L, Friedman JM Nature 372 (1994) 425-432
6. Halaas JL, Gajiwala KS, Maffei M, Cohen SL, Chait BT, Rabinowitz D, Lallone RL, Burley SK, Friedman JM Science 269 (1995) 543-546
7. Yoshimatsu H, Itateyama E, Kondou S, Hidaka S, Tajima D, Kurokawa M, and Sakata T Diabetes 48 (1999) 1342-1346
8. Masaki T, Yoshimatsu H, Chiba S, Watanabe T and Sakata T Diabetes (*in press*)

© 2001 Elsevier Science B.V. All rights reserved.
Histamine Research in the New Millennium
T. Watanabe, H. Timmerman and K. Yanai (Editors)

Chronic histamine treatment improves impaired energy intake and hyperinsulinemia in diet-induced obese mice

Hironobu Yoshimatsu, Daisuke Tajima, Takayuki Masaki, Seiichi Chiba, Hitoshi Noguchi and Toshiie Sakata

Department of Internal Medicine I, School of Medicine, Oita Medical University, 1-1 Idaigaoka, Hasama, Oita, 879-5593. Japan.

To examine functional roles of hypothalamic histamine neurons in regulation of energy homeostasis in obese and/or diabetic states, the present study aimed to investigate effects of central administration of histamine on food intake, body weight and glucose metabolism in diet-induced obese (DIO) mice. Chronic infusion of histamine into the cerebroventricle (icv) ($0.05\,\mu$ mol/ body weight g/day for 5 days) remarkably decreased food intake and body weight ($p<0.05$ for each). Hyperglycemia was not improved by the icv infusion, but was hyperinsulinemia compared with the pair-fed controls ($p<0.05$). Activation of hypothalamic histamine neurons is thus effective on not only weight reduction but also improvement of insulin resistance in obese mice.

1.INTRODUCTION

The pathophysiological basis of obesity is poorly understood and a number of approaches have been employed to study the roles of leptin and neuropeptides in regulation of feeding behavior and energy homeostasis in different models of rodents (1-3). Recent studies have demonstrated that neuronal histamine plays an important role in regulation of feeding behavior and energy metabolism as a target of leptin action in the brain (4). Central administration of leptin elevated histamine turnover rate. The suppressive effect of leptin on food intake was attenuated both in histamine-depleted mice due to α-fluoromethylhistidine and in histamine H_1 receptor knock out (H1KO) mice (4,5). The decrease in fat deposition and the increase in uncoupling protein (UCP) expression induced by leptin were found to be partially mediated through histamine H_1 receptor (5). The present study aimed to investigate roles of histamine neurons in regulation of energy metabolism in obese animals. To address the issue, we examined effects of histamine loading on food intake, body weight and glucose metabolism in diet-induced obese (DIO) mice.

2.RESEARCH DESIGN AND METHODS

2.1 Animals and diet.
Mature male C57BI/6J mice were used. For preparation of diet-induced obesity, mice were fed with high-energy diet for 6 weeks. They were housed in a room illuminated daily from 07:00 to 19:00 hr (a 12:12 hr light-dark cycle) with ambient temperature at $21\pm1°C$ and humidity $55\pm5\%$. Number of rats used was 5 in each group.

206

Daily food intake and body weight were measured at 09:00 hr throughout the experiment. All studies were conducted in accordance with the Oita University Guideline for the Care and Use of Laboratory Animals based on the NIH Guideline.

2.2 Surgery and histamine infusion.
Under nembutal anesthesia (1mg/kg, ip), mice used were placed in a stereotaxic apparatus and implanted with a 29-gauge stainless steel cannula into the left lateral cerebroventricle (icv). Subjects were allowed one week of postoperative recovery. Through a 30-gauge stainless steel injector, histamine solution was infused icv at a dose of $0.05\,\mu$ mol/g body weight with an infusion speed of $1.0\,\mu$ l/10min daily for 5 successive days. Phosphate buffered saline (PBS) was infused icv at the same volume.
2.3 Procedures for blood sampling and chemical assay.
Blood samples were collected at the end of experiment through a catheter implanted chronically in the atrium through the jugular vein (5). After separation of serum, all the samples were stored at $-80°C$. Serum glucose and insulin were measured using commercially available kits (Merckaut Glucose, Kanto Chemical Co, Tokyo, Japan, Insulin [^{125}I] assay system, Amersham, Buckinghamshire, England).

2.4 Statistical analysis.
All the data were expressed as mean±S.E.M. Statistical significance was assessed by one-way analysis of variance (ANOVA) followed by Scheffe's multiple comparison test and two-way ANOVA with repeated measures. Probability of 0.05 was used as the threshold for statistical significance.

3.RESULTS AND DISCUSSION

The present study demonstrated that icv infusion of histamine decreased 24-hr cumulative food intake (23.3 ± 2.6 %) and body weight (19.2 ± 1.5 %) in DIO rats that were more predominant than those in the PBS controls (p<0.01 for each). DIO mice showed higher serum glucose (193.5 ± 10.2 mg/dl) and insulin concentrations ($92.3\pm6.5\,\mu$ U/ml) than controls (122.4 ± 10.1 mg/dl for glucose, $62.2\pm4.9\,\mu$ U/ml for insulin) (p<0.05 for each). Histamine infusion decreased serum insulin ($57.5\pm5.2\,\mu$ U/ml) (p<0.05) leaving serum glucose unaffected. PBS infusion showed no remarkable changes in glucose or insulin concentration.

Activation of hypothalamic histamine neurons has been shown to suppress food intake through H_1 receptor in the ventromedial hypothalamic and the paraventricular nuclei (6). The present study provided evidence that sustained histamine treatment was effective on reduction of food intake and body weight in even obese animal models. Hypothalamic histamine neurons have been shown to play their roles as a target of leptin in control of feeding behavior in rodents (4,5). DIO mice used in the present study was found insensitive to exogenous leptin treatment (7). Histamine neurons thus regulate feeding behavior as well as body weight in even leptin-resistant mice. Another factor besides feeding suppression, which is important for histamine-induced weight reduction, is acceleration of peripheral energy expenditure induced by neuronal histamine.

Our previous study demonstrated that activation of histamine neurons up-regulated expression of UCP1 mRNA in brown adipose tissue, an essential marker for peripheral energy expenditure (8).

The findings are supportive of the concept that histamine neurons involve in maintenance of energy homeostasis as a down-stream signal message in brain leptin cascade. In other words, the effect of neuronal histamine on weight reduction in obese animal models is regulated by its dual actions of decrease in energy intake and increase in energy expenditure.

Another important result demonstrated in the present study is that chronic activation of hypothalamic histamine neurons improves hyperinsulinemia in DIO mice without affecting hyperglycemia. Histamine treatment, on the other hand, is thus efficient on recovery of insulin resistance. Together with these findings, besides the effect of neuronal histamine on body weight reduction, it seems most probable that increase in sympathetic nerve activity induced by activation of hypothalamic histamine neurons may improve insulin sensitivity since sympathetic nerve activation accelerates glucose uptake into the skeletal muscle. In summary, histamine-mediated anti-obesity and anti-diabetic actions may help in development of therapeutic strategies for human obesity, insulin resistance and diabetes mellitus.

REFERENCES

1. Y. Zhang, R. Proenca, M. Maffei, M. Barone, L. Leopold and J.M. Friedman, Nature, 372 (1994) 425.
2. J. K. Elmquist, E. Maratos-Flier, C. B. Saper and J. S. Flier, Nature Neuroscience, 1 (1998) 445. Review.
3. W. Fan, B. A. Boston, R. A. Kesterson, V.J. Hruby and R. D. Cone, Nature, 385 (1997) 165
4. H. Yoshimatsu, E. Itateyama, S. Kondou, S. Hidaka, D. Tajima, M. Kurokawa and T. Sakata, Diabetes, 48 (1999) 1342
5. T. Masaki, H. Yoshimatsu, S. Chiba, T. Watanabe and T. Sakata, Diabetes (in press).
6. T. Sakata, H. Yoshimatsu, Nutrition, 13 (1997) 403.
7. M. V. Heek, D.S. Compton, C.F. France, R. P. Tedesco, A. B. Fawzi, M. P. Graziano, E. J. Sybertz, C. D. Strader and H. R. Jr. Davis, J. Clin. Invest., 99 (1997) 385
8. T. Masaki, H. Yoshimatsu, S. Chiba, T. Watanabe and T. Sakata, Diabetes (in press).

Histamine Research in the New Millennium
T. Watanabe, H. Timmerman and K. Yanai (Editors)

Neurotransmitter inputs to the tuberomammillary neurons

K.S. Eriksson, D.R. Stevens, R.E. Brown and H.L. Haas

Department of Physiology II, Heinrich-Heine-Universität, Moorenstrasse 5, D-40225 Düsseldorf, Germany

The neurons in the tuberomammillary nucleus of the ventral posterior hypothalamus innervate most parts of the brain. They exhibit a regular slow firing which is correlated with activity, the firing rate being lowest during sleep. The TM neurons store histamine and the anatomy of this neuronal system has been mapped with an antiserum against histamine.

With anatomical methods adrenergic, noradrenergic, serotonergic, GABAergic inputs as well as peptidergic (NPY, substance P) inputs have been demonstrated. Electrophysiological studies have revealed excitatory actions on the TM neurons mediated by glutamatergic NMDA and non-NMDA, nicotinic ACh and $5\text{-}HT_2$ receptors, and the neurons are also excited by ATP and orexin. An excitation by morphine is a presynaptic effect. Inhibitory inputs include actions on $GABA_A$ receptors and hyperpolarization by galanin and nociceptin.

Histamine has an important role in the regulation of the TM neurones. Agonists of the H_3 autoreceptor slow their firing and H_3-antagonists increase their firing rate.

1. Introduction

The neurons of the tuberomammillary (TM) nucleus in the posterior hypothalamus send out varicose axons that innervate most parts of the central nervous system (CNS) and release histamine (HA), which acts as a neurotransmitter. This system is a part of the ascending projections that consists of several mutually interacting aminergic systems [1-3].

The physiological functions in which the HAergic system has been implicated include regulation of the states of arousal and waking, energy metabolism and body temperature, locomotor, feeding and drinking behavior, and nociception. The possible role of the HAergic system in the control of wakefulness and attention has received much interest, since the activity of the TM neurons is strongly associated with behavioral state. Thus, these neurons fire tonically during waking, little during slow wave sleep and not at all during rapid-eye-movement (REM) sleep. Apart from this, a considerable body of evidence has accumulated indicating a role for HA in the control of energy metabolism and feeding behavior [4-8]. In this paper we review the current knowledge about afferent inputs to the TM nucleus.

2. Inputs to the tuberomammillary neurons

2.1. Tracing studies

Retrograde tracing in the rat brain of markers injected into the TM nucleus identified about 70 cell groups in the forebrain and brainstem. The majority of labeled neurons were found in the forebrain and especially in the infralimbic cortex, lateral septal nucleus and preoptic region. Comparatively fewer neurons were found in the brainstem, but all parts of the TM nucleus receive inputs from the brainstem monoaminergic nuclei. Characteristic for these afferents is that they usually do not enter the core of the TM nucleus but terminate immediately adjacent to the cell group and apparently contact the dendrites of the TM neurons [9,10].

These results suggest that the activity of the TM neurons is under the influence of inputs from many brain regions. For some of these inputs the neurotransmitter is known, and these inputs will be dealt with in the reminder of this paper.

2.2.Histamine

Histamine has an important role in the regulation of the TM neurons. The inhibitory H_3-receptor is present on the soma and dendrites as well as presynaptically on the terminals of the TM neurons [11]. Activation by HA of the H_3-receptor inhibits the neuron and the HA-release is therefore regulated by an autoinhibitory feedback system [12-14]. The H_3-receptor was recently cloned and it is a G-protein coupled receptor which is able to inhibit adenylate cyclase [15].

During intracellular recording from TM neurons in slices we have seen that the H_3-receptor agonist (R)α-methylHA inhibits their firing. Furthermore, the antagonist thioperamide increases the firing rate of these cells, which shows that they are under tonic inhibition by endogenous HA (unpulished results) [16]. Experiments *in vivo* showed that (R)α-methylHA increased deep slow wave sleep in the cat and inhibited HA-release in the rat, while thioperamide enhanced wakefulness and enhanced HA-release in these animals [17;18]. The decreased firing rate after stimulation of the H_3-receptor would by itself be sufficient to explain the observed attenuation of HA-release. Furthermore, since the H_3-receptor is present on HAergic terminals, a local inhibition of presynaptic Ca^{2+}-currents may be another mechanism for inhibition of HA-release. The influx of Ca^{2+} through N- and P-type Ca^{2+}-channels in the presynaptic membrane trigger neurotransmitter release and these channels are inhibited by the H_3-receptor [19;20].

2.3. Acetylcholine

The K^+-induced release of HA from rat cortical slices and synaptosomes is inhibited by the cholinergic system via presynaptic muscarinic M_1 receptors. Acetylcholinesterase inhibitors also decreased HA-release and this effect could be blocked by the muscarinic antagonist atropine, suggesting a modulation by endogenous acetylcholine. The M_1 mediated inhibition of HA-release has also been demonstrated in the hypothalamus *in vivo* [18;21;22].

Nicotine enhances HA-release from hypothalamic slices of the rat and this effect can be blocked with the nicotinic antagonist hexamethonium. Whole cell recordings from TM neurons support this. Thus, both acetylcholine and nicotine elicit different inward, excitatory currents which would increase HA-release. The involved receptor is a α-bungarotoxin-sensitive cationic channel containing the $α_7$-subunit [23 24]. These results indicate that nicotinic and presynaptic muscarinic cholinergic receptors have antagonistic effect on the release of HA.

2.4. Catecholamines

All parts of the TM contain a dense network of noradrenergic fibers which make synaptic contacts with the dendrites, but not somata, of the TM neurons. Much fewer of these fibers appear to be dopaminergic or adrenergic. Retrograde tracing revealed that these fibers emanate mainly from the noradrenergic A1 and A2 and adrenergic C1, C2 and C3 groups in the ventrolateral and dorsomedial medulla, while the innervation from the locus coeruleus, substantia nigra and ventral tegmental area is much less prominent [9].

The release of HA in the rat is inhibited by the noradrenergic system and this inhibition has been demonstrated to be mediated by the $α_2$ receptor. Thus, noradrenaline inhibits the release of HA from K^+-depolarized cortical slices, indicating that $α_2$ receptors are located presynaptically on HAergic terminals. Noradrenaline also decreases HA-release from the hypothalamus *in vivo*. The $α_2$ antagonist yohimbine increases the basal release of HA from the hypothalamus, and this indicates that HA-release is tonically inhibited by noradrenaline [25-27].

Dopamine influences the release of HA in a dual way. Stimulation of D_2 receptors increases the release of HA, while D_3-receptors attenuate it [28]. Exactly where the involved receptors are located is not known, but the mammillary nuclei of both rat and human brain exhibit a high expression of the D_3-receptor, while the D_2-receptor binding and mRNA is dense in the human TM nucleus [29 30]. Although the D_2-receptor commonly has inhibitory actions, these results would suggest that the D_2-mediated excitation is postsynaptic and that the TM nucleus receives afferents from e.g. the mammillary nuclei expressing presynaptic D_3-receptors.

2.5. Serotonin

Both the medial and lateral parts of the TM nucleus receive serotonergic inputs which originate from the dorsal raphe, medial raphe, pontine tegmental reticular and the pontine raphe nuclei. The peripheral, dendritic, rather than the central regions of the subnuclei are innervated and the very few observed serotonergic synaptic contacts are restricted to the dendrites [9].

In vivo microdialysis studies have shown that serotonin (5-HT) increases HA release in rat hypothalamus and that the involved receptor belongs to the 5-HT$_2$ group [31]. During intracellular recording studies on rat hypothalamic slices we have demonstrated that 5-HT excites the TM neurons and increases their firing. It is a postsynaptic effect that appears to be mediated via 5-HT$_{2C}$ receptors that activate the Na$^+$/Ca^{2+}-exchanger which leads to depolarization[32].

A recent study done on mice showed that oral administration of 5-HT$_{2A}$ receptor antagonists increases the level of the HA-metabolite *tele*-methylHA in several brain regions [33]. That would indicate tonic inhibition of HA-release by 5-HT via 5-HT$_{2A}$ receptors. The location of these receptors is not clear but our present results show that, at least in the rat, they are not on the somata or dendrites of the TM neurons. One possibility is that they are presynaptically located on e.g. interneurons, where they might modulate the recently described GABAergic inputs to the TM neurons [34]. Another possibility is inhibition of HA-release by 5-HT$_{2A}$ receptors on the axon terminals of the TM neurons. An inhibitory action on HA turnover by the 5-HT$_{1A}$-receptor has also been suggested in both rat and mice [35]. In that study an agonist and an antagonist of 5-HT$_2$ receptors had no effect on HA turnover in the mouse, and a species difference is possible.

2.6 GABA

Injection of the GABA$_A$-receptor agonist muscimol into the TM region of the cat causes a strong hypersomnia, while the GABA$_A$ antagonist picrotoxin increases basal HA release in the hypothalamus. The TM neurons also exhibit postsynaptic potentials that can be blocked with the GABA$_A$-receptor antagonist bicuculline [34;36;37]. GABA-like immunoreactivity has been demonstrated in synapses contacting the TM neurons, and one of the regions that send a GABAergic projection into the TM nucleus is the ventrolateral preoptic nucleus. Sleep-active neurons in this nucleus provide a prominent innervation of the TM nucleus. About 80% of these neurons are immunoreactive to both the GABA-synthesizing enzyme glutamic acid decarboxylase and the neuropeptide galanin and therefore probably inhibitory. Electrical stimulation of this region leads to GABA$_A$-mediated responses in the TM nucleus [38 39-41]. These findings strongly suggest an important role for the TM nucleus in the induction or maintenance of sleep. Another region that provides the TM nucleus with GABAergic inputs is the diagonal band of Broca [41]. The GABAergic input to the TM neurons is under inhibitory control by presynaptic GABA$_B$-receptors which suppress the inhibitory GABAergic transmission [34].

2.7. Glutamate

Microdialysis studies in the rat *in vivo* have shown that glutamate increases the release of HA through NMDA-receptors located on HAergic terminals. Application of a NMDA antagonist, (AP-5) alone decreased the basal HA-release, which indicates that there is a tonic glutamatergic excitation of the TM neurons [42]. Electrical stimulation in horizontal slices of the lateral preoptic and anterior lateral hypothalamic area result in both inhibitory and excitatory responses in the TM neurons. The excitatory responses could be blocked with NMDA- (AP-5) and non-NMDA- (CNQX or NBQX) receptor antagonists [41]. Consistent with this, the NMDA1 receptor is expressed throughout the hypothalamus and in most neurons in the mammillary area, and the kainate-preferring glutamate receptor GluR6 is also present in the mammillary region [43]

2.8. Galanin

Galanin applied to hypothalamic slices hyperpolarized the TM neurons and decreased their firing rate. An increased input resistance indicated that the hyperpolarization was caused by a reduction of an inward current [44]. Galanin also reduced HA-release from hypothalamic and hippocampal preparations, suggesting presynaptic inhibition of HAergic nerve endings by galanin [45]. About half of the TM neurons in the rat contain galanin, and the galanin immunoreactivity is located in vesicles which also are present in axosomatic synapses on these neurons [46;47]. The GABAergic projection from the ventrolateral preoptic area also contains galanin [40].

2.9. Opioids

Increased release of HA in the periaqueductal gray and striatum has been demonstrated after subcutaneous or intracerebroventricular injections of the μ-receptor agonists morphine and DAMGO *in vivo* [48;49]. In a later study Chikai and Saeki (1995) saw a decreased cortical release of HA after injections of DAMGO into the TM nucleus [50]. There is convincing evidence that CNS HA plays a central role in the analgesic actions of morphine [51]. Studies *in vitro* on cortical slices have shown that κ-receptors, decrease HA-release from axons innervating the cortex [52]. In the mammillary region of the hypothalamus the μ-receptors are the most densely expressed opioid receptors but κ-receptors are also present [53]. We tested the effect of a μ-agonist, morphine, and a κ-agonist, dynorphin. Morphine increased the firing of TM neurons in slices while dynorphin lacked any effect. The excitation by morphine appears to be a presynaptic effect and the target may be GABAergic terminals on TM neurons. These findings are consistent with the earlier reports showing that μ-receptor agonists increase HA-release *in vivo*.

2.10. Nociceptin

The recently isolated neuropeptide nociceptin /orphanin FQ excerts strong inhibitory actions in all tested brain regions and it modulates many functions [54]. During intracellular recordings from TM neurons in hypothalamic slices we saw that nociceptin strongly inhibited the firing of the TM neurons and hyperpolarized them. It was a postsynaptic effect that was associated with a decreased input resistance. The current-voltage relation and sensitivity to Ba^{2+} and Cs^+ indicated the involvement of an inwardly rectifying K^+-channel[55].

2.11. Leptin

The peptide hormone leptin is secreted from white adipose tissue and suppresses food intake. There is evidence that leptin excerts its actions by enhancement of HA-release. A bolus injection of leptin elevates the turnover rate of HA and suppresses food intake in rats and mice. If the animals are pretreated with the irreversible inhibitor of histidine decarboxylase, α-fluoromethylhistidine, the effect of leptin is either strongly attenuated or abolished. In agreement with this, leptin has no effect on food intake in mice lacking H_1-receptors. In leptin-deficient obese mice the HA turnover is lower than in lean littermates and this can be corrected by leptin infusion [56;57]. Weak leptin receptor immunoreactivity is present in the TM nucleus [58].

2.12. Purines

TM neurons are excited by ATP and the underlying mechanism is opening of nonselective cation channels. The P2X2 receptor subunit of the ATP-gated ion channels is also present in the TM nucleus [59;60]. The TM neurons are immunoreactive for adenosine deaminase, the enzyme that catabolizes adenosine, and this suggests that these neurons are targets for neurotransmission involving this nucleoside [61]. Injection of CGS21680, an agonist for the adenosine A_{2A} receptor, into the posterior hypothalamus of the rat significantly promoted sleep, especially REM sleep [62].

2.13. Other compounds

Injections of the endogenous pyrogen interleukin-1β into the TM nucleus leads to increased release of HA in the anterior hypothalamus [63]. Treatment with the cyclooxygenase inhibitor indomethacin completely blocked this effect, indicating that the production of prostaglandins is involved in the mechanism. In keeping with this, icv injection of prostaglandin E_2 increased the HA turnover [64]. This suggests that interleukin-1β suppresses feeding via prostaglandin E_2-production, thereby increasing HA-release from the TM neurons.

Nitric oxide has been reported to inhibit HA-release. Studies *in vivo* have shown that hypothalamic superfusion of NO-donors decrease the extracellular HA-level. This effect can be blocked by atropin, indicating that NO acts on the cholinergic system which in turn affect muscarinic receptors on the TM neurons [65]. Other immunocytochemically characterized inputs to the TM neurons contain neuropeptide Y, substance P and thyrotropin releasing hormone [47;66].

3. Discussion

In comparison with other transmitter systems, such as monoamines and acetylcholine, the HAergic system has received less attention. There are several reasons for this, but the most important is probably the fact that reliable and sensitive methods for localization and quantitation of HA did not become available until the middle of the eighties [2;67;68], while such methods for studies of catecholamines and 5-HT were available 10-20 years earlier. It is obvious that the TM nucleus receives modulatory inputs from many brain regions and neurotransmitter systems and that the effect of any single input to the TM nucleus will be modulated by many others.

The firing rate of the individual neurons, and thereby the rate of HA-release, is controlled at least at two levels. First, the intrinsic firing rate of each individual TM neuron is very stable, even when the neuron is synaptically isolated. Secondly, the inhibitory feedback system mediated via the H_3-receptor should have a stabilizing effect on the excitability of the whole nucleus. This suggests that the rate of HA-release is under a very strict control and that very strong inputs are needed to change the HA-release. Recent findings suggest the involvement of the HAergic system in sleep-waking regulation. The projection from the ventrolateral preoptic area, containing the two inhibitory neurotransmitters GABA and galanin, may provide such a powerful input, and may be the factor that abolishes TM firing during REM sleep.

Eating disorders and obesity are rampant in western societies. A better understanding of the HAergic system, with its central involvement in the regulation of food-intake and activity may provide clues as to how these trends could be reversed. Much interest has focussed on the role of leptin, and recent studies which have been cited above indicate that leptin´s anorexic actions are mediated by HA. Thus we anticipate a greatly increasing interest in the HAergic system.

References

1. H. L. Haas and A. Konnerth, *Nature* 302, 432-434 (1983).
2. P. Panula, H. Y. Yang, E. Costa, *Proc.Natl.Acad.Sci.U.S.A* 81, 2572-2576 (1984).
3. P. Panula, U. Pirvola, S. Auvinen, M. S. Airaksinen, *Neuroscience* 28, 585-610 (1989).
4. R. Leurs, P. Blandina, C. Tedford, H. Timmerman, *Trends Pharmacol.Sci.* 19, 177-183 (1998).
5. J. S. Lin, K. Sakai, M. G. Vanni, M. Jouvet, *Brain Res.* 479, 225-240 (1989).
6. K. Onodera, A. Yamatodani, T. Watanabe, H. Wada, *Prog.Neurobiol.* 42, 685-702 (1994).
7. T. Sakata, H. Yoshimatsu, M. Kurokawa, *Nutrition* 13, 403-411 (1997).
8. J. C. Schwartz, J. M. Arrang, M. Garbarg, H. Pollard, M. Ruat, *Physiol Rev.* 71, 1-51 (1991).
9. H. Ericson, A. Blomqvist, C. Kohler, *J.Comp Neurol.* 281, 169-192 (1989).
10. H. Ericson, A. Blomqvist, C. Kohler, *J.Comp Neurol.* 311, 45-64 (1991).
11. H. Pollard, J. Moreau, J. M. Arrang, J. C. Schwartz, *Neuroscience* 52, 169-189 (1993).
12. J. M. Arrang, M. Garbarg, J. C. Schwartz, *Nature* 302, 832-837 (1983).
13. J. M. Arrang et al., *Nature* 327, 117-123 (1987).
14. Y. Itoh, R. Oishi, M. Nishibori, K. Saeki, *J.Neurochem.* 56, 769-774 (1991).
15. T. W. Lovenberg et al., *Mol.Pharmacol.* 55, 1101-1107 (1999).
16. H. L. Haas, in *The Histamine Receptor*, J. C. Schwartz and H. L. Haas, Eds. (Wiley-Liss Inc., New York, 1992) ,chap. 8.
17. J. S. Lin et al., *Brain Res.* 523, 325-330 (1990).
18. H. Prast, H. P. Fischer, M. Prast, A. Philippu, *Naunyn Schmiedebergs Arch.Pharmacol.* 350, 599-604 (1994).
19. P. Fossier, L. Tauc, G. Baux, *Trends Neurosci.* 22, 161-166 (1999).
20. Y. Takeshita et al., *Neuroscience* 87, 797-805 (1998).
21. C. Gulat Marnay, A. Lafitte, J. M. Arrang, J. C. Schwartz, *J.Neurochem.* 52, 248-254 (1989).
22. R. Oishi, N. Adachi, K. Okada, N. Muroi, K. Saeki, *J.Neurochem.* 55, 1899-1904 (1990).
23. J. Ono, A. Yamatodani, J. Kishino, S. Okada, H. Wada, *Methods Find.Exp.Clin.Pharmacol.* 14, 35-40 (1992).
24. V. V. Uteshev, D. R. Stevens, H. L. Haas, *Pflugers Arch.* 432, 607-613 (1996).

25. C. Gulat Marnay, A. Lafitte, J. M. Arrang, J. C. Schwartz, *J.Neurochem.* 53, 513-518 (1989).
26. S. J. Hill and R. M. Straw, *Br.J.Pharmacol.* 95, 1213-1219 (1988).
27. H. Prast, M. Heistracher, A. Philippu, *Naunyn Schmiedebergs Arch.Pharmacol.* 344, 183-186 (1991).
28. H. Prast, M. Heistracher, A. Philippu, *Naunyn Schmiedebergs Arch.Pharmacol.* 347, 301-305 (1993).
29. M. L. Bouthenet et al., *Brain Res.* 564, 203-219 (1991).
30. E. V. Gurevich and J. N. Joyce, *Neuropsychopharmacology* 20, 60-80 (1999).
31. K. S. Laitinen, L. Tuomisto, J. T. Laitinen, *Eur.J.Pharmacol.* 285, 159-164 (1995).
32. K. S. Eriksson, D. R. Stevens, H. L. Haas, *Neuropharmacology*, in press.
33. S. Morisset et al., *J.Pharmacol.Exp.Ther.* 288, 590-596 (1999).
34. D. R. Stevens, A. Kuramasu, H. L. Haas, *Eur.J.Neurosci.* 11, 1148-1154 (1999).
35. R. Oishi, Y. Itoh, K. Saeki, *Naunyn Schmiedebergs Arch.Pharmacol.* 345, 495-499 (1992).
36. K. Okakura-Mochizuki, T. Mochizuki, Y. Yamamoto, A. Horii, A. Yamatodani, *J.Neurochem.* 67, 171-176 (1996).
37. M. Sallanon et al., *Neuroscience* 32, 669-683 (1989).
38. H. Ericson, C. Kohler, A. Blomqvist, *J.Comp Neurol.* 305, 462-469 (1991).
39. J. E. Sherin, P. J. Shiromani, R. W. McCarley, C. B. Saper, *Science* 271, 216-219 (1996).
40. J. E. Sherin, J. K. Elmquist, F. Torrealba, C. B. Saper, *J.Neurosci.* 18, 4705-4721 (1998).
41. Q. Z. Yang and G. I. Hatton, *Brain Res.* 773, 162-172 (1997).
42. K. Okakura, A. Yamatodani, T. Mochizuki, A. Horii, H. Wada, *Eur.J.Pharmacol.* 213, 189-192 (1992).
43. A. N. van den Pol, I. Hermans-Borgmeyer, M. Hofer, P. Ghosh, S. Heinemann, *J.Comp Neurol.* 343, 428-444 (1994).
44. B. Schonrock, D. Busselberg, H. L. Haas, *Agents Actions* 33, 135-137 (1991).
45. J. M. Arrang, C. Gulat Marnay, N. Defontaine, J. C. Schwartz, *Peptides* 12, 1113-1117 (1991).
46. C. Kohler et al., *J.Comp Neurol.* 250, 58-64 (1986).
47. M. S. Airaksinen, S. Alanen, E. Szabat, T. J. Visser, P. Panula, *J.Comp Neurol.* 323, 103-116 (1992).
48. K. E. Barke and L. B. Hough, *J.Neurochem.* 63, 238-244 (1994).
49. T. Chikai, R. Oishi, K. Saeki, *J.Neurochem.* 62, 724-729 (1994).
50. T. Chikai and K. Saeki, *Neurosci.Lett.* 196, 137-139 (1995).
51. L. B. Hough and J. W. Nalwalk, *Brain Res.* 588, 58-66 (1992).
52. C. Gulat Marnay, A. Lafitte, J. M. Arrang, J. C. Schwartz, *J.Neurochem.* 55, 47-53 (1990).
53. A. Mansour et al., *J.Comp Neurol.* 350, 412-438 (1994).
54. T. Darland, M. M. Heinricher, D. K. Grandy, *Trends Neurosci.* 21, 215-221 (1998).
55. K. S. Eriksson, D. R. Stevens, H. L. Haas, *Neuropharmacology* 39, 2492-2498 (2000).
56. T. Morimoto et al., *Physiology and Behavior* 67, 679-683 (1999).
57. K. Yoshimatsu et al., *Diabetes* 48, 2286-2291 (1999).
58. M. L. Hakansson, H. Brown, N. Ghilardi, R. C. Skoda, B. Meister, *J.Neurosci.* 18, 559-572 (1998).
59. K. Furukawa, H. Ishibashi, N. Akaike, *J.Neurophysiol.* 71, 868-873 (1994).
60. R. Kanjhan et al., *J.Comp Neurol.* 407, 11-32 (1999).
61. E. Senba, P. E. Daddona, T. Watanabe, J. Y. Wu, J. I. Nagy, *J.Neurosci.* 5, 3393-3402 (1985).
62. S. Satoh et al., *Eur.J.Neurosci.* 11, 1587-1597 (1999).
63. M. Niimi, T. Mochizuki, Y. Yamamoto, A. Yamatodani, *Neurosci.Lett.* 181, 87-90 (1994).
64. M. Kang, H. Yoshimatsu, M. Kurokawa, R. Ogawa, T. Sakata, *Proc.Soc.Exp.Biol.Med.* 220, 88-93 (1999).
65. H. Prast, C. Lamberti, H. Fischer, M. H. Tran, A. Philippu, *Naunyn Schmiedebergs Arch.Pharmacol.* 354, 731-735 (1996).
66. R. Tamiya, *Osaka City Med.J.* 37, 107-122 (1991).
67. N. Takeda et al., *Proc.Natl.Acad.Sci.U.S.A* 81, 7647-7650 (1984).
68. A. Yamatodani, H. Fukuda, H. Wada, T. Iwaeda, T. Watanabe, *J.Chromatogr.* 344, 115-123 (1985).

© 2001 Elsevier Science B.V. All rights reserved.
Histamine Research in the New Millennium
T. Watanabe, H. Timmerman and K. Yanai (Editors)

The difference of leptin-histamine signaling in the hypothalamus of obese animal models.

Hironobu Yoshimatsu, Emi Itateyama, Katsuro Himeno, Toshiie Sakata

Department of Internal Medicine I, School of Medicine, Oita Medical University, 1-1 Idaigaoka, Hasama, Oita, 879-5593. Japan.

Leptin, an *ob* gene product, has been shown to regulate energy intake and expenditure partially through hypothalamic histamine (HA) neurons. The present study was designed to examine differential characteristics of leptin-HA signal message among leptin-receptor deficient Zucker fatty (*fa/fa*), Ootsuka Long Evans Tokushima Fatty (OLETF) and diet-induced obese (DIO) rats. Hypothalamic HA concentration was decreased in *fa/fa* rats ($p<0.05$) but remained at the control level in OLETF rats. Contrary, HA concentration was increased in DIO rats loaded with sucrose for 20 weeks ($p<0.05$), but not in those for 4 weeks. Plasma leptin concentrations were higher in all of those obese models except DIO rats for 4 weeks than those in corresponding controls ($p<0.01$ for each). Leptin-HA signal message in the hypothalamus was thus completely and partially disrupted in *fa/fa* rats and OLETF rats, respectively, but unaffected in DIO rats. These findings implicate that the involvement of HA neurons in development of obesity depends on difference in pathogenesis of obesity in each animal model.

Key words: hypothalamic histamine neurons, leptin, Zucker fatty (*fa/fa*) rat, OLETF rats, diet-induced obese (DIO) rats.

1. INTRODUCTION

Leptin, an *ob* gene product, secreted from the adipose tissue has been shown to regulate food intake and fat deposition through its actions in the hypothalamus (1,2). Recently, histamine (HA) neurons were found to play an essential role as one of leptin targets in the hypothalamus (3). Infusion of leptin into the cerebroventricle (icv) increased HA turnover assessed by accumulation of *tele*-methylhistamine (*t*-MH), a major HA metabolite. Suppressive effects of leptin on food intake and body weight were attenuated by depletion of neuronal HA using α-fluoromethylhistidine (FMH), a suicide inhibitor of HA synthesizing enzyme (3). Targeted disruption of HA H_1 receptor (H1KO) in mice mimicked those results (4). Accelerating effect of leptin on uncoupling protein 1 (UCP1) in the brown adipose tissue (BAT), a marker of peripheral thermogenesis and energy expenditure, was similarly attenuated in H1KO mice. These results indicate that hypothalamic HA neurons are involved through its H_1 receptor in regulation of energy intake and expenditure as downstream transduction of leptin actions in the brain.

The leptin-HA signal pathway may thus contribute to homeostatic regulation of energy balance. Disruption of this signal message is probable to disarrange maintenance of homeostatic energy metabolism that leads to obesity. Indeed, hypothalamic HA concentration was decreased in both leptin-deficient *ob/ob* mice and leptin-insensitive *db/db* mice (3) (E.I., H.Y., T.S., unpublished data). To examine whether the leptin-HA signal message may be essential for prevention from development of obesity, the present study was aimed to assess effects of leptin production on activity of hypothalamic HA neurons in a variety of obese animal models.

2. MATERIAL AND METHOD

2.1 Animals and diet

Male Zucker fatty (*fa/fa*) rats of 18-week (wk) of age weighing 582 ± 20g, their lean littermates (+/+) weighing 324 ± 16g, Ootsuka Long Evans Tokushima Fatty (OLETF) rats of 32-wk of age weighing 680 ± 11g, their lean littermate Long Evans Tokushima Otsuka (LETO) rats weighing 435 ± 8g and Wistar King A rats weighing 295 ± 15g were used. To produce diet-induced obesity (DIO), WKA rats were simultaneously exposed *ad libitum* to liquid diet containing 34% sucrose and standard rodent pellets. Measuring consumption of sucrose solution and rodent food, both parameters of total energy intake and body weight were recorded weekly. Number of rats used was 5 in each group. All studies were conducted in accordance with the Oita University Guideline for the Care and Use of Laboratory Animals based on the NIH Guideline.

2.2 Assay of plasma leptin

Blood samples were collected at the end of experiment through a catheter implanted chronically in the atrium through the jugular vein (4). After separation to plasma, all the samples were stored under deep freeze. All rats were killed under sodium pentobarbital anesthesia (45mg/kg) to dissect the hypothalamus. The samples from DIO rats were taken 4 and 20 weeks after sucrose loading. Plasma leptin concentration was quantitated using a radioimmunoassay (RIA) kit (Linco Co. Ltd., St. Louis, MO, USA).

2.3 HA measurement

The hypothalamus was separated immediately on an ice plate from the dissected brain. The tissue was immediately frozen on dry ice and stored at $-80°C$ until the assay. HA concentration was measured by high performance liquid chromatography (5). The details of the amine assay have been described elsewhere (6).

2.4 Statistics analysis

Statistical analysis for measurements of amines was carried out by the Mann-Whitney U test.

3. RESULTS

Calculating both sucrose and rat chaw intake, total energy intake in the 20-week DIO group was greater than that in their controls, while consumption in the 4-week group did not differ significantly from that in the controls (data not shown). Consequently, the 20-week DIO increased body weight (578 ± 15g) than the controls (521 ± 7g) (p<0.05), but not in case of the 4-week DIO groups (DIO, 390 ± 11g; the controls, 383 ± 12g). Plasma leptin concentration showed no significant difference between the 4-week DIO group and the controls (data not shown), but plasma leptin increased more in the 20-week DIO group than in their controls

(DIO, 12.6±3.3; controls, 1.6±0.3 ng/ml; p<0.01). Leptin levels in both *fa/fa* rats and OLETF rats were higher than those in their lean littermates (*fa/fa*, 45.4±5.6; lean, 5.6±1.3 ng/ml; p<0.01. OLETF, 46.3±4.1; LETO, 10.4±2.1ng/ml; p<0.01).

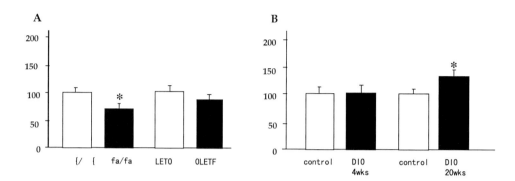

Figure. Percentage differences in concentrations of hypothalamic histamine in Zucker fatty (*fa/fa*) rats, OLETF rats (A) and diet-induced obese (DIO) rats with 4 or 20 weeks sucrose loading (B) Values, mean ± S.E. (n=5 for each), *=p<0.05.

Hypothalamic HA concentration did not differ between the 4-week DIO and the control groups, but elevated more in the 20-week DIO group than in the controls (p<0.05) (Fig. 1-A). In contrast to DIO rats, HA concentration in *fa/fa* rats was lower than that in their lean littermates (p<0.05). OLETF rats showed no significant difference of HA concentration compared with LETO rats (Fig. 1-B).

4. DISCUSSION

Obese animal models used in the present study showed hyperleptinemia in response to their fat accumulation. From the viewpoint of functional relation between leptin and HA, it seems quite probable that over-secretion of leptin may activate HA neurons. Unexpectedly, the effect of hyperleptinemia on hypothalamic HA concentration was dependent on each obesity model. These results indicate that obesity *per se* is not a main factor that regulates HA concentration. Rather, known and unknown factors that disrupt the leptin-HA signal message may be involved in those obese animal models. Leptin actions in the brain are disrupted by mutation of leptin receptor in *fa/fa* rats (7). For this reason, the present result that hypothalamic HA concentration decreased in *fa/fa* rats is consistent with our previous reports (8). Akin to the present result, our previous study showed that hypothalamic HA concentrations in leptin-deficient *ob/ob* and leptin-insensitive *db/db* mice (7, 9, 10) were decreased (3) (E.I., H.Y., T.S., unpublished observation). Obesity animals with disruption of leptin message are thus lowered in HA concentration because of deficit in leptin signaling toward HA neurons.

The present results revealed another type of unresponsiveness to leptin message as shown in OLETF rats. Regardless of hyperleptinemia, HA concentration was unaffected in OLETF rats. Secretion potency of leptin as well as its receptor is considered to be naive in OLETF rats, while its susceptible gene has not been identified to date. It seems probable that unknown factor(s) except leptin deficiency or leptin receptor abnormality may partially interrupt leptin-HA signal message in OLETF rats. One possible explanation for the query is leptin resistance.

218

The findings that plasma leptin levels are significantly higher in obese animals and humans have led to a concept that obese individual is relatively insensitive to endogenous leptin signal (11,12,13). If the concept would be accepted in OLETF rats, leptin resistance in the animals may disrupt transduction of leptin to HA neurons. Hyperleptinemia expressed as an indicator of leptin resistance was ascertained in OLETF rats in the present study. Difference in HA concentration between *fa/fa* rats and OLETF rats, moreover, implicates that disruption of leptin-HA signaling may be incomplete in OLETF rats compared with *fa/fa* rats.

The present DIO rats at 4-week sucrose loading showed no remarkable changes in either hypothalamic HA or plasma leptin. A key regulator affecting HA level in the hypothalamus may not be sucrose *per se*. Hypothalamic HA concentration was conversely increased in DIO rats with 20-week sucrose load when those rats gained body weight markedly (3). Elevation of plasma leptin concentration was similarly demonstrated in those rats, indicating existence of leptin resistance in DIO rats. Together with those findings, hypothalamic HA neurons in DIO rats seem to be ordinarily activated by leptin despite their leptin resistance. Development of leptin resistance is known to depend on how long dietary treatment was carried out, how much amount of calorie was loaded, and which species of animal were involved in (13). DIO animals treated with sucrose reveal an increase in food intake, but develop to mild and slowly progressive obesity (K.H., H.Y., M.K., T.S., unpublished observation). Hypothalamic NPY mRNA expression was over-expressed in *ob/ob* and *db/db* mice (14) and *fa/fa* rats (15) because of deficiency in leptin actions. In contrast, DIO rats loaded with sucrose for 20 weeks did not differ significantly in NPY mRNA (K.H., H.Y., S.H., M.K., T.S., unpublished observation). These findings lead us to an assumption that leptin resistance may not have been developed enough by sucrose load within 20 weeks. The assumption is supported by the present results that the grade of hyperleptinemia was milder in DIO rats than those in *fa/fa* and OLETF rats. Taken together, it is reasonable to imply that leptin-HA signal message may play one of essential roles to prevent mammals from development of obesity and still keep its function effective during progression of diet-induced obesity until the period when leptin resistance develops potently enough to disrupt its signaling. The concept is supported by the studies on H1KO mice. H1KO mice loaded with high fat diet developed obese more severely than wild type controls (4). Exogenous HA supplementation was found to be effective on reduction of food intake and body weight even in obese *db/db* and DIO mice (16).

In summary, we demonstrated that leptin-HA signal message was disrupted in a different way depending on obesity animal models. Suppression or acceleration of HA-neuron activity in turn affects feeding behavior and energy expenditure differently that determines development of obesity in those animal models.

Acknowledgements. This study was supported partly by Grant-in-Aid 07457225 from the Japanese Ministry of Education, Science and Culture and by Research Grants from the Japanese Fisheries Agency for Research into Efficient Exploitation of Marine Products for Promotion of Health, 1998-1999.

REFFERENCES
1. J.L. Halaas, K.S. Gajiwaka, M. Maffei, S.L. Cohen, B.T. Chait, D. Rabinowitz, R.L. Lallone, S.K. Burley and J.M. Friedman JM, Science, 269 (1995) 543.
2. L.A. Campfield, F.J. Smith, Y. Guisez, R. Devos and P.R. Burn, Science, 269 (1995) 546.
3. H. Yoshimatsu, E. Itateyama, S. Kondou, D. Tajima, K. Himeno, S. Hidaka, M. Kurokawa and T. Sakata, Diabetes, 48 (1999) 2286.
4. T. Masaki, H. Yoshimatsu, S. Chiba, T. Watanabe and T. Sakata, Diabetes, (2000) in press.

5. R. Oishi, Y. Itoh, M. Nishibori and K.Saeki, J. Neurochem., 49 (1987) 541.
6. A. Oohara, H. Yoshimatsu, M. Kurokawa, R. Ooishi, K. Saeki and T. Sakata,
    J. Neurochem., 63 (1994) 677.
7. S.C. Chua, W.K. Chung, X.S. Wu-Peng, Y. Zhang, S. M. Lui, L. Tartaglia and R.L. Leibel,
    Science, 271 (1996) 994.
8. H. Yoshimatsu, H. Machidori, T. Doi, M. Kurokawa, K. Ookuma, M. Kang and T. Sakata,
    Physiol. Behav., 54 (1992) 487.
9. G.H. Lee, R. Proenca, J.M. Montez, K.M. Carroll, J.G. Darvishzadeh, J.I. Lee and J.M.
    Friedman, Nature, 398 (1996) 632.
10. Y. Zhang, R. Proenca, M, Maffei, M. Barone, L. Leopord and J.M. Friedman, Nature, 372
    (1994) 425.
11. M. Maffei, J. Halaas, E. Ravussin, R.E. Pratley, G.H. Lee, Y. Zhang, H. Fey, S. Kim,
    R. Lallone, S. Ranganathan, P.A. Kern and J.M. Friedman, Nature Med, 1 (1995) 1155.
12. R.V. Concidine, M.K. Sinha, M.L. Heiman, A. Kuriauciunas, T.W. Stephens, M.R. Nyce,
    J.P. Ohanneisian, C.C. Marco, L.J. McKee, T.L. Bauer and J.F. Caro, N. Engl. J. Med.,
    334 (1996) 292.
13. M.V. Heek, D.S. Compton, C.F. France, R.P. Tedesco, A.B. Fawzi, M.P. Graziano,
    E.J. Sybertz, C.D. Strader and H.R.Jr. Davis, J. Clin. Invest., 99 (1997) 385.
14. T.W. Stephens, M. Basinski, P.K. Bristow, J.M. Bue-Valleskey, S.G. Burgett, L. Craft,
    J. Hale, J. Hoffmann, H.M. Halung, A. Kriauclunas, W. Mackellar, P.R. Jr. Rostack,
    B. Schoner, D. Smith, F.C. Tiasley, X. Zhang and M. Helman, Nature, 377 (1995) 530.
15. G. Sanacora, M. Kershaw, J.A. Finkelstein and J.D. White, Endocrinology, 127
    (1996) 216.
16. T. Masaki, H. Yoshimatsu, S. Chiba, T. Watanabe and T. Sakata, Diabetes, (2000) in press.

© 2001 Elsevier Science B.V. All rights reserved.
Histamine Research in the New Millennium
T. Watanabe, H. Timmerman and K. Yanai (Editors)

A possible involvement of the chorda tympani in the enhancement of the hypothalamic histamine release by leptin

T. Morimoto-Ishizuka, Y. Yamamoto, K. Yamamoto, T. Hashimoto, and A. Yamatodani

Department of Medical Physics, School of Allied Health Sciences, Faculty of Medicine, Osaka University, 565-0871 Osaka, Japan

Leptin is a satiety factor, which is secreted from the white adipose tissue. The anorectic effect of leptin is thought to be expressed by acting on the hypothalamus, but the mechanism of this effect is not fully understood. We previously showed that leptin, controls feeding through the histaminergic system via histamine H_1 receptors in mice. In the present study, we studied a possible pathway through which leptin activates the histaminergic system. Histamine release from the anterior hypothalamus of rats examined by *in vivo* microdialysis was significantly increased by the intraperitoneal administration of leptin (1.3 mg/kg), whereas the intracerebroventricular injection of leptin (10 μg/rat) did not cause any significant changes in the histamine release. In the rats whose the chorda tympani nerve, a branch of the facial nerve which mediates taste information, were transected bilaterally, leptin injection (1.3 mg/kg, i.p.) had no effect on the histamine release. These findings indicate that leptin activates the histaminergic system by peripheral signal inputs via the chorda tympani.

Keywords: Leptin; Histamine; Microdialysis; The chorda tympani; Food intake

1. INTRODUCTION

The *ob* gene product leptin, which is secreted from white adipose tissue, plays an important role in the control of energy homeostasis [1]. Since the intracerebroventricular (i.c.v.) injection of leptin can reduce food intake and increase energy expenditure resulting in a reduction of body weight [2], the actions of leptin are thought to be expressed by the activation of leptin receptors in the hypothalamus. However, the mechanism of this effect is not fully understood.

Histamine is suggested to be involved in the regulation of food intake. The findings that i.c.v. injection of histamine or H_1-agonist decreased food intake [3] and that infusion of H_1-antagonist into the ventromedial hypothalamus or the paraventricular nucleus increased food intake [4] indicate that the central histamine decreases food intake through H_1 receptors. We hypothesized that the central histaminergic system is a target for leptin in its control of feeding, and previously reported that the pretreatment of α-fluoromethylhistidine, a specific and irreversible inhibitor of histidine decarboxylase, can abolish the effect of leptin and the intraperitoneal (i.p.) injection of leptin had no effect on food intake in H_1-receptors knock-out mice [5].

However, Lecklin et al. [6] recently showed that i.c.v. injection of leptin did not affect the contents of histamine and *tele*-methylhistamine, the main metabolite of histamine, in the hypothalamus while leptin actually reduced food intake. Based on these results, some peripheral inputs seem to participate in the activation of the histaminergic system by leptin. The chorda tympani (CT), a branch of the facial nerve, distributes to the anterior tongue and has been considered an important nerve for taste sensation [7]. Kawai et al. [8] showed that i.p. Leptin suppressed a response of the CT to sweet substances and leptin receptors were expressed in taste cells. Therefore, the CT is a possible candidate for the regulation of food intake by leptin at the peripheral level.

Thus, to study a possible pathway through which leptin activates the histaminergic system, we examined the difference between the hypothalamic histamine releases when leptin was injected intraperitoneally or intracerebroventricularly using *in vivo* microdialysis in anesthetized rats. Moreover, we also investigated the involvement of the CT in mediating the effect of leptin on the histaminergic system.

2. MATERIAL AND METHODS

2.1. Experiment 1: The effect of leptin on histamine release

Male Wistar rats (180-260g) were housed individually with a 12:12-h light-dark cycle. All animals had free access to standard pelleted chow (Oriental Yeast Co., Osaka, Japan) and tap water except the day before experiment.

Overnight fasted rats were anesthetized with urethane (1.2 g/kg, i.p.) and placed on a stereotaxic apparatus (Kopf Instrument, Tujunga, CA, USA) for microdialysis. The microdialysis probe (CMA/10, membrane length 2mm, CMA/Microdialysis, Stockholm, Sweden) aimed at the anterior hypothalamus was inserted using the following coordinates: AP, -1.5; LM, -0.5; DV, 9.2mm relative to the bregma and the skull surface [9]. Probes were perfused with artificial cerebrospinal fluid (CSF) composed as described previously [10]. CSF was perfused at a rate of 1 μl/min. To achieve stabilization of the histamine release, dialysates obtained during the first 2 hours were discarded, thereafter dialysates were collected every 20 min. After first 3 fractions (baseline samples) had been collected, rats were injected with murine recombinant leptin (1.3mg/kg, i.p, n=5; Amgen Inc., Thousand Oaks, CA, USA) or saline (n=5). The dose of the leptin we used has been reported to be effective in activating neurons in the rat hypothalamus [11]. Dialysates were collected for 4 h after drug administration. Histamine levels in dialysate fractions were determined by an HPLC-fluorometric method [12] with slight modification [10].

For the i.c.v. Injection, the guide cannula was implanted before the dialysis probe was inserted, aimed above the third ventricle as follows: AP, -4.5; LM, 0; DV, 4.8 mm relative to the bregma and the skull surface [9]. The guide cannula was fixed to the skull with dental acrylic cement, and then the dialysis probe was inserted. After collecting baseline samples, an injection cannula was inserted through the guide cannula. The tip of the injection cannula extended 2.0 mm below that of the guide cannula. The injection cannula was connected to a Hamilton microsyringe via polyethylene tubing. Murine recombinant leptin (10 μg/rat, n=6) or saline (n=4) was intracerebroventricularly infused at a rate of 5 μl/min. The infusion volume was 10 μl. This dose of leptin has been reported to induce suppression of food intake [6]. After drug administration, dialysates were collected for 4h.

2.2. Experiment 2: The effect of i.p. Leptin on histamine release in the CT-transected rats

Rats (n=10) were anesthetized with sodium pentobarbital (50 mg/kg). The external reveal auditory meatus was widened, and the tympanic membrane were partially removed to the CT, which was then cut with forceps bilaterally (CTX).

After a minimum 3 days recovery period, the microdialysis procedure was carried out as described above. After baseline samples were collected, the CTX rats were injected with leptin (1.3 mg/kg, n=5) or saline (n=5) as the control. Dialysates were collected for 4h after injection.

2.3. Statistical Analysis

The statistical significance was analyzed using a one-way analysis of variance. If significant main effects were found, data were further analyzed by post-hoc Newman-Keuls test.

3. RESULTS

3.1. Experiment 1: The effect of leptin on histamine release

The mean basal histamine releases of rats injected with leptin and that of control were 0.07 ±0.01 pmol/ 20 min and 0.08 ±0.01 pmol/ 20 min, respectively. As shown in Fig.1A, infusion of leptin caused a significant increase in the histamine release over the basal release ($F(14, 56)=6.38$, $p<0.01$), while saline injection had no effect on the histamine release ($F(14, 56)=0.41$, $p=0.96$). The mean basal histamine releases of rats treated with i.c.v. leptin and that of controls were 0.05 ±0.001 pmol/20 min and 0.05 ±0.004 pmol/20 min, respectively. Unlike the i.p. injection, the i.c.v. infusion of leptin did not affect the histamine release over the basal release ($F(14, 70)=0.98$, $p=0.48$), which was similar to the saline injection ($F(14, 42)=0.95$, $p=0.52$) (Fig. 1A).

3.2. Experiment 2: The effect of i.p. leptin on histamine release to the CTX rats

In the CTX rats, the mean basal level of histamine was 0.08 ±0.010 pmol/20 min and 0.08

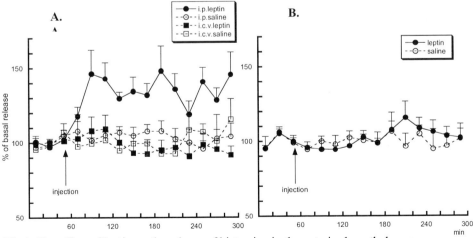

Fig.1. The effect of leptin on the release of histamine in the anterior hypothalamus.

The mean basal releases are taken as 100%. Values are presented as mean and SEM. ** $p<0.01$, * $p<0.05$ compared with the basal release of each group. (A) i.p. and i.c.v. injection, (B) i.p. injection in the CTX rats.

±0.007 pmol/20 min in leptin-injected rats and in the controls, respectively. No change was observed in the histamine level over the basal release in either leptin-injected rats (F(14, 56)=1.36, p=0.20) or in control rats (F(14, 56)=0.46, p=0.94) (Fig. 1B).

4. DISCUSSION

In this study, we could clearly show that i.p. leptin increased histamine release in the hypothalamus (Fig.1A). Thus, leptin is proved to be able to facilitate the hypothalamic histamine release. However, i.c.v. leptin did not increase histamine release (Fig. 1A). This finding is in agreement with an earlier observation that centrally administrated leptin did not affect the hypothalamic contents of histamine and *tele*-methylhistamine [6], and leptin is suggested to enhance histamine release via the peripheral nerve activity. As shown in Fig. 1B, i.p. leptin-induced elevation of the hypothalamic histamine level was completely abolished in the CTX rats. This finding shows that the peripheral inputs from the CT participate in the hypothalamic neurochemical change enhanced by leptin.

It has not yet been clarified how the leptin signaling via the CT activates the histaminergic system in the brain. There are direct projections from the A2/C1 group in the nucleus of the solitary tract, the termination of the CT [7], to the tuberomammillary nucleus (TM), a limited region where cell bodies of the histaminergic neurons are located [13]. From this morphological observation, the signal input from the CT to the nucleus of the solitary tract might affect the neuronal activity of the TM, followed by the increase in the hypothalamic histamine release. However, the more complicated pathway containing the gustatory system may be involved in this effect because the TM also receives projections from the brain areas which are important for taste information [7, 13].

In conclusion, leptin activates the histaminergic system via the peripheral signal inputs from the CT resulting in the suppression of food intake.

Acknowledgements

We are very grateful to Amgen Inc. (Thousand Oaks, CA, USA) for providing recombinant murine leptin.

References

[1] Friedman, J. M. and Halaas, J. L., Leptin and the regulation of body weight in mammals. Nature 395, (1998) 763-770.

[2] Schwartz, M.W., Seeley, R.J., Campfield, A., Burn, P., Baskin, D.G., Identification of targets of leptin action in rat hypothalamus. J. Clin. Invest., 98 (1996) 1101-1106.

[3] Lecklin, A., Etu-Seppala, P., Stark, H., Tuomisto, L., Effects of intracerebroventricularly infused histamine and selective H_1, H_2 and H_3 agonists on food and water intake and urine flow in Wistar rats. Brain Res., 793 (1998) 279-288.

[4] Ookuma, K., Yoshimatu, H., Sakata, T., Fujimoto, K., Fukugawa, K., Hypothalamic sites of neuronal histamine action on food intake by rats. Brain Res., 490 (1989) 268-275.

[5] Morimoto, T., Yamamoto, Y., Mobarakeh, J. I., Yanai, K., Watanabe, T., Watanabe, T., Yamatodani, A., Involvement of the histaminergic system in leptin-induced suppression of food intake. Physiol. Behav., 67 (1999) 679-683.

[6] Lecklin, A., Hermonen, P., Tarhanen, J., Mannisto, P. T., An acute i.c.v. infusion of leptin

has no effect on hypothalamic histamine and tele-methylhistamine contents in Wistar rats. Eur. J. Pharmacol., 395 (2000) 113-119.

[7] Norgren, R. The gustatory system in mammals. Am. J. Otolaryngol., 4 (1983) 234-237.

[8] Kawai, K., Sugimoto, K., Nakashima, K., Miura, H., Ninomiya, Y., Leptin as a modulator of sweet taste sensitivities in mice. Proc. Natl. Acad. Sci. USA, 97 (2000) 11044-11049.

[9] Paxinos, G. and Watson, C. The rat brain in stereotaxic coordinates 4th edn. (1998) Academic Press, Sydney.

[10]Mochizuki, T., Yamatodani, A., Okakura, K., Takemura, M., Inagaki, N., Wada, H., In vivo release of neuronal histamine in the hypothalamus of rats measured by microdialysis. Naunyn-Schmiedeberg's Arch. Pharmacol., 343 (1991) 190-195.

[11] Elmquist, J. K., Ahima, R. S., Maratos-Flier, E., Flier, J. S., Saper, C. B. Leptin activates neurons in ventrobasal hypothalamus and brainstem. Endocrinology,138 (1997) 839-842.

[12] Yamatodani, A., Fukuda, H., Wada, H., Iwaeda, T., Watanabe, T., High-performance liquid chromatographic determination of plasma and brain histamine without previous purification of biological samples: cation-exchange chromatography coupled with post-column derivatization fluorometry. J. Chromatogr., 344 (1985) 115-123.

[13] Ericson, H., Blomqvist, A., Kohler, C., Origin of neuronal inputs to the region of the tuberomammillary nucleus of the rat brain. J. Comp. Neurol., 311 (1991) 45-64.

H2 receptors and diseases

Histamine Research in the New Millennium
T. Watanabe, H. Timmerman and K. Yanai (Editors)

Functional and morphological abnormality of gastric mucosa in histamine H2 receptor (H2R)-deficient mice

Takeshi Watanabe[a], Takashi Kobayashi[a], Shunsuke Tonai[b], Yasunobu Ishihara[c], Ritsuko Koga[a] and Susumu Okabe[b]

[a]Department of Molecular Immunology, Medical Institute of Bioregulation, Kyushu University. 3-1-1 Maidashi, Higashi-ku, Fukuoka 812-8582, Japan [b]Department of applied pharmacology, Kyoto Pharmaceutical University. [c]Developmental Research Laboratories, Shionogi & Co., Ltd.

(Correspondence should be addressed to Takeshi Watanabe)

Histamine H2R-deficient mice were generated by gene targeting. Homozygous mutant mice were viable and fertile without apparent abnormalities and unexpectedly showed normal basal gastric pH. However, the H2R-deficient mice exhibited a marked hypertrophy with enlarged folds in gastric mucosa and an elevated serum gastrin level. Immunohistochemical analysis revealed increased numbers of parietal and enterochromaffin-like (ECL) cells. In spite of striking hypertrophic changes of the mucosa, the size of the parietal cells in mutant mice was significantly smaller than that of wild-type mice. Electron microscopic analysis revealed that the parietal cells in mutant mice contained enlarged secretory canaliculi with a lower density of microvilli and few typical tubulovesicles in the narrow cytoplasm. At older age, hypertrophy of gastric mucosa becomes more evident. There are numerous numbers of large vacuoles containing viscous and glossy fluid. Thus it resembles Menetrier disease. Gastric acid secretion induced by histamine or gastrin was completely abolished in the mutant mice, however, carbachol could induce acid secretion. The present study clearly demonstrates that H2R-mediated signal(s) are required for cellular homeostasis of the gastric mucosa and attainment of normal structure of the secretory membranes in parietal cells. Moreover, impairment of acid secretion due to the absence of H2R could be overcome by the signals from cholinergic receptors rather than by those from gastrin receptors on parietal cells.

230

1. Introduction

The gastric mucosa is composed of numerous blind tubular units containing various cell types. (a) the pit region containing surface mucous cells, (b) the isthmus containing stem cells, (c) the neck region containing mucous neck cells, and (d) the basal region containing chief cells and enterochromaffin-like (ECL) cells. Acid-producing cells, namely parietal cells, are scattered in the four regions. It has been well known that parietal cells secrete gastric acid from H^+,K^+-ATPase (gastric proton pump) on the membrane upon stimulation with gastrin, acetylcholine (ACh) and histamine through gastrin/cholecystokinin-B receptor (CCK-BR), muscarinic receptors (M1R and M3R) and histamine H2 receptor (H2R), respectively. The physiological significance of histamine signaling mediated by H2R in gastric acid secretion has been demonstrated by using selective antagonists such as cimetidine, ranitidine and famotidine which have a potent inhibitory effect on secretory response. By contrast, the acid secretion induced by ACh and gastrin is believed to involve two pathways; either directly by activating the parietal cells or indirectly by stimulating ECL cells which produce and release histamine, thus activating parietal cells in a paracrine fashion (1). The relative importance of these two modes of action remains to be clarified.

Parietal cells have unique structural properties to produce and secrete gastric acid. They are relatively large cells containing numerous mitochondria in their cytoplasm. The plasma membrane invaginates deep into the cytoplasm to form an interconnecting system of tortuous channels, termed secretory canaliculi, that are lined by numerous microvilli. Parietal cells contain intracellular vesicles, termed tubulovesicles, in the cytoplasmic region close to the canaliculi. In the resting state, H^+,K^+-ATPase is stored within cytoplasmic tubulovesicle. Upon stimulation, the tubulovesicles fuse with the apical membrane to form the extended secretory canaliculus and then functional pumps are recruited to the surface of canaliculus (1). The cessation of acid secretion is executed by means of endocytotic internalization of the H^+,K^+-ATPase and regeneration of the tubulovesicles. These events must be regulated by signal(s) from cAMP and/or Ca^{2+}-dependant pathways, however, there is little information on the mechanisms responsible for this regulated endocytosis and exocytosis.

2.1. Normal basal gastric pH in H2R-deficient mice

Mice with a disrupted histamine H2R gene (H2R$^{-/-}$ mice) was generated by gene targeting (2). In contrast to the H2R blockade by selective H2R antagonists which elevate gastric pH, basal gastric pH in H2R$^{-/-}$ mice was normal and less than 3.0. However, elevation of gastric pH by administration of a selective H2R antagonist, famotidine, was not observed in H2R$^{-/-}$ mice, even though a significant inhibition of gastric acid secretion occurred in the stomach of H2R$^{+/-}$ and wild-type littermates. This indicates that the H2R is functionally disrupted in the null mutant mice. In contrast, a selective M1R antagonist, telenzepine, blocked the secretion of gastric acid in H2R$^{-/-}$ mice as well as H2R$^{+/-}$ and wild-type littermates.

2.2 Gastric acid secretion in H2R-deficient mice is regulated by signal(s) from muscarinic receptors, but not from gastrin receptors.

The acid output induced by histamine was upregulated approximately 5 fold in wild-type mice (26.1 $\pm$ 2.65 µEq / hr) compared to the basal level (5.56 $\pm$ 0.74 µEq / hr), whereas it was not increased in H2R$^{-/-}$ mice (7.52 $\pm$ 1.02 µEq / hr). These results reconfirmed the complete absence of a functional H2R in the null mutant mice. In contrast, acid output induced by carbachol was increased in H2R$^{-/-}$ mice (25.1 $\pm$ 3.83 µEq / hr) similarly to that of wild-type mice (23.8 $\pm$ 3.23 µEq / hr). Surprisingly, there was no response to stimulation with gastrin in H2R$^{-/-}$ mice (5.31 $\pm$ 1.00 µEq / hr), even though marked elevation of the acid secretion was observed in heterozygous H2R$^{+/-}$ (25.9 $\pm$ 6.26 µEq / hr) and wild-type (26.4 $\pm$ 5.22 µEq / hr) littermates. These results strongly suggest that the muscarinic but not gastrin-induced signal could compensate the H2R-signal for gastric acid production, and also that an effect of gastrin on acid secretion is mainly mediated by H2R upon stimulation with histamine released from ECL cells which express CCK-BR.

2.3 Hypergastrinemia and gigantic hypertrophy of gastric mucosa in H2R-deficient mice.

It has been reported that treatment with anti-ulcer agents such as H2R antagonists and PPIs induced hypergastrinemia and hypertrophy of the gastric mucosa in rodents (3). The mean of serum gastrin level in 12-18-week-old H2R$^{-/-}$ mice was significantly elevated in comparison with that of wild-type mice (1528 $\pm$ 243 pg/ml versus 384 $\pm$ 42.3 pg/ml, p<0.001). To quantify the hypertrophy, wet weights and DNA contents of the stomach in 14-week-old female mice were measured. The mean wet weight in H2R$^{-/-}$ mice (11.19 $\pm$ 0.47 mg / g body weight) was higher than that of wild-type control (7.56 $\pm$ 0.22 mg / g body weight). The stomach DNA content in H2R$^{-/-}$ mice (71.94 $\pm$ 2.74 µg / g body weight) was also significantly higher than that of wild-type controls (44.49 $\pm$ 1.53 µg / g body weight). These data indicate that the increased stomach wet weight in the mutant mice resulted from the increased numbers of the cells rather than increased volume of each cell in the stomach. Therefore, genetic ablation of H2R leads to hypergastrinemia and gigantic hypertrophy of the gastric mucosa.

2.4 Increased numbers of parietal and ECL cells in H2R-deficienct mice.

Thickness of gastric mucosa in the glandular region was remarkably increased in 16-week-old H2R$^{-/-}$ mice compared with wild-type mice. The gigantic hypertrophic change resulted in a formation of enlarged gastric folds in the glandular region. The change in mucosal thickness was most prominent in the isthmus and neck region. In contrast, no significant change was found in the pit region. In H2R$^{-/-}$ mice, parietal cells were found throughout the hypertrophic oxyntic mucosa with increased cell numbers. ECL cells in H2R$^{-/-}$ mice were found not only in the basal region, but also in the neck region and isthmus with a marked increase in density. Histamine contents in the gastric mucosa were significantly elevated in H2R$^{-/-}$ mice. These findings suggest that the gigantic mucosal hypertrophy is resulted from the increased numbers of parietal cells, ECL cells and other H$^+$,K$^+$-ATPase negative cells. To determine whether the increase in the numbers of parietal cells and ECL cells resulted from enhanced proliferation, BrdU incorporation in the oxyntic mucosa was examined. BrdU incorporation in the oxyntic mucosa was significantly increased in young 4-week-old H2R$^{-/-}$ mice. Thus the gastric stem cells in the isthmus are highly proliferative in H2R$^{-/-}$ mice during the period prior to hypertrophy.

2.5 Morphological alteration of parietal cells in H2R-deficienct mice

The ultrastructure of the parietal cells in H2R$^{-/-}$ mice was quite distinct from that of wild-type mice. In normal parietal cells, secretory canaliculi with numerous microvilli were readily observed by electron microscopy. The mitochondria were very prominent and scattered throughout the cytoplasm and tubulovesicles were mainly located in the region close to the canaliculi. By contrast, the cytoplasmic volume was remarkably reduced in the parietal cells of H2R$^{-/-}$ mice, although the numbers of mitochondria in parietal cells appeared to be comparable with those of normal parietal cells. Moreover, many parietal cells contained enlarged secretory canaliculi with a lower density of microvilli and few typical tubulovesicles in the cytoplasm. These findings suggest that H2R deficiency caused the abnormal microstructure of secretory membranes of parietal cells.

3. Discussion:

3.1 Acid secretion by histamine, acetylcholine and gastrin

Acid secretion by histamine depends on direct stimulation of H2R expressed on parietal cells, while acid secretion by ACh or gastrin has been thought to occur either directly by activation of parietal cells or indirectly by triggering histamine release from ECL cells. There has been controversy concerning the relative significance of direct stimulation on parietal cells and indirect action through histamine release. The present results demonstrated that cholinergic signal(s) for acid secretion may act through both direct and indirect stimulation of parietal cells whereas gastrin signal(s) may act only indirectly through H2R by inducing histamine release from ECL cells.

3.2 Signal(s) from H2R play a role in negative regulation of gastric mucosal cell growth.

Similarly to the rodent model treated with H2R antagonists, the H2R deficient mice exhibited a marked hypertrophy of the gastric mucosa with an increase in numbers of parietal cells, ECL cells and other types of cells. Although gastrin has a powerful trophic effect on oxyntic mucosal cells (4), hypertrophy in H2R-deficient mice is more gigantic and prominent, compared to the report on the gastrin gene transgenic mice. Thus, the increased numbers of oxyntic mucosal cells in H2R-deficient mice may be in part a direct consequence of the deficiency of H2R-mediated signaling in addition to hypergastrinemia.

3.3 Involvement of H2R-mediated signal in regulation of endocytosis of H^+, K^+-ATPase and regeneration of tubulovesicles

The morphological change in parietal cells in the mutant mice may reflect the direct effect of H2R deficiency rather than the indirect effect of hypertrophic change of the gastric mucosa. Electron microscopic observation revealed structural alterations of the secretory membrane systems including secretory canaliculi and intracellular tubulovesicles. The abnormal parietal cells contained enlarged secretory canaliculi with a lower density of microvilli and few typical tubulovesicles. Secretory membrane transport is one of critical mechanism for regulation of acid secretion. The activation of acid secretion involves the exocytosis of H^+, K^+-ATPase to the cell surface by fusion of tubulovesicles with the apical membranes, while the cessation of acid secretion is associated with endocytosis of the H^+, K^+-ATPase and regeneration of tubulovesicles. Decreased numbers of tubulovesicles in H2R-deficient mice may be caused by impairment of generation or regeneration of tubulovesicles in the parietal cells (Fig. 1). A recent study has revealed that a tyrosine-based motif in the β subunit of H^+, K^+-ATPase is required for reinternalization of H^+, K^+-ATPase and regeneration of tubulovesicles. A mutation in the tyrosine-based motif of β subunit causes hypertrophic gastropathy resembling Menetrier's disease (5). The β subunit-deficient mice also exhibit abnormal structure of the secretory canaliculi in parietal cells and hypertrophy of gastric

234

mucosa (6). Interestingly, the gastric juice in the stomach with gigantic folds of H2R deficient mice was highly viscous and glossy, which also resembles Menetrier's disease. This is the first evidence that histamine signaling mediated by H2R may control the cellular size of parietal cells and preserve the normal structure of the secretory membrane in parietal cells. However, it is uncertain whether the morphological abnormality in the parietal cell is indeed functionally coupled to the potency of acid secretion.

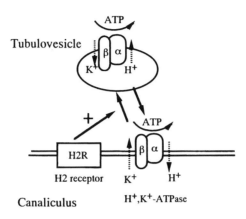

Fig.1 H2R-mediated signal(s) may regulate endocytosis of the H^+, K^+-ATPase and regeneration of tubulovesicles.

4. Conclusion

The present study demonstrates a physiological role of H2R signaling involved in crucial regulation of acid secretion, proliferation and attainment of normal secretory membrane structures of parietal cells. The H2R-deficient mouse provides an important tool for further understanding the molecular mechanisms for gastric function and morphological regulation of the oxyntic mucosa.

References
1. SJ. Hersey and G. Sachs.   Physiological Reviews. **75** (1995) 155.
2. T. Kobayashi et al.   J. Clin. Invest. **105** (2000) 1741.
3. TJ. Koh et al.   Gastroenterology. **113** (1997). 1015
4. N. Langhans et al.   Gastroenterology. **112** (1997) 280.
5. N. Courtois-Coutry et al.   Cell. **90** (1997) 501.
6. KL. Scarff et al.   Gastroenterology. **117**(1999) 605

New perspectives for histamine-mediated CNS functions

Histamine Research in the New Millennium
T. Watanabe, H. Timmerman and K. Yanai (Editors)

A Third Legacy for Burimamide: Discovery and Characterization of Improgan and a New Class of Non-Opioid Analgesics Derived From Histamine Antagonists[+]

L. B. Hough[a],[*], J. W. Nalwalk[a], R. Leurs[b], W. M. P. B. Menge[b] and H. Timmerman[b]

[a]Center for Neuropharmacology and Neuroscience, Albany Medical College, Albany, NY, USA

[b]Leiden/Amsterdam Center for Drug Research, Department of Pharmacochemistry, Vrije University, Amsterdam, The Netherlands

Burimamide, a histamine (HA) derivative with both H_2- and H_3- blocking properties, induces antinociception when injected into the rodent CNS. Several related compounds share this property, and structure-activity studies have shown that this new class of analgesics is distinct from known HA antagonists. The prototype drug, named improgan, shows the preclinical profile of a highly effective analgesic, with activity against thermal, mechanical and inflammatory nociception after doses that do not alter motor balance or locomotor activity. Improgan analgesia is not blocked by opioid antagonists and is observed in opioid receptor knock-out mice. Unlike morphine, improgan does not induce tolerance after daily dosing. Extensive in vitro pharmacology studies have excluded known histaminergic, opioid, serotonergic, GABAergic and adrenergic receptor mechanisms, as well as 50 other potential sites of action. The improgan-like analgesic activity of some HA congeners (e.g. impentamine) suggests an action on a novel HA receptor, but further studies are required to substantiate this. Recent work shows that improgan analgesia, like opioid analgesia, is reversed by the $GABA_A$ agonist muscimol, suggesting that improgan activates brain stem neurons to stimulate descending analgesic pathways. Studies in progress are characterizing the sites and mechanisms of action of improgan, and developing brain-penetrating derivatives for the treatment of clinical pain.

1. INTRODUCTION

Pain continues to be a worldwide health problem, despite many scientific advances in the field. An ideal agent for treating pain would be a morphine-like drug devoid of opioid side effects. This article will briefly review our discovery and characterization of a class of compounds derived from HA antagonists which have morphine-like analgesic properties after CNS administration. New results concerning the mechanism of action of these compounds are also presented.

[*]Corresponding author: Lindsay B. Hough, Neuropharmacology and Neuroscience, Albany Medical College MC-136, 47 New Scotland Ave., Albany, NY 12208. Phone: 518-262-5785; Fax: 518-262-5799; email: houghl@mail.amc.edu.
[+]This work was supported by the National Institute on Drug Abuse (DA-03816).

238

1.1. Improgan-Like Analgesics

Earlier investigations of the histaminergic modulation of pain transmission noted that some (but not all) H_2 antagonists induce analgesia when administered by intracerebroventricular (icv) injection (reviewed in [1]). Synthesis and testing of improgan (Fig. 1, previously known as SKF92374, a "chemical control" which lacks H_2 activity) showed that this analgesia was not due to H_2 receptor activity [2]. Burimamide, a compound with both H_2- and H_3- blocking activity, also has analgesic properties [2,3], as do several other compounds of similar structure (Fig. 1).

1.2. Characteristics of Improgan Analgesia

Table 1 summarizes some of the properties of improgan. As noted, this drug inhibits motor responses to several types of painful stimuli [4], suggesting a reduction in pain perception. However, some compounds reduce nociceptive responses because of motor impairment or alterations in locomotor behavior, so it was important to show that improgan does not alter these parameters [4]. Overall, the results suggest that improgan produces morphine-like pain relief, but not some of the undesirable opioid properties such as locomotor stimulation [4] and tolerance [5].

1.3. Structure-Activity Relationships (SARs) and the Search for Improgan's Receptor

Except for HA, the analgesic compounds in Fig. 1 have either H_2 or H_3-blocking properties, but detailed studies of the SARs of nearly 30 compounds have shown that neither of these receptors can account for improgan analgesia [6,7]. This conclusion is consistent with pharmacological studies, which concluded that neither the H_1, H_2, nor H_3 receptor seems to mediate improgan analgesia [2,8]. A role for the major opioid receptors has also been excluded by antagonist studies [1,8] and experiments with knock-out mice [9]. In vitro receptor screens have excluded more than 60 receptors as improgan targets (Table 2). Thus, the molecular site at which improgan acts to induce pain relief remains unknown.

1.4. Neuronal Circuits for Pain-Relieving Drugs

Many analgesics reduce spinal pain transmission by activating descending analgesic systems in the brain stem [10]. For example, morphine diminishes inhibitory GABAergic control of tonically active analgesic systems, accounting for: 1) reduction of opioid effects by $GABA_A$ the agonist muscimol [11], and 2) activation of these systems by bicuculline, a $GABA_A$ antagonist [12]. Because GABAergic mechanisms are significant in the brain's pain-relieving systems, and since improgan action is poorly understood, the present study examined the effects of the $GABA_A$ agonist muscimol on improgan and morphine analgesia.

2. METHODS

Male Sprague-Dawley rats (210-260 g) were maintained on a 12-hr light/dark cycle (lights on 07:00, lights off 19:00). The left lateral ventricle was chronically cannulated under anesthesia [13]. One week later, subjects received icv injections and were tested by the radiant heat tail flick test (see Fig. 2). All experiments were reviewed and approved by the appropriate Institutional Animal Care and Use Committees.

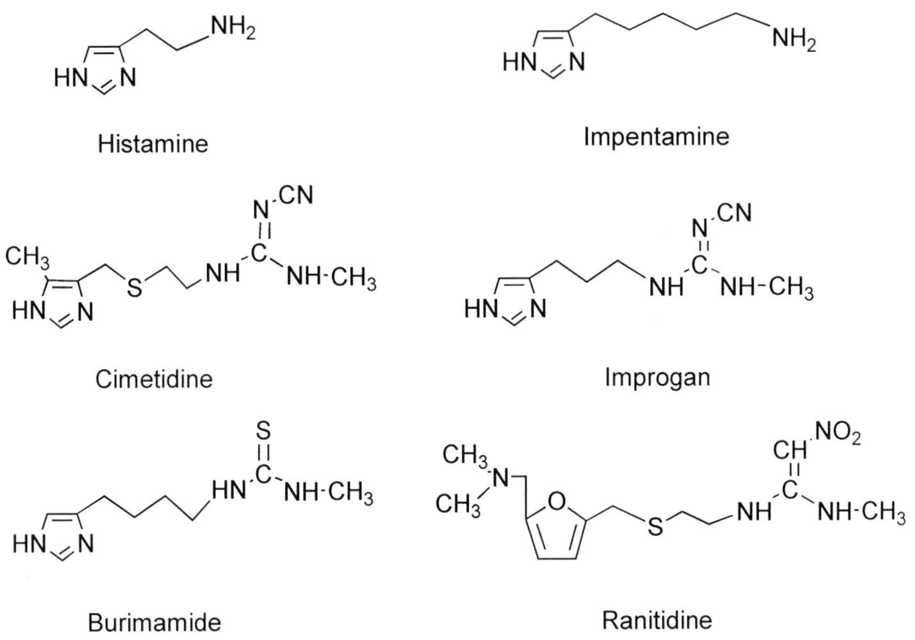

Figure 1 Chemical structures of HA and congeners. The compounds shown induce analgesia following icv injection in rodents. HA produces this effect through interactions with H_1 and H_2 receptors [1], but the receptor(s) mediating the effects of the other drugs remain unknown.

Table 1
Characteristics of Improgan Analgesia

Observations	Reference
Full activity on thermal and mechanical tests	1,2,4
Active in mice and rats	2,4
Inactive on spontaneous locomotor activity	4
Inactive on accelerated rotorod (balance) test	4
No tolerance with repeated daily dosing	5
Independent of μ, δ, κ opioid receptors	1,8,9
Independent of H_1, H_2, H_3 receptors	2,8
Novel structure-activity relationship	6,7
Unknown mechanism of action, possibly GPCR	1

Synopsis of the pharmacological properties of improgan.

240

Table 2
In Vitro Receptor Profile of Improgan

Class	Inactive Receptors [1]
HA	H1 [2], H2 [2]
Opioid	μ, μ1, μ2, δ [2] κ, κ1, κ3, OFQ
5-HT	5HT1A, 5HT1Dα, 5HT1Dβ, 5HT1E, 5HT2A, 5HT2C, 5HT5A, 5HT6, 5HT7
Muscarinic	M1, M2, M3, M4, M5
Nicotinic	α2/β2, α2/β4, α3/β2, α3/β4, α4/β2, α4/β2, α4/β4
Dopamine	D1, D2, D3, D4
Adrenergic	β1, β2, α1
GABA	GABA$_A$, GABA$_B$
Transporters	5HT, Norepinephrine, Dopamine, VMAT
Glutamate	NMDA, mGluR1A [2], mGluR2 [2], mGluR4 [2], mGluR5A [2], mGluR6 [2]
Other	PCP, Sodium Channel, Sigma1, Sigma2

[1] As an antagonist, improgan (10 μM) showed less than 30% inhibition of ligand binding or had a Kd of greater than 100 μM on these receptors. [2] Inactive as an agonist on this receptor: 10 μM showed less than 35% of maximal responses or had an EC50 of greater than 100 μM. Improgan was moderately active at 5HT$_3$, H$_3$ and α$_2$ receptors (not shown), but other analgesic congeners are inactive at these sites [1].

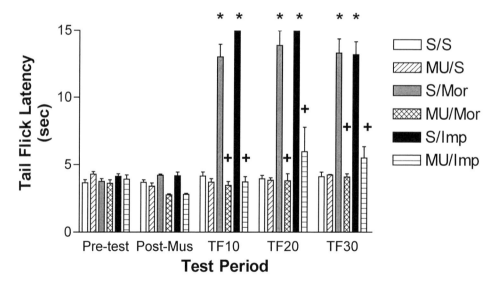

Figure 2. Effects of muscimol on improgan- and morphine-induced analgesia. Rats were tested for baseline responses ("Pre-test"), received icv muscimol (MU, 0.5 μg, 2 μl) or saline (S) and were re-tested 25 min later ("Post-Mus"). They then received morphine sulfate (Mor, 20 μg), improgan (Imp, 80 μg) or saline (S) and were re-tested 10, 20 and 30 min later. *P<0.01 vs S/S; +P<0.01 for effect of muscimol on respective analgesic treatment.

3. RESULTS

Both morphine and improgan induced 80-100% of maximal analgesia 10-30 min after icv administration (Fig. 2). The effects were reversible, since latencies returned toward baseline 60 min after dosing (not shown). Muscimol pretreatment completely abolished improgan antinociception 10-30 min after improgan treatment (Fig. 2). This muscimol treatment also completely attenuated morphine analgesia (Fig. 1), as found previously [11]. Baseline scores ranged from 3.65 ± 0.23 to 4.30 ± 0.19 sec and were not different across the groups. Muscimol had a slight, but significant ($P < 0.01$) hyperalgesic effect alone.

4. DISCUSSION

The finding that muscimol, a powerful inhibitor of neuronal activity, reverses improgan analgesia strongly suggests that improgan activates supraspinal analgesic circuits. A similar mechanism accounts for morphine analgesia in the brain stem [10,11,14].

4.1. Brain Stem Targets for Improgan Analgesia

Other preliminary findings in support of the descending analgesic mechanism for improgan include 1) antagonism of icv improgan analgesia by intrathecal administration of the α_2 antagonist yohimbine (unpublished results), 2) lack of analgesic activity of intrathecal improgan (unpublished results), and 3) antinociceptive activity of improgan administered in the periaqueductal grey [2] and raphe magnus (unpublished), brain regions known to participate in descending analgesic circuits [10,12,14]. However, further work is needed to map these targets and pathways.

4.2 Significance of GABAergic Transmission for Improgan Action

Morphine-like analgesics stimulate descending pathways by reducing the activity of GABAergic neurons [14], and improgan may have a similar effect through a non-opioid receptor. However, the fact that muscimol reverses improgan analgesia does not prove this hypothesis, and other mechanisms must be considered as well.

4.3 Muscimol – a Tool for Studying Improgan-Like Analgesics

Muscimol is the first drug discovered to antagonize improgan analgesia. Because improgan does not block $GABA_A$ receptors (Table 2 and [1],) the GABA agonist muscimol is functioning as a physiological (not pharmacological) antagonist of improgan. Many "improgan-like" compounds have already been described [6,7] and these have been assumed to act at a common receptor. This has not been proven, however, because no antagonists of improgan have been available. Thus, muscimol will be very useful tool in the classification of improgan-like analgesics. Early results with this approach already suggest the possibility that "improgan-like" drugs may be capable of relieving pain by more than one mechanism.

4.4 Is the Improgan Target a HA receptor?

Improgan analgesia is not mediated by known HA receptors (above), but the close resemblance to HA's structure and the analgesic properties of HA itself pose the possibility that undiscovered HA receptors might be improgan targets. The "improgan-like" activity of the HA congener impentamine (Fig. 1, [1]) may support this, but the idea remains unproven. Discoveries of new histamine receptors [15] will permit further assessment of this hypothesis.

242

REFERENCES

[1] Hough LB, Nalwalk JW, Barnes WG, Warner LM, Leurs R, Menge WMPB, Timmerman H, Wentland M. A Third Life for Burimamide: Discovery and Characterization of a Novel Class of Non-Opioid Analgesics Derived from Histamine Antagonists. In: Glick SD, Maisonneuve IM, editors: New Medications for Drug Abuse. New York: New York Acad. Sci., 2000. pp. 25-40.

[2] Li BY, Nalwalk JW, Barker LA, Cumming P, Parsons ME, Hough LB. Characterization of the antinociceptive properties of cimetidine and a structural analog. J. Pharmacol. Exp. Ther. 1996; 276:500-508.

[3] Lamberti C, Bartolini A, Ghelardini C, Malmberg-Aiello P. Investigation into the role of histamine receptors in rodent antinociception. Pharmacol. Biochem. Behav. 1996; 53:567-574.

[4] Li BY, Nalwalk JW, Finkel JM, Glick SD, Hough LB. SKF92374, a cimetidine analog, produces mechanical and thermal antinociception in the absence of motor impairment. Analgesia 1997; 3:15-20.

[5] Bannoura MD, Nalwalk JW, Tang Y, Carlile M, Leurs R, Menge WMPB, Timmerman H, Hough LB. Absence of antinociceptive tolerance to improgan, a cimetidine analog, in rats. Brain Res. 1998; 814:218-221.

[6] Hough LB, Nalwalk JW, Li BY, Leurs R, Menge WMPB, Timmerman H, Cioffi C, Wentland M. Novel qualitative structure-activity relationships for the antinociceptive actions of H_2 antagonists, H_3 antagonists and derivatives. J. Pharmacol. Exp. Ther. 1997; 283:1534-1543.

[7] Hough LB, Nalwalk JW, Leurs R, Menge WMPB, Timmerman H. Antinociceptive activity of derivatives of improgan and burimamide. Pharmacol. Biochem. Behav. 2000; 65:61-66.

[8] Li BY, Nalwalk JW, Hough LB. Effects of naltrexone and histamine antagonists on the antinociceptive activity of the cimetidine analog SKF92374 in rats. Brain Res. 1997; 748:168-174.

[9] Hough LB, Nalwalk JW, Chen Y, Schuller A, Zhu Y, Zhang J, Menge WMPB, Leurs R, Timmerman H, Pintar JE. Improgan, a cimetidine analog, induces morphine-like antinociception in opioid receptor-knockout mice. Brain Res. 2000; 880:102-108.

[10] Fields HL, Heinricher MM, Mason P. Neurotransmitters in nociceptive modulatory circuits. Annu. Rev. Neurosci. 1991; 14:219-245.

[11] Zonta N, Zambotti F, Vicentini L, Tammiso R, Mantegazza P. Effects of some GABA-mimetic drugs on the antinociceptive activity of morphine and β-endorphin in rats. Naunyn Schmiedebergs Arch. Pharmacol. 1981; 316:231-234.

[12] Roychowdhury SM, Fields HL. Endogenous opioids acting at a medullary μ-opioid receptor contribute to the behavioral antinociception produced by GABA antagonism in the midbrain periaqueductal gray. Neurosci. 1996; 74:863-872.

[13] Crane LA, Glick SD. Simple cannula for repeated intracerebral drug administration in rats. Pharmacol. Biochem. Behav. 1979; 10:799-800.

[14] Vaughan CW, Ingram MA, Connor MA, Christie MJ. How opioids inhibit GABA-mediated neurotransmission. Nature 1997; 390:611-614.

[15] Oda T, Morikawa N, Saito Y, Masuho Y, Matsumoto S. Molecular cloning and characterization of novel type of histamine receptor preferentially expressed in leukocytes. J.Biol.Chem. *in press*, 2000.

© 2001 Elsevier Science B.V. All rights reserved.
Histamine Research in the New Millennium
T. Watanabe, H. Timmerman and K. Yanai (Editors)

Involvement of central histamine in amygdaloid kindled seizures in rats

C. Kamei

Department of Pharmacology, Faculty of Pharmaceutical Sciences, Okayama University, Okayama 700-8530, Japan

The present study was undertaken to clarify the relationship between histaminergic neuron system in the brain and amygdaloid kindled seizures in rats. There was a high correlation between an inhibition of kindled seizures and an increase in histamine content of the amygdala. Not only post-synaptic histamine receptors (H_1-receptors) but also pre-synaptic histamine receptors (H_3-receptors) was responsible for an inhibition of amygdaloid kindled seizures.

Keywords: kindling, amygdala, histidine, metoprine, H_3-antagonist

1. INTRODUCTION

Since the discovery by Goddard et al. [1], kindling preparation is considered to be a very powerful tool for pathophysiological study of epilepsy and widely used as a useful model for estimating the effectiveness of antiepileptic drugs [2]. On the other hand, there are some findings that central histaminergic neuron system is related with epilepsy in pharmacological and clinical studies [3, 4]. The present study was undertaken to clarify the role of central histaminergic neuron system on amygdaloid kindled seizures in rats.

2. MATERIALS AND METHODS

2.1. Animals

Male Wistar strain rats 7-8 weeks old and weighing 200-250 g, were used. All animals were maintained in an air conditioned room controlled for temperature and humidity. The animals were given food and water *ad libitum*.

2.2. Surgery

Under sodium pentobarbital anesthesia, bipolar electrodes were implanted into the frontal cortex, dorsal hippocampus and amygdala according to the atlas of de Groot. Guide cannula was also implanted into the lateral ventricle. Electrodes were connected to a miniature receptacle and were fixed on the skull together with guide cannula by dental cement. At least 2 weeks were allowed for postoperative recovery. The procedure to cause kindled seizures was similar to that described in a previous paper [2].   EEG was recorded bipolary and electrical stimulation was applied to the amygdala bipolary.   Stimulating parameters were 60 Hz frequency, 1 msec pulse duration and 1 sec duration at an intensity just sufficient to induce after discharge (100-300 μA).

3.3. Experimental procedure in kindled seizures
The developmental stages of amygdaloid kindled seizures were classified using a method described by Racine [5].   That is, S-1 is jaw movement, S-2 is head nodding, S-3 is forelimb clonus, S-4 is kangaroo posture and S-5 is kangaroo posture & falling back.   After the animals developed the final stage of generalized seizures, stimulation was repeated for 5 more days and used for drug study.

3.   RESULTS AND DISCUSSION

A significant decrease in histamine contents in the amygdala was observed after development of amygdaloid kindling.   Histidine and metoprine an inhibitor of N-methyltransferase, inhibited amygdaloid kindled seizures at doses causing an increase in histamine contents of the brain.   In addition, intracerebro-ventricular (i.c.v.) injection of histamine resulted in an inhibition of amygdaloid kindled seizures. H_1-antagonists (diphenhydramine and chlorpheniramine) attenuated histidine-induced inhibition of amygdaloid kindled seizures, however no significant antagonism was observed with H_2-antagonists (zolantidine and ranitidine) [6].   Both i.c.v. and intraperitoneal (i.p.) injection of H_3-antagonists (thioperamide and clobenpropit) resulted in a dose-related inhibition of amygdaloid kindled seizures.   An inhibition induced by thioperamide was antagonized by an H_3-agonist [(R)-α-methylhistamine] and H_1-antagonists (diphenhydramine and chlorpheniramine).   On the other hand, an H_2-antagonists (cimetidine and ranitidine) caused no antagonistic effect.   Metoprine was also effective in inhibiting amygdaloid kindled seizures, and this effect was augmented by thioperamide treatment [7].   From these findings, not only post-synaptic H_1-receptors but also pre-synaptic H_3-receptors was responsible for an inhibition of amygdaloid kindled seizures.

GABA mimetic drugs, diazepam, sodium valproate and muscimol, which showed no significant effect on amygdaloid kindled seizures when used separately, significant potentiated the effect of clobenpropit.   In addition, bicuculline caused a significant antagonism of the inhibition of amygdaloid kindled seizures induced by clobenpropit.   These results suggest that inhibition of amygdaloid kindled seizures induced by histamine is closely associated with the action of GABA [8].   It is generally recognized that H_1 receptors are closely related with Ca ion.   Therefore, interaction between histamine and Ca ion on amygdaloid kindled seizure was studied.   Calcium chloride and A23187, which showed no significant effect on amygdaloid kindled seizures when used separately, significantly potentiated the effect of histamine.   An inhibition on amygdaloid kindled seizures induced by histamine was significantly antagonized by calcium chelater EGTA and EGTA/AM.

REFERENCES

1. G. V. Goddard, D.C. McIntyre and C. K. Leech, Exp. Neurol., 25 (1969) 295
2. C. Kamei, M. Oka, Y. Masuda, K.Yoshida and M. Shimizu, Arch. int. Pharmacodyn., 249 (1981) 164.
3. Y. Shimoda, A. Koizumi and K. Tanaka, Yonago Acta Med., 4 (1960) 99.
4. H. Yokoyama, K. Onodera, K. Maeyama, K.Yanai, K. Iinuma, L.Tuomisto and T. Watanabe, Naunyn-Schmiedeberg's Arch. Pharmacol., 346 (1992) 40.
5. R. J. Racine, Neurophysiol., 32 (1972) 269.
6. C. Kamei, K. Ishizawa, H. Kakinoki and M. Fukunaga, Epilepsy Res., 30 (1998) 187.
7. H. Kakinoki, K. Ishizawa, M. Fukunaga, Y. Fujii and C. Kamei, Brain Res. Bull., 46 (1998) 461.
8. K. Ishizawa, Z. Chen, C. Okuma, Y. Sugimoto, Y. Fujii and C. Kamei, Jpn. J. Pharmacol., 82 (2000) 48.

Histamine Research in the New Millennium
T. Watanabe, H. Timmerman and K. Yanai (Editors)

The role of histamine in a hypocretin (orexin)-deficient sleep disorder, narcolepsy

S. Nishino [a], K. Honda [b], N. Fujiki [a], S.W. Wurts[a], E. Sakurai [c], M. Kato [c], T. Watanabe [c], E. Mignot[a] and K. Yanai [c]

[a] Center for Narcolepsy, Stanford Sleep Research Center, Stanford, California, USA

[b] Department of Biocybernetics, Institute of Biomaterials and Bioengineering, Tokyo Medical and Dental University, Tokyo, Japan

[c] Department of Pharmacology, Tohoku University School of Medicine, Sendai, Japan

Growing evidence suggests that hypocretins/orexins, excitatory neuropeptides of hypothalamic origin, are critically involved in both the control of vigilance and in a sleep disorder, narcolepsy. Hypocretin-containing neurons project to the histaminergic tuberomammillary nucleus, and the histaminergic system may mediate some of the function of hypocretins. We found a decrease in global histaminergic neurotransmission in the brains of *hypocretin receptor 2* mutated canines, a genetic animal model of narcolepsy. We also found that central administration of a wake-promoting dose of hypocretin-1 increased brain histamine content in rats. Thus, involvement of a hypocretin-histamine interaction is suggested in the regulation of vigilance in both normal and pathological conditions.

1. Introduction

Narcolepsy is a chronic sleep disorder which affects 0.03-0.18% of the general population [1]. Recent animal studies in dogs and mice have led to the identification of genes (preprohypocretin and hypocretin receptor 2 *[Hcrtr-2]* genes) responsible for the disease [2, 3]. In humans, genetic mutations in the hypocretin-related genes are rare [4], but hypocretin deficiency is functionally involved in most cases [4, 5]. Hypocretins/orexins are primarily excitatory neuropeptides located exclusively in neurons of the lateral hypothalamic area, which send projections to most monoaminergic nuclei, such as adrenergic locus coeruleus, dopaminergic ventral tegmental area, and histaminergic tuberomammillary nucleus (TM) [6-8]. It is reported that intracerebroventricular (ICV) injection of hypocretin-1 enhances wakefulness in rats [9]. Considering the fact that Hcrtr-2 is enriched in the TM [10] (Eriksson et al, this issue), coupled with the fact that the histaminergic system plays an important role in the control of vigilance [11], it is likely that a deficit in histaminergic neurotransmission plays a role in the pathophysiology of narcolepsy. It is also possible that the wake-promoting action of hypocretin may be partially mediated by the histaminergic system.

In the current study, in order to test for a hypocretin/histamine interaction in the control of vigilance, we measured brain histamine levels in familial (*Hcrtr-2* mutated) narcoleptic and control Dobermans. We also measured changes in histamine content in the brains of rats 2 hours after ICV injection of a wake-promoting dose of hypocretin-1.

2. Materials and Methods

Brain tissue from 9 familial (*Hcrtr-2* mutated) narcoleptic and 9 control Dobermans was used. The brains of these animals were previously collected as described in Ripley et al [12]. The mean ages of narcoleptic and control animals were 26.0±21 months old, and 27.7±22.1 months old, respectively. Histamine content, as well as monoamine content (dopamine and norepinephrine and dopamine turnover), was measured in the cortex, thalamus and hippocampus with a fluorometric HPLC system [13] and with an HPLC with an electrochemical detector [14], respectively.

In order to evaluate whether the wake-promoting effect of hypocretin is mediated by the activation of the histaminergic neurotransmitter system, we also measured changes in histamine content in the brains (cortex, brainstem, cerebellum) of rats (control n=5, hypocretin n=4) 2 hours after an ICV injection of hypocretin-1 (5 nmol).

3. Results

We found that histamine content in the cortex (436±67 [SE] pmol/g) and thalamus (884±100 pmol/g) was significantly lower in narcoleptic Dobermans when compared to controls (733±93 pmol/g and 1749±227 pmol/g, respectively) (Fig. 1). The content in the hippocampus (602±132 pmol/g and 793±196 pmol/g, respectively) was also decreased, but was not statistically different.

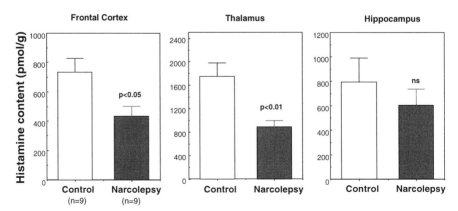

Figure 1. Measurement of histamine content in *Hcrtr 2*-mutated narcoleptic and control Dobermans. Histamine content in the cortex and thalamus was significantly lower in narcoleptic Dobermans than in controls (by student's t-test).

In the rat study, ICV injection of hypocretin-1 significantly enhanced wakefulness (169.9 % of that of the vehicle treatments) and increased histamine levels in the cortex (124 % of that of the vehicle treatments) and brainstem (130 %), but not significantly in the cerebellum (110%) (Fig. 2).

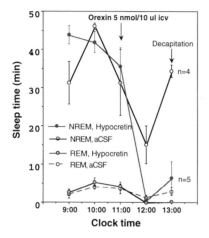
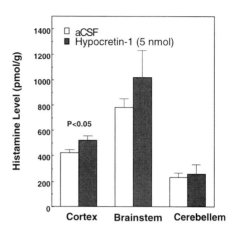

Figure 2. Measurement of histamine content after ICV administration of hypocretin-1 in rats. ICV injection of hypocretin-1 significantly reduced both non-REM sleep (NREM) and REM sleep, and increased histamine levels in the cortex and brainstem.

4. Discussion

In the genetic (*Hcrtr-2* mutated) canine model of narcolepsy, a decrease in global histaminergic neurotransmission is suggested. In contrast, DA and NE neurotransmission in the brain regions tested were not significantly altered. Since hypocretins excite TM histaminergic neurons through the activation of Hcrtr-2 (Eriksson et al, this issue), the decrease in histaminergic neurotransmission found in narcoleptic dogs may be due to the lack of hypocretin-mediated, excitatory input to TM histaminergic cell groups.

Genetically narcoleptic Dobermans have abnormal sleep patterns characterized by shorter sleep latencies, sleep onset REM sleep periods, and fragmented sleep patterns [15]. The 24 hour rest/activity pattern of these animals is also altered; affected animals are relatively inactive during the light period and do not show a clear rest-activity pattern [16]. Some of these characteristics are also observed in mice lacking histamine H1 receptors, such as a difficulty in staying awake during forced wake (i.e. sleep deprivation) (Mochizuki et al, this issue) and the disappearance of a clear rest-activity pattern [17]. Thus, it is possible that some aspects of the narcolepsy phenotype are mediated by impaired hypocretin/histamine interaction.

We previously demonstrated that H3 autoreceptor antagonists, such as GT-2331 and thioperamide, significantly reduce cataplexy and sleep in narcoleptic Dobermans [18]. Thus, compounds that enhance histaminergic neurotransmission may be a new choice in the treatment of narcolepsy.

Rat experiments also suggest that the wake-promoting effect of hypocretin may be partially mediated by the enhancement of histaminergic neurotransmission.

In conclusion, our results in rats and narcoleptic dogs suggest involvement of a hypocretin-histamine interaction in the regulation of vigilance in both normal and pathological conditions.

Acknowledgements

The authors thank Beth Ripley and Michael Chang for technical assistance. This work was supported by: NS 27710, NS23724, and MH01600.

References

1. Nishino, S., M. Okura, and M. Mignot, *Narcolepsy: genetic predisposition and neuropharmacological mechanisms.* Sleep Medicine Reviews, 2000. **4**(1): p. 57-99.
2. Lin, L., et al., *The sleep disorder canine narcolepsy is caused by a mutation in the hypocretin (orexin) receptor 2 gene.* Cell, 1999. **98**(3): p. 365-376.
3. Chemelli, R.M., et al., *Narcolepsy in orexin knockout mice: molecular genetics of sleep regulation.* Cell, 1999. **98**: p. 437-451.
4. Peyron, C., et al., *A mutation in a case of early onset narcolepsy and a generalized absence of hypocretin peptides in human narcoleptic brains.* Nat Med, 2000. **6**(9): p. 991-997.
5. Nishino, S., et al., *Hypocretin (orexin) deficiency in human narcolepsy.* Lancet, 2000. **355**(9197): p. 39-40.
6. De Lecea, L., et al., *The hypocretins: Hypothalamus-specific peptides with neuroexcitatory activity.* Proc Natl Acad Sci USA, 1998. **95**: p. 322-327.
7. Peyron, C., et al., *Neurons containing hypocretin (orexin) project to multiple neuronal systems.* J Neurosci, 1998. **18**(23): p. 9996-10015.
8. Sakurai, T., et al., *Orexins and orexin receptors: a family of hypothalamic neuropeptides and G protein-coupled receptors that regulate feeding behavior.* Cell, 1998. **92**(5): p. 573-585.
9. Hagan, J.J., et al., *Orexin A activates locus coeruleus cell firing and increases arousal in the rat.* Proc Natl Acad Sci U S A, 1999. **96**(19): p. 10911-10916.
10. Lu, X.Y., et al., *Differential distribution and regulation of OX1 and OX2 orexin/hypocretin receptor messenger RNA in the brain upon fasting.* Horm Behav, 2000. **37** (4): p. 335-344.
11. Lin, J.S., *Brain structures and mechanisms involved in the control of cortical activation and wakefulness, with emphasis on the posterior hypothalamus and histaminergic neurons.* Sleep Medicine Reviews, 2000. **4**(5): p. 471-503.
12. Ripley, B., et al., *Hypocretin levels in sporadic and familial cases of canine narcolepsy.* Neurobiology of disease, 2001, in press.

13.   Yamatodani, A., et al., *High-performance liquid chromatographic determination of plasma and brain histamine without previous purification of biological samples: cation-exchange chromatography coupled with post-column derivatization fluorometry.* J Chromatogr, 1985. **344**: p. 115-123.

14.   Yanai, K., et al., *Behavioral characterization and amounts of brain monoamines and their metabolites in mice lacking histamine H1 receptors.* Neuroscience, 1998. **87**(2): p. 479-487.

15.   Nishino, S., et al., *Is narcolepsy REM sleep disorder? Analysis of sleep abnormalities in narcoleptic Dobermans.* Neuroscience Research, 2000. **38**(4): p. 437-446.

16.   Nishino, S., et al., *Circadian distribution of rest/activity in narcoleptic and control dogs: assessment with ambulatory activity monitoring.* J Sleep Res, 1997, **6**: 120-127.

17.   Inoue, I., et al., *Impaired locomotor activity and exploratory behavior in mice lacking histamine H1 receptors.* Proc Natl Acad Sci U S A, 1996. **93**(23): p. 13316-13320.

18.   Tedford, C.E., et al., *Effects of a novel, selective, and potent histamine H3 receptor antagonist, GT-2332, on rat sleep/wakefulness and canine cataplexy.* Abstract: Soc Neurosci, 1999. **25**: p. 1134.

Histamine Research in the New Millennium
T. Watanabe, H. Timmerman and K. Yanai (Editors)

253

Central Histamine and Behavioral Respiration

I. Homma, M. Iwase, M. Kanamaru and M. Izumizaki

Department of Physiology, Showa University School of Medicine, 1-5-8 Hatanodai, Shinagawa-ku, Tokyo, 142-8555 Japan

Respiratory patterns are regulated by two systems, either metabolic respiration or behavioral respiration. We have been studying behavioral respiration histochemically, biochemically and physiologically using rabbits and mice to determine whether and how central histamine contributes to the regulation of respiration. The results indicate that central histamine may contribute to polypnea and a tracheal tension decrease induced by hyperthermia.

Key words; Central histamine, respiration, tracheal tension, sympathetic nerve, polypnea, hyperthermia

1. INTRODUCTION

Breathing is indispensable for us to live, and our chest is alternatively inflated and deflated without taking a rest. The center regulating the breathing pattern is located in the brain which is constituted by neural networks especially in the cerebral cortex, the limbic system and the brainstem. Even though the breathing movement looks like a simple rhythmic movement, the generator is controlled by various complex regulation systems. Respiratory output is regulated in the lower brainstem for metabolic demands of the body. Ventilation reflected on respiratory output consists of tidal volume and respiratory rate. These parameters increase when we inhale more oxygen and exhale more carbon dioxide under the chemical control system and also adjust the pH to maintain homeostasis of our body. This metabolic regulation system is always activated not only during the awake stage but also during the sleep stage. However, various inside or outside environmental factors influence our body, and our breathing pattern always changes during the awake stage. So-called behavioral breathing is believed to be generated in the higher center rather than the brainstem. The nervous system in the hypothalamus is especially important to adapt to the change in environment and plays a big role in the regulation of the autonomic nervous system.

Histaminergic neurons identified in the tuberomammillary nucleus (TMN) of the posterior hypothalamus are known to have a function in the nervous system related to sleep and awakening rhythms. Histamine secreted from this nervous system is called central histamine, named in order to distinguish between histamine secreted for the peripheral mast cells.
Recently it has become clear that histamine is related to various kinds of central nervous systems, such as feeding, learning, thermoregulation and autonomic functions [1]. We have been examining the role of central histamine on behavioral breathing during the past 10 years. We divide these studies into four parts as follows: 1. Physiological study, 2. Histochemical study, 3. Biochemical study, 4. Behavioral study.

254

2. RESULTS

2.1. Physiological study

Rabbits were intravenously anesthetized with urethane-chloralose, paralyzed with gallamine triethiodide and artificially ventilated through a tracheal canula. Administration of histamine into the fourth ventricle (IVth) dose-dependently decreased tracheal pressure (PT). The decrease of PT was blocked by pyrilamine, the H1-receptor antagonist, administered into the IVth. The administration of histamine into the IVth also increased the cervical sympathetic nerve activity simultaneously with the increase of PT. Electrical stimulation (0.5msec, 10-30Hz, 0.1-0.2mA) applied to the posterior hypothalamus caused PT to decrease, and the effect was reduced by the application of pyrilamine into the IVth. Administration of DL-homocysteic acid, which selectively stimulates cell bodies, into the TMN increased PT and the cervical sympathetic nerve activity. The effect was also blocked by pyrilamine into the bilateral rostroventrolateral medulla (RVLM).

2.2. Histological study

Rabbits were anesthetized with pentobarbital sodium; subsequently, Phaseolus vulgaris-leucoagglutinin (PHA-L) was applied into the TMN, an anterograde axonal tracer. After 10 to 21 days rabbits were perfused with 4% parformaldehyde and 0.4% glutaraldehyde in phosphate buffer. The medulla oblongata was sectioned into thin slices for histochemical study. PHA-L labeled fibers were identified in the C1, C2, A1 and A2 areas which were determined by tyrosine hydroxylase (TH)-immunohistochemistry (Fig.1). A double staining for PHA-L and TH-immunoreactivity was performed to find neurons projecting from the TMN. Some fibers labeled by PHA-L were in close contact with TH-immunoroactive neurons.

On the other hand, fluorogold (FG), a fluorescent tracer, was injected into the RVLM to examine retrograde labeling in the TMN. Cell bodies in the TMN were retrogradely labeled with FG from the RVLM and were immunoreactive with histamine.

Fig.1. Distribution of anterogradely labeled neuronal fibers (A) from the TMN and tyrosine hydroxylase-immunoreactive cell bodies (B) in the rostral medulla. A is ipsilateral to the PHA-L injection site [2].

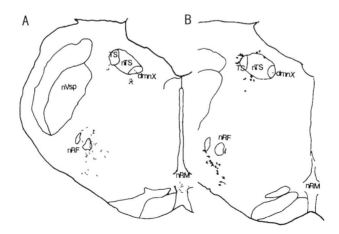

Fig. 2. Histamine release in the RVL induced by electrical stimulation of the posterior hypothalamus. Histamine concentrations are expressed as means ± SEM; underlining indicates samples during electrical stimulation; collection period 3 = 200μA and collection period 7 = 500μA, with 50Hz and 0.5ms pulses for 25min; HA, histamine concentration. *, Po=0.0129 for the repeated-measurement ANOVA with the Greenhouse-Geisser correction [3].

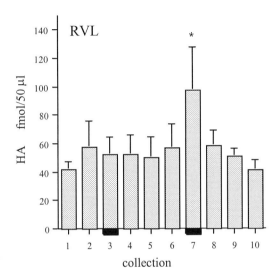

2.3. Biochemical study

Rabbits were anesthetized, paralyzed by gallamine triethiodide and artificially ventilated. Release of histamine from the RVLM, nR and nTs was investigated using microdialysis and high-performance liquid chromatography. Electrical stimulation of 0.5 mA applied to the posterior hypothalamus increased histamine release from these areas. Histamine release in the RVLM is shown in Fig. 2. Histamine release increased during perfusion of thioperamide, an H3-receptor antagonist, through a microdialysis probe. Moreover, histamine in the RVLM was significantly released during hyperthermia.

2.4. Hyperthermia and respiration

Mice were anesthetized with pentobarbital sodium for setting in a double-chamber body plethysmograph. Airflow of the head chamber was measured by a pneumotachograph. Tidal volume (VT), respiratory frequency (f), inspiratory time (TI) and expiratory time (TE) were measured. A raised body temperature induced by a heat lamp increased f with reduction in both TI and TE, and decreased VT. Application of S(+)-α-fluoromethylhistidine hydrochloride (α-FMH), which is a specific inhibitor of histidine decarboxylase, lowered f with a prolongation of TE at the raised temperature (Fig. 3).

Fig. 3 Comparison of respiratory frequency responses (top) to inspired CO2 with saline (●) and with α-FMH (○), VT (middle), and minute ventilation (bottom) at 36-37°C (A) and 39°C (B). Significant main effect for inspired CO2 (***p<0.001) ; significant main effect for α-FMH († P<0.05) [4].

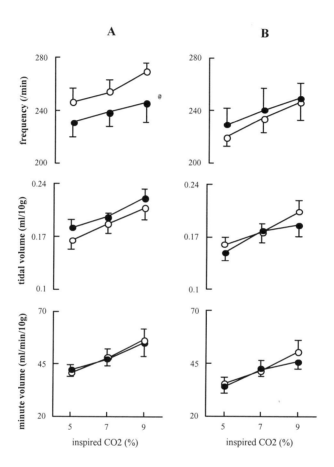

The same experiment was performed in mutant mice lacking the H1-receptors. Respiratory frequency in the mutant mice did not increase even though the body temperature was elevated (Fig. 4).

Fig. 4 Comparison of f responses (top) to inspired CO2 at 37-39°C (filled circle) and at 39°C (open circle), VT (middle), and VE (bottom) in wild (A) and histamine H1R deficient mice (B). Significant difference in f between at 37-38°C and at 39°C (*P < 0.05). Significant main effect for inspired CO2 (†† P < 0.01, ††† P < 0.001). Significant main effect for temperature († P < 0.05) [5].

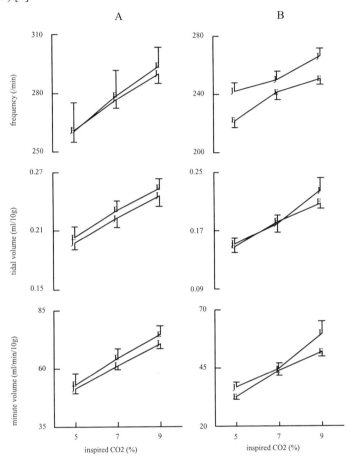

3. DISCUSSION

The neural networks regulating respiratory patterns for metabolic demands are located in the ventral part of the medulla oblongata, including the RVLM, and in the dorsal area, including nTs. In our study histaminergic neurons were determined to project from the TMN to C1 neurons in the RVLM. TMN neurons in the posterior hypothalamus have excitatory connections with the cervical sympathetic nerve [2]. Stimulation of the posterior hypothalamus releases histamine in the RVLM and decreases PT through the sympathetic nervous system.

258

Administration of histamine into the IVth also increases cervical sympathetic nerve activity and decreases the PT; furthermore, the H1-receptor antagonist into the IVth inhibits these effects [2]. Therefore, the PT is regulated by the hypothalamus through histamine H1-receptors in the RVLM and the cervical sympathetic nerve.

Stimulation of the posterior hypothalamus increased f but not VT (unpublished observation). This change of respiratory pattern, called polypnea, is similar to changes with increasing body temperature. A raised body temperature increased f, which was inhibited by the application of α-FMH. Temperature-induced polypnea could not be observed in the H1-receptor knockout mice. These results indicate that central histaminergic neurons in the TMN contribute to temperature-induced polypnea. Tracheal dilation controlled by central histaminergic neurons may be involved in the thermo-regulatory system.

REFERENCES

1. J.-C. Schwartz, J.-M. Arrang, M. Garbarg, H. Pollard and M. Ruat, Histaminergic transmission in the mammalian brain. Physiol. Rev., 71(1991) 1.
2. M. Iwase, M. Kanamaru, A. Kanamaru and I. Homma, Central histaminergic neurons regulate rabbit tracheal tension through the cervical sympathetic nerve. J. Auton. Ner. Sys.,74 (1998) 23.
3. M. Kanamaru, M. Iwase and I. Homma, Autoregulation of histamine release in medulla oblongata via H3-receptors in rabbits. Neurosci. Res., 31 (1998) 53.
4. M. Izumizaki, M. Iwase, H. Kimura, T. Kuriyama and I. Homma, Central histamine contributed to temperature-induced polypnea in mice. J. Appl. Physiol., 89 (2000) 770.
5. M. Izumizaki, M. Iwase, H. Kimura, K. Yanai, T. Watanabe, T. Watanabe and I. Homma, Lack of temperature-induced polypnea in histamine H1 receptor-deficient mice, Neurosci. Lett., 284 (2000) 139.

© 2001 Elsevier Science B.V. All rights reserved.
Histamine Research in the New Millennium
T. Watanabe, H. Timmerman and K. Yanai (Editors)

Peripheral neuronal histamine down regulates sympathetic activity and arterial pressure

H. Augusto Campos

Laboratory of origin: Laboratory of Functional Neurochemistry. Department of Pharmacology. Vargas Medical School. Central University of Venezuela. Caracas. Venezuela.

Mailing Address: H. Augusto Campos, M.D. P.O.Box 48269. Los Chaguaramos 1041-A. Caracas. Venezuela Telephones: +58-2-561-9871 (work). +58-2-241-5242 (private) Telefax: +58-2-241-5242 E-mail: hacampos@reacciun.ve

Abstract. The discovery of the peripheral reflex that down regulates sympathetic activity and arterial pressure, led to the notion that sympathetic activity is physiologically damped down in the intact rat and possibly in other animals and man. A histamine-containing neuron is involved in the peripheral short loop reflex. When sympathetic activity is enhanced, neuronal histamine is reflexly released to down regulate sympathetic activity via H-3 inhibitory receptors at sympathetic nerve terminals.

Keywords: Peripheral reflex, Sympathetic autoregulation, Neuronal histamine, Arterial pressure, Noradrenaline.

The concept that sympathetic activity in the intact rat is physiologically damped down by a peripheral inhibitory reflex, came from our studies on the relationship between a histamine (HA) pool and functionally intact sympathetic nerve terminals in the rat vas deferens. In the decade of the 1980s, we showed that chronic unilateral sympathectomy of the rat vas deferens causes a fall of HA levels in both the intact and the sympathectomized vas deferens. This bilateral effect was surprising and merited a more complete analysis. Following the anatomical distribution of the sympathetic system in the rat vas deferens, we performed surgical interruptions that we named preganglionic section (decentralization), ganglionectomy, interganglionic section and postganglionic axotomy. The changes of HA levels induced by these procedures suggested the presence of crossed HA-containing neuronal pathways adjacent to the sympathetic system of the rat vas deferens (Campos, 1983, 1988). These pathways are crossing over at the level of the sympathetic ganglionic clusters of both vasa deferentia. Then, we suggested that the cell bodies of neurons containing HA are located in the sympathetic ganglia. This proved to be true by using immunocytochemical techniques (Häppölä et, al., 1985). These authors showed the presence of HA-containing neurons in the superior cervical and caeliac ganglia of the rat. The neuronal system containing HA is structurally independent of the Central Nervous System as chronic decentralization does not modify its HA content.

260

The above mentioned distribution of HA-containing neurons was further sustained by the finding showing that chronic unilateral ganglionectomy causes a bilateral reduction of histidine decarboxylase (HD) activity in both vasa deferentia, as shown in Fig. 1. The fall of HA levels due to nerve degeneration parallels the reduction of HD activity, which suggests the presence of a decussation of HA-containing neuronal pathways at the level of the ganglionic clusters of both vasa deferentia.

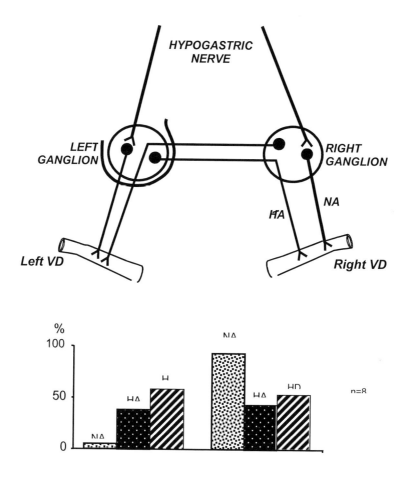

Fig 1. Effect of chronic unilateral sympathetic ganglionectomy on percentual changes of histamine (HA) levels and histidine decarboxylase (HD) activity in both rat vasa deferentia (Vs control, P< 0.005), NA noradrenaline; VD, vas deferens. After Campos, 1988, and Campos and Domínguez,1995.

At that time, we were wondering about the functional meaning of this novel system. We indirectly measured sympathetic activity in the rat vas deferens by following the time-course of noradrenaline (NA) depletion induced by reserpine in this organ, since the degree of depletion (NA release) is related to the traffic of impulses at the sympathetic nerve terminals (Karki et al., 1959; Hertting et al., 1962; Weiner et al., 1962; Benmiloud and Von Euler, 1963). Thus, we showed that unilateral sympathetic ganglionectomy causes a pronounced enhancement of reserpine- induced NA depletion (increase of sympathetic activity) in the contralateral vas deferens, as shown schematically in Fig. 2. When unilateral ganglionectomy is combined with contralateral decentralization, no enhancement of sympathetic activity is observed in the vas deferens contralateral to the ganglionectomy. This finding suggests that the peripheral inhibitory mechanism is evoked by the central sympathetic discharge, thus down regulating sympathetic activity. If the neuronal pathways involved in the decussation are interrupted (interganglionic section), facilitation of sympathetic activity occurs in both vasa deferentia. This bilateral facilitation is reverted when an i.v. infusion of HA (2 µg/kg/min) is given during the time of exposure to reserpine. All these findings suggest that a peripheral neuronal inhibitory mechanism, involving HA, is operating when sympathetic activity is enhanced in the vas deferens, thus regulating sympathetic activity. The neuronal system containing HA exerts a contralateral reciprocal inhibitory modulation of the vas deferens sympathetic activity (Campos and Briceño, 1992). Later on, an interaction between peripheral noradrenergic and HA-containing neurons was further shown in the vas deferens. In this respect, stimulation of sympathetic pathways to the vas deferens causes an increase in HD activity in the organ, and this increase is dependent on the functional integrity of the noradrenergic neuron, since it is blunted in the previously sympathectomized rat (Campos and Dominguez, 1995). Acute contralateral ganglionectomy subverts the increase in HD activity in the vas deferens whose sympathetic pathway was stimulated. Since the HA-containing neuronal pathways are relatively intact under these conditions, and if the interaction between noradrenergic and HA-containing neurons were direct, HD activity would have increased in the vas deferens whose sympathetic pathway was stimulated, but this did not occur. Therefore, the interaction requires the participation of an interneuron that conveys the message to the contralateral HA-containing ganglionic neuron, which, in turn, damps down sympathetic activity in the stimulated vas deferens (Fig. 3). The interneuron appears to be neuropeptidergic in nature since its destruction by neonatal administration of capsaicin causes facilitation of sympathetic activity (Campos et, al., 1998). These findings taken together depict a short loop reflex that down regulates sympathetic activity in the vas deferens.

Other findings referred below support the view that the peripheral reflex of sympathetic autoregulation found in the vas deferens is an overall mechanism that down regulates sympathetic activity:

a). A contralateral sympathetic ganglionic inhibitory mechanism that down regulates sympathetic activity was found in the dog heart, as facilitation of the tachycardia due to stimulation of the right sympathetic cardiac nerve occurs when left stellate ganglionectomy is performed (Campos and Briceño, 1992).

b). Footshock stress in the rat causes a rise of blood HA, which is dependent upon sympathetic activity because such a rise is blunted by previous ganglionic blockade or chronic sympathectomy (Campos and Montenegro, 1998).

c). The release of HA into the circulation due to enhancement of sympathetic activity, appears to be a compensatory phenomenon, wherein HA is inhibiting NA release from sympathetic nerve terminals through H-3 inhibitory receptors (Acuña et al.,1998).

262

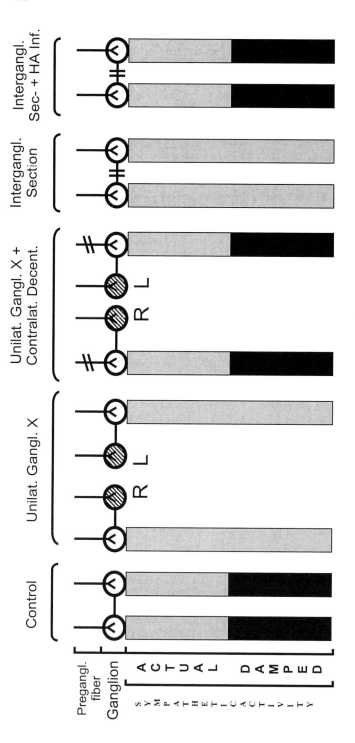

Fig 2. Schematic representation of changes of vas deferens sympathetic activity due to surgical interruptions of HA-containing neuronal pathways at the sites indicated. Unilat, unilateral. Gangl X, ganglionectomy. Contralat.decent, contralateral decentralization. Intergangl., interganglionic. HA INF., histamine infusion. Shaded circles: R, right ganglionectomy; L, left ganglionectomy. To assess sympathetic activity, reserpine was administered i.p. for 3 hours, 2mg/Kg. After Campos and Briceño, 1992.

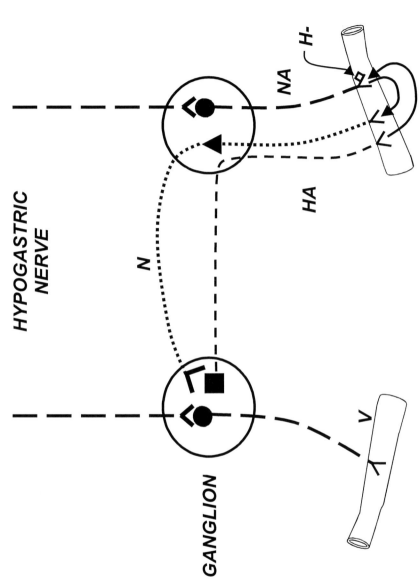

Fig 3. Scheme depicting the possible distribution of the three neurons involved in the peripheral reflex that down regulates sympathetic activity in the rat vas deferens. HA, histaminergic neuron. NA, noradrenergic neuron. NP, neuropeptidergic neuron. VD, vas deferens. H-3, histamine inhibitory receptor. The arrows indicate the direction of nerve impulses.

In this direction, alpha-methylhistamine, an H-3 receptor agonist, attenuates the hypertensive response to footshock stress, and thioperamide, an H-3 receptor antagonist, facilitates it.

d). Another finding indicating further the compensatory nature of the peripheral reflex is the following: Inhibition of neuronal HA biosynthesis in the rat by alpha-fluoromethylhistidine causes arterial hypertension and tachycardia. The enhancement of sympathetic activity could be the result of a relative absence of neuronal HA to be released and reach inhibitory H-3 receptors at the sympathetic nerve terminals (Domínguez et al.,1991; Campos et al., 1996).

e). In humans, some findings suggest that enhanced sympathetic activity is accompanied by a release of HA into the circulation, as it occurs in the rat. For example, mental arithmetic stress in children causes an increase in the urinary excretion of HA and NA (unpublished observations).

f). Treadmill exercise-induced enhancement of sympathetic activity causes a rise of blood HA in normotensive but not in primary hypertensive humans (Campos et al. , 1999), which indicates that the HA release that accompanies the enhancement of sympathetic activity is impaired in hypertensives. In addition, resting blood HA levels in hypertensives are half the ones of normotensives. We might speculate that peripheral neuronal HA is functionally deficient in hypertensives, and could be involved in the pathophysiology of the disease.

This brief analysis of the role of peripheral neuronal HA in the inhibitory modulation of sympathetic activity and arterial pressure allows us to conclude that a peripheral reflex, in which HA is involved, could be an important factor to consider in studies on the control of cardiovascular responses in animals and man.

Acknowledgements
This study was supported in part by grants from Consejo de Desarrollo Científico y Humanístico (09-11-3666-95) de la Universidad Central de Venezuela and Consejo Nacional de Investigaciones Científicas y Tecnológicas (SI-95000573), Caracas, Venezuela.

References
1. Campos HA. Histamine and the sympathetic system of the rat vas deferens. In: Velasco, M. (ed) Proceedings of the first Interamerican Congress of Clinical Pharmacology Therapy. Amsterdam: Excerpta Medica. International Congress Series, 1983; 119-120.
2. Campos HA. A possible crossed histamine containing pathway adjacent to the sympathetic system of the rat vas deferens. J Pharmacol Exp Ther 1988; 744: 1121-1127.
3. Häpölä O, Seinila S, Päivarinta H, Panula P, Eranko O. Histamine inmunoreacting cells in the superior cervical ganglion and the caeliac superior mesenteric ganglion complex of the rat. Histochemistry 1985; 82: 1-3.
4. Karki NT, Paasonen MK, Vanhakartano A. The influence of pentolinium, isoraunescine and yoimbine on the noradrenaline depleting actions of reserpine.
5. Hertting G, Potter LT, Axelrod J. Effect of decentralization and ganglionic blocking agents on the spontaneous release of H3-norepinephrine. J Pharmacol Exp Ther 1962; 136: 289-292.
6. Weiner N, Perkins M, Sidman RL. Effect of reserpine on noradrenaline content of innervated brown adipose tissue of the rat. Nature (Lond) 1962; 193: 137-138.

7. Benmiloud M, Von Euler US. Effects of bretylium, reserpine, guanethidine and sympathetic denervation on the noradrenaline content of the rat submaxillary gland. Acta Phisiol Scand 1963; 59: 34-42.

8. Campos HA, Briceño E. Two models of peripheral sympathetic autoregulation: Role of neuronal histamine. J Pharmacol Exp Ther 1992; 261: 943-950.

9. Campos HA, Domínguez J. Interaction between noradrenergic and histamine-containing neurons in the rat vas deferens. J Pharmacol Exp Ther 1995; 272: 732-738.

10. Campos HA, Losada M, Bravo C. Role of neuronal histamine and capsaicin-sensitive neurons in modulating peripheral sympathetic activity and arterial pressure. In: Velasco M., Hernandez R. (eds). New advances in Cardiovascular Physiology and Pharmacology. Amsterdam. Excerpta Medica International Congress Series, 1998; 217-221.

11. Campos HA, Montenegro M. Footshock-induced rise of rat blood histamine depends upon the activation of postganglionic sympathetic neurons. Eur J Pharmacol 1998; 347: 159-164.

12. Acuña Y , Mathison Y, Campos HA, Israel A. Thioperamide, a histamine H3-receptor blocker, facilitates vasopressor responses to footshocks. Inflamm res 1998; 47: 109-114.

13. Domínguez J, Sosa A, Campos HA, Hypertension in the rat induced by α-fluoromerhylhistidine. Abstract of the 9th Scientific Meeting of International Society of Hypertension. Rio de Janeiro. Hypertension 1991, 17:428

14. Campos HA, Acuña Y, Magaldi L, Israel A. Alpha-fluoromethylhistidine, an inhibitor of histamine biosynthesis, causes arterial hypertension. Naunyn- Schmiedeberg´s Arch Pharmacol 1996; 354: 627-632.

15. Campos HA, Montenegro M, Velasco M, Romero E, Alvarez R, Urbina A. Treadmill exercise-induced stress causes a rise of blood histamine in normotensive but not in primary hypertensive humans. Eur J Pharmacol 1999; 383: 69-73.

Histamine Research in the New Millennium
T. Watanabe, H. Timmerman and K. Yanai (Editors)

Changes in brain histamine H_1 receptors in chronic hepatic encephalopathy

V. Lozeva[a,b], D. Sola[a,c], C. Plumed[a,c], M. Attila[a,d], M. Hippeläinen[e], R. Butterworth[b], and L. Tuomisto[a]

[a]Department of Pharmacology and Toxicology, University of Kuopio, 70211 Kuopio, Finland

[b]Neuroscience Research Unit, Centre Hospitalier de l`Université de Montréal, Campus St-Luc, Montreal, Quebec, H2X 3J4, Canada

[c]Universitat Autonoma de Barcelona, Barcelona, Spain

[d]Department of Clinical Veterinary Sciences (Pharmacology and Toxicology), University of Helsinki, Helsinki, Finland

[e]Department of Surgery, Kuopio University Hospital, 70211 Kuopio, Finland

1. ABSTRACT

In order to assess the possible involvement of brain histamine in the pathogenesis of hepatic encephalopathy (HE), we have studied the binding properties and the regional distribution of histamine H_1 receptors in post-mortem brain tissue from cirrhotic patients with HE, as well as in an animal model of the disease, rats with portacaval anastomosis (PCA). Receptor binding studies and autoradiography were performed, employing the specific histamine H_1 receptor antagonist, [^{3}H]mepyramine. The results from the present study suggest a selective up-regulation of histamine H_1 receptors in the cortex of rats with PCA and patients with HE. In view of the fact that central histaminergic mechanisms are involved in the control of arousal and circadian rhythmicity and based on the previous observation of improved locomotor activity and circadian rhythmicity following blockade of central histamine H_1 receptors in PCA rats, these findings suggest that (1) cortical histaminergic hyperactivity could contribute to the neuropsychiatric symptoms characteristics of human HE and (2) that selective histamine H_1 receptor antagonists could be beneficial in the prevention and treatment of HE in cirrhotic patients.

2. BACKGROUND

The course of chronic liver failure can be complicated by the development of neurological symptoms, collectively known as hepatic encephalopathy (HE). Among the most common early symptoms of HE are sleep disturbances and altered circadian rhythms, which occur in approximately half of the cirrhotic patients without overt encephalopathy [1]. The exact mechanisms that underlie these changes are not well known. However, studies in an animal model of HE, the rat with portacaval anastomosis (PCA), have suggested that neurotransmission failure involving the serotonergic system is the most probable cause [2, 3]. We have recently shown that the histaminergic neurotransmitter system undergoes marked changes after PCA surgery [4, 5]. Histaminergic neurons in the mammalian brain participate in the regulation of a wide variety of functions, including vigilance, sleep, and circadian rhythmicity [6, 7]. Consequently, histaminergic synaptic imbalance could play a role in the development of the neurobehavioural changes in chronic HE, particularly the altered sleep-wake cycle and diurnal rhythms. Since histamine exerts these effects primarily through the activation of the post-synaptic histamine H_1 receptors [6, 7], and in view of the fact that the histamine H_1 blocker, mepyramine, improves the circadian rhythmicity scores in PCA rats [8], we hypothesised that changes in the central histamine H_1 receptors could be involved in experimental and human HE associated with chronic liver failure. Therefore, we studied the binding characteristics, the pattern of distribution and the regional density of these receptors in HE patients and in PCA rats.

3. MATERIAL AND METHODS

3.1. Material

Twenty-four male Han:Wistar rats, 250 - 300 grams, were used in this study. The rats were kept under constant conditions of light (12 hour light/12 hour dark) and temperature (20° ± 2°C) and received standard food pellet and tap water ad libitum. Twelve rats were subjected to end-to-side PCA surgery according to the method of Lee and Fisher, 1961 [9]. Control rats were sham-operated using the same procedure except for the anastomosis. All experiments were conducted six months after surgery. For the [³H]mepyramine saturation binding assay, the brains were dissected into cortex, cerebellum and rest of the brain. For the [³H]mepyramine autoradiographic procedure, serial coronal sections (15 μm thickness) from brains of sham-operated and PCA-operated rats were thaw-mounted on gelatine-coated glass slides. Post-mortem human brain tissue obtained from 6 cirrhotic patients who died in hepatic coma and 6 control subjects, matched for age, sex, and autopsy delay times were dissected into the following brain regions: frontal cortex, temporal cortex, insular cortex, parietal cortex, occipital cortex and caudate-putamen. All samples were kept at -80°C until use.

3.2. Histamine H_1 receptor binding.

Membrane suspensions prepared in 150 mmol/L Na^+/K^+ phosphate buffer, pH 7.5, were incubated for 60 min at 25°C with [³H]mepyramine in a final volume of 500 μL. For the saturation experiments, [³H]mepyramine was used at concentrations between 0.1 nmol/L and 15 nmol/L; the other experiments were performed with 2 nmol/L of the radioligand. Triprolidine, 1μmol/L concentration, was used for non-specific binding. The incubation was stopped by dilution with ice-cold buffer, followed by rapid filtration under vacuum through Whatman GF/B filters using a Millipore harvester. Filter-bound activity was counted by liquid scintillation spectrometry.

3.3. Histamine H_1 receptor autoradiography

Slides were incubated with 5 nmol/L [³H]mepyramine for 60 min at 4°C. Non-specific binding was determined by incubation of adjacent sections in the presence of 1 μmol/L triprolidine. Slides were drained, washed in buffer (2 x 5 min), rinsed briefly with ice-cold distilled water and dried quickly with an air blower. Slides and tritium standards were exposed to a tritium sensitive film (Hyperfilm-^{3}H, Amersham International) for 6 weeks. Regional optical densities were quantified by MCID image analysis device and program (Imaging Research Inc., St. Catharines, Canada). Brain structures were identified according to the stereotaxic atlas of Paxinos and Watson, 1986 [10].

3.4. Statistical analysis

Data are expressed as means ± SEM. All statistical analyses were performed using the computer software program GraphPad Prism. Data were analysed using two-factor ANOVA followed by the post-hoc Scheffe's F test. When two groups were compared, the unpaired two-tailed Student's t-test was used. A probability of less than 5% (p < 0.05) was considered to indicate statistical significance.

4. RESULTS AND DISCUSSION

4.1. Binding characteristics of central histamine H$_1$ receptors in rats with portacaval anastomosis and patients with HE.

The saturation binding study revealed a marked, ten-fold, difference in the maximal binding density (B$_{max}$) of [^{3}H]mepyramine binding between human and rat brain (Figure 1). Within the rat brain, binding was higher in the rest of brain compared with cortex in both sham and PCA-operated rats (Figure 1, A), whereas the binding affinity of approximately 10 nmol/L was similar in the two regions and did not change after PCA surgery. These results support the observation that histamine H$_1$ receptors show striking differences in their expression among various species and confirm the previously described 10-fold lower affinity of these receptors in rat brain compared with human brain (Kd = 7.4 ± 1.3 nmol/L and 0.5 ± 0.1 nmol/L for rat cortex and human frontal cortex respectively) [11]. Importantly, the present results show a significantly increased maximal binding density of [^{3}H]mepyramine binding in the cortex of PCA rats and HE patients.

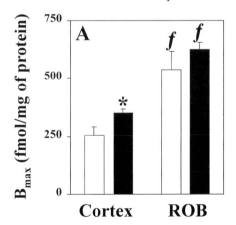 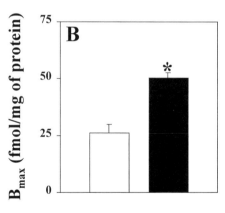

FIGURE 1. *Maximal binding density (B$_{max}$) for histamine H$_1$receptors in rat (A) and human (B) brain.* □ *Control;* ■ *HE/PCA. All values are group means ± S.E.M; all n=6. Statistics: ANOVA, followed by Sheffé's F-test. * p<0.05 vs. control; f p<0.05 vs. cortex.* **Abbreviations: PCA**=*portacaval anastomosis;* **ROB**= *rest of brain.*

4.2. Regional distribution of central histamine H₁ receptors in rats with portacaval anastomosis.

The regional distribution of histamine H₁ receptors in rat brain after PCA surgery was studied in detail with autoradiography (Figure 2). Histamine H₁ receptors were heterogeneously distributed in the brain of both sham- and PCA-operated rats. Binding was particularly high in the dentate gyrus and CA3-4 regions of the hippocampus, moderate in the hypothalamus, where the histaminergic neuron bodies are located, and low to moderate in cortex. The density of histamine H₁ receptors in the cerebellum was near the background level. These results support previous findings of heterogeneous distribution of histamine H₁ receptors in rat brain [12]. They also suggest that PCA surgery in the rat does not affect the pattern of distribution of the brain histamine H₁ receptors.

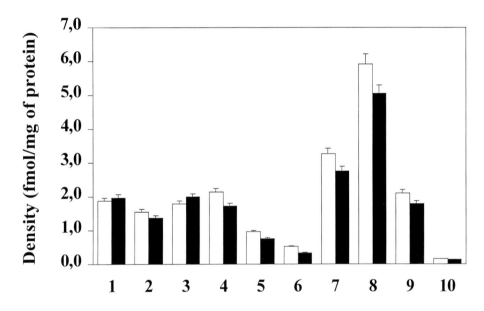

FIGURE 2. *Regional distribution of histamine H₁ receptors in brain of sham-operated ☐ or PCA-operated ■ rats. All values are group means ± S.E.M; both n=6. 1=Frontal cortex; 2=Temporal cortex; 3=Insular cortex; 4=Parietal cortex; 5=Occipital cortex; 6=Caudate-putamen; 7=Hippocampus, CA3-4; 8=Dentate gyrus; 9=Hypothalamus; 10=Cerebellum.*

4.3. Regional binding density of central histamine H₁ receptors in patients with HE.

The effect of HE on the density of histamine H₁ receptors in human brain was assayed in several cortical regions, as well as in caudate-putamen (Figure 3). Human parietal and temporal cortex showed the highest level of specific binding for [³H]mepyramine. Binding density in the caudate-putamen was very low. These findings are in good agreement with previous reports showing that the predominant location of the central histamine H₁ receptors in brain of primates is in cortex [13]. Importantly, there was a significantly higher [³H]mepyramine binding density in the frontal, parietal and insular cortex of patients with HE

(Figure 3). Taken together, the findings of increased [³H]mepyramine binding density in human cortex and the increased B_{max} for [³H]mepyramine in brain of PCA rats and HE patients suggest a moderate up-regulation of histamine H_1 receptors in chronic HE.

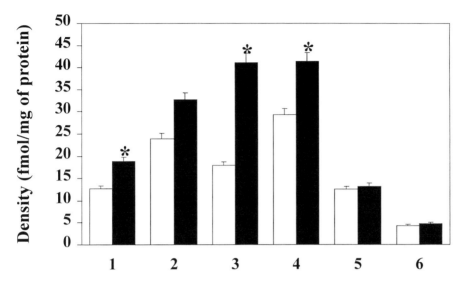

FIGURE 3. *Binding density of histamine H_1 receptors in brain of control* ☐ *or HE* ■ *patients. All values are group means ± S.E.M; both n=6. Statistics: Student`s t-test * p<0.05. 1=Frontal cortex; 2=Temporal cortex; 3=Insular cortex; 4=Parietal cortex; 5=Occipital cortex; 6=Caudate-putamen;*

Histamine has been implicated in the control of a wide range of physiological and behavioural functions, including sleep and arousal, and circadian rhythmicity. Activation of the post-synaptic histamine H_1 receptors suppresses the deep slow-wave sleep and promotes waking [14]. In addition, histamine H_1 receptors are important for the entrainment of circadian rhythms to the light-dark cycle in mammals [15, 16]. The clinical presentation of HE is dominated by the diminished total duration of slow-wave sleep and the disorganisation of the normal sleep cycle [1]. The neurological changes following PCA surgery in the rat are also manifested as disruptions of the sleep patterns and diurnal rhythms [8, 17]. The up-regulation of histamine H_1 receptors in cortex of PCA rats and HE patients, along with the selective changes in serotonin receptors found in autopsied brain tissue from patients with HE [18] may well account for the generation and maintenance of sleep disturbances in PCA rats and for the altered sleep patterns in cirrhotic patients with HE. The "classic" histamine H_1 receptor blocking antihistamines have long been known to exert significant effects on the sleep continuum in man. There is anecdotal evidence of the use of such drugs in patients with cirrhosis without apparent side effects [19]. Furthermore, we have previously reported a significant improvement in the circadian rhythmicity scores in PCA rats following mepyramine treatment [8]. Therefore, pharmacological blockade of the central histamine H_1 receptors may be of potential therapeutic value in cirrhotic patients with HE.

In conclusion, the findings from the present work support the idea that cortical histaminergic hyperactivity is a feature of experimental and human HE and give us grounds to suggest that selective histamine H_1 receptor antagonists could be beneficial in the prevention and treatment of HE in cirrhotic patients.

REFERENCES

1. J. Cordoba, J. Cabrera, L. Lataif, P. Penev, P. Zee, A.T. Blei, Hepatology 27 (1998) 339.

2. R.F. Butterworth, Semin Liver Dis., 16 (1996) 235.

3. R.F. Butterworth, J Hepatol., 32 (2000) 171.

4. V. Lozeva, E. MacDonald, A. Belcheva, M. Hippelainen, H. Kosunen, L. Tuomisto, J Neurochem., 71 (1998) 1450.

5. V. Lozeva, M. Attila, E. Anttila, K. Laitinen, M. Hippelainen, L. Tuomisto, Naunyn Schmiedebergs Arch. Pharmacol.,358 (1998) 574.

6. J.C. Schwartz, J.M. Arrang, M. Garbarg, H. Pollard, M. Ruat, Physiol. Rev. 71 (1991) 1.

7. A. Yamatodani, N. Inagaki, P. Panula, N. Itowi, T. Watanabe, H. Wada, Structure and functions of the histaminergic neurone system, Uvnäs B (ed.) Histamine and histamine antagonists, Springer-Verlag, Berlin, 1991, 243

8. V. Lozeva, A. Valjakka, A. Lecklin, H. Olkkonen, M. Hippelainen, M. Itkonen, C. Plumed, L. Tuomisto, Hepatology, 31 (2000) 336.

9. Lee SH, Fischer B. Porto-caval shunt in the rat. Surgery 1961;50:668-672

10. Paxinos G, & G. Watson (eds.) The rat brain in stereotaxic coordinates, 2nd edn. Academic Press, Sidney, 1986

11. J.C. Schwartz, J.M. Arrang, M.L. Bouthenet, M. Garbarg, H. Pollard, and M. Ruat, Histamine receptors in brain. In: Uvnäs B, (ed.) Histamine and histamine antagonists. Springer-Verlag, Berlin, 1991, 191

12. J.M. Palacios, W.S. Young 3d, M.J. Kuhar, Eur. J. Pharmacol. 58 (1979) 295.

13. B. Bielkiewicz, D.A. Cook, Can. J. Physiol. Pharmacol. 63 (1985) 756.

14. K. Tasaka. New advances in histamine research. Spinger Verlag, Tokyo, 1994

15. L. Tuomisto, Involvement of histamine in circadian and other rhythms. In: Watanabe T, Wada H (eds.) Histaminergic neurons: morphology and function. Boca Raton: CRC Press, 1991, 283.

16. E.H. Jacobs, A. Yamatodani, H. Timmerman, Trends Pharmacol. Sci. 21 (2000) 293

17. V. Lozeva, A. Valjakka, E. Anttila, E. MacDonald, M. Hippeläinen, L. Tuomisto, Hepatology 29 (1999) 340.

18. V.L. Rao, R.F. Butterworth, Neurosci. Lett., 182 (1994) 69.

19. C.G. Meredith, C.D. Christian Jr., R.F. Johnson, S.V. Madhavan, S. Schenker, Clin. Pharmacol. Ther. 35(1984) 474.

Histamine Research in the New Millennium
T. Watanabe, H. Timmerman and K. Yanai (Editors)

Activation of central histaminergic system induced by histamine H_3-receptor antagonists on anxiety and learning in mice.

K. Onodera[a], M. Imaizumi[b], S. Miyazaki[c], N. Sogawa[a] and H. Furuta[a]

[a]Department of Dental Pharmacology, Okayama University Dental School, Okayama, 700-8525, Japan

[b]Laboratory of Nutrition Chemistry, Division of Applied Life Sciences, Graduate School of Agriculture, Kyoto University, Kyoto, 606-8502, Japan

[c]Immunology Laboratory, Diagnostic Division, Yamasa Corporation, Choshi, 288-0056, Japan

We studied that effects of H_3 antagonists which could enhance release of histamine from presynaptic terminals on anxiety, and learning and memory in mice. Thioperamide, an H_3 antagonist, significantly decreased the locomotion and time spent in a light zone, and shuttle crossing, which means anxiogenic effects in a light/dark test, only when the animals were pretreated with zolantidine, an H_2 antagonist. The decreased parameters induced by the combination of thioperamide and zolantidine were reversed by pretreatment with pyrilamine, an H_1 antagonist. Further, thioperamide significantly ameliorated learning deficits induced by scopolamine when mice were pretreated with zolantidine in an elevated plus-maze test. The ameliorating effects of thioperamide plus zolantidine were also antagonized by pyrilamine. These results suggest that thioperamide induces the release of neuronal histamine, which produces the anxiogenic effect and the ameliorating effect on scopolamine-induced learning deficits via H_1-receptors.

The other H_3 antagonists, clobenpropit and FUB 181 also improved scopolamine-induced learning deficits in mice in a passive avoidance test and the elevated plus-maze test, respectively. The effects of cloenpropit were significant only when mice were pretreated with zolantidine but FUB 181 significantly improved without zolantidine.

These results suggest that central histaminergic systems are involved in anxiety, and learning and memory. Further, H_3 antagonists such as FUB 181 may be useful as a novel cognitive enhancer.

1. INTRODUCTION

Central histamine neurons are suggested various physiological roles such as thermoregulation, feeding behavior, circadian rhythms and so on (1). Classical H_1 antagonists being capable to penetrate brood brain barrier (BBB) are well known to induce sleepiness and recently non-sedative H_1 antagonists such as terfenadine are developed (2). Therefore, histaminergic neuronal systems in the brain may be involved in higher functions such as learning and emotion. We addressed this problem using animal model measuring anxiety, and learning and memory.

Histamine receptors are classically known as postsynaptic H_1 and H_2 subtypes. Arrang et al. reported existence of presynaptic autoreceptors, H_3, regulating histamine release and synthesis in 1983 (3). Histamine, an agonist of H_3 receptors, suppressed histamine release acting on these receptors and an antagonist enhanced its release and activated histamine neurons (4). Because histamine can not cross the BBB, peripherally injected histamine does not elicit a central action. Recently, centrally acting and specific H_3 antagonists have been developed and we got a tool activating central histamine neurons by a systemic injection. Therefore, we studied effects of several histamine H_3 antagonists on anxiety, and learning and memory in animal models to examine involvement of central histaminergic neuronal systems in these higher brain functions.

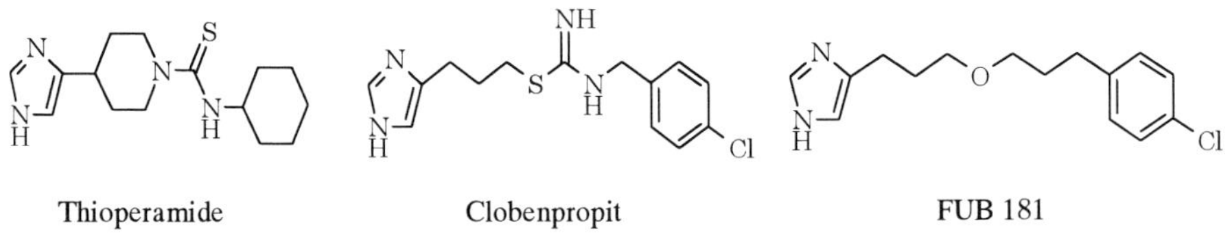

| Thioperamide | Clobenpropit | FUB 181 |

Figure 1. H_3 antagonists.

2. ANXIETY

We used a light/dark test to measure anxiety in mice (5). The light/dark test measures anxiety without punishing based on propensity of natural aversion to a light place in rodents and exploratory behaviors in the novel circumstances (6).

Namely, mice put in the unfamiliar light/dark box do exploration in the both boxes but spent more time in the dark box because of aversion to the light place and preference for the dark place. Anxiolytics are thought to relieve the rodents from aversion to the light place and increase time spent in the light box, and anxiogenics act vice versa.

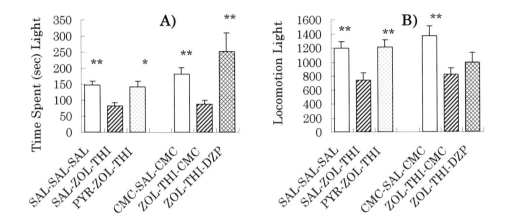

Figure 2. Antagonism of zolantidine (ZOL) plus thioperamide (THI)-induced anxiogenic effects by pyrilamine (PYR) and diazepam (DZP) in time spent (A) and locomotion (B) in the light zone in a light/dark test. PYR (6 mg/kg), ZOL (6 mg/kg), THI (20 mg/kg) and DZP (5 mg/kg) were ip injected 80, 70, 60 and 15 min before the test, respectively. Appropriate vehicles, saline (SAL) and saline containing 0.5% carboxymethylcellulose (CMC), were administered as control at the same manner. Each column and bar represent mean + S.E. * $p<0.05$, ** $p<0.01$ vs. a ZOL, THI and vehicle-treated group by the Mann-Whitney U test.

We examined effects of thioperamide, an H_3 antagonist, on the light/dark test in mice (7). Thioperamide decreased time spent and locomotion in the light zone, which meant anxiogenic effects in this test (Figure 2). These effects were antagonized by pretreatment with pyrilamine, an H_1 antagonist, but enhanced by zolantidine, an H_2 antagonist, and reached a significant level. Anxiogenic effects induced by zolantidine plus thioperamide were antagonized by pyrilamine before it and by diazepam, an anxiolytic, after it (8). These results suggested that histamine released from presynapses by thioperamide stimulated postsynaptically both H_1- and H_2-receptors to elicit anxiogenic effects. The stimuli to H_1-receptors mediated anxiogenic effects and the stimuli to H_2-receptors might mask the H_1-mediated anxiety. We also observed that betahistine, an H_1 agonist and H_3 antagonist, showed anxiogenic effects in combination with zolantidine and those were antagonized by pretreatment with pyrilamine, which supported the H_1-mediated anxiety (9).

3. LEARNING AND MEMORY

Learning and memory in mice were evaluated by an elevated plus-maze test (10) and a passive avoidance test (11). The both tests consist of one acquisition trial and one retention trial 24 h after it, and we disturb learning in mice by scopolamine, a muscarinic antagonist, which are well known to induce learning deficits. In the elevated plus-maze test, each mouse was placed on an end of the open arm and learned to escape to a closed arm from fear of the open space. We evaluated escape behavior by a transfer latency, a time taking until each mouse enter into the closed arm from start. In the retention trial, a day after the acquisition trial, the transfer latency was significantly reduced but pretreatment with scopolamine before the acquisition trial significantly suppressed its decrease in the retention trial, which meant scopolamine-induced learning deficits. If drugs ameliorate these deficits, the transfer latency in the retention trial becomes shorter than the scopolamine-treated deficient group. On the other hand, in a passive avoidance test, mice learned suffering from electric foot shocks in a dark box and avoid it by staying on the light box in spite of preference for a dark place.

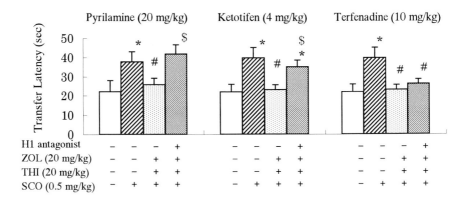

Figure 3. Ameliorating effects of zolantidine (ZOL) plus thioperamide (THI) on scopolamine (SCO)-induced learning deficits and antagonism by H_1 antagonists in an elevated plus-maze test. H_1 antagonists, ZOL, THI and SCO were ip injected 80, 70, 60 and 15 min before the test, respectively. Appropriate vehicle was administered as control at the same manner. Each column and bar represents a mean transfer latency in a retention trial + S.E. * p<0.05 vs. control, # p<0.05 vs. a SCO induced-deficient group, $ p<0.05 vs. a THI+ZOL induced amelioration by the Mann-Whitney U test.

Effects of thioperamide in the elevated plus-maze test (12)

Thioperamide significantly ameliorated learning deficits induced by scopolamine when the animals were pretreated with zolantidine. The ameliorating effects of thioperamide plus zolantidine were antagonized by pyrilamine and ketotifen, central acting H_1 antagonists but not terfenadine, an H_1 antagonist, which is hardly capable of passing the BBB (Figure 3). We further examined histaminergic contribution to learning and memory using the another animal model and another H_3 antagonist.

Effects of clobenpropit in the passive avoidance test (13)

Clobenpropit (10 mg/kg) also significantly ameliorated learning deficits induced by scopolamine (1 mg/kg) when the animals were pretreated with zolantidine (20 mg/kg) in the passive avoidance test. The ameliorating effects of thioperamide plus zolantidine were antagonized by pyrilamine (20 mg/kg), an H_1 antagonist and *(R)*-α-methylhistamine (20 mg/kg), an H_3 agonist.

These results suggested that the ameliorating effects were also mediated H_1-receptors and stimuli to H_2-receptors might act conversely to those to H_1-receptors in similar with the anxiogenic effects. This idea was supported by the findings which intracerebroventricularly injected 4-methylhistamine, an H_2 agonist, disrupted the passive avoidance like scopolamine and this effect was antagonized by zolantidine (14).

These findings suggested possible development of a cognitive enhancer (a nootropic drug) based on H_3 antagonists. However, both thioperamide and clobenpropit include a sulfur atom in their chemical structures (Figure 1) and hepatic adverse effects are afraid (15). Therefore, we examined that ameliorating effects of a newly developed H_3 antagonist without the sulfur atom on scopolamine-induced learning deficits in mice.

Effects of FUB 181 in the elevated plus-maze test (16)

FUB 181 (2.5 and 5 mg/kg) alone significantly ameliorated learning deficits induced by scopolamine (0.5 mg/kg). The ameliorating effects of FUB 181 (2.5 mg/kg) were antagonized by ketotifen (4 mg/kg) but not terfenadine (10 mg/kg). These effects were also blocked by BP 2.94 (10 mg/kg), an H_3 agonist. Moreover, zolantidine (20 mg/kg) enhanced the ameliorating effects of a lower dose (1.3 mg/kg) of FUB 181 which itself was not significant, and their effects reached significant level by the combination of treatments.

In the present study, we suggested that central histaminergic systems were involved in anxiety, and learning and memory using H_3 antagonists. Stimuli to H_1-receptors and those to H_2-receptors might elicit converse effects each other. Further, we showed that an H_3 antagonist, FUB 181, might be developed as a novel cognitive enhancer.

REFERENCES

1. K. Onodera, A. Yamatodani, T. Watanabe and H. Wada, Prog. Neurobiol. 42 (1994) 685.
2. M.J. Mattila and I. Paakkari, Eur. J. Clin. Pharmacol. 55 (1999) 85.
3. J.M. Arrang, M. Garbarg and J.C. Schwartz, Nature, 302 (1983) 832.
4. J.M. Arrang, M. Garbarg and J.C. Schwartz, Neuroscience, 15 (1985) 553.
5. M. Imaizumi, T. Suzuki, H. Machida and K. Onodera, Jpn. J. Psychopharmacol., 14 (1994) 83.
6. M. Imaizumi, Meth. Find. Exp. Clin. Pharmacol., 18 (Suppl. A) (1996) 31.
7. M. Imaizumi and K. Onodera, Life Sci., 53 (1993) 1675.
8. M. Imaizumi and K. Onodera, Annals Psychiat., 5 (1995) 239.
9. M. Imaizumi, S. Miyazaki and K. Onodera, Meth. Find. Exp. Clin. Pharmacol., 18 (1996) 19.
10. S. Miyazaki, M. Imaizumi and H. Machida, Meth. Find. Exp. Clin. Pharmacol., 17 (1995) 121.
11. S. Miyazaki, M. Imaizumi and K. Onodera, Meth. Find. Exp. Clin. Pharmacol., 17 (1995) 653.
12. S. Miyazaki, M. Imaizumi and K. Onodera, Life Sci., 57 (1995) 2137.
13. S. Miyazaki, K. Onodera, M. Imaizumi and H. Timmerman, Life Sci., 61 (1997) 355.
14. K. Onodera, S. Miyazaki and M. Imaizumi, Meth. Find. Exp. Clin. Pharmacol., 20 (1998) 307.
15. F.S. LaBella, G. Queen, G. Glavin, G. Durant, D. Stein and L.J. Brandes, Br. J. Pharmacol., 107 (1992) 161.
16. K. Onodera, S. Miyazaki, M. Imaizumi, H. Stark and W. Schunack. Naunyn-Schmiederberg's Arch. Pharmacol., 357 (1998) 508.

Mast cells, ECL cell and others:

2001 Elsevier Science B.V.
Histamine Research in the New Millennium
T. Watanabe, H. Timmerman and K. Yanai (Editors)

Role of Histamine and Mast Cells in Metabolic Encephalopathy

P.J. Langlais

Behavioral Neurobiology Section, Dept. of Psychology, SDSU, San Diego,CA 92021 and Neurology Service, VA San Diego Healthcare System, San Diego, CA 92121.

1.0 OXIDATIVE STRESS AND METABOLIC ENCEPHALOPATHY

Wernicke's encephalopathy is a metabolic disorder associated with thiamine (vitamin B1) deficiency. An important feature of thiamine deficiency-induced brain damage is the selective vulnerability of specific brain regions to pathologic changes. In humans, WE is characterized by bilateral lesions of the midline, medial, and intralaminar nuclei of the thalamus, the mammillary body, periacqueductal grey, brainstem periventricular regions, and the cerebellar vermis (1). Adjacent structures and other brain regions remain relatively unaffected. A second important feature of WE is that the lesions often develop 'silently', i.e., in the absence of detectable clinical features. This is particularly evident among alcoholics in whom WE is common and in many cases goes undiagnosed clinically (2).

Thiamine plays a key role in the utilization of glucose, acting as a coenzyme in the form of thiamine pyrophosphate (TPP), also known as thiamine diphosphate (TDP). Reductions in α-ketoglutarate dehydrogenase, a TPP-dependent enzyme of the Krebs cycle, occur in many neurodegenerative diseases but it is not known what relationship, if any, these reductions have to the selective lesions. Is TD an initiating event, part of a critical cascade, or merely a secondary phenomenon? Studies of experimental thiamine deficiency have suggested that changes in histamine release, mast cell degranulation and vascular disturbances may be initial and critical events in the pathogenesis of WE. These studies and a model of the pathogenesis of WE are the focus of this paper and described in the following sections.

2.0 PTD RODENT MODEL OF WERNICKE'S ENCEPHALOPATHY

Pyrithiamine is a potent and highly selective inhibitor of thiamine within nervous tissue. When combined with a thiamine deficient diet, daily pyrithiamine administration produces a reproducible sequence of clinical, biochemical and histological changes in the rat that occur over a period of several days (Figure 1). This latter feature offers a significant advantage over conditions such as ischemia in which the entire pathogenetic cascade can evolve and run its course within just a few minutes to hours. The selective distribution and nature of the lesions observed in the PTD rat bear a striking resemblance to that observed in human WE (3). Experimental PTD treatment results in both "delayed onset" apoptosis and fulminant necrosis within thalamus but not in other vulnerable brain regions (4,5). Rats with PTD-induced lesions, like patients with WKS, have significant anterograde cognitive impairments (3,6).

3.0 A WORKING MODEL OF THE LATE EVENTS UNDERLYING PTD-INDUCED THALAMIC DAMAGE

In recent years, a number of important events have been uncovered which appear to be the immediate causes of neuronal and tissue destruction within thalamus of the PTD rat. These changes appear to follow a temporal sequence, shown in Figure 1, and result in the appearance of both apoptosis and necrosis.

3.1 BBB Breakdown.

A breakdown in the blood-brain barrier (BBB) occurs after 12-13 days of PTD treatment and coincident with the onset of ataxia. A number of cellular changes also occur within or near microvessels of the thalamus. These changes include an increased activity of endothelial nitric oxide synthase (eNOS) and NADPH-diaphorase, presence of inducible NOS (iNOS) enzyme in microglia, and ferritin accumulation in microglia (7,8). Vascular changes, i.e., edema, perivascular leakage and dilated blood vessels, are among the first to occur within vulnerable thalamic regions of the PTD rodent (9). BBB breakdown is associated with extravasation of serum proteins within vulnerable brain regions, including thalamus and inferior colliculus (10). Similar early disruptions of the BBB have also been reported in the PTD mouse (11), guinea pig (12) and human WE (13).

BBB-Breakdown Endothelial *i*NOS, Increased eNOS	Increased ROS c-*fos*, c-*jun*, *fos*-B	TUNEL+Cells Increased ECF Glutamate Excitotoxic-type changes in Ge and AV nuclei	Necrosis & Apoptosis in VPL/VPM
DURATION OF THIAMINE DEFICIENCY			
Day 12-----------------→ **ATAXIA**	Day 13-----------------→ **LOSS OF RIGHTING REFLEXES**	Day 14-----------------→	Day 15 **OPISTHOT ONOS**

Figure 1.

3.2 Free Radical Production and IEG Activation

When animals reach the stage at which righting reflexes are impaired, increased tissue levels of reactive oxygen species (ROS)(14) are observed within the thalamus. This increase in ROS and free radicals may lead to lipid peroxidation, DNA damage, and eventual cell death. This hypothesis is supported by two recent observations. First, administration of the free radical scavenger, deprenyl, increases neuronal survival within PTD rats (15). Secondly, at this same stage of PTD, i.e., loss of righting reflexes, there is a marked increase in the expression of the immediate-early genes (IEG), c-*fos*, c-*jun*, and *fos*-B within neurons within the thalamus (16,17). The orchestrated activation of these IEGs is believed to be essential to the initiation of DNA fragmentation and apoptosis.

3.3 Elevated Extracellular Glutamate and NMDA-Mediated Excitotoxicity.

When righting reflexes are severely impaired (day 14), extracellular fluid (ECF) concentration of glutamate, measured by in vivo microdialysis, increases significantly within VPM/VPL region of thalamus but not within non-vulnerable brain regions such as the hippocampus and prefrontal cortex (18,19). Pretreatment with MK-801, a noncompetitive NMDA receptor antagonist, prevents the elevation of glutamate within thalamus (18) and dramatically reduces the extent of necrotic lesions within medial and lateral thalamus (20). However, MK-801 administration does not provide complete protection against PTD-induced neuronal loss within lateral thalamus (21). These observations suggest that mechanisms other than glutamate-NMDA mediated excitotoxicity may play a role in thiamine deficiency-induced neurodegeneration within thalamus.

3.4 Apoptosis and Necrosis

Shortly after the complete loss of righting reflexes, and when animals display a characteristic hunched posture called opisthotonus, neurons displaying excitotoxic-type cytopathological changes (4) and positive staining for apoptotic DNA fragmentation (5) are observed within thalamus. Ultrastructural analyses have provided definitive evidence of a sequence of pathologic changes within thalamus that are highly consistent with an excitotoxic process beginning on days 13-14 of PTD treatment (4). The onset of these excitotoxic-apoptotic changes occurs first within the gelatinosus, also known as the submedius nucleus, then within anterior nuclei, then the ventrolateral and ventrobasal nuclei (VPL/VPM) and lastly appears within the midline intralaminar nuclei. These DNA changes occur within thalamus and medial geniculate but not in other vulnerable regions such as the inferior colliculus and mammillary body.

4.0 ROLE OF HISTAMINE AND MAST CELLS IN VASCULAR DISTURBANCES AND CELL LOSS

4.1 Histamine Release in Early, Pre-Lesion Stages of PTD

Two studies have examined the hypothesis that changes in histamine release contribute to the early vascular changes in PTD treated rats. This hypothesis was prompted by several observations. First, histamine is a well-known regulator of both blood vessel diameter and vascular permeability and the histaminergic innervation of cerebral vasculature is well documented (22,23). Second, regionally selective increases in tissue histamine concentrations have been previously reported in the brains of thiamine deficient rats (24-26). The first study from our labs (27) using in vivo microdialysis demonstrated a significant increase in histamine release within thalamus but not hippocampus of PTD rats during the onset of histological lesions. Since prelesion stages of TD were not examined in this earlier study, it was unclear whether increased histamine release within thalamus was the result or the cause of the vascular changes that precede active neuronal degeneration.

A second study (28) demonstrated that compared to pairfed controls (PFC) histamine release is significantly increased within lateral and medial thalamus after only 9-10 days of PTD. At this duration of thiamine deficiency, there is enhanced vascular permeability, perivascular edema but no evidence of BBB breakdown or neuronal damage (4). These results suggest that enhanced histamine release may directly contribute to the early vascular changes. Interestingly, histamine release was also significantly increased within the hippocampus on day 9, declined progressively on days 10-12 and then increased on days 13-14 of thiamine deficiency (28). Neither vascular damage nor marked neuronal loss has been reported in the hippocampus. The observation of elevated histamine release in a brain region that is relatively resistant to PTD-induced damage suggests at least two possibilities: First, the effect of histamine on vascular changes is regionally specific. Second, the vascular changes within the thalamus are caused by factors other than increased histamine release.

4.2 Proliferation and Degranulation of Mast Cells

Within the brain, histamine is contained within two compartments, i.e., nerve terminals of the tuberomammillary (TM) nucleus of the hypothalamus and mast cells. As in several other parts of the body, mast cells are situated most frequently around blood vessels. Degranulation of mast cells locally opens the BBB, enhancing permeability and swelling of endfoot processes (29) and has been implicated in a variety of conditions leading to brain damage (30,31). After only 6 days of PTD treatment large clusters of mast cells, frequently associated with ED2 positive macrophages line thalamic blood vessels(28,32). A significant proportion of these mast cells are actively degranulating on day 7 within lateral thalamus and day 8 within medial thalamus of PTD treated rats. The percentage of degranulating mast cells increases steadily over subsequent days of PTD, reaching a maximum on days 9-10. Mast cells were not detected in hippocampus, lateral vestibular nucleus, inferior olivary complex, or facial nucleus in any of the controls or PTD-treated animals. These latter observations suggest that recruitment of mast cells is specific to thalamus and occurs much earlier in PTD and prior to any of the vascular changes reported to date in the PTD rat model. Ultrastructural electron microscopic analyses have confirmed the movement of mast cells from the blood into the parenchyma and the presence of large numbers of degranulating mast cells in regions of the thalamus in early, presymptomatic PTD-treated animals (33).

The presence of large numbers of degranulating mast cells could trigger the expression of cell adhesion molecules and attract additional mast cells into thalamus. This hypothesis is consistent with the recent report of increased expression of endothelial cell ICAM within thalamus of thiamine deficient mice (7). However, a significant increase in degranulation occurred on day 7, whereas an increase in mast cell number was observed as early as day 6 of TD. It is possible that the small and non-significant increases in rate of degranulation on day 6 was sufficient to trigger migration of blood born cells into thalamus. Alternatively, it is possible that some unique property of endothelial cells within thalamus causes them to produce adhesion molecules and possibly promote mast cell degranulation in response to TD. Exposure of rat brain endothelial cells in culture to TD produces increased glucose consumption and lactate production, cytotoxic effects, and increased permeability on a monolayer of these endothelial cells (34). In thiamine deficient mice, enhanced endothelial nitric oxide synthase and NADPH-diaphorase have been observed within microvessels in thalamus (7). Nitric oxide (NO•) not only produces enhanced permeability of BBB but also directly stimulates mast cell degranulation. The role of NO• in the early vascular changes and mast cell degranulation is currently under study in our laboratories.

5.0 A Working Model of TD-Induced Metabolic Encephalopathy

Our current model of the role of histamine and mast cells is shown in Figure 2 and suggests that TD triggers the release of histamine and cytokines from mast cells, macrophages and glia which in turn promote vascular permeability, release of NO and the production of free radicals. These series of biochemical changes subsequently lead to increase ECF glutamate and lipid peroxidation, breakdown of the BBB barrier and apoptotic and necrotic cellular destruction.

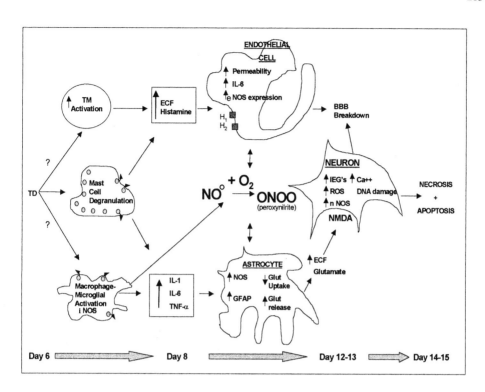

REFERENCES

1. Victor M, Adams RD, Collins GH <u>The Wernicke-Korsakoff's Syndrome and Related Neurologic Disorders due to Alcoholism and Malnutrition</u>, (1989): F.A. Davis:Philadelphia.

2. Harper CG, Giles M, Finlay-Jones R <u>J. Neurol Neurosurg Psychiat</u> 49 (1983) 341.

3. Langlais PJ In L.R. Squire & N. Butters (Eds), <u>Neuropsychology of Memory</u>, (1992)pp. 440-450, New York: Guilford Press

4. Zhang, S.X., Weilersbacher GS, Henderson SW, Corso T., Olney JW, Langlais PJ, <u>J Neuropathol Exp Neurol</u> 54(1995)255-267.

5. Matsushima K, MacManus JP, Hakim AM, <u>Neuro Report 8</u> (1997)867-870.

6.Langlais PJ, Savage LM, <u>Behav Brain Res, 68</u> (1995)75-89.

7.Calingasan NY, Park LCH, Calo LL, Trifiletti RR, Gandy SE, Gibson GE, <u>Amer J Pathol</u> 153 (1998) 599-610.

8.Calingasan NY, Park LCH, Uchida K, Gibson GE, <u>Soc Neurosci Abstr</u> 24(1998) 475.

9. Watanabe I, Kanabe S J, <u>Neuropathol Exp Neurol</u> 37 (1978) 401-413.

10. Calingasan NY, Baker H, Sheu K-FR, Gibson GE, <u>Exp Neurol</u> 134 (1995) 64-72.

11. Harata N, Iwasaki Y, <u>Metab Brain Dis</u> 10 (1995)159-174.

12. Calingasan NY, Park LCH, Gandy SE, Gibson GE <u>Dev. Neurosci.</u> 20 (1998) 454-461.

13. Schroth G, Wichmann W, Valavanis A, J Computer Assisted Tomography 15 (1991) 1059-1061.

14. Langlais PJ, Anderson G, Guo SX, Bondy SC, Metab Brain Dis 12 (1997) 137-143.

15. Todd KG, Butterworth RF, J Neurosci Res 52 (1998) 24-246.

16. Munujos P, Vendrell M, Ferrer I, J Neurol Sci 118 (1993) 175-180.

17. Hazell AS, McGahan L, Tetzlaff W, Bedard AM, Robertson GS, Nakabeppu Y, Hakim AM J Molec Neurosci, 10 (1998)1-15.

18. Langlais PJ, Zhang SX, J Neurochem 61 (1993) 2175-2182.

19. Hazell AS, Butterworth RF, Hakim AM J. Neurochem 61(1993) 1155-158.

20. Langlais PJ, Mair RG, J. Neurosci 10 (1990) 1664-1674.

21. Todd KG, Butterworth RF, Exp Neurol 149 (1998)130-138.

22. Steinbusch HM, Verhofstad AJ, In C. Owman and J.E. Hardebo (Eds), Neural Regulation of Brain Circulation, (1986) pp. 181-194. Elsevier:Amsterdam.

23. Tagaki H, Morishima T, Matsuyama T, Hayashi H, Watanabe T, Wada H, Brain Res. 364 (1986) 14-123.

24. Onodera K, Maeyama K, Watanabe T, Jap J Pharmacol 47 (1988) 323-326.

25. Onodera K, Shinoda H, Watanabe T, Jap J Pharmacol 54 (1990) 339-343.

26. Panula P, Tuomisto L, Karhunen T, Sarviharju M, Korpi ER Agents Actions (Special Conf. Issue) (1992) C354-C357.

27. Langlais PJ, Zhang SX, Weilersbacher G, Hough LB, Barke KE, J Neurosci Res 38(1994) 565-574.

28.McRee CR, Terry-Ferguson M, Langlais PJ,, Nalwalk JW, Hough L, Brain Res 58 (2000) 773-783.

29. Zhuang X., Silverman A-J, Silver R, J Neurobiol 31 (1996) 393-403.

30. Dines KC, Powell HC J Neuropathol Exp Neurol 56 (1997) 627-640.

31. Purcell WM, Atterwill CK, Neurochem. Res 20 (1995) 521-532.

32. Ferguson M, Dalve-Endres A, McRee RC, Langlais PJ, J Neuropath Exp Neurol 58 (1999) 773-783.

33. Langlais PJ, Anderson G, Powell H, Dimlich R, Brain Pathol 7 (1997) 1020.

34. Romero IA, Rist RJ, Aleshaiker A, Abbott NJ, Brain Res 756 (1997) 133-140.

Mast cell degranulation in the rat small intestine: role of endothelin-A receptors

Mihály Boros, László Szalay and József Kaszaki[*]

University of Szeged, Szent-Györgyi Albert Medical Center, Institute of Surgical Research, Pécsi u. 4, 6701 Szeged, Hungary

Background: Impairment of splanchnic perfusion is a key event in the development of the acute circulatory response in low-flow states. The production of vasoconstrictor endothelin-1 (ET-1) peptide increases significantly under these conditions. *Our objective* was to define the *in vivo* relation between ET-1 and the gastrointestinal mast cell (MC) system. *Methods:* Increasing doses of ET-1 (0.1, 1.0 and 3.0 nmol/kg i.v.) were administered to anesthetized Sprague-Dawley rats. In a second series, the animals were pretreated with equimolar doses of the ET-A receptor antagonist BQ 610, ETR-P1/fl peptide or the ET-B receptor antagonist IRL-1038, respectively. An additional group of animals served as ischemic control. Macrohemodynamics were recorded, the proportion of degranulated MCs was determined in ileal biopsies after alcian blue-safranine staining. The average mucosal thickness was measured with an image analysis system, and the degree of mucosal damage was established on a semiquantitative 0 to 5 grade scale. *Results:* ET-1 induced dose-dependent reduction in villus height (from the 0.34±0.04 mm baseline value to 0.27±0.02, 0.22±0.03 and 0.2±0.04 mm in the 0.1, 1.0 and 3.0 nmol/kg ET-1-treated groups, respectively). The ratio of degranulated MCs was similar in all ET-1-treated groups (77%, 82% and 86%) to that observed in control animals subjected to 15-min ischemia and 60-min reperfusion (85% degranulation). Pretreatment with the ET-A receptor antagonist ETR-P1/fl peptide decreased structural injury of the mucosa. Similarly, ET-1-induced MC degranulation was significantly inhibited by the ET-A receptor antagonists, but not by ET-B receptor antagonist IRL-1038 pretreatment. *We concluded* that elevated levels of circulating ET-1 might induce intestinal MC degranulation and tissue injury via the ET-A receptors. This raises the possibility that ET-A receptor antagonist administration could exert a potentially beneficial effect through a mechanism other than the blockade of vasoconstriction in pathologies associated with an increased ET-1 release.

1. INTRODUCTION

One of the early events in shock conditions is the production of activators for effector cells of secondary circulatory responses. The endothelins (ETs) embrace a family of 21-amino acid vasoactive peptides produced by the endothelial cells. Among the three active isoforms

[*] This study was supported by research grants OTKA 16889, ETT 606/96, OTKA T023089 and HHMI 75195-54150. M. B. is a Howard Hughes International Research Scholar.

ET-1 is the most powerful endogenous vasoconstrictor substance known to date [1]. The vasoconstrictive effects of ET-1 are mediated predominantly via the endothelin-A (ET-A) receptors present on the vascular smooth muscle cells. The ET-B receptors mediate vasoconstriction (ET-B_2) and vasodilation (ET-B_1), but ET-1 has a higher affinity for ET-A than for ET-B receptor subtypes.

There is a growing body of evidence that, in addition to the separate role of ET-1 as a dominant vasoconstrictor, the peptide may also influence the biological activity of other cell types in the cardiovascular system. The effect of ET-1 on the gastrointestinal MCs is of special interest, since it may be an important component of the tissue response that occurs in the mucosa during inflammation or reoxygenation injuries. The mucosal MC of the small intestine are a unique cellular source of both preformed and *de novo* synthesized mediators, and are located mainly around postcapillary venules from which they can influence local tissue reactions. Intestinal MCs have both ET-A and ET-B receptors on their membrane surface, and this suggests a possible crosstalk between endothelial cell-derived humoral mediators and the MC system [2, 3].

Our studies was directed to an examination of whether and how intestinal MCs respond to increasing doses of exogenously administered ET-1. To this end, the ET-1-induced mucosal morphological changes were correlated to the degrees of intestinal MC degranulation. Secondly, we used ET-A receptor and ET-B receptor-selective antagonist treatments to investigate the roles of these receptor subtypes in mediating ET-1-induced intestinal MC activation.

2. MATERIALS AND METHODS

2.1. Animals

The experiments were performed in adherence to the NIH guidelines on the use of experimental animals. 42 male Sprague-Dawley rats (weighing 200±20 g) were deprived of food but not water, for 12 h prior to the experiments. The animals were anesthetized with sodium pentobarbital (60 mg/kg i.p.). The left carotid artery and jugular vein was cannulated for the recording of mean arterial pressure and the injection of test compounds, respectively. Throughout the experiment, the animals received an infusion of Ringer's lactate at a rate of 40 ml/kg/h. After a transverse laparotomy, a segment of the terminal ileum perfused by a single artery was selected. The marginal vessels were divided and ligated, and the intestinal segment with intact neurovascular connections was covered by plastic sheets.

2.2. Experimental protocol

In the first series of experiments, dose responses to ET-1 (Alexis Corporation, Läufelfingen, Switzerland) were obtained. The animals were randomly allotted into the following groups: group 1, sham-operated (n=6), group 2, 0.1 nmol/kg ET-1 (n=5), group 3, 1 nmol/kg ET-1 (n=5), group 4, 3 nmol/kg ET-1 (n=6). In these groups, 30 min after the end of baseline measurements, a solution of 0.1 ml ET-1 or vehicle was infused i.v. into the systemic circulation over 15 min. In an additional group of animals (n=5) segmental intestinal ischemia was induced by a 15-min occlusion of the ileal artery. In the second series, the ET-A receptor antagonists ETR-P1/fl peptide (Kurabo Ltd. Osaka, Japan, 0.3 μmol/kg), BQ-610 (0.3

μmol/kg), (homopiperidinyl-carbonyl-Leu-D-Trp(CHO)-D-Trp-OH, Alexis Corp., Läufelfingen, Switzerland), or the ET-B receptor antagonist IRL-1038 (Cys11-Cys15-endothelin-1(11-21), 0.3 μmol/kg) was infused i.v. for 30 min, followed by a 15-min of ET-1 infusion into the systemic circulation after the end of BQ-610, ETR-P1/fl peptide, or IRL-1038 pretreatment, respectively. The circulatory changes were observed for 60 min, and at the end of the observation period, a tissue sample was taken from the intestinal segment.

2.3. Histology

Intestinal biopsy samples were placed into ice-cold Carnoy's fixative and trimmed along the longitudinal axis. The samples were embedded in paraffin, sectioned (6 μm) and stained with hematoxylin-eosin and alcian blue-safranin O (pH 0.4). An image analysis system system (IVM, Pictron Kft., Budapest, Hungary) was used to digitize the x and y coordinates of the sections. Three nonoverlapping fields were processed in each section and the average height of a single villus was measured from its origin to the villus tip. Mucosal damage was assessed according to the standard scale of Chiu et al. The grading was performed with the following criteria: grade 0, normal mucosa; grade 1, development of subepithelial space at the tip of the villus; grade 2, extension of the space with epithelial lifting; grade 3, massive epithelial lifting; grade 4, denuded villi; and grade 5, disintegration of the lamina propria. MC stained positively were quantitated in the villi of an average of 20 villus-crypt units. The counting was performed in coded sections at x400 optical magnification by one investigator. Loss of intracellular granules, stained material dispersed diffusely within the lamina propria was taken as evidence of MC degranulation.

2.4. Statistics

The Friedman test followed by Dunnett's method was applied for multiple comparisons with a control. Differences between groups were analyzed with the Kruskal-Wallis one-way analysis of variance on ranks. p values <0.05 were considered significant. Mean values ± SD are given.

3. RESULTS

The resting hemodynamic parameters were similar in each of the groups studied (data not shown). In the sham-operated group, the villus MC count was unchanged and no significant increase in degranulation was observed in biopsies taken at the end of the observation period. A significant, dose-dependent diminution of the villus height was induced by ET-1 infusion as compared to the control group. The shortening of the villi was statistically significant after the administration of 1 or 3 nmol/kg ET-1, and there was a significant difference in this parameter between the 0.1 and 3 nmol/kg ET-1-treated animals (Fig. 1). The MC degranulation ratio exhibited a significant increase after the ET-1 treatment. The ET-1 infusions elevated the proportion of degranulated MCs almost twofold in each of the ET-1-treated groups (Fig. 2). Simultaneously, the mucosal alterations as assessed on the Chiu scale were statistically different from the control in the 1 and 3 nmol/kg ET-1-treated groups (Fig. 3). The ET-A receptor antagonists ETR-P1/fl peptide and BQ-610 attenuated the ET-induced mucosal damage (Fig. 4).

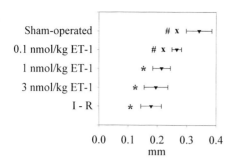

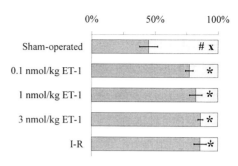

Figure 1. Changes in intestinal villus length in rats treated with 0.1, 1 or 3 nmol/kg ET-1 or following 15-min ischemia-reperfusion (I-R). * : $p<0.05$ vs. sham-operated group, # : $p<0.05$ vs. 3 nmol/kg ET-1-treated group, x : $p<0.05$ vs. I-R group.

Figure 2. Changes in mucosal MC degranulation as the percentage of intact MCs. Values are expressed as means ±SD. See Figure 1 for explanation of symbols.

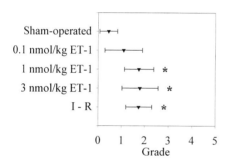

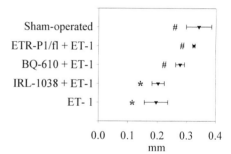

Figure 3. Grading of mucosal damage induced by 0.1, 1 or 3 nmol/kg ET-1 infusion or 15-min ischemia, respectively. * : $p<0.05$ vs. sham-operated group.

Figure 4. Changes in small intestinal villus length in animals that received ET receptor antagonist pretreatment. ETR-P1/fl, BQ-610 or IRL-1038 was administered in a 300 nM/kg dose.

Similarly, MC degranulation was significantly inhibited by the ET-A receptor antagonist pretreatment (Fig. 6). ET-B receptor antagonist IRL-1038 peptide administration did not influence the 3 nmol/kg ET-1-induced morphological alterations.

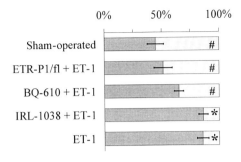

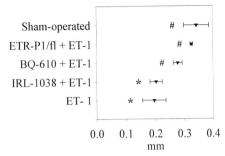

Figure 5. Changes in small intestinal mucosal MC degranulation as the percentage of intact MCs in rats treated with 3 nmol/kg ET-1 and ET receptor antagonist pretreatment.

Figure 6. Grading of mucosal damage induced by ET-1 infusion in animals that received ET receptor antagonist pretreatment

4. DISCUSSION

Previous studies have revealed that even a short period of intestinal arterial occlusion leads to structural damage to the mucosal layer and triggers the discharge of a variety of MC-derived inflammatory mediators into the mesenteric circulation [4]. The major finding of the present study is that the vasoconstrictor mediator ET-1 induces intestinal microcirculatory disturbances and mucosal damage, and concomitantly exerts significant effects on MC degranulation via the ET-A receptors. The ET-A receptor antagonist pretreatment was effective in reducing the morphological signs of ET-1-induced structural damage.

Depending on the localizations of the ET-A receptors, at least three possible mechanisms may be hypothesized. **1.** One possibility might be a direct effect of ET on MCs. This notion is supported by recent data demonstrating ET-A receptor expression on the surface of MCs in the rat [2, 3]. A direct interaction between MC degranulating peptide (MDP) and G-proteins in MCs [5] has also been reported. With regard to the very close structural similarities between ET-1 and MDP, a similar connection between ET-1 and G-proteins in MCs might be suggested. **2.** On the other hand, the profound ET-A receptor-mediated microvascular vasoconstriction and the ensuing ischemic injury could be another plausible explanation for the MC degranulation. In this case, the structural injury of the small intestinal mucosa may be directly connected with the hemodynamic consequences of ET administration. The mucosal lesions were similar to those described in animal models of intestinal ischemia-reperfusion or after nanomolar doses of exogenous ET-1 [6]. In this case, tissue hypoxia, or oxygen-derived free radicals generated during local ischemia-reperfusion injuries could also be MC-degranulating factors. **3.** Another explanation may be provided by the altered osmolarity of the intestinal mucosa as a result of localized perivascular edema. The fragility of the MC membranes to osmotic stress has been demonstrated. Indeed, Filep et al. have shown that ET-1 causes dose-dependent increases in vascular permeability through the activation of ET-A receptors as a consequence of the disruption of the endothelial barrier [7].

Following the decrease in arterial inflow, the declining energy supply for active membrane transport processes and the lack of removal of metabolites may be accompanied by a rapid fluid movement from the vascular lumen to the lamina propria. An acute circulatory breakdown may therefore rapidly cause perivascular edema, leading to MC degranulation.

In conclusion, exogenous ET-1 infusion significantly enhances degranulation of the intestinal MCs by an ET-A receptor-dependent mechanism. Recent data indicate that MCs and ET-1 may both be involved in the mechanism of endothelial cell-leukocyte interactions and neutrophil sequestration after ischemia [8, 9]. Our results demonstrate that ET-A receptor antagonism may have additional beneficial activity through the inhibition of MC reactions during intestinal pathologies. Similarly, these data suggest that an important connection exists between endothelial cell-derived humoral mediators and the perivascular MC system. If ET-1 acts as an amplifier of the process of leukocyte activation, any alteration in this mechanism could have important consequences in local tissue responses.

REFERENCES

1. Inoue A, Yanagisawa M, Kimura S, Kasuya Y, Miyauchi T, Goto K, Masaki T. The human endothelin family: three structurally and pharmacologically distinct isopeptides predicted by three separate genes. Proceedings of the National Academy of Sciences of the United States of America 1989;86(8):2863-7.
2. Yamamura H, Nabe T, Kohno S, Ohata K. Endothelin-1 induces release of histamine and leukotriene C4 from mouse bone marrow-derived mast cells. European Journal of Pharmacology 1994;257(3):235-42.
3. Liu Y, Yamada H, Ochi J. Immunocytochemical studies on endothelin in mast cells and macrophages in the rat gastrointestinal tract. Histochemistry and Cell Biology 1998;109(4):301-7.
4. Boros M, Takaichi S, Masuda J, Newlands GF, Hatanaka K. Response of mucosal mast cells to intestinal ischemia-reperfusion injury in the rat. Shock 1995;3(2):125-31.
5. Mousli M, Bronner C, Bueb JL, Landry Y. Evidence for the interaction of mast cell-degranulating peptide with pertussis toxin-sensitive G proteins in mast cells. European Journal of Pharmacology 1991;207(3):249-55.
6. Massberg S, Boros M, Leiderer R, Baranyi L, Okada H, Messmer K. Endothelin (ET)-1 induced mucosal damage in the rat small intestine: role of ET(A) receptors. Shock 1998;9(3):177-83.
7. Filep JG, Foldes-Filep E, Rousseau A, Fournier A, Sirois P, Yano M. Endothelin-1 enhances vascular permeability in the rat heart through the ETA receptor. European Journal of Pharmacology 1992;219(2):343-4.
8. Boros M, Massberg S, Baranyi L, Okada H, Messmer K. Endothelin 1 induces leukocyte adhesion in submucosal venules of the rat small intestine. Gastroenterology 1998;114(1):103-14.
9. Kanwar S, Kubes P. Mast cells contribute to ischemia-reperfusion-induced granulocyte infiltration and intestinal dysfunction. American Journal of Physiology 1994;267(2 Pt 1):G316-21.

© 2001 Elsevier Science B.V. All rights reserved.
Histamine Research in the New Millennium
T. Watanabe, H. Timmerman and K. Yanai (Editors)

Altered response of (isolated) placental vessels to histamine in diabetes complicated pregnancy

D. Szukiewicz[a,b], M. Gujski[a], D. Maslinska[c], A. Szukiewicz[a], K. Wypych[b] and S. Maslinski[a]

[a] Laboratory of Placental Research, Department of General and Experimental Pathology, University School of Medicine, ul.Krakowskie Przedmiescie 26/28, 00-928 Warsaw, Poland

[b] First Department of Obstetrics and Gynaecology, Second Faculty of Medicine, University School of Medicine, ul. Kondratowicza 8, 03-242 Warsaw, Poland

[c] Institute of Medical Research Centre, Polish Academy of Sciences, Warsaw, Poland

The role of placental mast cells and histamine in normal and pathological pregnancy is still under consideration. Total number of placental mast cells and mean histamine concentration in placental tissue are significantly increased in diabetes complicated pregnacies. In this study responses of isolated placental vessels to histamine in normal term pregnancy ($N = 36$; group II) and pregnancy complicated by diabetes class C ($N = 36$; group I) have been compared. Rings of placental vessels (4 mm in axial length) were prepared in vitro, mounted in tissue bath, plunged in Krebs-Ringer solution, buffered at pH = 7.4 and maintained at 37^0 C. Change in isometric tension of the vessels in both groups was recorded as a parameter of the vascular response to histamine (100 μmol/l) and calculated as a percentage of its reference potassium chloride contraction (100 mmol/l). Maximum response to histamine [%, $\pm$ SD] was significantly decreased ($p < 0.05$) in placental vessel rings from group I, and reached 77.31 ± 4.89 of the value obtained for group II, which was taken as 100%. Altered reactivity to histamine in pregnancy complicated by diabetes class C may be a consequence of decreased number of histamine H_1 receptors in placental vessels (the down-regulation phenomenon), increased number of histamine H_2 receptors, or altered endothelial nitric oxide production.

1. INTRODUCTION

In contrast to the systemic vasculature, there is no autonomic innervation in placental vessels [1]. For that reason, humoral stimuli are the most important in the regulation of umbilico-placental vascular tone. Among many vasoactive factors affecting maternal-fetal circulation the role of biogenic amines, especially histamine is widely discussed [3,4,5]. Human placental tissue contains a moderate amount of histamine in the vesicular structures of mast cells [6]. Histamine induces a vasoconstriction mediated via H_1 receptors and a vasodilation via H_2 receptors which exist in vascular smooth muscles [4]. In isolated perfused human placentas challenge with compound 48/80 induces an increase in perfusion pressure, which reflects the release of histamine from placental stores, and histamine H_1 receptors predominance [4,5]. Under physiological conditions the net effect (usually slight vasodilation) of histamine in placental circulation is related to secondary release of nitric oxide from endothelial cells [7]. The data from literature showed a statistically significant increase in histamine concentration in placental tissue after diabetes complicated pregnancies [8,9]. The class C of diabetes in pregnancy (by White) is the last stage without recognized vascular changes [10,11]. In our previous studies we found, that in diabetes class C both, total number of the placental mast cells and mean histamine concentrations are increased [12,13]. Moreover, in our another study, administration of compound 48/80 during in vitro perfusion of the placenta, produced a significantly higher increase in vascular resistance in diabetic placentas compared to control placentas [5]. Histamine should also be considered as an angiogenic factor. Since, it has been discovered that occupancy of intracellular histamine receptors (H_{IC}) by histamine inhibits mast-cell mediated angiogenesis, while binding of histamine to H_1- and H_2-membrane receptors stimulates mast-cell mediated angiogenesis the role of increased number of mast cells may be essential in vascular pathology of the diabetic placenta [14].

The aim of study was to investigate comparatively the responses of placental vessels to histamine in pregnancy complicated by diabetes and after normal-course pregnancy.

2. MATERIALS AND METHODS

Twenty four human placentae were obtained within 30 min of vaginal or cesarean section delivery from women (aged 22-30 years) after normal pregnancies (12 placentae) or from patients who had experienced pregnancies complicated by diabetes class C after White (12 placentae). Placentae from women with arterial blood pressure of > 140/90 mmHg or who had experienced an increase of > 20 mmHg diastolic pressure during pregnancy were not used, nor were those from women who smoked cigarettes or received antihypertensive vasodilator drugs. The courses of diabetic pregnancies were normal, without additional drug administration, except insulin. The control of glycemia in all cases was satisfactory: the levels of fraction of glycosylated hemoglobin (HbA_{1c}) in all trimesters of pregnancy were less than 7.5% ($6.5 \pm 0.5\%$). The maximal admissible level of HbA_{1c} for our diabetic pregnant patients was 7.5%. Our laboratory reference values (normal range) of HbA_{1c} for healthy population are 5.0 – 7.5%. In order to eliminate blood from the placental vascular system, each placenta was perfused in vitro for 30 min in standardized manner at 37^0 C [15].

The vessels (chorionic plate veins and arteries) were isolated from tertiary branch after insertion of the umbilical vessels into the placenta. From each placenta 3 vessels (2 veins and 1 artery) were dissected and analysed together. Rings of placental vessels (4 mm in axial length), obtained from pregnancies complicated by diabetes class C ($N = 36$; group I), and after normal pregnancies ($N = 36$; group II) were prepared in vitro, mounted in tissue bath, plunged in Krebs-Ringer solution, buffered at pH = 7.4 and maintained at 37 degrees Centigrade. The vessels were mounted on a micrometric manipulator and connected to isometric force-displacement transducers (Grass Instruments, USA). The study was conducted under 1.5 g of passive tension, and the tissues were equilibrated for 60 minutes. Isometric (active) tension of the isolated vessels was recorded as a parameter of the vascular response to histamine. Wall tension was expressed in millinewtons per millimeter of axial lenght of each ring (mN/mm). Using analysis of experimental concentration-response curves we determined histamine concentration as 100 μmol/l for initiation (approximately) 50% of maximum observed response. In each group the maximal response to 100 mmol/l potassium chloride was also evaluated in order to measure functional contractility of placental vessels. In the analysis of the data the contractile response of each ring to the histamine (100 μmol/l) was calculated as a percentage of its reference potassium chloride contraction (100 mmol/l).

Differences between values of the maximal response to 100 mmol/l potassium chloride in each group were evaluated using *t* test for unpaired data. Differences (mean percentage values) between control and experimental groups were verified by Student's *t*-test and considered to be significant if $p < 0.05$.

3. RESULTS AND CONCLUSIONS

Contractile response was observed after administration of both, potassium chloride and histamine. The response [mN/mm ± SD] to histamine compared to potassium chloride, was significantly stronger in group II (normal placental vessels) and amounted 8.59 ± 0.78 vs. 6.15 ± 1.09, while differences between intensity of contractile response to histamine and potassium chloride in group I (diabetic vessels; 6.64 ± 1.01 and 6.5 ± 0.95, respectively) did not achieve statistical significance (see Figure 1).

Maximum response to histamine [%, ± SD] was significantly decreased ($p < 0.05$) in placental vessel rings from group I, and reached 77.31 ± 4.89 of the value obtained for group II, which was taken as 100% (see Figure 2).

Our results indicate that diabetes class C reduces responsiveness to histamine in isolated placental vessels. Responsiveness to potassium chloride is not altered. This modification of vascular reactivity to histamine suggest that this amine may be implicated in pathological processes of the placental circulation. It must be noticed, that regulation of the blood flow in human placental tissue by changes of the vascular resistance is very particular and depends on humoral factors, because of the lack of sympathetic innervation in placental vessels [1,2]. Increased amounts of histamine in placental tissue from degranulated mast cells in diabetes complicated pregnancy may alter vasomotor reactivity in human placenta, increasing risk of pre-eclampsia, eclampsia, fetal anoxia or preterm delivery [16]. It has been proven, that HA contracts myometrial smooth muscle cells. The risk of spontaneous abortion and preterm delivery in diabetes is significantly increased [16]. It is very likely, but still under investigation, that mast cells control the invasion and growth of trophoblast, partly by release of angiogenic factors [6,12,17]. If histamine and other mast cell mediators (TNFα, IL-8, bFGF) are angiogenic, and neovascularization is increased in diabetic placentae, it is apparently in contradiction to intrauterine fetal anoxia, a well docu-

296

mented clinical observation in diabetes [16,18]. Increased nitric oxide synthase expression and hence increased NO production in the placental-fetal vasculature may be an adaptive response to the increased resistance and poor perfusion in diabetes [19].

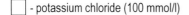 □ - potassium chloride (100 mmol/l)

▦ - histamine (100 μmol/l) on diabetic vessels

▨ - histamine (100 μmol/l) on normal vessels

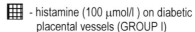 ▦ - histamine (100 μmol/l) on diabetic placental vessels (GROUP I)

▨ - histamine (100 μmol/l) on normal placental vessels (GROUP II)

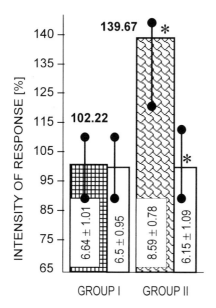

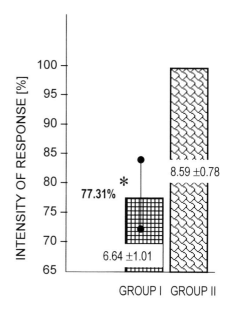

Figure 1. Contractile response to histamine in diabetic vessels (group I) and normal placental vessels (group II) as a percentage of of its reference potassium chloride contraction (taken as 100%). Columns show also mean values [mN/mm]. The line joining two dots shows SD. * p < 0.05

Figure 2. Maximal response [%, ±SD] to histamine in placental vessels in diabetes class C. The mean value obtained for group II (normal placental vessels) was taken as 100%. Columns show also mean values [mN/ mm]. The line joining two dots shows SD. * p < 0.05

There are at least two possible explanations for fetal anoxia in diabetes: first – decreased permeability to oxygen within the placental-fetal unit due to vascular pathologies, second – an increase in placental vascular resistance (vasoconstriction) as a result of histamine receptor stimulation. In contrast, it is believed that hypoxia can intensify degranulation of mast cells. However, gestational diabetes alters human placental vascular responses to changes in oxygen tension [20]. The pathophysiological meaning of reduced sensitivity to histamine in diabetic vessels is unclear. Altered reactivity to histamine in pregnancy complicated by diabetes class C may be a consequence of decreased number of histamine H_1 receptors in placental vessels (the down-regulation phenomenon to preserve normal blood supply to the fetus), increased number of histamine H_2, or altered endothelial nitric oxide production. It is important, that the vessels used in our study were morfologically unchanged (diabetes class C), and obtained after well controlled diabetes during pregnancy. We assume, that reactivity to histamine in placental vessels obtained after diabetes of more advanced stages (for example class D or F by White) may be different. In order to evaluate pregnancy age-related resposiveness of placental vessels to histamine in normal and diabetes complicated pregnancies, as well as the influence of placental mast cell heterogeneity in pregnancy complicated by diabetes class C [21] our another studies have been started.

Despite the limitations of the model used in this study, the results may have important implications in explaining the processes involved in the development of placental blood flow disorders in diabetes. Thus the elevated risk of spontaneous abortion, preterm delivery, placental insufficiency and fetal distress in the course of pregnancy in diabetic woman can be explained in part by histamine induced vasoconstriction (when adaptive mechanisms fail). Some authors however emphasize impairment of the vascular response to many compounds in diabetes mellitus [19,22,23].

REFERENCES

1. F.D. Reilly and P.T. Russell, Anat. Rec. No. 188 (1977) 277.
2. M.A. Read, A.L.A. Boura and W.A.W. Walters, Placenta, No. 16 (1995) 667.
3. C. Bertrand and J. St-Louis, Am. J. Obstet. Gynecol. No. 180 (1999) 650.
4. M.A. Cruz, C. Gonzalez, W.H. Sepulveda and M.I. Rudolph, Pharmacology No. 42 (1991) 86.
5. D. Szukiewicz, A. Szukiewicz, D. Maslinska, M. Gujski, P. Poppe and M. Markowski, J. Physiol. Pharmacol. No. 48 (suppl. 2; 1997) 86.
6. W.M. Purcell and T.H. Hanahoe, Agents Actions No. 33 (1991) 8.
7. N.M. Gude, R.G. King and S.P. Brennecke, Lancet No. 336 (1990) 1589.
8. M.R. Parwaresch, H.P. Horny and K. Lennert, Path. Res. Pract. No. 179 (1985) 439.
9. Y.Z. Diamant, Isr. J. Med. Sci. No. 27 (1991) 493.
10. P. White, Am. J. Obstet. Gynecol. No. 130 (1978) 228.
11. National Diabetes Data Group, Classification and diagnosis of diabetes mellitus and other categories of glucose intolerance, Diabetes, No. 28 (1979) 1039.
12. D. Szukiewicz, A. Szukiewicz, D. Maslinska and M.W. Markowski, Trophoblast Res. No. 13 (1999) 503.

13. D. Szukiewicz, D. Maslinska, J. Stelmachow and E. Wojtecka-Lukasik, Clin. Exp. Obstet. Gynecol. No. 22 (1995) 66.
14. K. Norrby, Int. J. Exp. Pathol. No. 76 (1995) 87.
15. L. Cedard, Acta Endocrinol. Scand. No. 69 (suppl. 158; 1972) 331.
16. L. Cousins, Obstet. Gynaec. Surv. No. 42 (1987) 140.
17. K. Norrby, A. Jakobsson, N. Simonsen and J. Sorbo, Experientia, No. 46 (1990) 856.
18. H. Fox, Obstet. Gynecol. No. 34 (1969) 792.
19. G. Schonfelder, M. John, H. Hopp, N. Fuhr, M. van der Giet and M. Paul, FASEB J. No. 10 (1996) 777.
20. R. Figueros, H.A. Omar and N. Tejani, Am. J. Obstet. Gynecol. No. 168 (1993) 1616.
21. D. Szukiewicz, D. Maslinska, P. Poppe, M. Gujski and A. Tomecki, Inflamm. Res. No. 49 (suppl. 1; 2000) 33.
22. R. Bradley, Br. J. Hosp. Med. No. 44 (1990) 386.
23. B.J. Trudinger, W.B. Giles and C.M. Cook, Br. J. Obstet. Gynaec. No. 92 (1985) 39.

© 2001 Elsevier Science B.V. All rights reserved.
Histamine Research in the New Millennium
T. Watanabe, H. Timmerman and K. Yanai (Editors)

Gastric submucosal microdialysis: A method to monitor ECL-cell histamine mobilization from rat stomach.

Masayuki Kitano[a], Per Norlén[b], Yosuke Kishimoto[c], Junichi Hasegawa[c], Hironaka Kawasaki[d], Masatoshi Kudo[a], Tadao Itoh[e], and Rolf Håkanson[b]

[a]Dept. of Gastroenterol. and Hepatol., Kinki Univ., School of Medicine, Osaka-Sayama, 589-8511 Japan, [b]Dept. of Pharmacol., Univ. of Lund, S-223 62 Lund, Sweden, [c]Dept. of Clin. Pharmacol. and [d]Second Dept. of Internal Medicine, Faculty of Medicine, Tottori Univ., Yonago,683-8503 Japan, [e]Osaka Pharmacology Research Clinic, Suita, 565-0853 Japan

ECL cells are histamine-forming endocrine cells in the oxyntic mucosa. Using a flexible microdialysis probe implanted in the gastric submucosa, we have monitored the mobilization of ECL-cell histamine under different experimental conditions.

I: Gastrin- and food-evoked mobilization of ECL-cell histamine in conscious rats.

Refeeding of fasted rats raised the microdialysate histamine concentration 3-fold. Exogenous gastrin raised the microdialysate histamine concentration in a dose-dependent manner. The food- or gastrin-evoked rise in microdialysate histamine was reduced by intravenous infusion of a CCK_2 receptor antagonist (YM022). Pretreatment with α-fluoromethylhistidine (α-FMH), which is known to deplete the ECL cells of histamine without affecting mast-cell histamine, greatly reduced the amount of histamine mobilized in response to food or gastrin. These results suggest that mobilized gastric histamine originates in the ECL cells and that exogenous and endogenous gastrin (food intake) mobilizes ECL-cell histamine via an effect on CCK_2 receptors.

II: Role of histamine in acute gastric mucosal damage induced by ischaemia-reperfusion.

Ischemia-reperfusion produces stress ulcer in the rat stomach. Clamping of the celiac artery (30 min) followed by removal of the clamp produced mucosal erosions, and raised the concentration of microdialysate histamine 50-fold. There were no significant differences in the area of erosion between wild type rats and rats deficient in mast cells. α-FMH reduced the rise in microdialysate histamine and protected the gastric mucosa from damage. Histamine H_1 and H_2 receptor antagonists dose-dependently reduced the total area of erosions induced by ischaemia-reperfusion. The results suggest that ECL-cell histamine plays a pivotal role in the pathogenesis of gastric mucosal damage induced by ischaemia-reperfusion.

Key words: histamine, ECL cell, microdialysis, gastrin, ischemia-reperfusion

There are several reports demonstrating gastrin-induced histamine mobilization in the stomach [1, 2, 3, 4]. However, studies of gastric histamine release have involved either anesthetized animals (often subjected to major surgery) or isolated cells. In no instance has the relationship between food intake and gastric histamine release been studied in intact, conscious animals.

Reperfusion followed by temporal clamping of the celiac artery can produce macroscopically apparent mucosal damage [5]. The histamine H_2 blockers have been shown to exert protective effect on acute gastric mucosal injury induced by ischemia-reperfusion [6]. The effect is thought to be exerted through suppression of gastric acid secretion, and there are no reports to demonstrate the role of ECL-cell histamine in the pathogenesis of the gastric mucosal damage.

In the past, *in vivo* microdialysis has been used to estimate the extracellular concentration of many substances, including histamine, in brain and other tissues. In the present study, we set out to measure histamine in the interstitial fluid by the use of microdialysis probes implanted into the gastric submucosa. The aim of the study was to investigate food- and gastrin-evoked ECL-cell histamine mobilization in intact conscious rats and the role of ECL-cell histamine in acute gastric mucosal injury induced by ischemia-reperfusion.

1. Materials and Methods

1.1 Implantation of the microdialysis probe and sampling of microdialysate

Flexible microdialysis probes (MAB3.8.10, AgnTho's AB, Stockholm, Sweden and Pt-200-08-PW, Eicom Co. Ltd., Kyoto, Japan) were used. Under chloral hydrate or pentobarbital anaesthesia, the serosa of the ventral aspect of the acid-producing part of the stomach was tangentially punctured by a needle and a tunnel (12-15 mm) was made in the submucosal layer from the greater to the lesser curvature. The probe was gently inserted into the tunnel and kept in place with sutures. The inlet and outlet tubes were tunneled under the skin to a point at the nape of the neck. The inlet tube was connected to a microinfusion pump and the outlet was allowed to drain into polystyrene vials. The microdialysis probes were perfused with degassed saline (1.2 µl min^{-1}). Microdialysate samples for histamine measurement were collected every 10, 20 or 60 min. Histamine was measured by RIA or ELISA using a commercially available kit (Immunotech, Paris, France).

1.2 Experimental design
1.2.1 Infusion of gastrin-17

Sprague-Dawley rats deprived of food for 48 h or fed freely were used. Sampling of microdialysate was performed 3 days after the implantation of the microdialysis probe. During perfusion of the microdialysis probes, they were kept in Bollman-type restraining cages. After 3 h of stabilization, microdialysate samples were collected hourly for 2 h. Synthetic human Leu^{15}-gastrin-17 was then infused at a dose of 0.05, 0.15, 0.5, 1.5, 5 or 50 nmol kg^{-1}h^{-1} for 4 h. Samples for histamine measurement were collected every 20 min during the first h of and then every h. Five rats received YM022 (CCK$_2$ receptor antagonist, a kind gift from Dr. K. Miyata, Yamanouchi Pharmaceutical Co. Ltd. Ibaraki, Japan) intravenously at a dose of 1 µmol kg^{-1} h^{-1} starting 1 h before gastrin infusion (5 nmol kg^{-1}h^{-1}). Ten freely fed rats received α-FMH (3 mg kg^{-1}h^{-1}) or vehicle via osmotic minipumps (24 h). This treatment is known to deplete histamine from the ECL cells without affecting mast-cell histamine [7].

1.2.2 Refeeding

Sprague-Dawley rats were deprived of food for 48 h but had free access to water at all times. After 3 h of stabilization and 2 h of basal sampling, rats were given standard rat food pellets. In a parallel experiment, YM022 was infused intravenously at a dose of 1 μmol kg^{-1}h^{-1} starting 1 h before refeeding. This dose is known to induce CCK$_2$ receptor blockade [8].

1.2.3 Ischemia-reperfusion

Wistar rats and Ws-RC rats were used. The subtype of Ws-RC rats (Ws/Ws) is known to be deficient in mast cells [9, 10]. Rats were fasted for 18 hours prior to the experiments, but were allowed free access to water. Under pentobarbital anesthesia, samples for histamine measurement were collected every 10 min throughout the whole experimental period. After collecting three fractions of microdialysate, the celiac artery was occluded for 30 min (ischemia) after which the clamp was removed (reperfusion). Rats were killed by exsanguination from the abdominal aorta 60 min after removal of the clamp. The stomach was removed and opened along the major curvature, and the injury score of the mucosa was calculated as the total area of erosions using the computer system of imaging analysis. Ws/Ws rats were compared with the wild type of rats (Ws-RC, +/+) in order to clarify the role of mast-cell histamine in the gastric mucosal damage. Some rats received α-FMH (3 mg kg^{-1}h^{-1} for 4days, via osmotic minipumps), cimetidine (1, 3, 10, 30 and 100 mg/kg, i.p. 70 min before ischemia) or diphenhydramine (1, 3, 10 and 30 mg/kg, i.p. 70 min before ischemia).

In one series of experiments, the histamine concentration in the portal vein was monitored by *in vivo* microdialysis technique. The microdialysis probe was inserted into the portal vein of anesthetized rats. Samples from the probe were collected every 10 min and the rats were subjected to ischemia-reperfusion (without pretreatment with any drugs).

2 Results

2.1 Microdialysate histamine in response to gastrin-17 and food intake.

Intravenous infusion of gastrin (4 h) raised the histamine concentration in the microdialysate in a dose-dependent manner. A maximum dose of gastrin (5 nmol kg^{-1}h^{-1}) produced a 4-fold increase in mobilized histamine. The concentrations of histamine reached maximum within the first h of gastrin infusion and remained elevated for the duration of the experiment (4 h). Intravenous infusion of YM022 (1 μmol kg^{-1}h^{-1}) to fasted rats the prevented gastrin-stimulated increase in microdialysate histamine. Pretreatment with α-FMH lowered the basal histamine concentration by more than 70 % and virtually prevented the gastrin-induced increase.

Refeeding promptly raised the serum gastrin level. Also the histamine concentration in the microdialysate increased rapidly and peaked within 20 min (3-fold increase) (Fig. 1A). The peak was followed by a slow and gradual decline. Intravenous infusion of YM022 (1 μmol kg^{-1}h^{-1}) reduced the post-prandial histamine response to only 20 % of that in rats not treated with YM022 (Fig. 1).

302

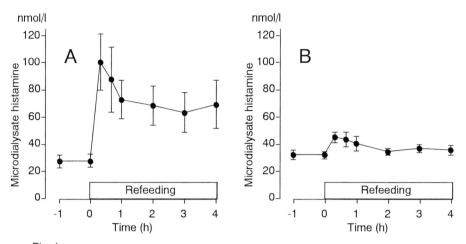

Fig. 1
Mobilization of histamine after refeeding in S-D rats treated with vehicle (A) or YM022 (B).
Mean±SEM, n=5

2.2 Microdialysate histamine in response to ischemia-reperfusion

Removal of the clamp after 30 min of ischemia was accompanied by macroscopically apparent mucosal damage. Immediately after the ischemia, the microdialysate histamine started to rise. After 30 min of ischemia, the concentration of microdialysate histamine increased 50-fold. Both cimetidine and diphenhydramine dose-dependently reduced the total area of erosions induced by ischemia-reperfusion without affecting the increase of microdialysate histamine. There were no significant differences in the area of erosion and the microdialysate histamine between rats deficient in mast cells (Ws/Ws) and wild type rats (+/+). On the other hand, α-FMH prevented the rise in microdialysate histamine (Fig. 2) and protected the gastric mucosa from damage.

In the rats to be used for monitoring histamine in the portal vein, the microdialysate histamine was found to increase 3-fold within 10 min after the start of ischemia, and then gradually declined.

3 Discussion

3.1 Gastrin- and food- evoked mobilization of histamine

. While oxyntic mucosal histamine in the rat occurs in both mast cells and ECL cells, approximately 80 % is in the ECL cells [7]. It appears to be generally accepted that mast cells do not respond to gastrin while gastrin mobilizes histamine from the ECL cells [11, 12]. In the present study, exogenous gastrin induced a dose-dependent rise in the concentration of histamine in the gastric submucosa (measured by microdialysis). CCK_2 receptor blockade prevented the response, in line with the view that gastrin mobilizes ECL-cell histamine through an action on CCK_2 receptors. α-FMH, an irreversible inhibitor of histidine decarboxylase, depletes histamine from the ECL cells while leaving mast-cell histamine unaffected [7]. Hence, the observations 1) that gastrin increased the microdialysate concentrations of histamine and 2) that α-FMH prevented the gastrin-evoked mobilization of gastric histamine support the view that mobilized oxyntic mucosal histamine derives from ECL cells rather than from mast cells. In the present study, food intake raised both the serum gastrin level and the microdialysate histamine concentration. This observation together with the fact that exogenous gastrin raised the microdialysate histamine, suggest that gastrin plays an important role in food-evoked mobilization of ECL-cell histamine.

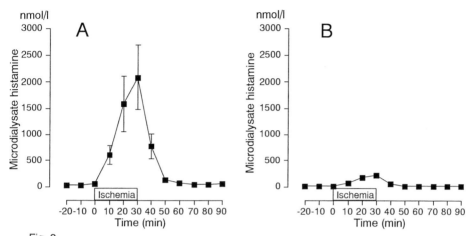

Fig. 2
Mobilization of histamine in response to ischemia-reperfusion in Ws/Ws rats treated with vehicle (A) or α-FMH (B). Mean±SEM, n=5

3.2 Mobilization of histamine in response to ischemia-reperfusion

Ischemia for 30 min led to a 50-fold rise in the microdialysate histamine concentration. From the observation that histamine H_1 and H_2 receptor antagonists inhibited the development of erosions, it is suggested that histamine released during ischemia plays a pivotal role in the pathogenesis of the mucosal damage. The inhibition by α-FMH of the increase of microdialysate histamine and of the total area of erosions supports this view. The increase in microdialysate histamine during ischemia in rats treated with histamine H_1 or H_2 receptor antagonist did not differ from that in control rats, suggesting that such agents did not inhibit the mobilization of histamine, but antagonized the action of histamine.

In order to find the source of the histamine mobilized, we used rats treated with α-FMH and rats deficient in mast cells. There were no significant differences in the area of erosions and the microdialysate histamine between rats deficient in mast cells and wild type rats. On the other hand, a remarkable reduction of the increase of microdialysate histamine during ischemia was observed in rats treated with α-FMH. These results suggest that the histamine mobilized during ischemia does not originate from mast cells but rather from ECL cells.

Accumulation of histamine in the stomach due to stagnant blood flow during ischemia may raise the microdialysate histamine concentration. If the increase in submucosal histamine concentration had been merely due to a reduced rate of wash-out of histamine from the stomach, the histamine concentration in the portal vein should have decreased during ischemia. However, the concentration of histamine in the portal vein during the ischemia was higher than before ischemia, suggesting that the increase in microdialysate histamine reflected release from ECL cells rather than accumulation of histamine because of stagnant blood supply.

3.3 Methodological considerations

There have been reports showing mobilization of gastric histamine in response to gastrin. Gastrin-stimulated mobilization of gastric histamine has been directly or indirectly demonstrated using intact rats [13, 14], or vascularly perfused rat stomachs [1], or by monitoring histamine in the portal vein of anaesthetized animals [2]. Release of histamine has also been demonstrated using isolated ECL cells [3, 4]. The present study makes use of *in vivo* microdialysis to examine gastric histamine release in response to gastrin, food intake or ischemia. *In vivo* microdialysis seems to have distinct advantages over previously employed techniques in that it can be used to monitor the time-course of release of histamine into the gastric submucosa in response to a great variety of physiological stimuli and pharmacological treatments. Another advantage is that the technique can be applied in conscious animals. It has been suggested that locally released histamine stimulates nearby parietal cells by way of diffusion [13]. The existence of such a paracrine histamine pathway is supported by our observation that mobilized histamine can be measured in the extracellular fluid.

In conclusion, gastric submucosal microdialysis appears to be a technique well suited for the study of ECL-cell histamine mobilization.

REFERENCES

1. Sandvik and H.L. Waldum, Am. J. Physiol., 260 (1991) G925-928.
2. J.G. Gerber and N.A. Payne, Gastroenterology, 102 (1992) 403-408.
3. C. Prinz, M. Kajimura, D.R. Scott, v. Mercier, F. Helander and G. Sachs, Gastroenterology, 105 (1993) 449-461.
4. E. Lindström, M. Björkqvist, Å. Boketoft, D. Chen, C.M. Zhao, K. Kimura and R. Håkanson, Regul. Pept., 71 (1997) 73-8.
5. K. Wada, Y. Kamisaki, M. Kitano , K. Nakamoto and T. Itoh Eur. J. Pharmacol., 294 (1995) 377-382.
6. M. Kitano, K. Wada, Y. Kamisaki, K. Nakamoto, Y. Kishimoto, H. Kawasaki and T. Itoh, Pharmacology, 55(1997) 154-164.
7. K. Andersson , D. Chen, R. Håkanson, H. Mattsson and F. Sundler, Cell. Tissue. Res., 270 (1992) 7-13.
8. X.Q. Ding and R. Håkanson, Pharmacol. Toxicol., 79 (1996) 124-130.
9. H. Onoue, K. Maeyama, S. Nomura, T.kasugai, H. Tei, H.M. Kim, T. Watanabe, Y. Kitamura, Am J Pathol. 1993 Apr;142(4):1001-7.
10. S. Nakamura, H. Watanabe, T. Yokota, H. Matsui, M. Onji and K. Maeyama, Eur. J. Pharmacol., 394 (2000) 9-16.
11. A.H. Soll, M. Toomey, D. Culp, F. Shanahan and M.A. Beaven, Am. J. Physiol. 254 (1988), G40-G48.
12. D.D. Metcalfe, D. Baram and Y.A. Mecori, Pharm. Rev. 77 (1997) 1033-1079.
13. G. Kahlson, E. Rosengren, D. Svahn and R. Thunberg, J. Physiol., 174 (1964) 400-416.
14. R. Håkanson, J. Hedenbro, G. Liedberg, H.A. El Munshid and J.F. Rehfeld, Experientia, 33 (1977) 1541-1542.

Histamine Research in the New Millennium
T. Watanabe, H. Timmerman and K. Yanai (Editors)

The interaction between histamine H_3 receptors and dopamine D_1 receptors in the regulation of [^{3}H]-γ-aminobutyric acid release in rat striatum[*]

[1]J.-A. Arias-Montaño, [1]B. Floran, [1]M. Garcia, [1]J. Aceves and [2]J.M. Young

[1]Department of Physiology, Biophysics and Neurosciences, Centro de Investigación y de Estudios Avanzados, Apartado Postal 14-740, Mexico, D.F., Mexico and
[2]Department of Pharmacology, University of Cambridge, Tennis Court Road, Cambridge, CB2 1QJ, U.K.

1. HISTAMINE H_3 RECEPTORS IN THE STRIATUM

The striatum is the main input nucleus of the basal ganglia, a group of nuclei involved in motor control (Gerfen and Wilson, 1996). The neuronal population of rat striatum is made up of one principal neurone cell type, the GABAergic spiny projection neurone (~95% of the cell population). These neurones can be further divided in two groups of approximately equal numbers, one with neurones expressing substance P and dopamine D_1 receptors, that project to the substantia nigra pars reticulata (SNr), and a second group of neurones projecting to the globus pallidus, which contain enkephalin and express dopamine D_2 receptors (Gerfen and Wilson, 1996).

We have reported previously that activation of histamine H_3 receptors located on the terminals of striatonigral projection neurones in rat SNr selectively inhibits the component of depolarisation-induced [^{3}H]-γ-aminobutyric acid ([^{3}H]-GABA) release that is dependent on concomitant dopamine D_1 receptor stimulation (Garcia et al., 1997). The striatonigral projection neurones have axon collaterals which remain within the striatum (Gerfen and Wilson, 1996), which is also rich in histamine H_3 receptors (Pollard et al., 1993; Lignaeu et al., 1994).

Striatal quinolinic acid lesions result in a parallel decrease in the numbers of ipsilateral D_1 and H_3 receptors, both in SNr and striatum (Ryu et al., 1994), suggesting that both receptors are colocalised on the same terminals in the striatum as in SNr and, hence, that depolarisation-induced, D_1 receptor-dependent release of [^{3}H]-GABA in striatum may be regulated by H_3 receptor activation in the same way as in SNr.

---

[*] This project was supported by Grant 28276N from CONACyT (Mexico). Part of the work was carried out during the tenure by JMY of an Exchange Fellowship between the Royal Society and the Mexican Academy of Sciences.

2. METHODS

2.1 Measurement of [³H]-GABA release from slices of rat striatum.

Striatal slices were dissected from vibratome-cut slices (300 µm) of rat brain (Wistar strain, males, 250-300 g). Labelling with [³H]-GABA (80 nM) and superfusion was carried out as described in detail elsewhere (García et al., 1997). It has been shown that >90% of the tritium released by a depolarising stimulus from rat striatal slices is [³H]-GABA (Kuriyama et al., 1984; Harsing & Zigmond, 1997). Sulpiride (10 µM) or SCH 23390 (1 µM) were added 4 min before the first basal fraction was collected. Histamine, immepip, clobenpropit and thioperamide were present from 12 min before the change to the medium containing 15 mM K^+. For experiments in dopamine-depleted slices, rats were treated with reserpine (5 mg kg^{-1}, i.p.) 24 h before preparation of striatal slices. The reserpine treatment reduces striatal dopamine levels by 95% (Garcia et al., 1997).

2.2 Analysis of data.

Fractions were collected at 4 min intervals (2-ml fractions). [³H]-GABA release (1000-7000 dpm per sample; 0.3-2% of the total amount of [³H]-GABA remaining in the tissue) was normalised by expressing the amount of tritium as a fraction of [³H]-GABA present in the fraction collected immediately before depolarisation. The effect of drugs on the release of [³H]-GABA was obtained by comparing the areas under the appropriate release curves between the first and last fractions collected after the change to high K^+. The K_d for clobenpropit was calculated from the curves for immepip and clobenpropit using the method of Lazareno and Roberts (1987; Dickenson & Hill, 1993). To test for statistical differences between treatments, the area under the release curve in the presence of elevated K^+ was calculated for each individual chamber and the data then analysed as described previously (Garcia et al., 1997).

3. RESULTS

3.1 Effect of D_2 and D_1 dopamine receptor blockade on [³H]-GABA release.

Increasing the K^+ concentration in the superfusion medium to 15 mM caused only a small increase in the release of [³H]-GABA from striatal slices. However, the D_2 antagonist sulpiride (10 µM) markedly enhanced the effect of depolarisation, to 2.9 ± 0.2 fold of basal (n = 3) without any significant effect on basal release. The depolarisation-induced release of [³H]-GABA in the presence of sulpiride was strongly Ca^{2+}-dependent (84 ± 6% inhibition in medium with no added Ca^{2+}, n = 3) and was markedly reduced by the dopamine D_1 receptor antagonist SCH 23390 (1 µM; mean inhibition 84 ± 6%, n = 3) (Arias-Montaño et al., 2000).

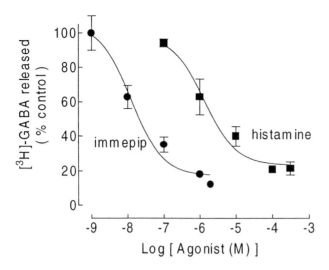

Figure 1. Concentration-dependence of the inhibition by histamine and immepip of depolarisation-induced [³H]-GABA release. Values are means ± SEM from 3-6 independent determinations at each concentration, except for 300 μM histamine, which is from a single experiment. The curves drawn are best-fit lines to an hyperbola.

3.2 Effect of histamine and immepip on [³H]-GABA release.

Depolarisation-induced [³H]-GABA release was strongly inhibited by 100 μM histamine and by the selective histamine H_3 receptor agonist immepip (1 μM), with mean inhibitions of 78 ± 3% and 81 ± 5% respectively. The inhibitory effect of the agonists was concentration-dependent (IC_{50} values of 1.3 ± 0.2 μM for histamine and 15.5 ± 2.3 nM for immepip; Fig. 1) and was blocked by the H_3 receptor antagonist thioperamide (1 μM; Fig. 2). The potency of immepip is similar to that reported for inhibition of electrically-evoked twitches of guinea-pig jejunum, IC_{50} 10 nM (Leurs et al., 1995a,b), 0.03 nM (Harper et al., 1999) and 0.08 nM (Valentine et al., 1999).

The action of H_3 agonists appears to be selective for the D_1 receptor-dependent component of release since the extent of the inhibition of depolarisation-induced [³H]-GABA release in the presence of 1 μM SCH 23390 (84 ± 6%) was not significantly different from that in the presence of 1 μM SCH 23390 + 1 μM immepip (88 ± 9% inhibition, n = 3).

The selective H_3 receptor antagonist clobenpropit (1 μM) had no significant effect on either basal or depolarisation-induced release of [³H]-GABA, but reversed in a concentration-dependent manner the inhibition of depolarisation-induced [³H]-GABA release by 1 μM immepip. The calculated K_d, 0.11 ± 0.04 nM, is in good accord with the reported value of 0.13 nM (Leurs et al., 1995a).

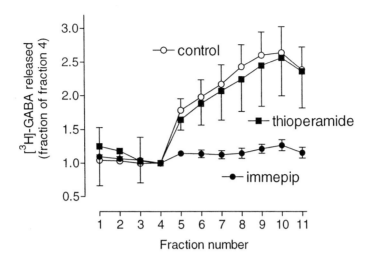

Figure 2.   Reversal by 1 μM thioperamide of the inhibition by 1 μM immepip of depolarisation-induced [³H]-GABA release. Values are expressed as a fraction of the release of [³H]-GABA in fraction 4, at which point the K^+ in the medium was increased to 15 mM. The points are means ± SEM from a single experiment, which was repeated twice further. Sulpiride (10 μM) was present throughout.

3.3 Effect of SKF 38393 and immepip on depolarisation-induced [³H]-GABA release in striatum from reserpinised rats

To establish whether there is an interaction at GABA terminals between H_3 receptors and dopamine D_1 receptors, measurements were made on depolarisation-induced [³H]-GABA released from striatal slices from animals treated with reserpine. Sulpiride was omitted from the superfusion medium in these experiments.

In the absence of added drugs depolarisation with raised K^+ had a minimal effect on the release of [³H]-GABA. However, in the presence of the D_1 receptor agonist R(+)-SKF 38393 (1 μM), the depolarisation-induced release was markedly stimulated. Immepip (1 μM) reduced the depolarisation-induced release in the presence of SKF 38393 to control levels.

4. DISCUSSION

Our results show that histamine causes the same inhibition of dopamine-dependent [³H]-GABA release in rat striatal slices as we have previously reported in slices of rat substantia nigra pars reticulata (SNr) (Garcia et al., 1997) and provide strong evidence that this action of histamine is mediated by H_3 receptors. The mechanism of the inhibitory effect remains to be determined, but the evidence from the slices from reserpinised rats suggests strongly that H_3 and D_1 receptors are located on the same GABA terminals. This is consistent with the reports that striatal quinolinic acid lesions result in a parallel decrease in the numbers of ipsilateral D_1 and H_3 receptors (Ryu *et al.*, 1994). Presumably H_3 receptor activation inhibits the cyclic AMP signalling pathway activated by D_1 receptors. H_3 receptors appear to be able to couple to both G_o and G_i, since there is evidence that H_3 receptors produce inhibition of N-type voltage-sensitive Ca^{2+} channels (reviewed in Leurs *et al.*, 1995a; Hill *et al.*, 1997) and a cloned human H_3 receptor transfected into mouse L cells has been shown to be coupled to the inhibition of forskolin-stimulated cyclic AMP accumulation (Lovenberg *et al.*, 1999).

Exactly which neurones in the striatum are innervated by the recurrent collaterals is of particular interest, but remains to be established. Inhibition of GABA release in the SNr implies an inhibitory action of histamine on the so-called direct pathway through the basal ganglia (Gerfen and Wilson, 1996). It would be inconsistent with an overall inhibitory action if the recurrent collaterals served to provide feedback inhibition of the parent or neighbouring GABA projection neurones: in this case histamine would be pro-excitatory by preventing the negative feedback. It is therefore more likely that the collaterals synapse on striatal interneurones. Cholinergic interneurones are one probable target (Prast *et al.*, 1999). It would be particularly interesting to know whether one or more of the GABA-containing interneurones (Kawaguchi et al., 1995) is also innervated. Indeed, we cannot rule out at this stage the possibility that some of the observed GABA release is from interneurones and it is notable that the pattern of depolarisation-induced [^{3}H]-GABA release observed in striatal slices differs from the pattern observed in SNr (Garcia *et al.*, 1997). However, whether any of the interneurones possess both H_3 and D_1 receptors, which the marked D_1-dependence of the [^{3}H]-GABA release demands, is not established.

In summary, histamine H_3 receptors have a potentially important role in regulating signal processing in the direct GABAergic pathway through the basal ganglia. There is every prospect that we shall eventually know enough about the inter-relationships of striatal neurones to understand exactly how H_3 receptors in the striatum contribute to this regulation.

REFERENCES

Arias-Montaño, J.-A. et al., Br. J. Pharmacol., 129 (2000) 66P.
Dickenson, J.M. and S.J. Hill, Br. J. Pharmacol., 108 (1993) 85.
García, M. et al., Neuroscience, 80 (1997) 241.
Gerfen, C.R. and C.J. Wilson, Integrated Systems of the CNS, Part III (Handbook of Chemical Neuroanatomy, Vol. 12. A. Björklund, T. Hökfelt and L. Swanson (eds., Elsevier, Amsterdam, 1996, pp. 369-466.
Harper, E.A. et al., Br. J. Pharmacol., 128 (1999) 881.
Harsing, L.G., Jr and M.J. Zigmond, Neuroscience, 77 (1997) 419.
Hill, S.J. et al., Pharmacol. Rev., 49 (1997) 253.
Kawaguchi, Y. et al., Trends Neurosci., 18 (1995) 527.
Kuriyama, K. et al., J. Neurochem., 42 (1984) 943.

Lazareno, S. and F.F. Roberts, Br. J. Pharmacol., 92 (1987) 677P.
Leurs, R.et al., Pharmacol. Ther., 66 (1995a) 413.
Leurs, R. et al., Br. J. Pharmacol., 116 (1995b) 2315.
Ligneau, X. et al., J. Pharmacol. Exp. Ther., 271 (1994) 452.
Lovenberg, T.W. et al., Mol. Pharmacol., 55 (1999) 1101.
Pollard, H. et al., Neuroscience, 52 (1993) 169.
Prast H.et al., Naunyn Scmiedeberg's Arch. Pharmacol., 360 (1999) 558.
Ryu, J.H. et al., NeuroReport, 5 (1994) 621.
Valentine, A.F. et al., Eur. J. Pharmacol., 366 (1999) 73.

© 2001 Elsevier Science B.V. All rights reserved.
Histamine Research in the New Millennium
T. Watanabe, H. Timmerman and K. Yanai (Editors)

Immunohistochemical localization of histamine N-methyltransferase in the bovine central nervous system.

M. Nishibori, A. Tahara , K. Sawada , J. Sakiyama , H. Kohka, N. Nakaya and K. Saeki

Department of Pharmacology and School of Health Science, Okayama University Medical School. 2-5-1 Shikata-cho, Okayama 700-8558, Japan.

    Histamine N-methyltransferase (HMT)(EC 2.1.1.8) plays a crucial role in the inactivation of the neurotransmitter histamine in the CNS. However, the localization of HMT remains to be determined. In the present study, we investigated immunohistochemical localization of HMT in the bovine CNS using a polyclonal antibody against bovine HMT. The HMT-like immunoreactivity (HMT-LI) was observed mainly in neurons. The strong immunoreactive neurons were present in the oculomotor nucleus and ruber nucleus in the midbrain, the facial nucleus in the pons, the dorsal vagal nucleus and hypoglossal nucleus in the medulla oblongata and in the anterior horn as well as intermediolateral zone of the spinal cord. The tuberomammillary nucleus, where histaminergic neurons are present, were weekly positive. The other immunoreactive structures in the CNS were blood vessels. Almost all of the blood vessel walls, irrespective of arterial or venous, were variably stained. The GFAP-immunoreactive astrocytes were not stained. These findings indicated that histamine released from histaminergic nerve terminals or varicose fibers is methylated mainly in postsynaptic or extrasynaptic neurons rather than in astrocytes. The localization of HMT in the blood vessel wall may mean that blood-borne histamine and histamine released from mast cells associated with the blood vessels are catabolized in this structure.

1. INTRODUCTION

    Histamine functions as a neurotransmitter in the central nervous system (CNS) (1). Although methylation and oxidative deamination are two pathways of histamine catabolism in the mammalian tissues (2), methylation of histamine by histamine N-methyltransferase (EC 2.1.1.8.)(HMT) seems to be the sole pathway in the CNS (1). Since the resultant catabolite tele-methylhistamine is inactive for three subtypes of histamine receptors (2) and the high affinity reuptake system for histamine has not been demonstrated using brain slices (1), the process of methylation appears to be a crucial step for the inactivation of histamine in the CNS. It was demonstrated that the extracellular level of histamine in the rat hypothalamus measured by in vivo microdialysis increased significantly after the systemic administration of HMT inhibitor (3,4), especially in the combination with H_3-receptor antagonist thioperamide (3).

The finding indicates that the simultaneous regulation of both HMT activity and H3-autoreceptor stimulation can synergistically contribute to the elevation of extracellular histamine levels in the brain. Thus, HMT may be an important target molecule in modulating histaminergic transmission in the brain, in addition to histamine receptors.

At present the cellular localization of HMT, neuronal or glial, remains unclear. The findings from lesion studies and expression experiments using culture cells have not been conclusive (1). In the present study, we raised a specific antibody against bovine HMT in the rabbit and investigated the immunohistochemical localization of HMT in the bovine CNS. We report here that HMT is localized mainly in neurons and the vascular walls in the bovine CNS.

2. MATERIALS AND METHODS

2.1 Immunohistochemical studies

Bovine brain HMT was purified as described previously (5). The antibody against bovine HMT was obtained as described (6).The blocks of bovine brain regions 5 mm thick were fixed in 10 % formalin in 0.01 M phosphate buffered saline. The fixed tissue pieces were dehydrated, embedded in paraffin and cut into 5-7 μm thin sections. After blocking, rabbit anti-HMT antiserum (diluted to 1: 1500), preimmune rabbit serum (1: 1500) or anti-HMT antiserum preabsorbed with purified HMT was applied to the sections for 24 h at 4 ℃. after washing, the sections were incubated with biotinylated anti-rabbit IgG goat IgG, washed and reacted with streptoavidin-peroxidase. The peroxidation reaction was developed using DAB as a substrate in the presence of NiCl2. When the immunoreactive cells for HMT and GFAP were

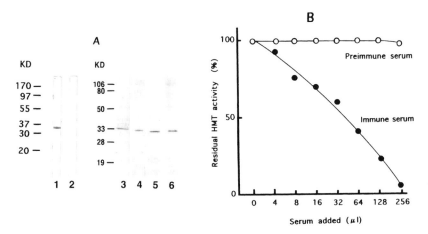

Fig. 1 (A) Western immunoblotting of HMT using anti-HMT serum. Whole bovine brain (lanes 1 and 2) and brain regions (lane 3, cerebral cortex; lane 4, hypothalamus; lane 5, midbrain; lane 6, pons) were electrophoresed and blotted with anti-HMT antiserum (lanes 1, 3-6, 1: 1500) and preimmune serum (lane 2, 1: 1500).
(B) Immunoprecipitation of HMT activity by anti-HMT antiserum (●) and preimmune serum (○). (Reproduced from ref. 6 with the permission of Blackwell Science)

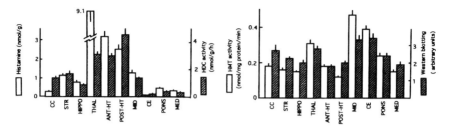

Fig. 2 The regional distribution of histamine, histidine decarboxylase and HMT in the bovine brain. The findings represent the means of at least four samples. CC, cerebral cortex; STR, striatum; HIPPO, hippocampus; THAL, thalamus; ANT-HT, anterior hypothalamus; POST-HT, posterior hypothalamus; MID, midbrain; CE, cerebellum; PONS, pons; MED, medulla oblongata. (Reproduced from ref. 6 with the permission of Blackwell Science)

compared, the adjacent sections were used for the staining with each antibody.

2.2 Determination of histidine decarboxylase activity, histamine and tele-methylhistamine contents in the bovine brain regions

The activities of histidine decarboxylase (HDC) and HMT and the contents of histamine and tele-methylhistamine were determined as described previously(7).

3. RESULTS AND DISCUSSION

As shown in Fig. 1A, antiserum against bovine HMT recognized a single band on Western blotting using brain supernatants, which had the same molecular size, 33 KDa, as the purified HMT (5). Increasing concentrations of antiserum immunoprecipitated HMT activity in a concentration dependent manner while the preimmune serum did not (Fig. 1B). These findings indicated that antiserum specifically recognized bovine HMT. The regional distribution of histidine decarboxylase in the bovine brain was highest in the posterior hypothalamus (P <0.01 as compared with other brain regions by Student's t-test) (Fig. 2) where the histaminergic neurons are present in the tuberomammillary nucleus in mammals (12, 13). The HDC activity in the pons, medulla oblongata and cerebellum were low as compared with other brain regions (P < 0.01). In the thalamus, extraordinary high levels of histamine were observed while the HDC activity was comparable to that in the anterior hypothalamus. This strongly suggested the presence of considerable numbers of mast cells in this region of the bovine brain. The regional distribution of HMT was examined by the determination of enzymatic activity and Western blotting (Fig. 2). The findings from the quantification of Western blotting were compatible with the determination of HMT activities. The levels of HMT activity in the brain regions were variable; highest in the midbrain and lowest in the posterior hypothalamus where the HDC activity was highest. In contrast to the low levels of HDC and Fig. 3 Fig.

histamine in the brain stem and cerebellum, the HMT levels were relatively higher in these regions (P < 0.01, posterior hypothalamus vs. midbrain, cerebellum and pons). Inconsistency in the distribution of HMT activity with those of histidine decarboxylase activity or histamine content strongly suggests that the histaminergic cell bodies do not contain much HMT and that cells other than histaminergic neurons show large levels of HMT activity as estimated in the rat brain (1).

The immunohistochemical studies revealed that there are several nuclei strongly immunoreactive for HMT. Fig. 3 shows immunoreactive neurons in the upper levels of the medulla oblongata. The large neurons in the hippoglossal nucleus(Fig. 3A) were strongly immunoreactive. Preimmune serum and immune serum preabsorbed with purified HMT did not stain any structure, indicating the specificity of the staining using polyclonal antibody against bovine HMT. At the same level of the medulla oblongata, the neurons in the dorsal nucleus of the vagal nerve were identified as another strongly immunoreactive structure (Fig. 3B). The dendrites as well as cell soma of these neurons were immunostained. In the pons the neurons in the facial nucleus were strongly immunoreactive. Also, the relatively small neurons in the inferior olive nucleus had intermediate HMT-LI . In the midbrain, the neurons in the oculomotor nucleus (Fig. 3C) and red nucleus (Fig.3D) were strongly immunoreactive. The axon bundles originating from the oculomotor nucleus and passing through the red nucleus were clearly stained (Fig. 3D).

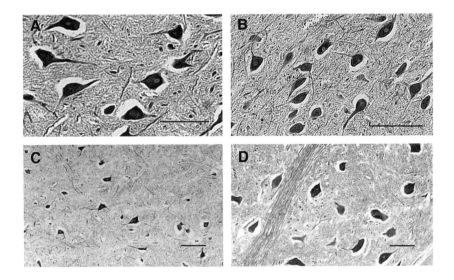

Fig. 3 Photomicrographs of the HMT-immunoreactive neurons in the hypoglossal nucleus (A) and the dorsal nucleus of the vagal nerve (B) in the upper medulla oblongata, and the oculomotor nucleus (C) and red nucleus (D) in the midbrain. Bar= 50 μm. (Reproduced from ref. 6 with the permission of Blackwell Science)

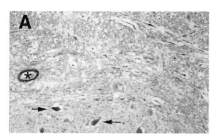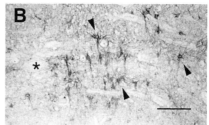

Fig. 4 Photomicrographs of the adjacent sections of ventromedial part of the bovine pons immunostained with anti-HMT antiserum (A) or anti-GFAP antibody (B). Asterisk in each figure shows the same blood vessel which was immunoreactive only for HMT. The arrows in (A) represent HMT-immunoreactive neurons. The arrowheads in (B) represent GFAP-immunoreactive astrocytes. GFAP-immunoreactive astrocytes were not stained by anti-HMT antiserum at all. Bar= 50 μm. (Reproduced from ref. 6 with the permission of Blackwell Science)

In the cervical spinal cord, α-motor neurons in the anterior horn were strongly immunoreactive. In addition to the α-motor neurons, some of neurons in the intermediolateral zone were strongly positive. The tuberomammillary nucleus, where histaminergic neurons are present (8, 9), was weakly positive. This finding was consistent with the lowest level of HMT activity in the posterior hypothalamus. In contrast with the presence of the strong HMT-LI neurons from the brain stem to the spinal cord, there are few such neurons in the forebrain regions. The adjacent sections of the ventral pons were immunostained by anti-HMT or anti-GFAP antibody. Astrocytes stained with anti-GFAP antibody (Fig. 4) were not immunoreactive for HMT. It is apparent, from the present study, that the contribution of astroglial components to the catabolism of histamine, if any, may be small compared with that of neurons and the blood vessel walls in the bovine CNS.

There were other immunoreactive structures in the CNS. The vascular walls, both arterial and venous, were stained. The intensity of the staining was variable depending on the blood vessels. This observation is consistent with the finding that blood vessels prepared from bovine brain contained high levels of histamine (10) and that there are blood vessel-associated mast cells in the mammalian brain (11). These findings taken together suggest that localization of HMT in the vascular wall is for the catabolism of histamine released from mast cells embedded in blood vessels.

In conclusion, it was demonstrated that HMT was localized in diverse neurons with variable levels and in vascular walls in the bovine CNS. Since many of the histaminergic axon varicosities were reported not to form typical synaptic contacts (12), histamine released from the varicosities appeared to be methylated in extrasynaptic as well as postsynaptic neurons rather than in astrocytes.

REFERENCES

1. J.-C. Schwartz, J.-M. Arrang, M. Garbarg, H. Pollard and M.Ruat, Physiol. Rev., 71 (1991) 1.
2. C.R. Ganellin and M.E. Parsons (eds.), Pharmacology of Histamine Receptors. Wright, Bristol, 1982.
3. Y. Itoh, R. Oishi, M. Nishibori and K. Saeki, J. Neurochem., 58 (1992) 884.
4. N. Adachi, Y. Itoh, R. Oishi and K. Saeki, J. Cereb. Blood Flow Metab., 12 (1992) 477.
5. M. Nishibori, R.Oishi, Y. Itoh and K. Saeki, Neurochem. Int., 19 (1991) 135.
6. M. Nishibori, A. Tahara, K. Sawada, J. Sakiyama, N. Nakaya and K. Saeki, Eur J. Neurosci., 12 (2000) 415.
7. M. Nishibori, R.Oishi, Y. Itoh and K. Saeki, J. Neurochem., 52 (1989) 1375.
8. T. Watanabe, N. Taguchi, S.Shiosaka, J. Tanaka, H. Kubota, Y. Terao, M. Tohyama and H. Wada, Brain Res., 295 (1984) 13.
9. P. Panula, H.Y.T. Yang, and E. Costa, Proc. Natl. Acad. Sci. U.S.A., 81 (1984), 2572.
10. B. Jarrott, J.T. Hjelle and S. Spector, Brain Res., 168 (1979) 323.
11. L. Edvinsson, J. Cervos-Navarro, L.-I. Larsson, C.H. Owman and A.-L. Ronnberg, Neurology, 27 (1977) 878.
12. H. Takagi, Y. Morishima, T. Matsuyama, H. Hayashi, T. Watanabe and H. Wada, Brain Res., 364 (1986) 114.

Histidine decarboxylase

Histamine Research in the New Millennium
T. Watanabe, H. Timmerman and K. Yanai (Editors)

Histidine decarboxylase activity in hematopoietic progenitors as a marker for basophil potentiality. Evidence for the existence of a common progenitor for megakaryocytes and basophils.

Michel Dy[1], Elke Schneider[1], Najet Debili[2], Dominique Dumenil[2], Maria Pacilio[1], Malvyne Rolli-Derkinderen[1], Jean Marie Launay[3], Anne Arnould[1], François Machavoine[1], Michel Arock[4].

[1] CNRS UMR 8603 -Université Paris V, Hopital Necker, 161,rue de Sèvres. 75743 Paris Cedex 15 France. [2] INSERM U362- Villejuif, France. [3] Service de Biochimie et de Biologie moléculaire, Hôpital Lariboisière, Paris, France. [4] Lab. d'Hématologie cellulaire et moléculaire Faculté de Pharmacie, Paris France

1. INTRODUCTION

Histamine, a well-known mediator synthesized from histidine by L-histidine decarboxylase (HDC: EC 4.1.1.22) is produced by murine hematopoietic precursors in response to various stimuli including IL-3, GM-CSF or calcium ionophore (1-3). These agents induce *de novo* synthesis of histidine decarboxylase rather than release of stored histamine (2). Histamine-producing cells can be enriched from the low-density bone marrow fraction by sorting the subset with the highest rhodamine retention (Rh-bright). Among sorted cells, around 40% express the transcripts for HDC in response to IL-3 which induces a concomitant production of IL-6 and IL-4 (1). Confirming previous evidence against the participation of mature hematopoietic components and mast cell precursors in this biological activity (4), we have recently identified the producer cells as basophil precursors (1).

In humans, both bone marrow and cord blood cells respond to IL-3 or GM-CSF by increased histamine production resulting from enhanced HDC activity (5). In the present study, by examining various human leukemia cell lines for their capacity to express HDC, we provide evidence for the existence of a common megakaryocyte/basophil precursor.

2. Histamine synthesis by normal cord blood progenitor cells during basophil or mast cell differentiation

We previously demonstrated that histamine synthesis by human cord blood cells is increased in response to IL-3 during the first days of culture(5). Since IL-3 acts as a basophilopoietin in the human system, our data suggest that, similarly to our observations in murine, rapid increase in histamine synthesis by progenitors could be related to basophil differentiation. However, it was not known if a similar increase could be observed during mast cell differentiation. For this purpose we cultured human cord blood cells in conditions leading either to basophil (IL-3+ TGFβ) or to mast cell (SCF+IL-6) differentiation.

While both conditions resulted in an almost pure population of either basophils or mast cells after 30-40 days of culture, only basophil conditions induce a rapid increase in histamine synthesis during the first 7 days of culture. In this case, HDC expression is never accompanied by increased tryptase conversely to HDC expression observed later in differentiated mast cells (after more than 20 days of culture)(data not shown).

3. Histamine synthesis by UT7 and UT7-derived cell lines

Constitutive histamine synthesis in UT7 and UT7D1 cell lines

UT7 cells were capable of producing substantial amounts of histamine when maintained in GM-CSF. From this parental cell line, we derived a stable subpopulation called UT7D1 (for UT7-Derived 1), with considerably enhanced spontaneous histamine production (6). This capacity to synthesize histamine is associated with the transcription of all three FcεRI chains, as well as CCR3, IL-5Rα and IL-4RαmRNAs. These features are shared by the well-known basophilic leukemia cell line KU812F and by mature basophils (7-12). They are consistent with a possible basophil differentiation potential of the UT7D1 cell line. This conclusion is further supported by the spontaneous expression of MBP (major basic protein) mRNA (personal unpublished data), which is shared by eosinophils and basophils (9). Yet, conversely to KU812F cells, only few UT7D1 cells display spontaneaously the basophil-specific antigen recognized by the Bsp-1 mAb when cultured in GM-CSF. This might be explained by their arrest at an early differentiation stage, when the expression of this basophil-specific antigen has not yet taken place whereas HDC mRNA is already transcribed.

PMA strinkingly increases histamine synthesis in UT- derived cell lines

In response to PMA, a striking increase in histamine synthesis occurs in UT7D1 cells as well as another UT7 derived cell line (110C1), with a maximum on day 1. Northern blot analysis (figure 1) as well as *in situ* hybridization revealed an increase in HDC mRNA expression upon exposure to PMA which varies depending on cell lines while histamine syntheis were equivalent in both cells. This increase in HDC activity was hardly affected by actinomycin D suggesting that HDC gene transcription in response to PMA accounts only partially for HDC activation which seems to result mainly from a post-transcriptional event, as already described in some other cell lines (13). The rapid enhancement of HDC activity in response to PMA is not accompanied by an increase in tryptase content but is concomitant with several other modifications: 1/ appearance of the specific basophil antigen recognized by Bsp-1 mAb (14,15) on a small UT7D1 subpopulation. 2/ transient increase in FcεRIα chain mRNA transcription. 3/ induction of cytokine genes whose expression is associated with the basophil lineage (16-18). Indeed, PMA induced both IL-6 and IL-4 mRNA expression in UT7D1 cells, a feature reminiscent of the previously characterized "basophil-like" murine hematopoietic precursor cells whose growth factor-induced increase in histamine synthesis is always associated with IL-6 and IL-4 production (1,19). In addition, UT7D1 cells respond to PMA by expressing IL-13 mRNA, as previously reported for the basophil precursor cell line KU812 (16). Taken together, these findings suggest that PMA can drive at least some UT7D1 cells towards basophil differentiation.

Basophil differentiation is not sustained in long-term cultures since a striking decrease in the expression of these molecules takes place within 4 days, suggesting that once PMA has induced some early steps towards basophil commitment, it cannot maintain survival, maturation and proliferation.

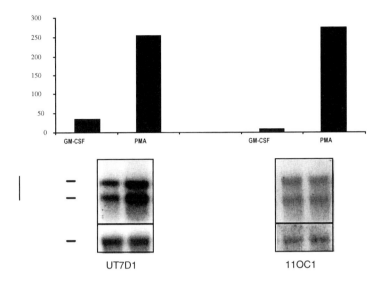

Figure 1: HDC mRNA expression in UT7D1 and 11OC1 cells (after a16h-incubation with or without PMA) is respectively slightly or not increased following PMA stimulation (as shown by Northern blot analysis) while histamine synthesis is greatly enhanced in both cell lines .

4. Histamine synthesis and megakaryocytopoiesis

At this point our data supported a relationship between histamine synthesis and basophil potentiality. However since phorbol myristate is a major inducer of megakaryocytic differentiation, as judged by the induction of CD41 and PDGF A and B mRNA expression, and has been claimed to increase the histamine content of platelets (20), its effect on UT7D1 cells could also reflect the commitment to this lineage. It should however be noted that the presence of HDC in platelets is controversial (21) and that the PMA-induced increase in platelet HDC activity is not affected by cycloheximide (22), indicating that it does not rely on newly synthesized enzyme. Conversely, UT7D1 cells fail to produce histamine in the presence of the inhibitor, as previously reported for RBL 2H3 cells (23).

In addition, to prove that PMA-induced HDC activation is not associated with megakaryocytopoiesis, we cultured CD34[+] cells from normal bone marrow for 9 -10 days with TPO and then purified CD61+ megakaryocytes. No transcripts for HDC were detectable in these purified cells by RT-PCR analysis, in contrast with the well-known basophil leukemia cell line KU812F, as well as UT7D1, HEL or 11OC1 cells. Conversely to the cell lines, megakaryocytes expressed both PDGF A and B transcripts. Furthermore, the lack of HDC mRNA expression in megakaryocytes was confirmed by in situ hybridization and purified megakaryocytes produced histamine neither spontaneously nor upon stimulation with PMA.

5. Histamine synthesis in other megakaryocytic leukemic cell lines

The study with UT7D1 cells suggests the existence of precursor cells with dual megakaryocyte/basophil differentiation potential. To confirm such a possibility we have examined various other leukemic cell lines for their spontaneous or PMA-induced histamine synthesis. As shown in table I, all the other megakaryocytic cell lines tested synthesized histamine either spontaneously or after PMA stimulation. This is true for the HEL, CMK, LAMA 84, whose basophil potentiality has already been reported (9). In addition, the megakaryocytic leukemic cell line MTT95 has also recently been shown to be a basophil precursor (24). The only exception is the K562 cell line which does not share this property. However it is well established that these cells are more engaged into the erythroid differentiation pathway, as attested by their expression of specific markers of this lineage (25). It could be argued that histamine production by these leukemic cells may simply reflect an aberrant expression pattern in transformed cell lines adapted to cell culture. However, this does not seem to be the case because only cells with megakaryocytic potential synthesize histamine and for some of them express Bsp1 while this fails to occur in other cells such as U937, HL60 and lymphoid cell lines.

Another argument in favor of the basophil potentiality of some of these cell lines is provided by the generation of antibodies recognizing specifically basophil following immunization with a megakaryocytic leukemic cell line. Thus, Bsp-1 mAb was prepared by immunizing mice against the human leukemic cell line HEL and turned out to be specific for human basophils (14). These cells have been described as erythro-megakaryocytic rather than basophilic, and their ability to transcribe the three FcRI c h a ins and to synthesize histamine, comes as a surprise (6). Similarly, immunization against UT7 cells has led to the generation of 97A6 antibodies which recognize basophils (26). In these two cases our data explain at length why basophil specific antibody could be raised following these immunization.

Table I. Histamine production by various leukemic cell lines.

HISTAMINE PRODUCTION (NG/10^6 CELLS) FOLLOWING 48 H OF INCUBATION WITH

	Culture medium	PMA
Megakaryocytic Cell lines		
UT7	307 ±40	1142±317
UT7D1	1129± 67	4812±658
HEL	135±49	1376±529
CMK	341±56	1377±359
LAMA 84	364	884
K562	Not Det.	Not Det.
Other cell lines		
U937	Not Det.	Not Det.
HL60	Not Det.	Not Det.
Jurkat	Not Det.	Not Det.

(Not Det.: Not detectable, less than 10ng/10^6cells)

As far as the leukemic cell lines examined in this study are concerned, there is no correlation between their ability to produce histamine either spontaneously or in response to PMA and their expression of the basophil-specific antigen recognized by Bsp-1 mAb. Indeed, the antibody labels the majority of unstimulated KU812F and HEL cells, even though they produce less histamine than the UT7D1 cell line. This lack of correlation between Bsp-1 expression and histamine-producing capacity is also evident among the UT7 population itself. Bsp-1⁺ cells are actually more numerous in the parental (10 to 15%) than in the derived cell line (around 2%), although histamine synthesis (spontaneous or PMA-induced) is much higher in the latter.

6. PMA-induced histamine synthesis is inhibited by the simultaneous presence of ERK and PKC inhibitors

Knowing that PMA increases PKC and ERK activities in various cells, We tested the effect of their specific inhibitors on PMA-induced histamine synthesis. GF109203X, a PKC inhibitor markedly diminished histamine synthesis induced by PMA ($60\pm6\%$ at a dose of $3\mu M$), while ERK inhibitor, U0216 ($10\mu M$) had less pronounced effect ($31\pm4\%$ of inhibition). Maximal inhibition occurred in the presence of both inhibitors ($81\pm4\%$).

As shown by Kuramasu et al , alteration of DNA methylation of the HDC gene promoter explains the specificity of its expression in basophils and mast cells (27,28). The variations of response to PMA in terms of HDC activity in different cell lines could thus depend on its status concerning basophil differentiation. Cells with high basophil potentiality would be the better responder because of a freely accessible HDC promoter while those unrelated to the basophil lineage would be unresponsive because of the methylation of their HDC gene.

7. Conclusion

The study of HDC activity in conjunction with other basophil markers in leukemic cell lines suggest the existence of a common precursor for basophil and megakaryocyte. The relevance of this finding to normal hematopoiesis remains to be confirmed with human bone marrow progenitor cells. However, in favor of such a possibility it should be noted that basophils very often contaminate megakaryocytes generated during culture of normal bone marrow CD34+ cells with TPO .

This is the first evidence for a factor-dependent cell line, UT7D1, with basophil potentiality in which early events in basophil differentiation, maturation and proliferation can be evaluated. Basophil commitment estimated by the induction of several markers, and especially HDC and Bsp1 expression, is induced by PMA. The striking decline in the expression of these markers during long-term culture might eventually be explained by the lack of a basophil-specific growth factor ensuring survival, maturation and proliferation. Indeed, although various cytokines have been shown to affect basophil differentiation, a specific "basophilopoietin", analogous to other lineage-specific factors (M-CSF, G-CSF, IL-5, EPO, TPO) has yet to be discovered. This particular situation has even led to the assumption that basophil differentiation is a default pathway taking place when no other growth factor is available (29). We are presently investigating this hypothesis.

References

1. E. Schneider, F. Lemoine, I. Breton-Gorius, F. Machavoine, A. Arnould, J. Guichard, E.M. Cramer and M. Dy, Exp. Haematol., 27 (1999) 1010.
2. E. Schneider, H. Pollard, F. Lepault, D. Guy-Grand, M. Minkowski and M. Dy , J. Immunol., 139 (1987) 710.
3. M. Dy, A. Arnould, F.M. Lemoine, F. Machavoine, H. Ziltener and E. Schneider , Blood, 87 (1996) 3161.
4. E. Schneider, R.E. Ploemacher, B. Nabarra, N.H.C. Brons and M. Dy , Blood, 81 (1993) 1161.
5. M.A. Minkowski, B. Lebel, A. Arnould and M. Dy , Exp. Hematol., 18 (1990) 1158 .
6. M.Dy, M. Pacilio, A. Arnould, F. Machavoine, P. Mayeux, O. Hermine, M. Bodger, E . Schneider, Exp. Hematol., 27 (1999) 1295.
7. M. Uguccioni, C.R. MacKay, B. Ochensberger, P. Loetscher, S. Rhis, G.J. Larosa, P. Rao, P.D. Ponath , M. Baggiolini and C.A. Dahinden, J. Clin. Invest., 100 (1997) 1137.
8. J.A. Denburg, M.D. Imman, B. Leber, R. Sehim and O'Byrne P.M., Allergy, 51 (1996) 141.
9. T. Blom, G. Nilsson, C. Sundstrom, K. Nilsson and L. Hellman, Scand. J. Immunol., 44 (1996) 54.
10. T. Blom, R. Huang, M. Aveskogh, K. Nilsson and L. Hellman, Eur. J. Immunol., 22 (1992) 2025.
11. P. Valent, and P. Bettelheim, Adv. Immunol., 52 (1992) 333.
12. P. Valent, J. Besemer, K. Kishi, F. Di Padova, K. Geissler and P. Bettelheim, Blood, 76 (1990) 1734.
13. K. Maeda, H. Taniguchi, J. Ohno, H. Ohtsu, K. Yamauchi, E. Sakurai, Y. Tanno, J.M. Butterfield, T. Watanabe and K. Shirato, Exp. Hematol., 26 (1998) 325.
14. M.P. Bodger, G.L. Mounsey, J. Nelson and P.H. Fitzgerald, Blood, 69 (1987) 1414.
15. M.P. Bodger and L.A. Newton, Br. J. Haematol., 67 (1987) 281.
16. Y. Yanagihara, K. Kajiwara, Y. Basaki, K. Ikizawa, K. Akiyama, H. Saito, Clin. Exp Immunol., 108 (1997) 295.
17. A.C. Redrup, B.P. Howard, D.W. MacGlashan, A. Kageysobotka, L.M. Lichtenstein and J.T. Schroeder , J. Immunol., 160 (1998) 1957.
18. G.F. Zhu, K. Gomi and J.S. Marshall, J. Immunol., 161 (1998) 2541.
19. M. Dy, D. Jankovic, R. Ploemacher, J. Theze and E. Schneider, Exp. Hematol., 19 (1991) 934.
20. S.P. Saxena, C. Robertson, A.B. Becker and J.M. Gerrard, Biochem. J., 273 (1991) 405.
21. D.S. Gill, M.A. Barradas, V.A. Fonseca and P. Dandona, Metabolism, 38 (1989) 243.
22. S.P. Saxena, L.J. Brandes, A.B. Becker, K.J. Simons, F.S. Labella and J.M. Gerrard, Science, 243 (1989) 1596.
23. K. Maeyama, Y. Taguchi, M. Sasaki, H. Wada, M.A. Beaven and T. Watanabe, Biochem. Biophys. Res. Commun., 151 (1988) 1402.
24. N. Mizobuchi, I. Takahashi, S. Yorimitsu, T. Horimi, K. Hamada, M. Matsuoka, H. Sonobe, M. Hiroi and I. Kubonishi, Acta Med. Okayama, 53 (1999) 95.
25. T. Tani, J. Ylanne and I. Virtanen, Exp. Hematol., 24 (1996) 158.
26. H.J. Buhring, P.J. Simmons, M. Pudney, R. Muller, D. Jarrossay, A. Van Agthoven, M. Willheim, W. Brugger, P. Valent and L. Kanz, Blood, 94 (1999) 2343.
27. A. Kuramasu, H. Saito, S. Suzuki, T. Watanabe, H. Ohtsu, J. Biol. Chem. 273 (1998) 31607.
28. S. SuzukiIshigaki, K. NumayamaTsuruta, A. Kuramasu, E. Sakurai, Y. Makabe, S. Shimura, K. Shirato, K. Igarashi, T. Watanabe and H. Ohtsu, Nucleic Acids Res., 28 (2000) 2627.
29. S. Tsai, S. Bartelmez, R. Heyman, K. Damm, R. Evans, Collins S.J., Genes Dev., 6 (1992) 2258.

Histamine Research in the New Millennium
T. Watanabe, H. Timmerman and K. Yanai (Editors)

Endogenous histamine and allergic eosinophil infiltration into the airways

A. Koarai[a], M. Ichinose[a], S. Ishigaki[b], S. Yamagata[a], H. Sugiura[a], E. Sakurai[b], A. Kuramasu[b], T. Watanabe[b], T. Hattori[a], K. Shirato[a] and H. Ohtsu[b]

[a] First Department of Internal Medicine, and [b] Department of Cellular Pharmacology, Tohoku University School of Medicine, 1-1 Seiryo-machi, Aoba-ku, Sendai 980-8574, Japan.

Histamine is thought to have an important role in the acute phase of the allergic airway inflammatory response rather than in the late phase. Recently, De Bie, *et al.* showed that a selective histamine H_2 receptor antagonist inhibited the eosinophil infiltration into the airway in an ovalbumin (OVA) sensitized challenged mice model, suggesting that endogenous histamine might also have important effects on the late phase of allergic inflammation. In the present study, we aimed to examine the role of histamine in allergic airway inflammation using OVA-sensitized wild type mice and knockout mice deficient in L-Histidine decarboxylase (HDC), which catalyzes the formation of histamine from L-histidine. In HDC-knockout mice, the histamine levels in the airway and lung were significant lower than those in the wild type mice ($p < 0.05$). OVA sensitized animals were challenged with aerosolized 0.5% OVA for 1 hr on two occasions 4 hr apart. In the wild type mice, OVA challenge increased eosinophil infiltration in the bronchoalveolar lavage fluid (BALF) 3 days after challenge. In HDC-knockout mice, OVA challenge-induced eosinophil accumulation in BALF was significantly reduced. Total IgE levels were not significantly different between the wild type and HDC-knockout mice.

These findings suggest that endogenous histamine may play an important role in the eosinophil infiltration into the airway during allergic reactions.

1. INTRODUCTION

Histamine [2-(4-imidazole)ethylamine] is formed by decarboxylation of the amino acid histidine by L-histidine decarboxylase (HDC). Histamine is stored in granules within mast cells and basophils, and is released when these cells degranulate in response to various stimulations, such as, IgE and cytokines.

Histamine has been thought to be one of the important proinflammatory mediators and to play a key role in the pathophysiology of asthma. In an acute allergic reaction, histamine induces various responses such as, contraction of airway smooth muscles, vasodilation, plasma exudation, and mucus production, mainly mediated by H_1 receptors [1]. However, histamine has been thought to be less important for the late phase of allergic airway inflammation. Recently, De Bie, *et al.* [2] have shown that a selective histamine H_2 receptor antagonist inhibits the eosinophil infiltration into the airways in an ovalbumin (OVA) sensitized challenged mice model, suggesting that histamine might also have important effects on the late phase of allergic inflammation.

However, pharmacological studies have used antagonists which might have nonspecific effects on the whole body. Recently, we have developed HDC-knockout mice, in which the levels of histamine in various tissues were much lower than those in wild type mice [3]. In this study, we examined the role of histamine in the eosinophil infiltration into the airway during the late allergic response using OVA sensitized HDC-knockout and wild type mice.

2. MATERIAL AND METHODS

2.1. Animals

HDC-knockout mice of the 129Sv strain was prepared as previously reported [3]. The mice were maintained in conventional animal housing under specific pathogen-free conditions at a constant temperature and humidity with regular 12 hr cycles of light and darkness. Only male mice were used for these studies and were examined at 8 weeks of age. All of the experiments performed in this study were conducted with the consent of the Ethics Committee for the Use of Experimental Animals of the Tohoku University School of Medicine.

2.2. Measurement of histamine

Non-sensitized wild and HDC-knockout mice were sacrificed. After that, lung tissues were isolated and divided into two portions, the trachea and main bronchus, and the lungs. The tissues were homogenized with a Polytron homogenizer (Kinematica, Luzern, Switzerland) at maximal speed for 15 s. Then, 20 l of 60% perchloric acid were added to the homogenates, which were then centrifuged at 10000 g for 20 min. Histamine was determined fluorimetrically by high performance liquid chromatography [4]. An aliquot of 70 l of each supernatant was injected into an HPLC system, and fluorescence was determined by a fluoromonitor (F-1100, Hitachi, Tokyo, Japan).

2.3. Sensitization and allergen challenge

Mice were sensitized by an intraperitoneal injection of 0.5 ml solution containing 50 g of ovalbumin (OVA) and 4 mg of aluminum hydroxide in saline on day 0 and 5. Twelve days later, the mice were placed in a plexiglas chamber (10 cm × 15 cm × 25 cm) and challenged with aerosolized saline or 0.5% OVA in saline for 1 hr on two occasions 4 hrs apart. The aerosolized OVA was produced by an ultrasonic nebulizer (NE-12, Omron, Tokyo, Japan; output 0.8 mL/min). At 3 days after challenge, the mice were anesthetized by intraperitoneal injection of pentobarbital (70 mg/kg body weight) and used for the following experiments.

2.4. Bronchoalveolar lavage

3 days after challenge, the mice were sacrificed. To collect bronchoalveolar lavage fluid (BALF) cells, the lungs were dissected and the trachea was cannulated with a polyethylene tube (1.1 mm outer diameter). The lungs were lavaged twice with PBS (0.25, 0.20 ml each time) and approximately 0.4 ml of instilled fluid were consistently recovered.

Total cell numbers were counted with a hemocytometer. After centrifugation, cell pellets were resuspended in 100 l of PBS and the preparations were processed using a Shandon cytocentrifuge (Shandon III Southern Instruments, Seuekley, PA) at 300 rpm for 5 min. All preparations were stained with Diff-Quik stain (Baxter, McGraw Park, IL). Differential cell counts in BALF were performed with at least 300 leukocytes.

2.5. Measurement of serum concentration of IgE

3 days after challenge, blood was drawn from the right ventricule, and serum was obtained by centrifugation at $1500 \times g$ for 10 min. Serum IgE levels were determined with a commercial ELISA kit (Yamasa, Chiba, Japan).

3. RESULTS

3.1. Histamine level

In HDC-knockout mice, the histamine levels in the airway and the lung were significantly lower than in the wild type mice ($p < 0.01$).

3.2. Cell differentiation in BALF after allergen challenge

OVA-challenged mice showed increases in the numbers of eosinophils in the bronchoalveolar lavage fluid (BALF) 3 days after challenge ($p < 0.01$). In HDC-knockout mice, OVA-challenged mice showed a significant decrease in eosinophils in the BALF compared to the wild type mice ($p < 0.05$).

3.3. Serum total IgE level

Because it might be supposed that histamine directly affects the sensitization level in this system, therefore we measured the total IgE level. There was no difference between the serum total IgE level of the wild type mice and that of the HDC-knockout mice 3 days after OVA challenge.

4. DISCUSSION

In the HDC-knockout mice, the histamine levels in the airway and the lung were significantly lower than those in the wild type mice, suggesting that HDC-knockout mice could be used as a histamine-deficient mice model of the airway and the lung. Therefore, in this study, we use such mice for elucidating the role of histamine in the eosinophil infiltration into the airway during the late allergic response.

In the present study, we showed that the eosinophil counts in the BALF of HDC-knockout mice 3 days after allergen challenge decreased significantly compared to those of wild type mice, which is compatible with the result of a selective histamine H_2 receptor antagonist study [2]. These results suggest that endogenous histamine may be an important molecule in eosinophil infiltration into the airway in the late allergic reaction.

We propose three possible mechanisms by which histamine may contribute to the eosinophil infiltration into the airway in the allergic late response.

Firstly, histamine has been found to influence the release of cytokines and inflammatory mediators from a variety of inflammatory and immune cells [5]. Accordingly, histamine might affect T cells and change the balance between T helper 1 (Th1) and T helper 2 (Th2) cytokines. Th1 cytokines such as interferon (INF)-gamma and interleukin (IL)-2 are thought to decrease in allergic reactions, and Th2 cytokines such as IL-4 and IL-5 to increase, which may be important in eosinophil infiltration into the airway [6]. Recently, it has been reported that Th2 cells have HDC and could make histamine [7], and that histamine inhibits the lymphocyte functions of producing IL-2 and INF-gamma and, in contrast, increases anti-CD3-induced IL-5 production in Th2 cells via H_2 receptors [8].

Secondly, histamine could increase the amounts of adhesion molecules, such as P-selectin. It has been reported that P-selectin contributes to eosinophil infiltration. In P-selectin-deficient mice, eosinophilia was inhibited in allergic airway inflammation [9]. Also, histamine has been reported to increase the expression of P-selectin [10]. Thirdly, histamine might increase the ability of eosinophils to migrate. Raible et al. have reported that histamine activates human eosinophils, which is mediated by a rise in $[Ca^{2+}]_i$ [11]. Further studies are needed to clarify the underlining mechanism of the histamine-related eosinophil infiltration in this allergic model.

In summary, we have shown that eosinophil infiltration into the airway after allergic reaction is significantly reduced by HDC genetic depletion. This evidence suggests the important role of endogenous histamine in allergic airway inflammation.

ACKNOWLEDGMENT

The writers thank Miss. Makabe for maintaining the mice and Mr. Brent Bell for reading the manuscript.

REFERENCES

1. P.J. Barnes, K.F. Chung, C.P. Page. Inflammatory mediators of asthma: an update. Pharmacol Rev 1998;50(4):515.
2. J.J. De Bie, P.A. Henricks, W.W. Cruikshank, G. Hofman, E.H. Jonker, F.P. Nijkamp, et al. Modulation of airway hyperresponsiveness and eosinophilia by selective histamine and 5-HT receptor antagonists in a mouse model of allergic asthma. Br J Pharmacol 1998;124(5):857.
3. H. Ohtsu, S. Tanaka, Y. Hori, Y. Makabe, G. Pejler, E. Tchougounova, et al. Mice lacking histidine decarboxylase exhibit multiple phenotypes due to diet-dependent histamine deficiency. EMBO. J. (submitted)
4. A. Yamatodani, H. Fukuda, H. Wada, T. Iwaeda, T. Watanabe. High-performance liquid chromatographic determination of plasma and brain histamine without previous purification of biological samples: cation-exchange chromatography coupled with post-column derivatization fluorometry. J Chromatogr 1985;344:115.
5. A. Falus, K. Meretey. Histamine: an early messenger in inflammatory and immune reactions. Immunol Today 1992;13(5):154.
6. K.G. Lim, P.F. Weller. Lymphokines. In: Barnes PJ, Grunstein MM, Leff AR, Woolcock AJ, editors. Asthma. vol 1. Philadelphia: Lippincott-Raven Publishers; 1997: 663.
7. Y. Ohuchi, H. Ohtsu, E. Sakurai, K. Yanai, A. Ichikawa, Z. Radvany, et al. Induction of histidine decarboxylase in type 2 T helper lymphocytes treated with anti-CD3 antibody. Inflamm Res 1998;47(Suppl 1):S48.
8. J. Schmidt, S. Fleissner, I. Heimann-Weitschat, R. Lindstaedt, I. Szelenyi. Histamine increases anti-CD3 induced IL-5 production of TH2-type T cells via histamine H2-receptors. Agents Actions 1994;42(3-4):81.
9. G.T. De Sanctis, W.W. Wolyniec, F.H. Green, S. Qin, A. Jiao, P.W. Finn, et al. Reduction of allergic airway responses in P-selectin-deficient mice. J Appl Physiol 1997;83(3):681.
10. H. Asako, I. Kurose, R. Wolf, S. DeFrees, Z.L. Zheng, M.L. Phillips, et al. Role of H1 receptors and P-selectin in histamine-induced leukocyte rolling and adhesion in postcapillary venules. J Clin Invest 1994;93(4):1508.
11. D.G. Raible, E.S. Schulman, J. DiMuzio, R. Cardillo, T.J. Post. Mast cell mediators prostaglandin-D2 and histamine activate human eosinophils. J Immunol 1992;148(11):3536.

Histamine Research in the New Millennium
T. Watanabe, H. Timmerman and K. Yanai (Editors)

Role of histamine in gastric acid secretion: L-hitidine decarboxylase deficient mice

S. Tanaka[a], K. Hamada[a], H. Ohtsu[b], T. Watanabe[b], A. Falus[c], A. Nagy[d], S. Okabe[e] and A. Ichikawa[a]

[a]Department of Physiological Chemistry, Graduate School of Pharmaceutical Sciences, Kyoto University, Kyoto, Japan
[b]Department of Pharmacology, Tohoku University School of Medicine, Sendai, Japan
[c]Department of Genetics, Cell- and Immunology, Semmelweis Medical University, Budapest, Hungary
[d]Samuel Lunenfeld Research Institute, Mount Sinai Hospital, Toronto, Canada
[e]Department of Applied Pharmacology, Kyoto Pharmaceutical University, Kyoto, Japan

Histamine is one of the primary secretagogues for gastric acid secretion, but it remains to be clarified how its roles are shared with other ones, such as gastrin and acetylcholine. We evaluated the role of histamine in acid secretion using L-histidine decarboxylase (HDC) deficient mice. HDC deficient mice exhibited a response of high acid secretion upon exogenous histamine, mild to carbachol, and negligible to gastrin. Higher acid secretion induced by histamine appears to be resulted from enhanced signal transduction of H_2 receptors and from cooperation of H_2 with muscarinic receptors.

1. INTRODUCTION

The central role of histamine in gastric acid secretion has been studied by many investigators [1] In 1972, Black et al. reported for the first time that histamine stimulated gastric acid secretion via histamine-2 (H_2) receptor and successfully developed antagonists that were selective for the receptor [2]. These antagonists have potent effects in the treatment of peptic ulcer and gastroesophageal reflux diseases. Regarding the peripheral regulation of gastric acid secretion, it is now considered that the major stimuli acting on parietal cells are histamine, acetylcholine (ACh) and gastrin [1]. It must be noted, however, that the interaction between these secretagogues in acid secretion is complex and not fully understood. With *in vivo* study, it is difficult to evaluate the function of one secretagogue separately from that of another, because one secretagogue often induces another and efficacy of antagonists is incomplete and not last for very long. In this study, we developed a L-histidine decarboxylase (HDC) deficient mouse strain by gene targeting in embryonic stem cells. We analyzed the effect of exogenously administrated histamine, gastrin and carbachol in the gastric acid secretion in HDC deficient mice.

2. MATERIALS AND METHODS

2. 1. Materials

YM-022 and YF-476 were kindly provided by Yamanouchi Pharmaceutical Industries, Ltd. (Tokyo, Japan). The following materials were purchased from the sources indicated: Histamine dihydrochloride from Wako Pure Chemicals (Osaka, Japan), famotidine, [Leu^{15}] human gastrin I and atropine from Sigma (St. Louis, MO), carbachol from CARBIOCHEM (San Diego, CA), tiotidine from TOCRIS (Bristol, UK). All other chemicals were commercial products of reagent grade.

2.2. Generation of HDC deficient mice

We replaced exons 6-8 of HDC gene with an inverted PGK promoter-driven neomycin phosphotransferase (*neo*) gene. This replacement should result in the loss-of-function mutation since exon 8 contains the coding sequence for the putative binding site (TFNPSKW) to which pyridoxal 5'-phosphate, the coenzyme of HDC protein, is thought to bind [3]. The mutant mice have a mixed genetic back ground (129/ ICR). Eight to 12-week-old wild type and HDC$^{-/-}$ mice, bred and maintained independently, were used in all experiments. Mice were fasted for 24 hours before each experiment with free access to tap water.

2. 3. Gastric acid secretion

Each mouse was fasted for 24 hours, with free access to tap water, and anesthetized with intraperitoneal injection of urethane at 1.25 g/kg. After tracheotomy, a polyethylene tube was inserted into the trachea to ensure a patent airway. A gastric acute fistula was made by the insertion of a polyethylene tube toward the antrum through an incision of the duodenum. Four hundred μl of saline was injected and collected every 15 minutes and acid output (μmol H⁺/15 min) was determined by titration with 10 mM NaOH. Mice were injected with 100 μl of each reagent solution subcutaneously. Drugs were prepared as follows; histamine dihydrochloride, [Leu^{15}] human gastrin I, carbachol and atropine in saline, famotidine in 0.1 % carboxymethyl cellurose, YF-476 and YM-022 in polyethylene glycol #300. Control animals were injected with vehicle solution simultaneously.

2. 4. Histidine decarboxylase assay

The stomach of each mouse was minsed, suspended in a lysis buffer (10 mM HEPES, pH 7.3 containing 1.5 mM MgCl$_2$, 10 mM KCl, 0.5 mM dithiothreitol, 1 % Triton X-100, 1 mM EDTA, 1 mM EGTA, 0.2 mM phenylmethylsulfonyl fluoride (PMSF), 0.1 mM benzamidine, 10 μg/ml leupeptin, 10 μg/ml aprotinin, 10 μg/ml E-64 and 1 μg/ml pepstatin A) and homogenized. The homogenate was centrifuged at 1,000 x g for 10 minutes at 4˚C to remove the debris. The supernatant was recentrifuged at 100,000 x g for 1 hour at 4˚C. The resultant supernatant was assayed for HDC activity as described previously by the o-phtalaldehyde method [4]. The protein concentration was determined by the method of Bradford with bovine serum albumin as standard.

2. 5. Northern blot analysis

Stomachs were collected from each mouse and immediately frozen in liquid nitrogen and stored at -80˚C until use. Total RNA was extracted by the acid guanidium thiocyanate-phenol-chloroform method.[18] Poly(A⁺) RNA was further purified from total RNA by oligo (dT) Latex (TaKaRa, Kyoto, Japan). Poly(A⁺) RNA (5 μg) was separated by electrophoresis on a 1.5 % agarose gel and transferred onto a nylon membrane (Biodyne-A, Pall, Port Washington, NY). Hybridization was performed with a [^{32}P]-labeled cDNA fragment specific for mouse HDC (PvuII fragment) or other genes. The filters were then rehybridized with a [^{32}P]-labeled cDNA fragment specific for glyceraldehyde-3-phosphate dehydrogenase (GAPDH) (CLONTECH, Palo Alto, CA).

2. 6. Immunoblot analysis

Stomachs of each mouse were collected and homogenized in 25 mM sodium phosphate, pH 7.4 containing 10 mM HEPES-NaOH, pH 7.3, 5 mM MgCl$_2$ and 0.1 mM PMSF. The homogenate was centrifuged at 800 x g for 15 minutes at 4˚C. The supernatant was recentrifuged at 30,000 x g for 30 minutes at 4°C. The resultant precipitate was resuspended in the same buffer. The immunoblot analysis was performed as described previously [4]. The membrane was incubated with anti-α subunit of H^+, K^+-ATPase antibody (1:200) (MBL, Nagoya, Japan), anti-chromogranin A antibody (1:200), anti-Gsα antibody (1:200) (Santa Cruz Biotechnology, Santa Cruz, CA), or anti-Giα antibody (1:1000) (NEN Research Products, Boston, MA). Then, the membrane was incubated with anti-mouse (goat, or rabbit) IgG antibody conjugated with horse radish peroxidase (DAKO, Glostrup, Denmark) and then stained with ECL staining kit (AmershamPharmacia, Uppsala, Sweden).

3. RESULTS

3. 1. General appearance

Northern blot analysis demonstrated the absence of HDC transcripts (2.7 kb) in the stomach of HDC deficient mice. HDC deficient mice showed no HDC activity and a negligible amount of histamine (<50 ng/g tissue) in the gastric mucous homogenates. The level of basal acid secretion in the mutants was slightly lower than in the wild type mice (0.59 ± 0.02 vs. 0.52 ± 0.01 μmolH$^+$/15 min, n=38, p<0.01). Although the mutants demonstrated mild hypergastrinemia (302 ± 31.2 vs. 100 ± 24.5 pg/ml, n=4, p<0.01), no significant changes of general histological appearance were observed in the gastric mucosal cells.

3. 2. Gastric acid secretion induced by histamine

The maximal acid output was about two folds higher in the mutants than in the wild type mice (10 mg/kg histamine, 3.63 ± 1.39 vs. 7.59 ± 1.20 μmolH$^+$/15 min, n=7, p<0.01). Histamine-stimulated acid secretion both in the wild type and in the mutants was completely abolished by pretreatment with 10 mg/kg famotidine 1 hour before the stimulation.

3. 3. Gastric acid secretion in response to gastrin

Whereas [Leu^{15}] human gastrin I at a dose of 1 mg/kg stimulated acid secretion in the wild type mice, even at a dose of 3 mg/kg, it could not stimulate acid secretion in the mutants.

3. 4. Gastric acid secretion in response to carbachol

It was found that 0.1 mg/kg carbachol induced biphasic acid secretion responses in the wild type mice. The early phase was characterized by famotidine-insensitive secretion within

30 min of treatment, while the late phase was characterized by famotidine-sensitive secretion. Both phases were completely abolished by pretreatment of 3 mg/kg of atropine. In contrast, when the mutant mice were treated with carbachol, acid secretion was induced only in the early phase, but not in the late phase.

3. 5. Effect of atropine or gastrin CCK-B antagonists on histamine-induced acid secretion

The histamine-induced (10 mg/kg) acid secretion in the mutants treated with atropine (3 mg/kg) remained higher than that in the wild type mice, but not significant in the cumulative acid output. On the other hand, subcutaneous injection of YF-476 (10 μmol/kg) did not suppress the histamine-induced acid secretion in the mutants although YF-476 treatment resulted in considerable inhibition of the acid secretion induced by histamine in the wild type mice. The YM-022 (10 μmol/kg) treatments resulted in the same effect on the histamine-induced acid secretion in both mice strains.

3. 6. Expression of genes and proteins involved in gastric acid secretion

Quantification of the accumulation of transcripts in the gastric mucosa, such as H_2, M_3, gastrin/CCK-B receptors, gastrin, and H^+, K^+-ATPase α subunit demonstrated that the expression levels of all the genes investigated were unchanged in the mutants. Similarly, the expression of the H^+, K^+-ATPase α subunit and chromogranin A was unchanged in the mutants at the level of protein expression. Nevertheless, the expression in the gastric membranes of Gsα, but not that of Giα, was significantly increased in the mutants.

3. 7. Binding analysis for gastric H_2 receptors

Scatchard plot analysis demonstrated a lower binding affinity and a higher binding maximum for [^{3}H]tiotidine, a specific H_2 antagonist in the gastric membrane fraction of HDC deficient mice. *Kd* and *Bmax* values were as follows: *Kd*, 3.24 (wild type mice) vs. 17.5 nmol/L (mutant mice), *Bmax*, 1.09 (wild type mice) vs. 1.88 pmoles/mg protein (mutant mice).

4. DISCUSSION

This report demonstrated that HDC deficient mice acquire a high sensitivity to exogenous histamine in the gastric acid secretion. Since the mutants maintained their responses to carbachol, but not to gastrin, the basal acid secretion appears to be partially compensated for by the muscarinic pathway. In the presence of atropine, the histamine-induced acid secretion in the mutants was no longer higher significantly than in the wild type mice. These observations indicate that cholinergic effect should have some contribution to the enhancement of histamine-induced acid secretion in the mutant mice. In addition, an increase in Gsα expression was obtained in the gastric membranes of the mutant mice, suggesting that enhancement of the efficiency in the histamine-mediated signaling should occur in parietal cells. It is likely that the signal transduction pathway via H_2 receptors is converted to the highly sensitive state in the mutants. The analysis of certain phenotypes in HDC deficient mice might contribute to the development for the therapy for 'rebound' acid hypersecretion, which is observed after abrupt withdrawal of prolonged H_2 receptor blockade by H_2 antagonists. This study also demonstrated that [Leu^{15}] human gastrin I could not stimulate the acid secretion in the mutant mice, which indicates that gastrin-induced acid secretion is solely mediated by endogenous histamine formation in ECL cells. The hypergastrinemia in the mutants, which may resulted from the lower basal secretion, might result in the tolerance of gastrin/CCK-B receptors in ECL cells. In summary, we demonstrated that the enhanced acid secretion induced by histamine in HDC-deficient mice is caused both by the increase in H_2 receptor signaling efficiency and by cholinergic stimulation. Gastrin/CCK-B receptor pathway has little contribution to this phenotype and the acid secretion induced by gastrin in mice might be solely mediated by histamine.

REFERENCES

1.   S. J. Hersey and G. Sachs, Physiol. Rev., 75 (1995) 155.

2.   J. W. Black, W. A. Duncan, C. J. Durant, C. R. Ganellin and E. M. Parsons, Nature, 236 (1972) 385.

3.   J. Yamamoto, K. Yatsunami, E. Ohmori, Y. Sugimoto, T. Fukui, T. Katayama, A. Ichikawa, FEBS Lett., (1990) 276.

4.   S. Tanaka, K. Nemoto, E. Yamamura, A. Ichikawa, J. Biol. Chem., 273 (1998) 8177.

Histamine and allergic disease

Histamine Research in the New Millennium
T. Watanabe, H. Timmerman and K. Yanai (Editors)

Histamine as a Mediator of Allergic Airway Disease

Stephen T. Holgate.

RCMB Research Division, School of Medicine, University of Southampton

The recognition by Dale and Laidlaw that histamine could be released from anaphylactically challenged lung tissue (1) provided the first concrete evidence for the involvement of a specific chemical entity that could interact with specific tissues in chronic inflammatory diseases associated with allergic reactions, such as asthma. The identification of other contractile substances in the anaphylactically challenged perfusate of sensitised tissues was suggested in further experiments and Dale and Schultz, but it was not until 1938 that a second pharmacologically active substance designated slow reacting substance (SRS) was identified by Feldberg and Kellaway in tissue exposed to cobra venum (2). Kellaway and Trethewie, and later Brocklehurst (3), showed that SRS was also released during anaphylactic tissue responses (SRS-A) (3) which in 1978 and was subsequently identified by Bengt Samuelsson and his group in Stockholm as the cysteinyl leukotrienes comprising LTC_4 (and later identified LTD_4 and LTE_4) (4). The cysteinyl leukotrienes are approximately one thousand times more potent than histamine as smooth muscle contractile and vasoactive mediators. However, in an allergic reaction involving IgE-dependent mast cell activation, histamine is released in amounts far exceeding that of the cysteinyl leukotrienes. In the latter half of this century a third class mediator released during IgE-dependent responses, the prostanoids, e.g. prostaglandin (PG) D_2 (from mast cells) and thromboxane A_2 (from mast cells and macrophages) was added to histamine and SRS as an explanation to account for most of the immediate constrictor response experienced by allergic asthmatic individuals when they inhaled allergen to which they are sensitised (5).

There is currently overwhelming evidence to incriminate the mast cell as a source of histamine, PGD_2 and LTC_4 in all forms of asthma, but especially that associated with atopy. However, the role of the basophil as a source of mediators in asthma remains controversial. Using a basophil specific monoclonal antibody BB-1 (6), McEuen et al have shown that low numbers of basophils are present in biopsies from patients with mild to moderate disease. However, following allergen provocation, they are recruited into the airway wall along with eosinophils (7). It is likely that the presence of CCR-3 chemokine receptors on the surface of basophils (and eosinophils) partly accounts for their selective recruitment into the airway wall through an interaction with eotaxin, MCP-3, MCP-4 and RANTES. Monoclonal antibody BB-1 identifies a granule product called basogranulin with a mw of 5×10^6 daltons which is highly basic (p I, 9.6) and is released upon IgE-dependent basophil activation. In being susceptible to proteolysis but not ABC chondroitinase, it is likely to be a protein with some as yet unidentified mediator functions.

Although mast cells are found in most human tissues, they appear to be especially concentrated at mucosal surfaces where they adopt a particular phenotype.

Although at one time thought to be a static cell, mast cells are now known to migrate in response to chemoattractants, such as laminin, especially after exposure to a sensitising allergen. The majority of mast cells that are found in the epithelium and submucosa of normal and, to a greater extent, asthmatic airways, belong to the tryptase only type and originate from $CD34^+$ precursors in the presence of both stem cell factor and a number of mast cell growth factors derived from Th2-like lymphocytes, including interleukin (IL)-4, -6 and –9. Both the bronchial epithelium and the adjacent attenuated fibroblast sheath, which make up the epithelial mesenchymal trophic unit in asthma, provide an ample source of stem cell factor which is critical for mast cell maturation and priming. In addition, these cytokines are also involved in the regulation of the expression of the high affinity IgE receptor (FcεR1). The high affinity receptor is maintained in an active form on the mast cell surface when IgE is bound to the α chain. Thus, removal of IgE following treatment with the blocking monoclonal antibody E-25 results in a dramatic loss of expression of FcεR1 on circulating basophils (and, by implication, mast cells) which may contribute to the efficacy of this new treatment (8).

There have been many studies documenting the presence of elevated levels of histamine in bronchoalveolar lavage and broncho-wash fluid as well as induced sputum from patients with asthma of varying severity (9,10), indicating that these cells are not only present in the asthmatic airway but, even in the absence of allergen provocation, are in an activated state. The increased histamine concentration in lavage fluid is accompanied by other mast cell mediators, such as prostaglandin D_2, leukotriene C_4 and the unique mast cell protease, tryptase. Thus, it seems highly likely that histamine released from these cells will be acting in concert with other mast cell-derived products and, in this way, contribute to disordered airway function in ongoing disease.

In addition to histamine and neutral proteases, the mast cell is an important source of other mediators, including heparin and an array of cytokines, chemokines and growth factors. These important signalling molecules are released both preformed and newly generated upon IgE dependent activation of mast cells with secretion continuing for up to 72 hours following stimulation (11-13). The signalling mechanisms that are involved in the explosive release of mast cell mediators diverge from those that lead to the generation and persistent release of newly formed cytokines.

The Role of Histamine and other Mast Cell Mediators in Allergen Induced Bronchoconstriction

It has been recognised for many years that inhalation of allergen in sensitised asthmatic subjects leads to both early and late phase bronchoconstrictor responses with an acquired increase in bronchial hyperresponsiveness. This early asthmatic reaction is accompanied by the release of histamine which can be detected in the circulation whereas it's principal metabolite, N^T-methyl histamine, in the urine (14-16). Thus, it is hardly surprising that pre-treatment of asthmatic patients with a range of histamine H_1 receptor antagonists attenuates to varying degrees the early asthmatic response, confirming the contribution of histamine acting through H_1 receptors on airway smooth muscle and the microvasculature (17-19). Using selective antagonists or inhibitors against prostaglandin D_2 and cysteinyl leukotrienes, it would seem that release of these two mediators follow that of histamine in order.

Thus, all three of these autacoid mediators can account for the majority of the early asthmatic reaction with possible small additional contributions being made by bradykinin and neurokinins.

It has frequently been stated that the late asthmatic reaction results from the recruitment of inflammatory leukocytes, especially eosinophils with release of cysteinyl leukotrienes and other bronchoconstrictor mediators (22). However, the availability of potent and selective histamine H_1 receptor antagonists has enabled contribution of histamine to the late reaction to be clearly defined. This adds to the view that basophils are recruited into the asthmatic airway during the late asthmatic reaction (23,24). Roquet and colleagues have recently shown that the histamine H_1 receptor antagonist, loratadine, and the cysteinyl LT_1 receptor antagonist, zafirlukast, both attenuate to varying degrees the early and late asthmatic response to allergen challenge but the combination of the two drugs almost entirely inhibit both responses (25). Similar observations have been observed in the nasal response to allergen provocation where the principal target is the nasal microvasculature.

The fact that histamine, prostanoids and cysteinyl leukotrienes can interact to cause greater than additive effects on target tissues in allergic responses provides a strong case for combination therapy using mediator selective inhibitors and antagonists. Indeed, clinical trials, both in rhinitis and, more recently, asthma, have shown that a combination of an antihistamine and a cysteinyl leukotriene antagonist is almost as effective as a topical corticosteroid in the treatment of these disorders. The use of non-corticosteroid oral therapies achieves good compliance with treatment which is enhanced above inhalers by convenience and simultaneous treatment of co-morbidities. Indeed, rhinitis is now known to exist in up to 70% of asthmatic patients and its effective treatment along with asthma is likely to contribute to the improved quality of life that patients experience when treated with a combination of mediator antagonists and inhibitors.

The Role of Histamine and other Mast Cell Mediators in Exercise-Induced Asthma

Exercise- and cold air-induced airway responses in patients with asthma are also effectively inhibited by histamine and cysteinyl leukotriene antagonists. As with the immediate response to inhaled allergen, antihistamines are most effective in attenuating the initial phase of bronchoconstriction, provoked by exercise or cold air (26,27), whereas cysteinyl leukotriene antagonist are more effective against the recovery phase of the bronchoconstriction (28,29).

The mechanism whereby exercise or cold air activates mast cells in the asthmatic airway is probably through the inability of the bronchial epithelium to adequately condition the increased volume of respired air associated with exercise to full humidity (27,30,31). The precise mechanisms responsible for this are not known but seem most likely to relate to an inability of the bronchial epithelium to transport chloride ions and water to the airway surface, thereby creating a hyperosmolar environment (27,32). As water is evaporated from the airway surface liquid, it becomes hyperosmolar and provides an osmotic stimulus for water to move from any cell nearby resulting in cell volume loss (33). Anderson suggests that the regulatory volume increase after cell shrinkage is the key event resulting in release of inflammatory mediators from mast cells to cause airway smooth muscle to contract (27). In the upper airways of humans with allergic rhinitis, Togias et al have reported that the osmality of the nasal secretions increases with breathing of hot, dry air (34). Experiments in dogs also revealed that breathing dry air results in loss of water from the lower airways and a significant increase in osmolarity of the airway lining fluid (32).

There is now strong evidence to suggest that the bronchial epithelium itself is abnormal in asthma. For example, in the epithelium, it is a major source of proinflammatory mediators and cytokines as well as exhibiting features of premature programmed cell death and an impaired ability to proliferate in response to injury. We have suggested that abnormal signalling between the epithelium and the underlying attenuated fibroblast sheath (the epithelial mesenchymal trophic unit) is responsible for providing the microenvironment for persistent inflammation as well as driving an airway wall remodelling response (35). In relation to exercise-induced asthma, we have observed an enhanced expression of the glucose transporter, GLUT-1, in the bronchial epithelium of asthmatics, which would have the effect of increasing the glucose concentration of the airway lining fluid. In turn, this would lead to the formation of advanced glycosylated end products (AGE) in the epithelium and basement membrane which accumulate according to ambient glucose levels and form intermolecular cross links that are resistant to lysis. Thus, the hyperosmolar environment created by hyperventilation in asthma may be a combination of abnormal water and ion transport and an increase in glucose concentration.

Mast Cells in Asthma are Primed for Mediator Secretion

It appears that the microenvironment in which the mast cell finds itself in the asthmatic airway is an important factor that increases the "releasability" of these cells in response to environmental stimuli. One agent that we have shown is able to enhance lung mast cell responsiveness is TNFα which, through specific receptors, leads to the activation of the transcription factor NFκB with the induction of genes capable of enhancing activation secretion coupling. The enhanced releasability of mast cells can be demonstrated with the purine nucleoside, adenosine, which drives mast cell secretion via and A$_{2B}$ receptor on the cell surface linked to the activation of phosphatidylinositol generating pathway (36-38). In asthma, either down regulation of the A$_{2A}$ linked adenylate cyclase coupled GS protein activation or selective upregulation of Gv protein activation could explain the selected degranulation of mast cells that occurs with this stimulus. The absence of any late reaction with adenosine following bronchial provocation in asthma suggests that, different from allergen which triggers mast cells via IgE-dependent signalling, adenosine is restricted in its capacity to release histamine prostaglandin D$_2$ and cysteinyl leukotrienes but probably not pro-allergic cytokines. As would be expected from this profile of mediator release (39,40), adenosine-provoked bronchoconstriction is markedly attenuated by H$_1$-blockade (41). Similarly, exercise-, cold air- and hypertonic aerosol-induced bronchoconstriction in asthma also produces a single early but not a late response. Of interest in this regard is the cross refractoriness that occurs between exercise and adenosine challenge suggesting that these two stimuli might share either a similar mast cell activation mechanism or both generate an inhibitory mediator such as prostaglandin E$_2$ (37).

Interaction of Histamine with other Mediators in the Pathophysiology of Asthma and Rhinitis

Until recently the myriad of mediators that have been identified in allergic disorders have in large part been considered in isolation. While for autacoid mediators these interact with highly specific seven transmembrane G-protein coupled receptors on specific target cells, it is also becoming increasingly clear that different mediators are able to interact. For example, it is known that histamine is a powerful stimulus for the transportation of P-selectin from the Weibel Palisade bodies in endothelial cells to the cell surface (42). This adhesion molecule plays an important function as a lectin by interacting with its carbohydrate ligand expressed on migrating leukocytes, including neutrophils, eosinophils, basophils and T-cells, to initiate rolling and modulation. The cytokine induced expression of E-selectin and ICAM-1 by TNFα, IL-1β and interferon-γ and VCAM-1 by TNFα, IL-4, and IL-13 provides a secondary stimulus originating from mast cells and other inflammatory cells leading to tight binding of the leukocyte to endothelial cells followed by their migration into the airway wall, a key feature observed in the late asthmatic response (43).

There may also be direct ways in which histamine is able to interact with other mediators although simple studies of inhaling combinations of histamine, PGD$_2$ and LTD$_4$ have so far not revealed this. However, at the cell level, it has recently been demonstrated that different seven transmembrane receptors, such as the H$_1$ histamine and the M3 muscarinic receptor, may exist on "rafts" on the surface of smooth muscle cells and, when activated together, may generate an interactive intracellular signalling that potentiates contractile responses. This has led to a re-evaluation of combination of selective mediator inhibitors or antagonists for the management of allergic disease. Thus, in allergic rhinitis, the combination of a cysteinyl leukotriene antagonist (montelukast) and an H$_1$ histamine antagonist (loratadine) produced greater clinical benefit than either of the agents alone. Although only the whole selective inhibition of the lower airway effects of released histamine has been clinically disappointing in asthma (44), further clinical trials are needed to see whether this can be improved using combinations of mediator antagonists.

References

1. Dale HH, Laidlaw PP. The physiological action of β-iminazolyethylamine. J Physiol 1910; 41:318-41
2. Feldberg W, Holden HF, Kellaway CH. The formation of lysocithin and of a muscle stimulating substance by snake venoms. J Physiol 1938; 94:232-48
3. Brocklehurst WE. The release of histamine and formation of a slow reacting substance (SRS-A) during anaphylactic shock. J Physiol 1960; 151:416-35
4. Murphy RC, Hammarström S, Samuelsson B. Leukotriene C: A slow reacting substance from murine mastocytoma cells. Proc Natl Acad Sci USA 1979; 76:4275-9
5. Liu MC, Bleecker ER, Lichtenstein LM et al. Evidence for elevated levels of histamine, prostaglandin D$_2$ and other bronchoconstricting prostaglandins in the airways of subjects with mild asthma. Am Rev Respir Dis 1990; 142:126-32
6. McEuen AR, Buckley MG, Compton SJ, Walls AF. Development and characterisation of a monoclonal antibody specific for human basophils and the identification of a unique secretory product of basophil activation. Lab Invest 1999; 79:27-38
7. McEuen AR, Backley MG, Compton SJ, Walls AF. Development and characterisation of a monoclonal antibody specific for human basophils and the identification of a unique secretory product of basophil activation. Lab Invest 1999; 79:27-38
8. MacGlashan D, Bochner B, Adelman J, Jardieu P, Togias A et al. Down-regulation of FcϵR1 expression on human basophils during *in vivo* treatemnt of atopic patients with angi-IgE antibody. J Immunol 1997; 158:1438-45

9. Liu MC, Calhoun WJ. Bronchoalveolar lavage studies in asthma. In: Holgate ST, Busse WW (eds) Inflammatory Mechanisms in Asthma, New York, Marcel Dekker 1998, pp 39-74

10. Broide DH, Gleich GJ, Cuomo AJ et al. Evidence of ongoing mast cell and eosinophil degranulation in symptomatic asthmatic airways. J Allergy Clin Immunol 1991; 88:637-48

11. Bradding P, Roberts JA, Britten KM et al. Interleukin-4, -5, -6 and TNFα in normal and asthmatic airways: evidence for the human mast cell as an important source of thes cytokines. Am J Respir Cell Mol Biol 1994; 10:471-80

12. Bradding P, Okayama Y, Church MK, Holgate ST. Heterogeneity of human mast cells based on their cytokine content. J Immunol 1995; 155:297-308

13. Okayama Y, Petit-Frére C, Kassel O et al. Expression of messenger RNA for IL-4 and IL-5 in human lung and skin mast cells in response to FCε receptor cross-linkage and the presence of stem cell factor. J Immunol 1995; 155:1796-808

14. Wenzel SE, Westcott HY, Larsen GL. Bronchoalveolar lavage mediator levels 5 minutes after allergen challenge in atopic subjects with asthma: relationship to the development of the late asthmatic response. J Allergy Clin Immunol 1991; 87:540-8

15. Howarth PH, Durham SR, Lee TH, Kay AB, Church MK, Holgate ST. Influence of albuterol, cromolyn sodium and ipratropium bromide on the airway and circulating mediator responses to antigen bronchial provocation in asthma. Am Rev Respir Dis 1985; 132:986-92

16. Dahlén S-E, Kumlin M. Can asthma be studied in the urine? Clin Exp Allergy 1998; 28:129-33

17. Wasserfallen JB, Leuenberger P, Pecoud A. Effect of cetirizine, a new H_1-antihistamine, on the early and late allergic reactions in a bronchial provocation test with allergen. J Allergy Clin Immunol 1993; 91:1189-97

18. Holgate ST, Finnerty JP. Antihistamines in asthma. J Allergy clin Immunol 1989; 83(Suppl.):537-47

19. Howarth PH. Histamine and asthma: an appraisal based on specific H_1-receptor antagonism. Clin Exp Allergy 1990; 20(Suppl.2):31-41

20. Beasley CRW, Featherstone RL, Church MK et al. The effect of the thromboxane receptor antagonist on PGD_2- and allergen-induced bronchoconstriction. J Appl Physiol 1989; 66:1685-93

21. Taylor IK, O'Shaughnessy KM, Fuller RW et al. Effect of the cysteinyl-leukotriene receptor antagonist ICI 204,219 on allergen-induced bronchoconstriction and airway hyper reactivity in atopic subjects. Lancet 1991; 337:690-4

22. Liu MC, Hubbard WC, Proud D et al. Immediate and late inflammatory responses to ragweed antigen challenge of the peripheral airways in allergic asthmatics. Am Rev Respir Dis 1991; 144:51-8

23. Rafferty P, Ng WH, Phillips GD et al. The inhibitory actions of azelastine hydrochloride on the early and late bronchoconstrictor response to inhaled allergen in atopic asthma. J Allergy Clin Immunol 1989; 84:649-57

24. Guo C, Liu M, Galli S et al. Identification of IgE-bearing cells in the late phase response to antigen in the lung as basophils. Am J Resp Cell Mol Biol 1994; 10:384-90

25. Roquet A, Dahlén B, Kumlin M et al. Combined antagonism of leukotrienes and histamine produces predominant inhibition of allergy-induced early and late phase airway obstruction in asthmatics. Am J Respir Crit Care Med 1997; 155:1856-63

26. Patel KR. Terfenadine in exercise-induced asthma. Br Med J 1984;288:1496-7

27. Anderson SD, Daviskas E. The mechanism of exercise-induced asthma is ellipsis. J Allergy Clin Immunol 2000; 106:453-9

28. Finnerty JP, Wood-Baker R, Thomson H, Holgate ST. Role of leukotrienes in exercise-induced asthma: inhibitor effect of ICI 204219, a potent leukotriene D_4-receptor antagonist. Am Rev Respir Dis 1992; 145:746-9

29. Manning PJ, Watson RM, Margolskee DJ et al. Inhibition of exercise-induced bronchoconstriction by MK-571, a potent leukotriene D_4-receptor antagonist. N Engl J Med 1990; 323:1736-9

30. Makker HK, Holgate ST. Mechanisms of exercise-induced asthma. Eur J Clin Invest 1994; 24:571-85

31. Makker HK, Holgate ST. Relation of the hypertonic saline responsiveness of the airways to exercise-induced asthma symptom severity and to histamine or methacholine reactivity. Thorax 1993; 48:142-7

32. Freed AN, Davis MS. Hyperventilation with dry air increases airway surface fluid osmolality in canine peripheral airways. Am J Respir Crit Care Med 1999; 159:1101-7

33. Eveloff JL, Warnock DG. Activation of ion transport systems during cell volume regulation. Am J Physiol 1987; 252:F1-10

34. Togias AG, Proud D, Lichtenstein LM et al. The osmolarity of nasal secretions increases when inflammatory mediators are released in response to inhalation of cold, dry air. Am Rev Respir Dis 1988; 137-625-9

35. Holgate ST, Davies DE, Lackie PM, Wilson SJ, Puddicombe SM, Lordan JL. Epithelial-mesenchymal interactions in the pathogenesis of asthma. J Allergy Clin Immunol 2000; 105:193-204

36. Cushley MJ, Tattersfield AE, Holgate ST. Inhaled adenosine and guanosine on airway resistance in normal and asthmatic subjects. Br J Clin Pharmacol 1983; 15:161-5

37. Polosa R, Holgate ST. Adenosine bronchoprovocation: a promising marker of allergic inflammation in asthma? Thorax 1997; 52:919-23

38. Feoktistov I, Polosa R, Holgate ST, Biaggioni I. Adenosine A_{2B} receptors: a novel therapeutic target in asthma? Trends Pharmacol Sci 1998; 19:148-53

39. Phillips GD, Ng R, Church MK, Holgate ST. The response of plasma histamine to bronchoprovocation with methacholine, adenosine 5'-monophosphate, and allergen in atopic non-asthmatic subjects. Am Rev Respir Dis 1990; 141:9-13

40. Polosa R, Ng WH, Crimi N et al. Release of mast-cell-derived mediators after endobronchial adenosine challenge in asthma. Am J Respir Crit Care Med 1995; 151:624-9

41. Rafferty P, Beasley CR, Holgate ST. The contribution of histamine to bronchoconstriction produced by inhaled allergen and adenosine 5'-monophosphate in asthma. Am Rev Respir Dis 1987; 136:369-373

42. Kubes P. Mast cell activation and leukocyte rolling responses. In: Bochner BS (ed) Adhesion Molecules in Allergic Disease, Marcel Dekker, NY, 1997, pp 229-6

43. Montefort S, Gratziou C, Goulding D, Polosa R, Haskard DO, Howarth PH, Holgate ST and Carroll MP. Bronchial biopsy evidence for leucocyte infiltration and upregulation of

leucocyte endothelial cell adhesion molecules 6 hours after local allergen challenge of sensitised asthmatic airway. J Clin Invest 1994; 93:1411-1421

44. Van Ganse E, Kaufman L, Derde MP et al. Effects of antihistamines in adult asthma: a meta-analysis of clinical trials. Eur Respir J 1997; 10:2216-24

Histamine Research in the New Millennium
T. Watanabe, H. Timmerman and K. Yanai (Editors)

Histamine and skin allergic diseases

T. Koga, F. Kohda, M. Furue

Department of Dermatology, Graduate School of Medical Sciences, Kyushu University, Fukuoka, 812-8582, Japan

Correspondence author: Tetsuya Koga, M. D. Department of Dermatology Graduate School of Medical Sciences Kyushu University 3-1-1, Maidashi, Higashi-ku J-812-8582 Fukuoka. Japan. TEL: 81-92-642-5584 FAX: 81-92-642-5600 E-mail: tekoga@dermatol.med.kyushu-u.ac.jp

Abstract

Histamine is an important mediator in allergic skin diseases such as atopic dermatitis (AD) and urticaria, and antihistamine are used for the treatment of these skin diseases. Urticaria is characterized by a transient dermal edema, and histamine, released from dermal mast cells, plays a major role on its pathogenesis. The histamine iontophoresis is a non-invasive procedure that induces constant and strong skin response, mimicking clinical urticaria.   We examined the inhibitory effects of the second generation antihistamines on the histamine-induced flare and wheal responses using iontophoresis. The potent and long-lasting antihistamine activity of these drugs on the skin responses and itch sensation by iontophoretically-inoculated histamine was confirmed by our study.

While there is a growing interest in the role of histamine on the immunological reactions of AD, there are relatively few reports that explored the potential positive interaction between histamine and keratinocytes. Keratinocytes can synthesize and release a number of proinflammatory cytokines. We examined the effect of histamine on IL-6 and IL-8 production by keratinocytes in vitro. The results showed that histamine enhanced the IL-6 and IL-8 production and the effect of histamine was inhibited by H1 receptor antagonist and H2 receptor antagonist.   This suggested a contributory role of histamine on AD through increase of IL-6 and IL-8 production by keratinocytes.

1. Histamine and urticaria

Urticaria is a common skin disorder and a cutaneous reaction pattern for which there are multiple potential causes. Its physiopathology is poorly defined. The vascular changes observed in urticarial lesions can be attributed to the release of mediators: histamine plays an essential role but others mediators, such as serotonin, neuropeptides, may also be involved. These mediators are synthetized by mast cells which are the major effector cell type. During immediate hypersensitivity reaction, mast cells and basophils are activated by allergens through cross linking of cell-surface-bound IgE. However, more often than not, these cells are stimulated by non-immunological mechanisms. Release of mast cell mediators can cause inflammation and accumulation and activation of other cells, including eosinophils, neutrophils, and possibly basophils.

1.1 Antihistamine in the treatment of urticaria

Histamine is one of the major mediators of most forms of urticaria although in some cases, especially physical urticaria, other mediators seem to play a role. Therefore antihistamines, and mainly H1 antihistamines, are widely used in the treatment of urticaria. More than 50 years after the first introduction of an antihistamine into urticaria therapy, antihistamines still represent modern and exciting agents contributing to the continuous improvement of urticaria. Antihistamine therapy can be performed with either the classical or second generation antihistamines. Classical antihistamines are connected with considerable side-effects especially sedation and anticholinergic effects. New non-sedating antihistamines have been developed that do not cross the blood-brain barrier.

1.2 Histamine-induced skin response

The histamine-induced skin response is a reliable method to evaluate the effects of antihistamines. The histamine challenge is usually performed by prick test, however, the flare and wheal responses are relatively small and weak. Intradermal injection of histamine is painful. The histamine iontophoresis is a non-invasive procedure that induces more constant and stronger skin responses, mimicking clinical urticaria. Although the inhibitory capability on histamine-induced skin response is not necessarily correlated with the clinical anti-urticaria activity of the drug (1), the histamine iontophoresis is an useful method to investigate the pharmacodynamic aspects of antihistamines.

1. 3 Effects of antihistamines on the skin response to histamine iontophoresis

Epinastine and cetirizine are second-generation, nonsedating and long-lasting antihistamines that are now frequently used for the allergic disorders. We have examined the inhibitory effects of these 2 drugs on the histamine-induced flare and wheal responses using iontophoresis at 1, 2, 4, 8 and 24h after the oral administration by a double-blind, cross-over and placebo-controlled study (2). Both drugs significantly inhibited the histamine-induced flare and wheal responses at 2h after the oral administration when compared with placebo. The inihibitory effects on the flare response lasted long until at 24h. The inhibitory effects on the wheal response was also clearly and significantly evident at 2h through 8h. The histamine-induced itch sensation was also markedly or completely suppressed. Thus, both drugs exhibited the potent and long-lasting antihistamine activity on the skin responses induced by histamine iontophoresis.

2. Histamine and atopic dermatitis

Atopic dermatitis (AD) results from the interaction between allergen and allergen-specific IgE bound to the mast cell surface receptors. This process triggers mast cell degranulation and accounts at least for early phase reaction. Histamine, an important mediator in immediate-type hypersensitivity, is elevated in the skin of AD patients and is considered to play a pathogenic role in AD. The AD patients showed a high level of basal plasma histamine compared to that in non-allergic patients (3).

2.1 Histamine and itching in atopic dermatitis

While histamine is the crucial mediator of pruritus in immediate-type allergic reactions, its role in AD is unclear. Itching is an important factor in AD and can have a significant impact on the sufferer's quality of life. The pathophysiology of itch in AD is still not understood. Unlike in urticaria, histamine is not considered to be a major pruritogen in AD (4).

Various treatments are used to relieve itching in AD patients, but no specific antipruritic therapy is available. Although antihistamines are often used in the treatment of AD, little objective evidence exists to demonstrate relief of pruritus.

2.2 Proinflammatory cytokines from keratinocytes
Keratinocytes can synthesize and release a number of proinflammatory cytokines such as IL-6 and IL-8, which have been described to play a crucial role in the initiation and development of many inflammatory skin disorders including AD.

2.3 Histamine-induced exacerbation of skin lesions in atopic dermatitis
While there is a growing interest in the role of histamine on the immunological reactions of AD, there are relatively few reports that explored the potential positive interaction between histamine and keratinocytes (5). In order to elucidate the mechanism of histamine-induced exacerbation of skin lesions in AD, we examined the effect of histamine on proinflammatory cytokine production of keratinocytes (manuscript in preparation). Cultured human keratinocyte cell lines were incubated with histamine and the IL-8 and IL-6 released into the medium were measured using an ELISA. Histamine stimulated these cytokine production and had a dose-dependent effect. The effect of histamine was significantly blocked by pyrilamine, an H1 receptor antagonist. The H2 receptor antagonist, cimetidine, slightly inhibited the effect of histamine. These results suggest that the degranulation of mast cells induces the enhancement of cytokine release from keratinocytes probably via histamine. This indicates a contributory role for histamine in the exacerbation of atopic dermatitis induced by proinflammatory cytokine production of keratinocytes.

References
1. E.W. Monroe, AF. Daly, RF. Shalhoub, J. Allergy. Clin. Immunol., 99 (1997) s798.
2. M. Furue, H. Terao, T. Koga, J. Dermatol. Sci., in press.
3. K. Kimura, M. Adachi, K. Kubo, Y. Ikemoto, Fukuoka Acta Medica, 90 (1999) 457.
4. C.F. Wahlgren, J. Dermatol., 26 (1999) 1522.
5. S. Shinoda, Y. Kameyoshi, M. Hide, E. Morita, S. Yamamoto, Arch. Dermatol. Res. 290 (1998) 429.

2001 Elsevier Science B.V.
Histamine Research in the New Millennium
T. Watanabe, H. Timmerman and K. Yanai (Editors)

Effects of a selective H$_1$-receptor antagonist, epinastine, on airway inflammation in asthmatics

Keiji Kimura[a], Masakazu Ichinose[b], Masato Hayashi[a], Gen Tamura[b], Toshio Hattori[b], and Kunio Shirato[b]

[a] Second Department of Internal Medicine, Hiraka General Hospital,
1-1 Ekimae-machi, Yokote 013-8610, Japan

[b] First Department of Internal Medicine, Tohoku University School of Medicine,
1-1 Seiryo-machi, Aoba-ku, Sendai 980-8574, Japan

We evaluated the effects of epinastine on the clinical symptoms, lung function, airway hyperresponsiveness, and airway inflammation in adult asthmatics. Fourteen stable adult asthmatics took part in the study. After a 2 wk observation period, epinastine (20mg once daily) was administered orally for 4 weeks. Throughout the 6 weeks the patients described on daily diary cards the asthma symptoms, drug use, and measurements of peak expiratory flow (PEF). Measurement of forced expiratory volume in 1 sec (FEV$_1$) and airway responsiveness to methacholine as well as sputum induction were performed before and after the administration of epinastine. As inflammatory indices, the concentrations of eosinophil cationic protein (ECP), myeloperoxidase (MPO), substance P (SP), and bradykinin (BK) in the sputum were measured by radioimmunoassay. Epinastine treatment caused a significant decrease in the need for β_2-stimulant usage ($p<0.05$). The concentrations of ECP, SP, and BK in the induced sputum were also significantly decreased after epinastine treatment (all $p <0.05$). In contrast, the total asthma symptom score, FEV$_1$, PEF, airway responsiveness, and the concentration of MPO in sputum were not affected by epinastine. These data suggest that H$_1$-receptor blockade by epinastine ameliorates the asthmatic airway inflammatory changes, however, the effects on airway caliber and responsiveness were negligible.

1. Background

The histamine H$_1$-receptor mediates airway smooth muscle contraction, the increase in vascular pemeability, vagal afferent nerve stimulation, dilatation of bronchial artery, and increases in ion transport in the airway epithelium (1). These pharmacological actions cause bronchoconstriction, airway edema, mucous secretion, and cough, which mimic the pathophysiology of asthma. Moreover, histamine can provide an upregulatory signal on the immune system via H_1-receptors (1). For instance, histamine can act as a chemotactic agent for eosinophils (2) and interleukin-6 production in B cells is increased in response to histamine. Therefore, H_1-receptor antagonists are thought to be useful in the treatment of asthma. Until now many kinds of H_1-receptor antagonists have been used for the treatment of asthma, although the effects are small compared with other kinds of agents such as leukotriene receptor antagonists (3). There has been little evidence of improvement on lung function or airway hyperreactivity (4), and the effects on airway inflammation have not yet been studied.

Epinastine is one of the most effective peripherally acting H_1-receptor antagonists which lack significant CNS side effects (5). This study evaluated the effects of 4 weeks epinastine administration on the clinical symptoms, drug usage, lung function, airway hyperreactivity, and airway inflammation in adult asthmatics.

2. Methods

2.1. Subjects

14 patients with mild to moderate asthma entered the study. 13 patients completed the trial. 1 patient was withdrawn because of an exacerbation of asthma due to upper respiratory tract infection. The clinical details of the 13 patients were as follows: 10 males and 3 females with a mean age of 51 ± 17.0 yr, 11 atopic and 2 non-atopic, 12 moderate persistent, and 1 mild persitent. Their asthma was controlled by a combination of oral theophyllin and inhaled corticosteroids (9 used beclomethasone dipropionate (mean 533 μ g/day, range;400-800)) as well as on demand β_2-agonist usage.

All subjects were adult patients with a history of chronic asthma of at least 2 years who required daily treatment. Patients with asthma symptoms or with diurnal peak expiratory flow (PEF) variability over 20% in the observation period were selected. The age, sex, or severity of asthma was not limited. A signed informed consent document was required before the observation period. Patients who had an upper respiratory tract infection within 1 month before the observation period, pregnant women, and patients who needed oral corticosteroids daily were excluded.

2.2. Study design

Patients who satisfied the study inclusion criteria began a 2-week observation period. This was followed by a 4-week period during which epinastine, 20mg once daily, was administered orally. Before and after the administration of epinastine, mesurements of forced expiratory volume in one second (FEV_1) using a dry rolling-seal spirometer (OST 80A, Chest Co., Tokyo, Japan) and airway responsiveness to methacholine (6) as well as sputum induction were performed. β_2-agonists were stopped 12 h before each study day (Fig. 1).

Throughout the study, patients recorded the amount of backup medication used, PEF twice daily, and asthma symptoms in a diary. The total asthma symptom score consists of the degree of dyspnea (0 = none, 1 = chest tightness, 3 = mild dyspnea with wheeze, 6 = moderate dyspnea, 9 = severe dyspnea) and cough (0 = none, 0.5 = weak, 1 = strong). These symptoms were recorded

Figure 1. Study design

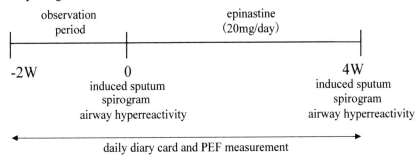

4 times a day (each 6 hours; morning, daytime, evening, and night), and the sum of the scores was calculated each week. The total asthma symptom score was the mean score per day.

2.3. Sputum induction and examination

Sputum induction was performed with an aerosol of 4% hypertonic saline generated by an ultrasonic nebulizer (MU-32, Sharp Co. Ltd., Osaka, Japan) with an output of 2.2 ml/min and particle size of 5.4 μ m aerodynamic mass median diameter. After inhalation of saline for 5 minutes, the subjects were instructed to cough sputum. This technique was repeated for up to 30 minutes until sputum was induced (7).

Sputum was processed within 1 hour. Sputum that macroscopically appeared free of salivary contamination was treated with 4 times the volume of 0.1% dithiothreitol (Sputasol; Kanto Chemical Co., Tokyo, Japan) in a 10-ml polystyren tube. The mixture was vortexed for 15 seconds and divided into two pieces. One was centrifuged at 3000 rpm for 5 minutes. The supernatant was aspirated and stored in -80°C for later assay of eosinophil cationic protein (ECP) and myeloperoxidase (MPO). The pellet was resuspended in a volume of PBS and recentrifuged at 3000 rpm for 5 minutes. The pellet was smeared on a slide glass. 400 nonsquamous cells were counted in a Papanicolaou-stained slide and expressed as a percentage of the total nonsquamous count. Sputum in which the percentage of squamous cells was less than 10% was used for the data analysis.

Another mixture was boiled with an alcohol lamp for 15 seconds to inhibit the degradation of substance P (SP) and bradykinin (BK) by proteases such as neutral endopeptidase or kinase II . After boiling the mixture was recentrifuged at 3000 rpm for 5 minutes. The supernatant was aspirated and stored in -80°C for later assay of SP and BK.

The concentrations of ECP, MPO, SP, and BK in the supernatant of induced sputum were measured by radioimmunoassay (7). ECP and MPO were measured at Otsuka Assay Institute (Tokushima, Japan). The radioimmunoassy of SP and BK was done at SRL Co. (Tokyo, Japan).

2.4. Statistical analysis

Data are expressed as mean ± SD. All comparisons were made with Student paired t test

352

(two-tailed). A p value below 0.05 was considered significant.

3. Results

13 of 14 patients completed the trial. No side effect of epinastine was observed. The clinical efficacy of epinastine was evaluated in daily diary cards. Epinastine treatment caused a significant decrease in the need for β_2-stimulant usage (Fig.2). However, epinastine did not affect the total asthma symptom score (Fig.3).

The effects of epinastine on pulmonary function were negligible. FEV$_1$ and PEF upon waking and before sleeping were not changed before and after epinastine administration (2.45 ± 1.02 versus 2.47 ± 0.87 L, 480 ± 148 versus 490 ± 137 L/min, 485 ± 140 versus 487 ± 131 L/min, repectively). Further, the airway responsiveness to methacholine was not changed before and after epinastine (Geometric mean of PD$_{200}$ of methacholine; 0.394 versus 0.184 Unit, repectively).

All subjects produced sputum during the observation period. However, 3 patients could not produce sputum after epinastine administration. Another 4 subjects produced inadequate sputum either before or after epinastine. 6 pairs of sputum were analyzed. Cell counts of leukocytes in the induced sputum were not changed before and after epinastine administration (eosinophil, neutrophil, and lymphocyte; 32.2 ± 31.5 versus 32.5 ± 26.5 %, 63.5 ± 32.8 versus 61.0 ± 31.1 %, 4.3 ± 3.5 versus 6.5 ± 5.6 %, repectively).

4 weeks epinastine administration significantly decreased the ECP levels (Fig.4). However, activated neutrophil marker MPO levels (Fig.5) were not affected by epinastine administration. The concentrations of both SP (Fig.6) and BK (Fig.7) in the induced sputum were also significantly decreased.

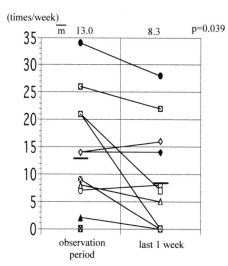

Figure 2. On demand β_2-agonists use
Bars indicate mean values. n=13

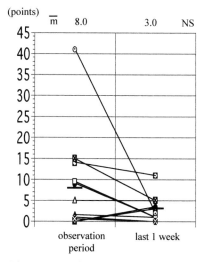

Figure 3. total asthma symptom score
Bars indicate mean values. n=13

Figure 4. Eosinophil cationic protein (ECP)
concentration in induced sputum. n=6

Figure 5. Myeloperoxidase (MPO)
concentration in induced sputum. n=6

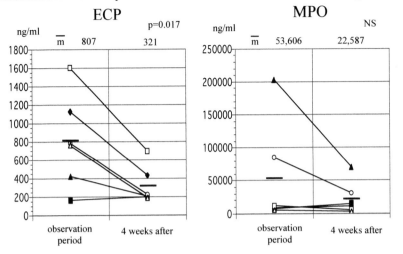

4. Discussion

In this study, we showed that the amount of on demand β_2-agonist use after four weeks administration of epinastine significantly decreased .The concentrations of ECP and SP as well as BK in the supernatants of the induced sputum after the treatment were significantly reduced. However, the effects on airway caliber, airway responsiveness, and astmatic symptom score were negligible by 4 weeks administration of epinastine.

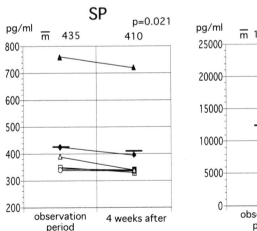

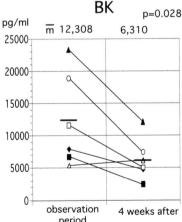

Figure 6. Substance P (SP) concentration
in induced sputum. n=6

Figure 7. Bradykinin (BK) concentration
in induced sputum. n=6

It has been reported that histamine can act as a chemotactic agent for eosinophils via the H_1-receptor (2). In this study, 4 weeks epinastine administration significantly decreased the ECP levels, although the cell counts of leukocytes including eosinophils were not affected. Epinastine might inhibit the activation of eosinophils. The mechanism of the decrease in SP in induced sputum is not known. Epinastine might inhibit SP release from the excitatory NANC system. Histamine H_1-receptor mediates the increase in vascular permeability (1). The decrease in BK in induced sputum might result from the inhibition of vascular leakage directly by H_1-receptor antagonism and indirectly by the decrease in SP levels in the airway.

Until now many kinds of H_1-receptor antagonists have been used for the treatment of asthma, although the effects are small (3, 4). Also in this study, the effects on airway caliber, airway responsiveness, and astmatic symptom score were not improved by epinastine. However, epinastine treatment caused a significant decrease in the need for β_2-agonist usage.

In conclusion, our epinastine trial showed that specific H_1-receptor antagonism reduces ECP, BK, and SP levels in asthmatic airways and causes a significant decrease in the need for β_2-stimulant usage. However, the magnitude of clinical efficacy was very small. If we could predict the degree of airway inflammation, in other words, if we can measure the mediators in asthmatic individuals, the subgroup of patients who respond to H_1-receptor antagonists may be predicted.

REFERENCES

1. MB Hogan and PA Greenberger. PJ Barnes et al (eds), Asthma, Lippincott-Raven Publishers, Philadelphia, 1997
2. LW Turnbull and AB Kay. Immunology, 31 (1976) 797
3. ST Holgate. Clin. Rev. in Allegy, 12 (1994) 65
4. E Van Ganse, L Kaufman, MP Derde et al. Eur. Respir. J. 10 (1997) 2216
5. JC Schilling, WS Adamus and H Kuthan. Int. J. Pharmacol. Ther. Toxicol., 28 (1990) 493
6. T Takishima, W Hida, H Sasaki et al. Chest, 80 (1981) 600
7. M Tomaki, M Ichinose, M Miura et al. Am. J. Respir. Crit. Care Med., 15 (1995) 613

Mast cells and inflammation

© 2001 Elsevier Science B.V. All rights reserved.
Histamine Research in the New Millennium
T. Watanabe, H. Timmerman and K. Yanai (Editors)

Suppression of MAP kinase pathways in mast cells by glucocorticoids; mechanisms and consequences

Michael A. Beaven, David S. Cissel, and Thomas R. Hundley

Laboratory of Molecular Immunology, National Heart, Lung, and Blood Institute, National Institutes of Health, Bethesda, Maryland

1. Introduction

Mast cells are the major source of histamine in most tissues and its release along with other inflammatory mediators is responsible for immediate hypersensitivity reactions to antigens. The signalling events that promote this release include activation of Lyn and Syk, two tyrosine kinases that interact with the IgE-receptor (Fc RI) in mast cells (1). The subsequent phosphorylation of LAT and other proteins by Syk leads to activation of diverse signalling pathways such as mobilization of calcium ions via phospholipase C, activation of protein kinase C by calcium and diglycerides, and the activation of the ERK, JNK, and p38 MAP kinases. The ensuing physiological responses include secretion of histamine-containing granules via a protein kinase C/calcium-dependent process of exocytosis (2), generation of arachidonic acid from membrane phospholipids through an ERK/calcium-dependent activation of cytosolic phospholipase A_2 (3), and the production of various inflammatory cytokines through gene transcription as a consequence of the activation of MAP kinases (4-6). The communicating links between Fc RI and phospholipase C or the MAP kinases are largely, but not completely, defined in molecular detail (1, 7). The linkages to the MAP kinases are of particular relevance here and will be discussed in further detail.

The MAP kinase pathways consist of a hierarchy of three kinases, the initiating kinase (i.e. MAP kinase kinase kinase), an intermediate MAP kinase kinase, and the MAP kinase itself (see Fig. 1). In the case of ERK1/2, the upstream kinases are Raf-1 and MEK. Phosphorylation and activation of the initiating kinase, Raf-1, occurs when it is recruited to the plasma membrane from cytosol by binding to Ras-GTP. Conversion of Ras from its inactive GDP-bound form to its active GTP-bound is dependent on the guanine nucleotide exchange factor, Sos. Further upstream and not shown in Figure 1, Sos activity is regulated by its interaction with the adaptor protein, Grb2, and the phosporylated form of the receptor-docking protein, Shc. The tyrosine phosphorylation of Shc by Syk is thought to allow formation of multiumeric complexes, which allow transduction of signals from F cRI via Syk/Shc/Grb2/Sos/Ras to Raf-1 (8). Pathways for activation of other MAP kinases in mast cells are less well-established but may include the guanine nucleotide exchange factor,Vav, the GTP-binding proteins, Cdc42/Rac, and the kinase PAK for the activation of MEKK1 and hence JNK (Fig.1).

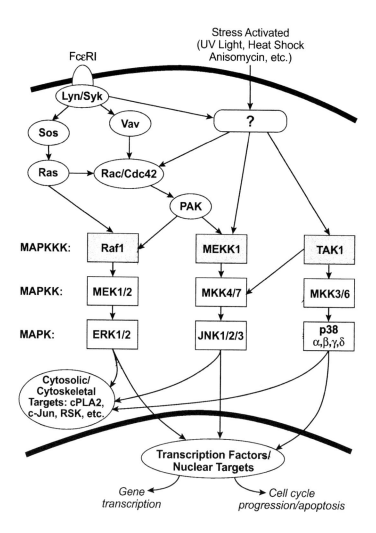

Figure 1. Activation pathways for the MAP kinases. Shaded boxes indicate enzymes targeted in dexamethasone treated cells (see text).

The signalling events that lead to the activation of p38 MAP kinase via TAK-1 and MKK3 are unknown. This pathway in mast cells regulates expression of enzymes involved in the synthesis of eicosanoids from arachidonic acid. The production of eicosanoids is thus regulated not only by ERK (for the activation of phospholipase A_2 as noted above) (3) but also by p38 MAP kinase for expression and induction of enzymes such as cyclooxygenase-2 and 5-lipoxygenase (Hundley, T. R. and Beaven, M. A., unpublished data).

The starting point for this study was the accumulation of data indicating that in the rat (RBL-2H3) mast cell line the signalling pathways described above varied in their sensitivity to glucocorticoid, dexamethasone.

Production of arachidonic acid and the cytokine, TNF, as well as the activation of ERK was suppressed at much lower concentrations of dexamethasone (IC_{50} 7 nM) than was secretion of granules and phospholipase C-mediated events (IC_{50} 50-100 nM). Our work had also indicated that production of arachidonic acid via phospholipase A_2 and TNF was linked to activation of ERK-2 as noted above.

2. RESULTS AND DISCUSSION

2.1 Disruption of the ERK pathway at the level of Raf-1

In view of the sensitivity of ERK related events to dexamethasone we determined where signalling was disrupted by examining each signalling step in the Fc RI/ERK pathway in RBL-2H3 cells. These studies showed that early antigen-stimulated events such as the phosphorylation of Syk and Shc, the association of Shc with Grb-2, and the activation of Ras were unaffected in dexamethasone-treated cells (9, 10). The phosphorylation, translocation, and activation of Raf-1 as well as the ensuing phosphorylation and activation of MEKK1 and ERK2 were suppressed, however. The suppression Raf-1activation was dependent on dose ($EC_{50} \sim 7$ nM) and duration of exposure of cells to dexamethasone with maximal effects being observed after 15 hrs. Also, the inhibitory actions of dexamethasone were not restricted to antigen-stimulation. Activation of Raf-1 was still blocked when dexamethasone-treated cells were stimulated by phorbol 12-myristate 13-acetate, thapsigargin, or carbachol in RBL-2H3 cells transfected with the gene for the muscarinic m1 receptor (10). Dexamethasone thus appears to target a process common to all stimulants and one closely associated with Raf-1 activation.

2.2 Dexamethasone causes loss of heat shock proteins (Hsp70 and Hsp90) from Raf-1 complexes

We next examined the integrity of the Raf-1 complex to find possible explanations for the loss of function of Raf-1. This kinase was known to exist as a multimeric complex with Hsp90, protein 14-3-3, $p50^{cdc37}$, and the immunophilin, FKBP65 (11, 12). These proteins were thought to allow translocation of Raf-1 to sites of action within the cell and, in the case of 14-3-3, to stabilize Raf-1 in its inactive and active conformations. Analogous scenarios have been proposed for other kinases and steroid receptors (13, 14). These scenarios prompted us to test Raf-1 immunoprecipitates for the presence of HIP, HOP, Hsp 40, and p23 in addition to the proteins noted above. Except for Hsp40 and p23, all these proteins co-immunoprecipitated with Raf-1 whether or not cell lysates were treated with chemical cross linking agents before immunoprecipitation. Additional observations were these. Antigen stimulation caused a consistent increase (~50%) in the amount of Hsp90 associated with Raf-1 and prior treatment with dexamethasone blocked this increase and reduced the amount Hsp90 associated with Raf-1 (~60%) in unstimulated cells. This apparent loss of Hsp90 from the Raf-1 complex correlated with loss of functional response of Raf-1 whether dose or exposure to drug was altered (10). An even more dramatic effect was noted with Hsp70. The amount of Hsp70 associated with Raf-1 decreased by ~80% in dexamethasone-treated cells although antigen had little effect on this association in treated or untreated cells (Cissel, D. S. and Beaven, M.A., unpublished data). Other proteins were unaffected by dexamethasone and there was no significant change in expression of any Raf-1-associated protein including Hsp70, Hsp90, and Raf-1 itself in whole cells. These findings are summarized in the Table.

Table 1
Effect of dexamethasone on Raf-1 associated proteins*

Protein	Association with Raf-1	Expression in cells
Hsp90	Decreased ~50%	No change
Hsp70	Decreased ~80%	"
Hsp40	N.D.	"
14-3-3	No change	"
p50^{cdc37}	"	"
FKBP65(immunophilin)	"	"
HIP	"	"
HOP	"	"
p23	N.D.	"

* Dexamethasone, 100 nM, or vehicle were added to cultures 18 hr before assay of the indicated protein in cell lysates and immunoprecipitates of Raf-1. N.D., not detectable and presence in Raf-1 complex is uncertain.

2.3 Potential role of Hsp70/90 in Raf-1 signalling

The net result of treatment with dexamethasone appears to be the selective loss of Hsp 70 and 90 from Raf-1 complex or complexes (Table 1). Hsp90 forms the core of an assembly of proteins that interact with steroid receptors and various protein kinases including Raf-1 and such complexes undergo continuous assembly and disassembly (14). This dynamic state is presumed to allow appropriate localization and functioning of the chaperoned protein. HIP and HOP are essential for early stages in the assembly of Hsp90 complex with steroid receptors while Hsp70, which has intrinsic ATPase activity, regulates Hsp90 function. Hsp90 exists in an ADP or ATP bound form which determines the conformational/functional state of the molecule. We may assume, therefore, that the partial disassembly of the Hsp90/Raf-1 complex in dexamethasone-treated cells occurs through loss of Hsp70 as the amounts of HIP, HOP, and other proteins retained by Raf-1 remain unchanged. Both Hsp70 and Hsp 90 are constitutively phosphorylated in RBL-2H3 cells and since both proteins are largely dephosphorylated in dexamethasone-treated cells we are exploring the possibility that dexamethasone induces synthesis of a phosphatase or suppresses production of a Hsp kinase (unpublished data). Regardless of mechanism, our results strongly suggest that Hsp 70 and 90 have an essential role in Raf-1 signalling and that this role is impaired in dexamethasone-treated cells.

2.4 JNK and p38 MAP kinase pathways are similarly blocked by dexamethasone

In the meantime, additional studies had shown that activation of all three MAP kinases were inhibited in dexamethasone-treated cells (10, 15, and our unpublished data). Like ERK, the activation of JNK and p38 MAP kinase by antigen was partially inhibited in cells treated with as little as 1 nM dexamethasone and was largely suppressed in the presence of 10 nM dexamethasone. The initiating kinases, Raf-1, MEKK1, and TAK-1 were inhibited along with ERK, JNK, and p38 MAP kinase (10 and Cissel, D. S. and Beaven M. A., unpublished data).

Of particular significance, MEKK1 and TAK-1, like Raf-1, were found to be associated with Hsp70 and 90 and this association was similarly affected by dexamethasone.

2.5 Involvement of the glucorticoid receptor

The suppression of the Raf-1/ERK pathway by dexamethasone was clearly mediated through the glucocorticoid receptor. First, this suppression was blocked by the glucocorticoid-receptor antagonist, RU486. Second, other glucocorticoids (i.e., methylprednisolone and triamcinolone), but not irrelevant steroids (i.e., 17 -estradiol and aldosterone), showed similar suppressive activities. Finally, the inhibitory actions of dexamethasone were not apparent in mast cells derived from human peripheral blood pluripotent cells which do not express glucocorticoid receptors (Cissel, D. S. and Beaven, M. A., unpublished data).

2.6 Consequences and implications

Loss of Hsp70 and 90 from the Raf-1 complex seems the most likely explanation for loss of Raf-1 function in dexamethasone-treated cells. As our studies also indicate that association of MEKK1 and TAK-1 with Hsp70 and 90 is similarly disrupted by dexamethasone, we assume that dexamethasone acts in common on all three kinases but the precise mechanism remains undefined. Interestingly, geldanamycin which binds to the ATP-binding pocket of Hsp90 blocks (16) also blocks activation of all three MAP kinase pathways (Cissel, D. S. and Beaven, M. A., unpublished data). In contrast to dexamethasone, however, geldanamycin causes loss of Hsp90 but not Hsp70 from the Raf-1 complex. Therefore, dexamethasone must act through a mechanism which is both novel and different from that of geldanamycin.

The disruption of the MAP kinase pathways in dexamethasone-treated cells should have specific consequences. These pathways are essential for activation of various transcription factors and production of cytokines (see 10 for citations) and, as noted earlier, the activation of cytosolic phospholipase A_2 and expression of enzymes involved in eicosanoid synthesis. The actions described here provide a plausible explanation for the immunosuppressive actions of glucocorticoids, especially in relation to production of inflammatory cytokines and eicosanoids, and thus provide an additional window for viewing the effects of glucocorticoids downstream of the known interactions of the glucocorticoid receptor with gene promoter elements and transcription factors (17).

REFERENCES

1. H. Turner, and J.-P. Kinet, Nature 402:B24 (1999).
2. K. Ozawa, Z. Szallasi, M. G. Kazanietz, P. M. Blumberg, H. Mischak, J. F. Mushinski, and M. A. Beaven, J. Biol. Chem. 268:1749 (1993).
3. N. Hirasawa, A. Scharenberg, H. Yamamura, M. A. Beaven, and J.-P. Kinet, J. Biol. Chem. 270:10960 (1995).
4. C. Zhang, R. A. Baumgartner, K. Yamada, and M. A. Beaven, J. Biol. Chem. 272:13397 (1997).
5. T. Ishizuka, N. Terada, P. Gerwins, E. Hamelmann, A. Oshiba, G. R. Fanger, G. L. Johnson, and E. W. Gelfand, Proc. Natl. Acad. Sci. USA. 94:6358 (1997).
6. N. Hirasawa, Y. Sato, Y. Fujita, and K. Ohuchi, Biochim. Biophys. Acta 1456:45 (2000).
7. M. A. Beaven, and R. A. Baumgartner, Curr. Opin. Immunol. 8:766 (1996).
8. B. Jabril-Cuenod, C. Zhang, A. M. Scharenberg, R. Paolini, R. Numerof, M. A. Beaven, and J.-P. Kinet, J. Biol. Chem. 271:16268 (1996).

9. L. G. Rider, N. Hirasawa, F. Santini, and M. A. Beaven, J. Immunol. 157:2374 (1996).
10. D. S. Cissel, and M. A. Beaven, J. Biol. Chem. 275:7066 (2000).
11. D. K. Morrison, and R. E. Cutler Jr., Curr. Opin. Cell Biol. 9:174 (1997).
12. M. C. Coss, R. M. Stephens, D. K. Morrison, D. Winterstein, L. M. Smith, and S. L. Simek, Cell Growth Differentiation. 9:41 (1998).
13. D. F. Smith, I. Whitesell, and E. Katsanis, Pharmacol. Rev. 50:493 (1998).
14. W. B. Pratt, Ann. Rev. Pharmacol. Toxicol. 37:297 (1997).
15. N. Hirasawa, Y. Sato, Y. Fujita, S. Mue, and K. Ohuchi, J. Immunol. 61:4939 (1998).
16. L. Neckers, T. W. Schulte, and E. Mimnaugh, International New Drugs. 17:361 (1999).
17. P. J. Barnes, Nature. 402:B31 (1999).

Histamine Research in the New Millennium
T. Watanabe, H. Timmerman and K. Yanai (Editors)

Antiasthmatic Indonesian Medicinal plants:
Their tracheospasmolytic activity against histamine induced contractions

Subagus Wahyuono[a], Gemini Alam[b], Ibnu G. Ganjar[a], Lukman Hakim[a], H. Timmerman[c]

[a]Faculty of Pharmacy, Gadjah Mada University, Yogyakarta, Indonesia

[b]Dept. of Pharmacy, Faculty of Science, Hasanudin University, Makasar, Indonesia

[c]LACDR, Dept. of Pharmacochemistry, Vrije Universiteit, Amsterdam, the Netherlands

ABSTRACT

"JAMU", Indonesian traditional medicine preparations are widely consumed in Indonesia. Jamu is a multiple preparation, consisting of plant materials. Various pharmacological activities have been reported for jamu, including antiasthma although there is no complete scientific prove for these mentioned activities. Therefore, this study is intended to prove potential antiasthmatic activity and eventually to isolate, identify the compounds responsible for this activity. Ten medicinal plants material traditionally utilized in Indonesia to treat respiratory disorders have been screened for their ability to inhibit trachea contractions induced by histamine (10^{-7}–10^{-3} M).

The plant materials are initially extracted with n-hexane, followed by ethanol to give n-hexane and ethanol extracts respectively. Those extracts are then tested for their tracheospasmolytic activity at the dose of 0.25 and 0.50 mg/ml. The test result indicates that some medicinal plant materials (the leaves of *Vitex trifolia*, *Thymus vulgaris*, *Eucalyptus globulus*, *Eugenia caryophyllata*, the fruit of *Piper cubeba* and *Curcuma xanthorrhiza* rhizomes) indeed inhibit the contractions induced by histamine. On the other hand, some medicinal plant materials (the fruit of *Foeniculum vulgare*, the leaves of *Justicia gendarusa* and the hull of *Garcinia mangostana*) rather increase the trachea contraction and one extract (the leaves of *Centella asiatica*) does not show any effect.

From the n-hexane extract of *V. trifolia*, two active tracheospasmolytic compounds are isolated and identified as (8R,10S)-6β-acetoxy-9α-hydroxy-labda-13Z-en-15,16-olide (compound **1**) and 3',5'-dihydroxy-3,4',6,7-tetramethoxyflavone (compound **2**) on the basis of spectroscopic data. Compound **1** (dose 0.05 mg/ml) inhibits contraction (by histamine) by 27%, compound **2** (equal dose) inhibits the trachea contraction stronger than **1** (64%). Furthermore, compound **2** is up to the minimum dose of 5 µg/ml also active in a model using the trachea sensitized guinea pigs (stimulated by ovalbumin) and is more potent than **1**.

INTRODUCTION

Most of Indonesians have been practicing "Jamu", a traditional preparation consisting of medicinal herbs to treat their illness, to maintain their wellness and their beauty. Based on the experiences or stories told, various medical indications have been labelled on each case of jamu although the reported activities are not proved completely. One of those reported activities that is not thoroughly
studied is jamu for antiasthma or respiratory disorders. Therefore, this study is aimed to prove potential antiasthmatic activity and eventually to isolate, identify the compounds responsible for this activity. In this study, tracheospasmolytic assay using male guinea pig trachea is used as antiasthmatic bioassay model, and this bioassay is utilized to monitor the successful processes in the extraction, fractionation and isolation of the active principals.

MATERIALS AND METHODS

Materials: Ten medicinal plant materials, obtained from Office of Medicinal Plant Research Center (BPTO), Indonesia. The powdered plant materials are macerated with n-hexane followed by ethanol to give n-hexane (H) and ethanol (E) extracts. The voucher specimens are deposited at the BPTO.
Tracheospasmolytic test: The tracheospasmolytic bioassay (Anonim, 1990) uses isolated male guinea pigs (250-550 g) trachea in a Krebs buffer. The trachea contraction is induced by histamine ($10^{-7} - 10^{-3}$ M). The extract (H or E) (0.25 & 0.50 mg/ml) is added to the organ bath, and their ability to inhibit trachea contraction is measured. Contraction obtained by histamine induction is calculated as 100%.
Isolation of the active compounds: The active extract (n-hexane of *Vitex trifolia* leaves) was subjected into bioassay-guided fractionation, partition and isolation. The structures of the active compounds are identified based on UV, IR, MS and NMR and comparison with reported data.
Analysis: The log dose-respond curves are expressed in Excel Microsoft Windows; and the structures of those 2 active compounds are determined on the basis of their spectroscopic (UV, IR, MS and NMR) and comparison with reported data.

RESULTS AND DISCUSSION

There are 6 medicinal plant materials tested shows tracheospasmolytic activity (Table 1). These are the leaves of *V. trifolia, T. vulgaris, E. globulus, E. caryophyllata*, the fruit of *P. cubeba* and rhizome of *C. xanthorrhiza*. The leaves of *T. vulgaris* have been used clinically to treat cough and respiratory disorder, and flavonoids have been identified as the principal active compound present in the leaves (Van den Broucke and Lemli, 1983). Euglobals are identified as the main active compounds in the leaves of *E. globulus*, as they inhibit the granulation (Kozuka et al., 1982a, 1982b; Sawada et al., 1980), and macrocarpals. Eugenol, the main component of *E. caryophyllata* leaves is the antispasmodic active principal.

TABLE 1

TRACHEOSPASMOLYTIC TEST RESULTS OF N-HEXANE AND ETHANOL
EXTRACTS OF SOME INDONESIAN MEDICINAL PLANT MATERIALS (n=3)
[H = Histamine ; M = Metacholine, as the spasmogen. (-) = Induces contraction, (+) = Inhibit
contraction]

No. !	Plant Materials	Dose (mg/ml)	Spasm inhibition (%)
	Ethanol 50 µl in 20 ml bath (Kreb's buffer)		+ 2.25
	100 µl in 20 ml bath (Kreb's buffer)		- 2.22
1.	The Hull *Garcinia mangostana*		
	n-hexane ext.	0.25	- 7.64
		0.50	+ 1.16
	Ethanol ext.	0.25	- 10.25
		0.50	- 19.12
2.	*Foeniculum vulgare* fructus		
	n-hexane ext.	0.50	- 34.81
	Ethanol ext.	0.25	- 30.12
		0.50	- 56.25
3.	The leaves of *Vitex trifolia*		
	n-hexane ext.	0.25	+ 1.14
		0.50	+ 41.65
	Ethanol ext.	0.25	+ 14.59
		0.50	+ 42.49
4.	The leaves of *Justicia gendarusa*		
	n-hexane ext.	0.25	- 17.98
		0.50	- 31.72
	Ethanol ext.	0.25	- 12.67
		0.50	- 17.35
5.	*Curcuma xanthorrhiza* Rhizoma		
	n-hexane ext.	0.25	+ 42.97
		0.50	+ 69.71
	Ethanol ext.	0.25	+ 46.34
		0.50	+ 87.03
6.	The leaves of *Thymus vulgaris*		
	n-hexane ext.	0.25	+ 46.22
		0.50	+ 64.08
	Ethanol ext.	0.25	+ 94.21
7.	The leaves of *Eucalyptus globulus*		
	n-hexane ext.	0.25	+ 22.92
		0.50	+ 67.14
	Ethanol ext.	0.25	+ 54.97
		0.50	+100.00
8.	*Piper cubeba* fructus		
	n-hexane ext.	0.25	+ 49.37
		0.50	+ 67.14

	Ethanol ext.	0.25	+ 35.26
		0.50	+100.00
9.	The leaves of *Centela asiatica*		
	n-hexane ext.	0.50	+ 19.77
	Ethanol ext.	0.25	- 1.64
		0.50	- 2.48
10.	The leaves of *Eugenia caryophyllata*		
	n-hexane ext.	0.25	+ 98.51
		0.50	+100.00
	Ethanol ext.	0.25	+ 2.58
		0.50	- 16.70

The n-hexane extract of *V. trifolia* is selected for this study. The **J** fraction that is tracheospasmolytic active contains two main compounds. These two compounds are separated by preparative tlc using SiO_2 GF 254 as the stationary phase and $CHCl_3$-EtOAc (12:1 v/v, developed 2 times) as the mobile phase. Compound **1** is identified as (8R, 10S)-6β-acetoxy-9α-hydroxy-labda-13Z-en-15,16-olide (vitexin) on the basis of its spectroscopic data and comparison with that of the reported data (Ono et al., 1998). Based on the spectroscopic and comparison to the reported data (Zheng et al., 1996), compound **2** is identified as 3',5-dihydroxy-3,4',6,7-tetramethoxyflavone (vitexicarpin).

1   **2**

Compound **1** (0.05 mg/ml, n=3) inhibits 18.5% the trachea contraction to 81.5% [contraction induced by histamine $(10^{-7} - 10^{-3}$ M)], and when the dose is raised to 0.15 mg/ml (n=3), compound **1** inhibits 50.5% the trachea contraction to 49.5% (Figure I). Compound **2** inhibits the trachea contraction better than compound **1** as **2** is able to inhibit 38.8% the contraction to 61.2% at the dose of 0.05 mg/ml. When the dose is raised to 0.15 mg/ml the inhibition also increases to 7.9% (inhibit 92.1% contraction) (Figure II). In addition, the mechanism of both **1** and **2** seems to be antagonist non-competitive to the agonist used (histamine).

Further test on a model using the trachea sensitized [stimulated by ovalbumin (5, 50, 5000 ng/ml) male guinea pigs of compounds **1** and **2** (each at the dose of 5 µg/ml) indicates that **2** inhibits trachea contraction better than **1** (Figure III). In order to see the reversibility of the organ after the test, the trachea is reinduced with carbachol at the dose of 2×10^{-3} M; and with saturated solution of KCl. Optimum trachea contraction (100% response) is obtained by both and the result indicates that no harmful effect on organ observed due to compounds **1** and **2**.

SUMMARY

Six tested medicinal plant materials (the leaves of *Vitex trifolia*, *Thymus vulgaris*, *Eucalyptus globulus*, *Eugenia caryophyllata*, the fruits of *Piper cubeba* and *Curcuma xanthorrhiza* rhizomes) inhibit trachea contraction induced by histamine. Three other materials (the fruit of *Foeniculum vulgare*, the leaves of *Justicia gendarusa* and the hull of *Garcinia mangostana*) rather increase trachea contraction while the leaves of *Centella asiatica* does not show any effect. Two active compounds are isolated and identified as (8R,10S)-6β-acetoxy-9α-hydroxy-labda-13Z-en-15,16-olide (**1**) and 3',5'-dihydroxy-3,4',6,7-tetramethoxyflavone (**2**). Compound **2** inhibits better than **1** on trachea contraction (induced by histamine) and also in a model using trachea sensitized guinea pigs.

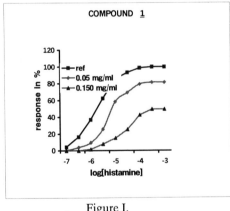

Figure I.

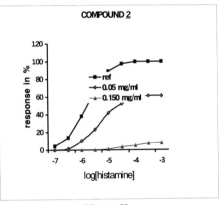

Figure II.

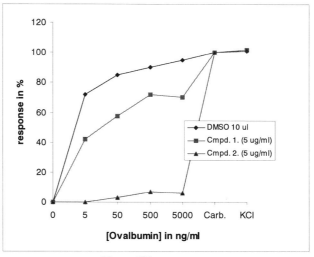

Figure III.

REFERENCES

Anonim, Practical Training Pharmacodynamics, Mid Career Training in Pharmacochemistry, Vakgroep Farmacochemie Vrije Universiteit-Faculty of Pharmacy,1990

Van den Broucke, C. O.;   and Lemli, J. A., Spasmolytic activity of the flavonoids from *Thymus vulgaris*, Pharm. Weekbl., Sci. Ed. 1983, 5(1), 9-14

Kozuka, M., Sawada, T., Kasahara, F., Mizuta, E., Amano, T., Komiya, T., Goto., M., The granulation-inhibiting principles from *Eucalyptus globulus* Labill., 2. The structures of euglobals 1A1, 1A2, 1B, 1C, 2A, 2B, 2C, Chem. Pharm. Bull., 1982a, 30, p. 1952-1963

Kozuka, M., Sawada, T., Mizuta, E., Kasahara, F., Amano, T., Komiya, T., Goto, M., The granulation-inhibiting principles from *Eucalyptus globulus* Labill. 3. The structures of euglobal-I, II, IVB and VIII, Chem.Pharm. Bull., 1982b, 30, 1964-1973

Sawada, T., Kozuka, M., Komiya, T., Amano, T., Goto, M., Euglobal-III, A novel granulation inhibiting agent from *Eucalyptus globulus* Labill., Chem. Pharm. Bull., 1980, 28, 2546-2548

Ono, M., Ito, Y., Nohara, T., A labdane diterpene glycoside from fruit of *Vitex rotundifolia*, Phytochemistry, 1998, 48(1), 207-209

Zheng, W. F., Tan, R. X., Yang, L., and Liu, L., Two flavones from *Artemisia giraldii* and their antimicrobial activity, Planta Medica, 1996, 62, 160-162

© 2001 Elsevier Science B.V. All rights reserved.
Histamine Research in the New Millennium
T. Watanabe, H. Timmerman and K. Yanai (Editors)

MAST CELLS IN RHINITIS

Pawankar R , Yamagishi S, Takizawa R, Yagi T.

Department of Otolaryngology, Nippon Medical School, 1-1-5, Sendagi, Bunkyo-ku, Tokyo 113-8603.

ABSTRACT :

Conventional knowledge tells us that mast cells are only important in the immediate phase allergic reaction. Yet, in recent years, much evidence has accumulated on the versatile role of mast cells in allergic inflammation. Here, we describe the novel roles of mast cells in allergic inflammation, especially in the light of local IgE synthesis and the IgE-IgE receptor mast cell network. Nasal mast cells (NMC) in allergic rhinitics are an important source of Th2 type cytokines, can induce IgE synthesis, and IgE itself can enhance the FceRI expression and subsequent mediator release from NMC thus perpetuatiing on-going allergic inflammation. Again, mast cells can interact with the extracellular matrix proteins as well as structural cells like epithelial cells to enhance cytokine release. Thus, it is increasingly evident that mast cells act not only in the genesis of the allergic reaction, but also contribute to the various aspects of the allergic inflammation.

INTRODUCTION :

Since the discovery of the granule laden mast cell (Mastzellen) in 1879 by Paul Ehrlich, and the description by Riley et al about the presence of the pre-formed mediator, histamine, in the mast cell, much has been learnt about its biochemical characteristics and functional properties. Enerback first classified mast cells (in rats) based on the morphology, size, and density of granules as well as their staining properties. Subsequently, in humans, Irani et al classified mast cells into phenotypically distinct subpopulations based on the neutral proteases they express, namely $MC_{(T)}$ mast cells that contain only tryptase, and the $MC_{(TC)}$ mast cells that contain chymase, cathepsin G and carboxypeptidase in addition to tryptase (1).

In humans and many other mammalian species, the numbers of mast cells in normal tissues vary considerably based on the anatomic site. The numbers of mast cells also vary in based on the underlying inflammatory or immunologic condition (2-8). Infact in allergic rhinitics, an increase in the number of MC $_{(T)}$ mast cells in the nasal epithelium has been well documented (9).

Mast cells are known to play a central role in the immediate phase allergic reaction through the allergen and IgE-dependent release of a variety of inflammatory mediators. Yet, recent studies have shown that the mast cell is an important source of a variety of cytokines.

Thus the mast cell cannot be be simplistically assigned a role in the immediate phase allergic response and recent studies suggest a more versatile role for the mast cell in regulating on-going allergic inflammation.

DISCUSSION :

MAST CELLS AS A SOURCE OF MULTIFUNCTIONAL CYTOKINES :

Mast cells can synthesis and release a variety of cytokines via IgE-dependent mechanisms (9-12). In humans, mast cells are a potential source of IL-4, IL-5, IL-6, IL-7, IL-8, IL-10, IL-13, TNF-α, and basic fibroblast growth factor (13). Bradding et al, first reported the expression of IL-4, IL-5, IL-6 in bronchial mast cells of atopic asthmatics and it is well known now that bronchial and nasal mast cells from atopic asthmatics and allergic rhinitics are an important source of Th2 type cytokines IL-4, IL-5, IL-6, and IL-13 (9-11). In fact, nasal mast cells from patients with perennial allergic rhinitis to house dust mite can release the protein of IL-4, IL-6 and IL-13 when stimulated by specific allergen (mite antigen) (13,14).

MAST CELLS AND IGE SYNTHESIS :

Recent studies have shown that not only T cells but also mast cells can induce IgE synthesis in B cells (13,15). In fact, nasal mast cells from PAR patients not only released sufficient amounts of IL-4 or IL-13 on stimulation with specific mite antigen, but also expressed the CD40L and induced IgE synthesis in B cells (13). Interestingly, the nasal mast cell-induced IgE synthesis was more IL-13 dependent (13) bringing us to our earlier observations of a strong correlation between the levels of IL-13 expression in the nasal mucosa of PAR patients and the levels of serum IgE (10). Again, while it is well known that allergen activated Th2 cells can produce IL-4 and IL-13 and induce IgE synthesis in B cells, the findings that mast cells can induce IgE synthesis not only suggest novel roles for mast cells in perpetuating chronic allergic inflammation, but also suggests that IgE may be produced locally in the shock organ itself.

MAST CELL - EXTRACELLULAR MATRIX INTERACTIONS :

In addition to cytokines, a number of cell surface molecules are involved in the recruitment of inflammatory cells into specific sites of inflammation (16). Lymphocytes and mast cells in the tissues are surrounded by other cells like fibroblasts and mucosal cells as well as extracellular matrix (ECM) proteins (eg. collagen, fibronectin and laminin). Therefore, the interaction of these inflammatory cells with fibroblasts and ECM may be important in the perpetuation of chronic inflammation. It has been reported that b1 integrins like VLA-4, 5, and the vitronectin receptor integrin are involved in mast cell activation, upregulation of cytokine expression in mast cells and in mast cell survival (17). Recently, we demonstrated an upregulation of the expression of VLA-4 and VLA-5 in nasal mast cells from PAR patients, and that IgE-mediated activation of mast cells induced the release of greater levels of IL-4, IL-13 and TNF-α when cultured on fibronectin (18). Thus mast cell-ECM interactions may contribute to the enhancement of mast cell activation especially when the levels of IgE and Ag in the microenvironment are rather low. This in fact may explain in part the phenomenon of hypersensitivity seen in patients with allergic rhinitis.

MAST CELL -EPITHELIAL CELL INTERACTIONS :

Mast cell activation may directly or indirectly promote the release of cytokines from other resident cells in the respiratory tract, such as macrophages, epithelial cells, vascular endothelial cells, fibroblasts, and nerves; cytokines released in these responses then contribute to the vascular and epithelial changes and to the angiogenesis that are so prominent. At certain points in the natural history of these complex processes, cytokines derived from mast cells (TGF-β) may also contribute to the down-regulation of the response. In fact, our most recent studies show that mast cell mediators like histamine and tryptase upregulated RANTES and GM-CSF production in cultured nasal epithelial cells (CNEC) whereas IL-4 and IL-13 when added to TNF-α upregulated Eotaxin production in CNEC. Pre-treatment with an H1 antihistamine, Cetirizine inhibited the histamine-induced upregulation of RANTES and GM-CSF production in CNEC in a dose-dependent manner. Moreover, the levels of tryptase in nasal secretions of allergic rhinitics treated with cetirizine was also downregulated.

VERSATILE ROLES OF MAST CELLS IN IGE-MEDIATED ALLERGY :

Immediate phase response : It is conventionally believed that mast cells when activated via the high affinity IgE receptor react by undergoing several morphological changes including swelling of the cytoplasmic granules and subsequent solubilization of its granule contents. Histamine, tryptase, PGD$_2$ and LTC$_4$ are among the mast cell products that can be detected immediately after exposure to allergens. Histamine induces vasodilatation, increased vascular permeability and increased glandular secretion in the ipsilateral as well as contralateral sides through neural reflexes. Prostaglandins like PGD$_2$ also cause edema by vasodilatation, and increased vascular permeability.

Late phase response : The late phase allergic reaction occurs as a result of the infiltration of a variety of inflammatory cells like eosinophils, basophils and T cells and the subsequent release of a number of soluble products like prostaglandins, leukotrienes, PAF, ECP, MBP and so on. Tissue eosinophilia is an important aspect of the late phase allergic reaction. Mast cells can orchestrate the late phase ereaction by inducing the infiltration of eosinophils not only through the upregulation of VCAM-1 (TNF-α, IL-4, IL-13) on endothelial cells but also through release of eosinophil-chemotactic factors like platelet activating factor and Leukotriene B4. In addition, mast cells can also enhance eosinophil survival through the release of granulocyte-macrophage colony-stimulating factor and IL-5. Interestingly, strong correlations were reported to exist between the numbers of IL-4+, IL-5+ and TNF-α+ mast cells and the number of tissue eosinophils in atopic asthma and allergic rhinitis (9) These recruited eosinophils (also basophils and T cells) then promote the further progression of the inflammatory response by providing additional sources of certain cytokines (that can also be produced by mast cells stimulated by ongoing exposure to allergen), as well as new sources of cytokines and other mediators that may not be produced by mast cells. In fact, time-kinetics of cytokine secretion from purified lung or nasal mast cells from PAR patients have shown that upon IgE-mediated stimulation induces the secretion of IL-13, TNF-α and IL-4 as early as from 2-6 hrs and peaked at 24-48 hours (19, 20) Again, TNF-α is constitutively expressed in mast cells and can be released within 2 hours of IgE-mediated stimulation. In fact, Klien et al (21) have shown that activation of mast cell products in fragments of human skin in vitro, resulted in the upregulation of E-selectin expression in adjacent vascular endothelial cells and this was attributed to the release of TNF-α. Moreover, interaction of mast cells with

372

extracellular matrix further enhances the IgE-mediated cytokine release from mast cells (18). Mast cells can contribute to the eosinophil/ T cell infiltration in the late phase allergic reaction through the histamine-induced upregulation of Eotaxin, RANTES, and GM-CSF production from nasal epithelial cells. Taken together, these studies strongly suggest that the mast cell is a key effector cell in the late phase reaction.

Chronic allergic inflammation : Most recent studies also suggest that the mast cell has the potential to regulate allergic inflammation by inducing IgE synthesis in B cells. Under allergic inflammatory conditions, "primed" mast cells express high levels of the high affinity receptor for IgE and the ligand for the surface antigen CD40, involved in T/B cell interactions leading to immunoglobulin production, as well as Th2-type cytokines, IL-4 and IL-13 (13). The critical role of these cells in the induction of IgE synthesis is supported by the findings that anti-ligand for the surface antigen CD40, anti-IL-4, and anti-IL-13 monoclonal antibodies inhibit IgE production. Mast cells also have the potential to function as antigen presenting cells with the ability to shift T cells into Th2 subtypes.

These recent findings suggest that mast cells can modulate the allergic response by acting directly on B cells and inducing IgE synthesis. Furthermore, the locally synthesized IgE itself can upregulate the FcεRI expression in mast cells. The augmented FcεRI in mast cells can bind increased number of IgE-Ag complexes which in turn can enhance the sensitivity of mast cells to allergen resulting in the enhancement of the production of immunomodulatory cytokines and chemical mediators, forming an important positive-feedback amplification loop involving the IgE-IgE receptor mast cell cascade (Figure 1) (13,14).

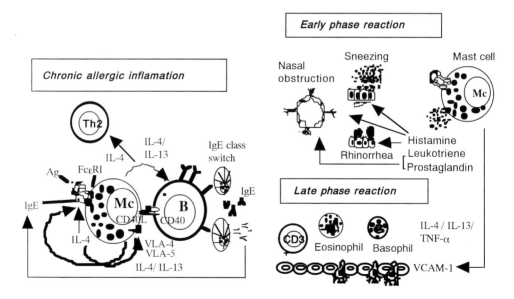

Figure 1. Versatile roles of mast cells in allergic diseases

REFERENCES

1.Irani AMA, Schecter NM, Craig SS, DeBlois G, and Schwartz LB. Two types of human mast cells that have distinct neutral protease compositions. Proc. Natl .Acad. Sci.. USA. 83(1986) 4464-4469.

2. Galli SJ, Zsebo KM, Geissler EN. The kit ligand, stem cell factor. Adv. Immunol. 55 (1994) 1-96.

3. Galli SJ. New insights into 'the riddle of the mast cells. Lab. Invest. 62 (1990) 5-33.

4. Kitamura Y. Heterogeneity of mast cells and phenotypic changes between subpopulations. Annu. Rev. Immunol. 7 (1989) 59-76.

5. Stevens RL, Austen KF. Recent advances in the cellular and molecular biology of mast cells. Immunol. Today. 10 (1989) 381-386.

6. Church MK, Benyon RC, Rees PH, et al. Functional heterogeneity of human mast cells. In: Galli SJ, Austen KF, eds. Mast Cell and Basophil Differentiation and Function in Health and Disease. New York, NY: Raven Press; (1989) 161-170.

7. Bienenstock J, Befus AD, Denburg JA. Mast cell heterogeneity. In: Befus AD, Bienenstock J, Denburg JA, eds. Mast Cell Differentiation and Heterogeneity. New York, NY: Raven Press; (1986) 391-402.

8. Enerback L, Pipkorn U, Olofsson A. Intraepithelial migration of mucosal mast cells in hay fever. Int. Arch. Allergy Appl. Immunol. 80 (1986) 44-51.

9. Bradding P, Feather IH, Wilson S, et al. Immunolocalization of cytokines in the nasal mucosa of normal and perennial rhinitic subjects. J. Immunol. 151 (1993) 3853-3865.

10. Pawankar R, Okuda M, Hasegawa S, et al. Interleukin-13 expression in the nasal mucosa of perennial allergic rhintics. Am. J. Resp. Crit. Care Med. 152 (1995) 2059-67.

11. Pawankar R, and Ra C. Heterogeneity of mast cells and T cells in the nasal mucosa. J. Allergy Clin. Immunol. 98 (1996) 249-62.

12. Gordon JR, Burd PR, Galli SJ. Mast cells as a source of multifunctional cytokines. Immunol. Today. 11 (1990) 458-464.

13. Costa JJ, Church MK, Galli SJ. Mast cell cytokines in allergic inflammation. In: Holgate ST, Busse W, eds. Inflammatory Mechanisms in Asthma. New York, NY: Marcel Dekker Inc; (1997) 111-127.

14. Pawankar R, Okuda M, Yssel H, Okumura K and Ra C. Nasal mast cells exhibit increased expression of the FcεRI, CD40L, IL-4 and IL-13 and can induce IgE synthesis in B cells. J. Clin Invest. 99 (7) (1997) 1492-1499.

15. Pawankar R, and Ra C. IgE-IgE receptor mast cells axis in allergy. Clin. Exp. Allergy. 28 (1998) 28: 6-11.

16. Gauchet JF, Henchoz S, Mazzei G, Aubry JP, Brunner T, Blasey H, Life H, Talabot T, Flores-Romo L, Thompson J, Kishi K, Butterfield J, Dahiden C, Bonnefoy J-F. Induction of human IgE synthesis in B cells by mast cells and basophils. Nature. 365 (1993) 340-343

17. Montefort S, Feather IH, Wilson SJ, Haskard DO, Lee TH, Holgate ST and Howarth PH. The expression of leukocyte-endothelial adhesion molecules is increased in perennial allergic rhinitis. Am. J. Respir. Mol. Biol. 7 (1992) 393-398.

18. Ra, .C., M. Yasuda, H. Yagita and K. Okumura. Fibronectin receptor integrins are involved in mast cell activation. J. Allergy Clin. Immunol. 94 (1994) 625-628, 1994.

19. Pawankar R, Yamagishi S, Nipapan D, Yagita H, Ra C, Okumura K. Nasal mast cells in perennial allergic rhinitics express increased levels of b1 integrins. Arerugi (Japanese) 49 (1999) 134 (abstract)

20. Kobayashi H, Okayama Y, Ishizuka T, Pawankar R, Ra C, and Mori M. Production of IL-13 by human lung mast cells in response to Fcereceptor crosslinkage. Clin. Exp. Allergy. 28 (1998) 1219-27.

21. Klien LM, Lavker RM, Mais WL, Murphy GF. Degranulation of human mast cells induces an endothelial antigen central to leukocyte adhesion. Proc. Natl. Acad Sci. USA. 86 (1989) 8972-8976.

Address for correspondence :

Ruby Pawankar, M.D., Ph.D
Dept. of Otolaryngology
Nippon Medical School
1-1-5, Sendagi,
Bunkyo-ku
Tokyo 113

Tel/Fax : 81-3-5685-0830
e.mail : Pawankar_Ruby/ent@nms.ac.jp

Poster Sessions

Molecular biology and application:

© 2001 Elsevier Science B.V. All rights reserved.
Histamine Research in the New Millennium
T. Watanabe, H. Timmerman and K. Yanai (Editors)

Characterization of splicing variants of histamine H3 receptor

Kenichi Tanaka, Takao Nakamura, Hiraku Itadani, Tetsuo Takimura, Yusuke Hidaka and Masataka Ohta

Tsukuba Research Institute, Banyu Pharmaceutical Co., Ltd., 3 Okubo Tsukuba, 300-2611, Japan

We found several splicing variants of the histamine H3 receptor (H3R) mRNA in human and rat. We characterized their profiles in the ligand binding and functional responses. All splicing variants-expressing cells, except one type, bound to $[^3H]$-N-α-methylhistamine (NAMHA) and responded to histamine (HA), inhibiting forskolin-induced cAMP accumulation. Marked differences of binding and functional profiles between the splicing variants were not observed.

1. Introduction

Histamine has important physiological roles, and its function is mediated via three histamine receptors, H1, H2, and H3, which belong to the superfamily of G protein-coupled receptors (GPCRs) (1). The histamine H1 receptor was cloned from cattle in 1991 (2), and then from humans in 1993 (3). The histamine H1 receptor is expressed in smooth muscle, endothelial cells, the adrenal medulla, the heart, and the central nervous system (CNS); it is mainly involved in smooth muscle contraction and increased vascular permeability. The histamine H1 receptor is an important therapeutic target for allergic conditions. The histamine H2 receptor was cloned from dogs and from humans in 1991 (4, 5). The histamine H2 receptor is expressed in gastric parietal cells, vascular smooth muscle, suppressor T cells, neutrophils, the CNS, and the heart; it is mainly involved in stimulation of gastric acid secretion. The histamine H2 receptor is an important therapeutic target in the treatment of gastric ulcers. The human histamine H3 receptor was recently cloned by Lovenberg *et al.* in 1999 (6). Cell clones expressing the human H3R responded to histamine, inhibiting forskolin-induced cAMP accumulation via the inhibition of adenylate cyclase. The H3R is expressed in the CNS and peripheral nerves. The H3R is a presynaptic autoreceptor on histamine neurons and controls histamine release (7). Several therapeutic targets for the H3R have been suggested: for example, sleep, wakefulness, cognition, memory processes, attention-deficit/hyperactivity disorder, obesity, and so on (8, 9). Many kinds of H1 antagonists and H2 antagonists have been developed and are currently used in medical care. Thus, histamine receptors are thought to be promising as therapeutic targets in the medical field.

To find new therapeutic targets, we attempted to clone orphan G protein-coupled receptors (oGPCRs) and identify their ligands. We cloned the oGPCR gene which we named BG2 and we identified it as the H3R independently, prior to the publication of the report by Lovenberg et al. (6). In the process of the cloning of BG2, we found 5 splicing variants of the H3R. In this study, we compared the pharmacological profiles of these splicing variants. We revealed that one splicing variant did not function as histamine receptor, and that marked differences of the phramacological profiles between the splicing variants were not observed.

2. Material and Methods

2.1. Bacteria, cells, vectors and reagents

Escherichia coli strains, JM109 and XL1-BlueMRF' were grown in Bacto LB agar, Millar or Bacto LB broth, Miller (Difco and Life Technologies). COS-7 cells and HEK293 cells were grown in Dulbecco's modified Eagle's medium (D-MEM, Asahi Techno Glass) and D-MEM/F-12 (1:1) mixture (Life Technologies), respectively, with 10 % fetal bovine serum (FBS) in a 95 % air/5 % CO_2 humidified atmosphere at 37 °C. The vector pEF1x was constructed by Itadani *et al.* (10). Poly-L-lysine-coated 24-well plate and poly-D-lysine cellware 96-well black/clear were obtained from Sumiron and Becton Dickinson, respectively. [^{3}H]-NAMHA (82 Ci/mmol) was the product of NEN Life Science Products. Histamine agonists and antagonists were obtained from Research Biochemicals Incorporated.

2.2 cAMP accumulation assay

We constructed the vectors using plasmid pEF1X for transient expression of each variant. The HEK293 cells (2.0 x 10^6 cells) were transfected with 2 μg of plasmid DNAs per 100-mm dish using Effectene Transfection Reagent (Qiagen) and grown for 18 hrs. The transfected HEK293 cells were plated on a 24-well plate (2.5 x 10^4 cells per well). After overnight cultivation, cells were incubated in FBS-free D-MEM/F-12 mixture for 15 min, further incubated with D-MEM/F-12 mixture containing 5 mM 3-ishobutyl-1-methylxanthine (a phosphodiesterase inhibitor) for 15 min, and then treated with or without forskolin (10 μM) and histamine (or agonists) for 15 min. The cells were lysed with 200 μl of lysis buffer, and then 20 μl of the mixture was tested for measurement of cAMP concentration. cAMP accumulation levels were determined using the cyclic AMP enzyme immunoassay (EIA) system (Amersham Pharmacia Biotech).

2.3. [^{3}H]-NAMHA binding assay

The COS-7 cells were washed twice using Opti-MEM (Life Technologies). Then the cells were transfected with 10 μg of plasmid DNAs per 100-mm dish with LipofectAMINE PLUS reagent (Life Technologies) and grown for 24 hrs. The membrane fraction was prepared according to described procedures with some modifications (11). The binding assay of [^{3}H]-NAMHA to the membrane fraction was performed in 0.2 ml of 50 mM Tris-HCl (pH 7.5), 2 nM [^{3}H]-NAMHA with or without 2 μM cold histamine at 30 °C for 40 min. Bound and free radioligand was separated by filtration using 0.5 % polyethylenimine-presoaked unifilter plate GF/C (Packard) and counted for radioactivity.

3. Results and Discussion

3.1. The structural characters of the histamine H3 receptor splicing variants

In the process of the cloning of BG2, we found 2 human H3R splicing variants, designated BG2 long (BG2L) and BG2 short (BG2S), and 3 rat H3R splicing variants, designated MP5, MP21, and MP22 (Fig. 1). The structural characters are as follows:

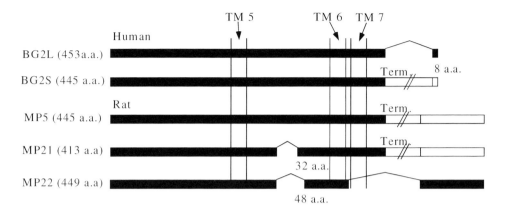

Fig. 1. Structure of the splicing variants forms of H3R. Filled boxes indicate coding sequence, open boxes indicate non-coding sequence. Term.: termination of open reading frame.

(1) The C-terminus amino acid sequence of BG2L was 8 amino acids longer than that of BG2S.
(2) MP5 is the counterpart of BG2S in rat.
(3) As compared with the amino acid sequence of MP5 between the fifth transmembrane domain (TM5) and TM6, these of MP21 and MP22 were deleted 32 amino acids and 48 amino acids, respectively.
(4) The amino acid sequence of MP22 were quite different from these of other splicing variants in the region including TM 7 and the C-terminus intracellular domain.
(5) The amino acid sequence of MP22 did not harbored two hallmarks of the biogenic amine subfamily of GPCRs: an asparagine residue and an NPXXY motif in TM 7.

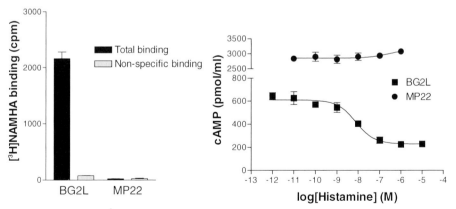

Fig. 2. Binding of [³H]-NAMHA to the membrane fraction of BG2L- or MP22-expressing cells and inhibition of forskolin-induced cAMP accumulation in BG2L- or MP22-expressing cells by histamine. Error bars represent SEM.

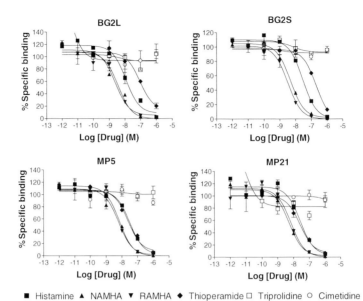

■ Histamine ▲ NAMHA ▼ RAMHA ◆ Thioperamide □ Triprolidine ○ Cimetidine

Fig. 3. Competitive binding of [³H]-NAMHA with histamine receptor agonists and antagonists to each variant. IC$_{50}$ values (data not shown) were determined by a single site curve fitting program and converted to Ki values (Prism). Error bars represent SEM.

To confirm that MP22 function as the H3R, we examined that the binding of [³H]-NAMHA, which is one of the H3R-specific agonists, to MP22-expressing cells. The binding was determined using a filtration assay (Fig. 2). We detected significant specific binding of [³H]-NAMHA to BG2L-expressing cells, but not to MP22-expressing cells. We then examined the capability of MP22-expressing cells to respond to histamine (Fig. 2). The forskolin-induced cAMP accumulation was inhibited in response to histamine in BG2L-expressing cells, but not in MP22-expressing cells. These results suggest that MP22 did not function as the H3R.

3.2. The comparison of the pharmacological profiles of the splicing variants

To study the functional implications of these splicing variants, we first compared the pharmacological profiles of these splicing variants. We first examined the binding of [³H]-NAMHA to each variant. We detected significant specific binding of [³H]-NAMHA to each variant (data not shown). The Kd values of each variant for [³H]-NAMHA are 0.55 nM for BG2L, 0.33 nM for BG2S, 0.58 nM for MP5, and 0.50 nM for MP21. Marked differences of the Kd values of each variant for [³H]-NAMHA were not observed.

We then examined the effects of histamine receptor agonists and antagonists on the binding of [³H]-NAMHA (Fig. 3). Histamine, H3 agonists (NAMHA and R(-)-α-methylhistamine (RAMHA)) and an H3 antagonist (thioperamide (THIO)) were found to compete out the binding of [³H]-NAMHA to each variant, while an H1 antagonist (triprolidine) and an H2 antagonist (cimetidine) did not. The Ki values for each compound are showed in Table 1. West et al. have suggested the existence of the receptor subtypes of H3R and reported the thioperamide binds to both high affinity site (H3a; Ki = 5nM) and low

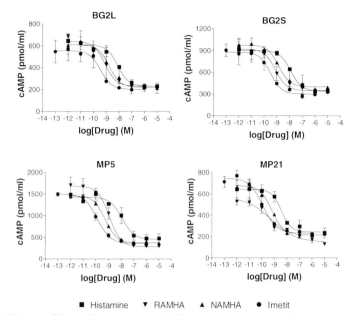

■ Histamine ▼ RAMHA ▲ NAMHA ● Imetit

Fig. 4. Inhibition of forskolin-induced cAMP accumulation in each variant-expressing cells by H3 agonists. EC_{50} values were determined by a single curved fitting program (Prism). Error bars represent SEM.

affinity site (H3b; $Ki = 68$ nM), in the rat brain (10). The Ki values of MP5 and MP21 for thioperamide are almost the same as that of H3a. These results suggest that both MP5 and MP21 may not be the histamine H3b receptor. To determine whether H3 agonists can act as agonists for each variants, we also examined the effects of H3 agonists on the inhibition of forskolin-induced cAMP accumulation (Fig. 4). Histamine and H3 agonists produced a reduction in forskolin-induced cAMP accumulation in each variant-expressing cells. The EC_{50} values for each compound are shown in Table 1.

Table 1
The summary of the pharmacological profiles of the H3R-splicing variants for H3 compounds.

	Ki values (nM)				EC_{50} values (nM)			
	HA	NAMHA	RAMHA	THIO	HA	NAMHA	RAMHA	Imetit
Human								
BG2L	2.5	0.51	0.78	20	7.7	1.6	0.79	0.36
BG2S	4.0	0.67	0.46	30	12	1.4	0.76	0.32
Rat								
MP5	7.1	1.4	1.5	5.4	6.9	0.47	1.8	0.12
MP21	5.3	1.0	1.4	5.1	5.1	0.63	2.1	0.13

Ki values were determined by competition binding with [³H]-NAMHA to each variant-expressing cells.

The pharmacological profiles of each variant were summarized in Table 1. The species differences of the pharmacological profiles between human and rat were observed: for examples, the potency of thioperamide on human variants was 4 to 6 times less than that on rat variants. However, marked differences of the pharmacological profiles were not observed in each species. The differences of the physiological functions of each variant are not yet clear. Further studies, including the development of the specific and potent agonists/antagonists and the conformation of the tissue distribution of each variant, would be necessary to elucidate the physiological functions of each variant.

REFERENCES

1. S. J. Hill, C. R. Ganellin, H. Timmerman, J. C. Schwartz, N. P. Shankley, J. M. Young, W. Schunack, R. Levi and H. L. Haas, Pharmacol. Rev., 49 (1997) 253
2. M. Yamashita, H. Fukui, K. Sugama, Y. Horio, S.Ito, H. Mizuguchi and H. Wada, Proc. Natl. Acad. Sci. USA, 88 (1991)11515
3. M. D. De Backer, W. Gommeren, H. Moereels, G. Nobels, P. Van Gompel, J. E. Leysen and W. H. M. L. Luyten, Biochem. Biophys. Res. Commun., 197 (1993) 1601
4. I. Gantz, M. Schaffer, J. DelValle, C. Logsdon, V. Campbell, M. Uhler and T. Yamada, Proc. Natl. Acad. Sci. USA, 88 (1991) 429
5. I. Gantz, G. Munzert, T. Tashiro, M. Schaffer, L. Wang, J. Del Valle and T. Yamada, Biochem. Biophys. Res. Commun., 178 (1991) 1386
6. T. W. Lovenberg, B. L. Roland, S. J. Wilson, X. Jiang, J. Pyati, A. Huvar, M. R. Jackson and M. G. Erlander, Mol. Pharmacol., 55 (1999) 1101
7. J. M. Arrang, M. Garbarg and J. C. Schwartz, Nature, 302 (1983) 832
8. R. Leurs, P. Blandina, C. Tedford and H. Timmerman, Trends Pharmacol. Sci., 19 (1998) 177
9. C. Sanmon, Drug Discovery Today, 5 (2000) 94
10. H. Itadani, T. Nakamura, J. Itoh, H. Iwaasa, A. Kanatani, J. Borkowski, M. Ihara and M. Ohta, Biochem. Biophys. Res. Commun. 250 (1998) 68
11. R. E. West, Jr., A. Zweig, N. -Y. Shin, M. I. Siegel, R. W. Egan and M. A. Clark, Mol. Pharmacol., 38 (1990) 610

© 2001 Elsevier Science B.V. All rights reserved.
Histamine Research in the New Millennium
T. Watanabe, H. Timmerman and K. Yanai (Editors)

Molecular cloning and characterization of a new subtype of histamine receptor, H4

Takao Nakamura, Hiraku Itadani, Yusuke Hidaka, Masataka Ohta and Kenichi Tanaka.

Tsukuba Research Institute, Banyu Pharmaceutical Co., Ltd., 3 Okubo Tsukuba, 300-2611, Japan

1.Abstract

A new subfamily member of histamine receptor gene, H4R, was isolated from human. The H4R was about 40% homologous to histamine H3 receptor (H3R) and expressed in leukocytes and other peripheral tissues, but not in brain according to the RT-PCR analysis. The cAMP accumulation in H4 expressing cells was inhibited in response to histamine. $[^3H]$-N-α-methyl-histamine (NAMHA) can bind to H4R specifically. These results suggested that H4R is a new subtype of histamine receptor.

2.Results and Discussion

To identify novel GPCRs, we performed homology searches on the GenBank database using known GPCR sequences as templates and found a partial sequence homologous to the H3R gene from the GenBank entry sequence (accession no. AC007922). We named this gene BG26 and defined the initiation and termination for the translation by more detailed homology analysis with H3R. To clone the complete open reading frame (ORF) of this gene, we designed the PCR primers, which were based on the upstream or downstream sequences of the putative ORF, and performed RT-PCR using human leukocyte cDNA as a template. The sequence of BG26 had a 1170 bp ORF that is able to encode a 44 kDa protein with 390 amino acids. The deduced amino acid sequence showed homology to several biogenic amine subfamilies of GPCRs, particularly the human histamine H3 receptor, with about 40 % identity.

To confirm that BG26 is a new member of the subfamily of histamine receptor gene, we first examined the capability of BG26-expressing cells to respond to histamine, which can affect the level of cAMP. When cells were treated with forskolin, the forskolin-induced cAMP accumulation was inhibited in response to histamine in BG26-expressing cells (Fig. 1A). It has been confirmed repeatedly that the original HEK293 cells did not show any response to histamine (not shown). We then examined the binding of histamine analogues to BG26-expressing cells. The binding of $[^3H]$-NAMHA and $[^3H]$-R-α-methyl-histamine (RAMHA) were determined using a filtration assay (Fig.1B). We detected significant specific binding of $[^3H]$-NAMHA and $[^3H]$-RAMHA to BG26-expressing cells, but not to mock cells (not shown). Furthermore, $[^3H]$-pyrilamine and $[^3H]$-cimetidine, which bind to histamine H1 and H2 receptors, respectively, did not bind to BG26-expressing cells. These results indicate that BG26 has the capacity to transmit the histamine signal into cells, reducing the intracellular cAMP level and is able to bind to histamine analogues which can also bind to H3R, therefore suggesting a new subtype of histamine receptor, H4R.

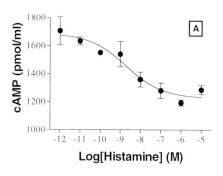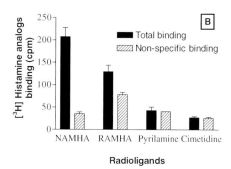

Figure 1. In BG26 expressing cells, inhibition of forskolin-induced cAMP accumulation by histamine (A) and binding of histamine analogues on membrane fraction (B).

To collect any functional implication of H4R, we were investigated its expression in different tissues and characterization of physiological functions. H4R mRNA was detected by RT-PCR in a wide variety of peripheral tissues, including the heart, kidney, liver, lung, pancreas, skeletal muscle, leukocyte, prostate, small intestine, spleen, testis, bone marrow, fetal liver, and lymph node, but not in brain. It is worth nothing that H4R mRNA was not detected in the brain by RT-PCR, in contrast with the histamine H3 receptor which is abundantly expressed in the brain.

We also examined the effects of histamine agonists and antagonists on the binding of [^{3}H]-NAMHA to H4R and compared this binding with that of H3R (table 1). Histamine, H3 agonists (NAMHA and RAMHA) and an H3 antagonist (thioperamide) were found to compete out the binding of [^{3}H]-NAMHA to H4R and H3R, while an H1 antagonist (triprolidine) and an H2 antagonist (cimetidine) did not. These IC$_{50}$ values of NAMHA and RAMHA for H4R were markedly different from those for H3R.

To determine whether H3 agonists can act as agonists for H4R, we performed the cAMP accumulation assay (table 2). The EC$_{50}$ values of the H3 agonists for H4R were markedly different from those for H3R. These results indicate that the pharmacological profiles of H4R are different from those of H3R and suggest that H4R may not be a subtype of H3R.

In summary, we suggest that H4R could mediate the histamine signals in peripheral tissues, thus its physiology should be different from H3R. This conclusion suggests that H4R could be a new therapeutic target and that specific and potent agonists/antagonists would be useful in the elucidation of the physiological roles of H4R.

Table 1 IC$_{50}$ values of known histamine agonists and antagonists (nM)

	histamine	NAMHA	RAMHA	thioperamide	cimetidine	tripolidine
H4R	2.31	92.4	123	52.1	>1000	>1000
H3R	11.5	2.38	3.61	92.3	>1000	>1000

Table 2 EC$_{50}$ values of known histamine agonists (nM)

	histamine	NAMHA	RAMHA	imetit
H4R	1.9	16	940	18
H3R	19	0.26	0.71	1.2

Genomic structure of histamine *N*-methyltransferase in mammals.

M. Takemura[a], T. Tanaka[b], Y. Tada[a], T. Oue[a], N. Kitanaka[a], and J. Kitanaka[a]

[a]Department of Pharmacology, Hyogo College of Medicine, Nishinomiya 663-8501, Japan

[b]Central Laboratory for Research and Education, Osaka University Graduate School of Medicine, Suita 565-0871, Japan

We have cloned guinea pig and mouse histamine *N*-methyltransferase cDNA. The predicted amino acid sequences of guinea pig and mouse enzyme shared 79.1 - 94.2% homology with that of human and rat. Two alternative putative polyadenylylation consensus sequences were found to be functional in guinea pig and mouse. We also cloned rat and mouse gene for this enzyme. The translated region and 3'-untranslated region was coded by 6 exons. The mouse gene had additional exon which encodes a part of 5'-untranslated region.

Keywords: methyltransferase, inactivation, cDNA, gene structure

1. INTRODUCTION

Histamine *N*-methyltransferase (HMT; EC 2.1.1.8) is one of the key enzymes in inactivation of histamine. The tissue distribution of this enzyme activity and also immunoreactivity [1] varies substantially from species to species. To elucidate the mechanisms underlying this species difference in the expression pattern of HMT, we have cloned HMT cDNA and HMT genome from several mammals.

2. MATERIAL AND METHODS

2.1 Cloning of guinea pig and mouse HMT cDNA

Total RNAs were extracted from the guinea pig brain and mouse liver with acidic guanidinium isothiocyanate-phenol-chloroform method and reverse transcribed with either HMT specific primer designed from rat [2] and human cDNA sequences [3,4] or "anchored" oligo(dT). cDNA transcribed with anchored oligo(dT) served as a template in two cycles of "nested" PCR with primers with rat and human HMT sequence and complementary to the anchor sequence. Amplification products were cloned into plasmid and their sequences were analyzed. cDNA with HMT specific primer was ligated with a single strand DNA "anchor" and served as a SLIC-RACE template [5]. Guinea pig HMT mRNA in the small intestine was visualized by *in situ* hybridization histochemistry.

2.2 Cloning of rat and mouse HMT genomic DNA

Genomic libraries (purchased from either Clontech Laboratory Inc, Palo Alto, CA or Stratagene, La Jolla, CA) were screened with rat and mouse HMT cDNA.

3. RESULTS and DISCUSSION

3.1 guinea pig and mouse HMT cDNA

The guinea pig HMT cDNA consisted of 1320 bp and encoded 879-bp ORF, whereas the mouse HMT cDNA consisted of 1631 bp and encoded 888-bp ORF. The predicted amino acid sequence of guinea pig HMT was 75.6% and 79.1% identical with that of rat and human, and that of mouse HMT was 94.2 and 82.9% identical with that of rat and human,

386

respectively. The homology between guinea pig and mouse HMT was 79.5%. Thus, HMT cDNA shared high homology among species and we could not find out the regions with especially high homology which might be important for the enzyme activity. Two putative polyadenylylation signal consensus sequences were found in both mouse and guinea pig HMT cDNA, and on 3'-RACE, it was found that these two sites were functional in both these two species.

We visualized HMT mRNA in the small intestine of the guinea pig. HMT mRNA seemed to be expressed throughout the tissue, but Auerbach's plexus and epithelial cells gave stronger signals than the surrounding tissue. This distribution pattern coincides well with the result of immunohistochemical staining of HMT [6].

3.2 mouse and rat HMT genome

The rat and mouse HMT gene was cloned except for intron 3. The entire length of HMT gene in human [7], rat, and mouse is 34, >28, and >34 kb, respectively. The translated regions and 3'-untranslated regions (UTR's) were composed of 6 exons and all their boundaries are conserved in these three species. The 5'-UTR of human HMT gene is reported to be 252 bp long and composes one exon together with 137 bp of tranlated region. We have decided transcription initiation site of rat HMT gene by primer extension and *S1* nuclease mapping to be 76 bp upstream from translational initiation site. The 5'-UTR of mouse HMT gene was predicted to be 66-bp long from the longest clone of 5'-RACE, of which 56 bp of 5' portion was encoded by a different exon than that encodes 3' region of 5'-UTR and 137 bp of coding region. No TATA or CAAT consensus sequence was found in the 5' flanking region of HMT gene in these three species.

Acknowledgements

This work was supported in part by a Grant-in Aid for Scientific Research from the Uehara Memorial Foundation and the Ministry of Education, Science and Culture of Japan.

REFERENCES

1. M. Takemura, I. Imamura, H. Mizuguchi, H. Fukui and A. Yamatodani. Tissue distribution of histamine *N*-methyltransferase-like immunoreactivity in rodents, Life Sci., 54, 1994, 1059.
2. M. Takemura, T. Tanaka, Y. Taguchi, I. Imamura, H. Mizuguchi, M. Kuroda, H. Fukui, A. Yamatodani and H. Wada. Histamine *N*-methyltransferase from rat kidney: Cloning, nucleotide sequence, and expression in *Escherichia coli* cells, J. Biol. Chem., 267, 1992, 15687.
3. K. Yamauchi, K. Sekizawa, H. Suzuki, H. Nakazawa, Y. Ohkawara, D. Katayose, H. Ohtsu, G. Tamura, S. Shibahara, M. Takemura, K. Maeyama, T. Watanabe, H. Sasaki, K. Shirato and T. Takishima. Structure and function of human histamine *N*-methyltransferase: critical enzyme in histamine metabolism in airway, Am. J. Physiol., 267, 1994, L342.
4. B. Girard, D. M. Otterness, T. C. Wood, R. Honchel, E. D. Wieben and R. M. Weinshilboum. Human histamine *N*-methyltransferase pharmacogenetics: cloning and expression of kidney cDNA , Mol. Pharmacol., 45, 1994, 461.
5. H. Oda, Y. Nakabeppu, M. Furuichi and M. Sekiguchi. Regulation of expression of the human *MTH1* gene encoding 9-oxo-dGTPase: Alternative splicing of transcription products, J. Biol. Chem., 272, 1997, 17843.
6. A. Tahara, M. Nishibori, A. Ohtsuka, K. Sawada, J. Sakiyama and K. Saeki. Immuno-histochemical localization of histamine *N*-methyltransferase in guinea pig tissues, J. Histochem. Cytochem., 48, 2000, 943
7. S. Aksoy, R. Raftogianis and R. Weinshilboum. Human histamine *N*-methyltransferase gene: Structural characterization and chromosomal localization, Biochem. Biophys. Res. Commun., 219, 1996, 548.

2001 Elsevier Science B.V.
Histamine Research in the New Millennium
T. Watanabe, H. Timmerman and K. Yanai (Editors)

In situ hybridization analysis of gene expression of histamine H1-receptor in murine dorsal root and trigeminal ganglia

M. Itoh[a], T. Andoh[a], E. Senba[b], and Y. Kuraishi[a]*

[a]Department of Applied Pharmacology, Faculty of Pharmaceutical Sciences, Toyama Medical and Pharmaceutical University, 2630 Sugitani, Toyama 930-0194, Japan,

[b]Department of Anatomy and Neurobiology, Wakayama Medical College, 811-1 Kimiidera, Wakayama 641-8509, Japan

We investigated the distribution of H1-receptor (H1R) mRNA the dorsal root and trigeminal ganglia of mice. The positive signals were detected almost all the neurons in these ganglia in BALB/c, C57BL/6, ddY, and ICR mice. The results suggest that H1R is involved in many functions of primary sensory neurons.

1. INTRODUCTION

Pharmacological studies have suggested that subgroups of primary sensory neurons are responsive to histamine via histamine H1 receptor (H1R). In guinea-pigs, H1R mRNA is expressed in small, non-peptidergic neurons in sensory ganglia (1), and these neurons are implicated in the transmission of histamine-induced itch. But it is still unknown whether H1R mRNA is expressed in the mouse ganglia. We have previously shown that histamine injected intradermally into the rostral back elicited prominent scratching, a behavior associated with itch, in ICR mice, but not at all in other strains of mice. Therefore, in the present study, we investigated the gene expression of H1R mRNA in sensory ganglia in various strains of mice by means of in situ hybridization (ISH) histochemistry.

2. MATERIAL & METHODS

Male BALB/c, C57BL/6, ddY and ICR mice of 5 weeks of age were used. The animals were transcardially perfused with 4% paraformaldehyde under deep anaesthesia. Frozen sections (8 μm thickness) of dorsal root ganglia (L4-L6) and trigeminal ganglia were hybridized with ^{35}S-labeled cRNA probe (antisense probe, 327 bp / sense probe, 361 bp) for mouse H1R mRNA. Emulsified sections were exposed in the dark for 3 weeks.

---

*Corresponding author. Tel.: +81 76 4347510; fax: +81 76 4345045

388

3. RESULTS

Almost all the neurons in dorsal root ganglia were intensely labeled with signals for H1R mRNA (Fig.1). There were no apparent differences in populations or intensity of labeled neurons between BALB/c, C57BL/6, ddY, and ICR strains. The corresponding sense probe did not show positive signals (data not shown), suggesting that the antisense probe recognised H1R mRNA in the murine sensory neurons. H1R mRNA in trigeminal ganglia were also expressed both small and large cells (data not shown).

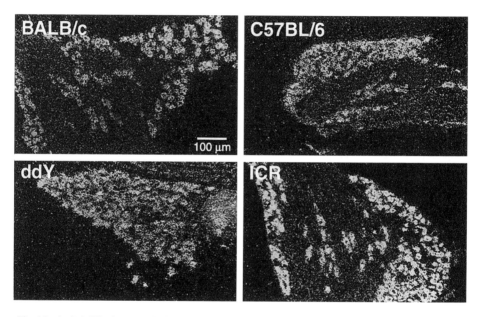

Fig. 1 In situ hybridization analysis for H1-receptor mRNA in the dorsal root ganglia of BALB/c, C57BL/6, ddY, and ICR mice. Sections from dorsal root ganglia were hybridized with a ^{35}S-labeled antisense probe.

4. DISCUSSION

The present results that H1R mRNA is expressed in many and all types of sensory neurons in mice of all the strains examined are inconsistent with the results of ISH study in guinea-pigs and scratching behavioral study in mice. At least in mice, H1R may be involved in many functions of primary sensory neurons

REFERENCES

1. H. Kashiba, H. Fukui, Y. Morikawa, and E. Senba. Mol. Brain Res. 66 (1999) 24.

Histamine Research in the New Millennium
T. Watanabe, H. Timmerman and K. Yanai (Editors)

L-Histidine decarboxylase protein and activity in rat brain microvascular endothelial cells

E. Sakurai[a], J. Yamakami[b], Y. Tanaka[a], A. Kuramasu[c], E. Sakurai[c], K. Yanai[c] and T. Watanabe[c]

[a]Department of Pharmaceutics I, Tohoku Pharmaceutical University,
4-4-1 Komatsushima, Aoba-ku, Sendai 981-8558, Japan

[b]Department of Pharmacy, Sapporo National Hospital,
4-2 Kikushui, Shiroishi-ku, Sapporo 003-0804, Japan

[c]Department of Cellular Pharmacology, Tohoku University School of Medicine,
2-1 Seiryo-machi, Aoba-ku, Sendai 980-8575, Japan

Brain microvascular endothelial cells (BMEC) are major structural and functional components of the blood-brain barrier (BBB) that maintain the homeostasis of the central nervous system. Histamine has been shown to increase BBB permeability and induce parenchymal cell swelling. Therefore, it is of interest to investigate the transport mechanism of L-histidine across the blood to brain of BBB and metabolism of L-histidine uptaken by rat BMEC. L-Histidine decarboxylase (HDC: EC4.1.1.22) catalyzes the formation of histamine from L-histidine. In the present study, we examined the uptake system of L-histidine in cultured rat BMEC. Moreover, this study was carried out to examine whether the BMEC have the ability to form histamine, and whether HDC mRNA is expressed in rat BMEC.

Male, 3-week-old Wistar rats were used. For in vitro studies, rat BMEC were isolated from rat brains, and subculture cells were grown on collagen-coated culture flask. The uptake rate of L-histidine, HDC assay, immunofluorescence analysis and expression of HDC mRNA by RT-PCR were performed in rat BMEC.

L-Histidine uptake was a saturable process. A decrease in incubation temperature from 37 to 0 °C or the addition of metabolic inhibitors (DNP and rotenone) reduced the uptake rate of L-histidine. Ouabain, an inhibitor of (Na^+, K^+)-ATPase, also reduced uptake of L-histidine. Moreover, the substitution of Na^+ with choline chloride and choline bicarbonate in the incubation buffer decreased the initial L-histidine uptake rate. The results suggested that L-histidine is actively uptaken by a carrier-

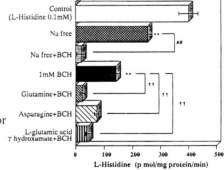

Figure 1. Rate of uptake of L-histidine into rat BMEC.
**, ##, † † $P < 0.01$

mediated mechanism into the BMEC, with energy supplied by Na^+. However, L-histidine uptake at 0 ℃ was not completely inhibited, and it was reduced in the presence of an Na^+-independent System-L substrate, BCH, suggesting facilitated diffusion (the Na^+-independent process) by a carrier-mediated mechanism into the BMEC. L-Histidine uptake in rat BMEC also appeared to be System-N mediated since uptake was inhibited by glutamine, asparagine and L-glutamic acid γ-monohydroxamate (Figure 1). System-N mediated transport was not pH sensitive.

The HDC activity in rat BMEC was estimated to be 0.14 $\pm$ 0.05 pmol/min/mg protein. This activity was completely inhibited by 1.0 μ M of (S)-α-Fluoromethylhistidine (FMH), a specific inhibitor of HDC (Figure 2). Rat BMEC contained L-histidine of 3.00 $\pm$ 0.14 nmol/mg protein and histamine of 2.18 $\pm$ 0.10 pmol/mg protein. Moreover, when rat BMEC were cultured with FMH (50 μ M), the concentration of histamine decreased 97.8 %. These results suggested that HDC is present in the endothelial cells of rat microvessels. Using a polyclonal anti HDC antibody and immunofluorescence microscopy, we confirmed the presence of HDC protein in rat BMEC. Moreover, RT-PCR products of RNA amplified with specific primers of rat HDC cDNA in rat BMEC are shown in Figure 3. Rat HDC cDNA plasmid was used as a positive control template. In this cell, HDC mRNA was expressed. However, the expression of HDC mRNA in rat BMEC extracts was low compared with that in the rat basophilic leukemia cells (RBL-2H3).

Conclusion: Our study demonstrated that L-histidine uptaken by both System-N and –L transporters into rat BMEC was shown to be converted histamine, suggesting that HDC in BMEC plays an important role in BBB (1,2).

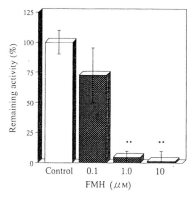

Figure 2. Inactivation of HDC by FMH
** P < 0.01, compared with control.

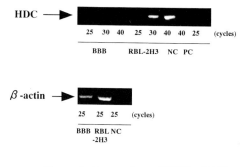

Figure 3. Expression of HDC mRNA in rat BMEC and rat basophilic leukemia cells (RBL-2H3)

REFERENCES
1. J. Yamakami, E. Sakurai, T. Sakurada, K. Maeda and N. Hikichi, Brain Res., 812 (1998) 105
2. J. Yamakami, E. Sakurai, A. Kuramasu, E. Sakurai, K. Yanai, T. Watanabe and Y. Tanaka, Inflamm. Res., 49 (2000) 231.

Allergy, Inflamation and Immunology

Histamine Research in the New Millennium
T. Watanabe, H. Timmerman and K. Yanai (Editors)

Participation of histamine H1 and H2 receptors in the induction of scratching behavior in ICR mice caused by IgE-mediated passive cutaneous anaphylaxis

N. Inagaki, M. Nagao, N. Nakamura, K. Igeta, J.F. Kim and H. Nagai

Department of Pharmacology, Gifu Pharmaceutical University,
5-6-1 Mitahorahigashi, Gifu 502-8585, Japan

ICR mice produced frequent scratching behavior and vascular permeability increase upon induction of passive cutaneous anaphylaxis (PCA), injection of compound 48/80 or histamine. Histamine H1 receptor antagonists inhibited the scratching behavior and vascular permeability increase. In contrast, histamine H2 receptor antagonists inhibited histamine-induced scratching behavior but not vascular permeability increase. Combination of histamine H1 and H2 receptor antagonists resulted in a synergism and histamine-induced scratching behavior could be abrogated. Histamine H1 and H2 receptors seem to participate in scratching behavior caused by PCA in ICR mice.

1. INTRODUCTION

Scratching behavior in some experimental animals such as rats, guinea pigs and monkeys has been employed as a model for investigating the mechanism of itch. In 1995, Kuraishi et al. reported that mouse scratching behavior could also be useful for studying itch [1]. Histamine is an important mediator for causing itch in humans. Intradermal injection of histamine at up to 50 nmol, however, fails to induce scratching behavior in many strains of mice except for a few strains including ICR [2]. ICR is the best responder strain among them. Similar results have been obtained in the case of serotonin at 1 nmol and substance P at 50 nmol. Therefore, ICR mice may be sensitive for stimuli causing scratching behavior. PCA established by Ovary involves mast cell activation and vascular permeability increase by mast cell mediators. Histamine and serotonin are the major vasoactive mediators released from rodent mast cells. ICR is a good responder strain for PCA.

2. METHODS

Mouse behavior was recorded in the absence of an observer using a video camera and then scratching behavior to the reaction site with the hindpaws was counted. Vascular

394

permeability increase was evaluated by measuring the extravasated dye.

3. RESULTS AND DISCUSSION [3,4]

Elicitation of IgE-mediated PCA, intradermal injection of compound 48/80 or histamine induced frequent scratching behavior and vascular permeability increase in ICR mice. Cetirizine and terfenadine inhibited the vascular permeability increase almost completely, whereas they could not inhibit scratching behavior completely. Similarly, oxatomide and epinastine inhibited the vascular permeability increase by PCA completely but scratching behavior partially. These results indicate that histamine is the major vasoactive mediator released from activated mast cells. It is also indicated that histamine increases vascular permeability predominantly through histamine H1 receptors, but that scratching behavior is induced not only through histamine H1 receptors but also through other types of histamine receptors. On the other hand, famotidine and ranitidine, histamine H2 receptor antagonists, partially inhibited the histamine-induced scratching behavior without affecting the vascular permeability increase. Furthermore, the histamine-induced scratching behavior was abolished by the simultaneous treatment with cetirizine and ranitidine. Therefore, histamine is considered to induce scratching behavior in ICR mice through both histamine H1 and H2 receptors. In contrast, although ranitidine also inhibited the scratching behavior induced by PCA, the simultaneous treatment with cetirizine and ranitidine failed to abolish it. This suggests a possibility that different mediators other than histamine also participate in the scratching behavior by PCA, although the participation is small.

In humans, many attempts have been made to find an additional benefit of simultaneous treatment with histamine H1 and H2 receptor antagonists for the treatment of itch. Among them, Davies et al. [5] and Monroe et al. [6] have shown some merit. Therefore, histamine H2 receptors may also be involved in the mediation of pruritus in humans. The role of histamine H2 receptors in the human itch, however, has not yet been established.

REFERENCES

1. Y. Kuraishi, T. Nagasawa, K. Hayashi and M. Satoh, Eur. J. Pharmacol. 275 (1995) 229.
2. N. Inagaki, M. Nagao, K. Igeta, H. Kawasaki, J.F. Kim and H. Nagai, Skin. Pharmacol. in press.
3. N. Inagaki, N. Nakamura, M. Nagao, K. Musoh, H. Kawasaki and H. Nagai, Eur. J. Pharmacol. 367 (1999) 361.
4. N. Inagaki, M. Nagao, N. Nakamura, H. Kawasaki, K. Igeta, K. Musoh and H. Nagai, Eur. J. Pharmacol. 400 (2000) 73.
5. M.G. Davies, R. Marks, R.J. Horton and F.E. Storari, Arch. Dermatol. Res. 266 (1979) 117.
6. E.W. Monroe, S.H. Cohen, J. Kalbfleisch and C.I. Schulz, Arch. Dermatol. 117 (1981) 404.

Histamine Research in the New Millennium
T. Watanabe, H. Timmerman and K. Yanai (Editors)

Immediate-type hypersensitivity and helper T cell function in histamine H1 receptor- and H2 receptor-deficient mice.

Takashi Kobayashi, Ritsuko Koga, Yasmin Banu and Takeshi Watanabe

Department of Molecular Immunology, Medical Institute of Bioregulation, Kyushu University, Fukuoka 812-8582, Japan

It is well known that histamine is one of major chemical mediators of immediate-type hypersensitivity. Pharmacological studies have been also suggested that histamine may affect function of Th1 and Th2 helper T cells via a signal(s) from their receptors. Histamine receptors are classified into three subclasses, termed H1, H2 and H3. To evaluate the significance of H1 and H2 receptors on anaphylaxis and regulation of helper T cell function, we analyzed mice lacking histamine H1 receptor (H1R) or histamine H2 receptor (H2R), which were produced by gene targeting. Our results clearly indicate that the increased vascular permeability in cutaneous anaphylaxis induced by histamine, IgE and allergens is exclusively regulated by H1R-mediated signaling(s) but not by H2R or H3R. Moreover, the signals from H1R positively regulate cytokine production by Th1 cells, whereas those from H2R negatively regulate cytokine production by Th2 cells.

1. Methods

The histamine H1 receptor (H1R) knockout mice and the histamine H2 receptor (H2R) knockout mice were established in our lab and described previously (1-3). These mutant 129 x C57BL/6 mice were maintained by brother-sister interbreeding and white-coat color lines were segregated and used in the skin reaction tests. These mutant mice were also backcrossed to C57BL/6 and used in the cytokine assay. The mice were maintained in our animal facility under pathogen free conditions with proper aeration, light and temperature. Cutaneous anaphylaxis was assessed by three types of test; Mediator Skin Reaction (MSR), Passive Cutaneous Anaphylaxis (PCA) and Active Cutaneous anaphylaxis (ACA). Briefly, MSR was elicited by intradermal injection of either histamine or serotonin into the ear followed by an intravenous injection of Evans Blue dye saline solution. PCA was elicited by injection of anti-DNP IgE mAb followed by an intravenous injection of a mixture of TNP and dye four hours later. ACA was elicited in the ear of OVA-immunized mice by injection of antigen followed by an intravenous

Correspondence should be addressed to Dr.Takeshi Watanabe, Medical Institute of Bioregulation, Kyushu University. 3-1-1 Maidashi, Higashi-ku, Fukuoka 812-8582, Japan.

injection of dye. Production of IL-2, IL-4, IL-13 and IFN-γ by spleen T cells from the mutant mice upon stimulation with antigen or anti-CD3 mAb was measured by ELISA.

2. Results

2.1 H1R but not H2R or H3R is obligatory for elicitation of cutaneous anaphylaxis.

Increased vascular permeability was assessed by three types of test; Mediator Skin Reaction (MSR), Passive Cutaneous Anaphylaxis (PCA) and Active Cutaneous Anaphylaxis (ACA). The allergic reactions induced by histamine, anti-DNP IgE and antigen (OVA) were markedly suppressed in H1R-deficient mice, but normal responses were elicited in H2R-deficient mice. Double deficient mice of H1R and H2R also exhibited reduced vascular permeability.

Our results strongly indicate that H1R is solely obligatory for elicitation of the cutaneous anaphylaxis. Serotonin increased vascular permeability in H1R-deficient mice, however the intensity was lesser than that of wild-type mice, indicating that histamine-H1R signaling is partially involved in cutaneous anaphylaxis induced by serotonin.

2.2 Signal(s) from H1R up-regulate cytokine production by Th1 helper T cells, whereas signal(s) from H2R down-regulate cytokine production by Th1 and Th2 cells

Spleen T cells from wild type, H1R- and H2R-deficient mice were cultured in anti-CD3ε antibody-coated plates or in the presence of antigen. The amounts of secreted cytokines were determined by ELISA. Production of IFNγ was greatly reduced in H1R-deficient mice, whereas that was rather increased in H2R-deficient mice. IL-13 production was remarkably enhanced in H2R-deficient mice. These results suggest that signal(s) from H1R positively regulate Th1 activation, and histamine acts as a co-stimulator for Th1 cells. In contrast, signal(s) from H2R play a role in negative regulation in activation of Th2 helper T cells.

3. Conclusion

Histamine plays a crucial role in the induction of immediate-type hypersensitivity through histamine H1 receptor (H1R), but also in the cease of allergic reaction through H2R on Th2 type helper T cells and H1R on Th1 cells by down-regulating cytokine production such as IL-13 and IL-4 and up-reguting IFNγ production.

References:

1.I. Inoue et al., Proc. Nat. Acad. Sci. USA. 93 (1996) 13316.
2.Y. Banu and T. Watanabe, J. Exp. Med. 189 (1999) 673.
3.T. Kobayashi, S. Tonai, Y. Ishihara, R. Koga, S. Okabe and T. Watanabe, J. Clin. Invest. 105 (2000) 1741.

Histamine Research in the New Millennium
T. Watanabe, H. Timmerman and K. Yanai (Editors)

IL-18 production induced by histamine in human PBMCs through H2 receptor stimulation

H. Kohka[a,b,c], M. Nishibori[a], H. Iwagaki[b], T. Yoshino[c], N. Nakaya[a], K. Saeki[a], T. Akagi[c] and N. Tanaka[b]

[a]Department of Pharmacology, [b]Department of Surgery I and [c]Department of Pathology, Okayama University Medical School, 2-5-1 Shikata-cho, Okayama 700-8558, Japan

Histamine concentration-dependently stimulated the production of IL-18 and IFN-γ, and inhibited those of IL-2 and IL-10 in human peripheral blood mononuclear cells (PBMCs). Histamine caused cytokine responses solely through the stimulation of H2-receptors.

1. Introduction

Histamine is a well-known mediator of inflammation and allergic response. The estimated functional roles of histamine as immunomodulator were often controversial probably due to the differences in the cell preparations used and the complexity of the involvement of histamine in immunomodulation (1,2). In the present study, we investigated the effects of histamine on cytokine production in human PBMCs and found that histamine is a potent inducer of IL-18 production in this preparation.

2. Materials and Method

PBMCs (5×10^5 cells/ ml) were incubated with histamine or H1-, H2-, H3-receptor agonist in the presence or absence of H1-, H2-, H3-receptor antagonists. After culture, the cell-free supernatant fractions were assayed for IL-18, IL-12, IL-2, IFN-γ and IL-10 protein, which were measured using Elisa employing the multiple Abs sandwich principle.

3. Results and Discussion

Histamine (10^{-7}- 10^{-4} M) concentration-dependently stimulated the production of IL-18 and IFN-γ, and inhibited those of IL-2 and IL-10 in human PBMCs. The stimulatory or inhibitory effects of histamine on the cytokine production were all antagonized by H2-receptor antagonists ranitidine and famotidine concentration-dependently, but not by H1- and H3-receptor antagonists. Selective H2-receptor agonists, 4-methylhistamine and dimaprit mimicked the effects of histamine on five kinds of cytokine production. The EC50 values of histamine, 4-methylhistamine and dimaprit for the production of IL-18 were 1.5,

398

1.0 and 3.8 μM, respectively. These findings indicated that histamine caused cytokine responses through the stimulation of H2-receptors. All effects of histamine on cytokine responses were also abolished by the presence of either anti-IL-18 antibody or IL-1β-converting enzyme/ caspase-1 inhibitor, indicating that the histamine action is dependent on mature IL-18 secretion and that IL-18 production is located upstream of the cytokine cascade activated by histamine. Addition of recombinant human IL-18 to the culture concentration-dependently stimulated IL-12 and IFN-γ production and inhibited the IL-2 and IL-10 production. IFN-γ production induced by IL-18 was inhibited by anti-IL-12 antibody, showing the marked contrast of the effect of histamine. Histamine thus is a very important modulator of Th1 cytokine production in PBMCs and is quite unique in triggering IL-18-initiating cytokine cascade without inducing IL-12 production.

REFERENCES

1. K. Hellstrand, A. Asea, C. Dahlgren, and S. Hermodsson J. Immunol. 153 (1994) 4940.
2. S. Laberge, W. W. Cruikshank, H. Kornfeld, and D. M. Center, J. Immunol. 155 (1995) 2902.
3. H. Kohka, M. Nishibori, H. Iwagaki, N. Nakaya, T. Yoshino, K. Kobashi, K. Saeki, N. Tanaka, and T. Akagi, J. Immunol. 164 (2000) 6640.

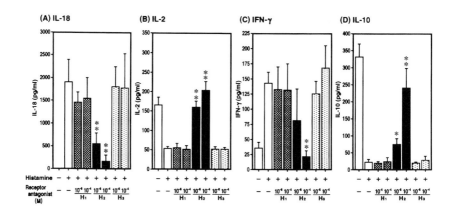

Fig. 1 Effects of histamine receptor antagonists on modulatory effects of histamine on cytokine production in PBMCs. PBMCs were cultured with 100 μM histamine in the presence of d-chlorpheniramine (H1 antagonist), famotidine (H2 antagonist) , or thioperamide (H3 antagonist) for 24 h. At the end of the culture, the concentrations of IL 18, IL-2, IFN-γ and IL-10 in the conditioned media were determined by Elisa. The results are the means ± SEM of three different donors. *P < 0.05, **P < 0.01 as compared with the value in the presence of histamine alone. (Reproduced from ref. 3 with the permission of the American Association of Immunologists)

Histamine Research in the New Millennium
T. Watanabe, H. Timmerman and K. Yanai (Editors)

Regulatory mechanism of eosinophil peroxidase release from guinea pig eosinophils

Y. Kirino, M. Mio and C. Kamei

Department of Pharmacology, Faculty of Pharmaceutical Sciences, Okayama University, Okayama 700-8530, Japan

A23187 stimulated eosinophil peroxidase (EPO) release from eosinophils. β-Agonists, such as isoproterenol, salbutamol and fenoterol, effectively inhibited A23187-induced EPO release mediated through β_2-adrenoceptor. Theophylline, rolipram, a selective phosphodiesterase (PDE) IV inhibitor, and dibutyryl-cAMP (db-cAMP) also significantly inhibited A23187-induced EPO release. The inhibition of EPO release induced by db-cAMP was attenuated by pretreatment with KT5720, a protein kinase A inhibitor. These results suggest that an increase in intracellular cAMP level may lead to activation of protein kinase A, which contributes to inhibition of EPO release. Calphostin C and cytochalasin D effectively inhibited A23187-induced EPO release, indicating that protein kinase C and microfilaments were involved in EPO release from eosinophils

Keywords : eosinophils, eosinophil peroxidase, β-agonists, phosphodiesterase

1.INTRODUCTION

It has been suggested that activated eosinophils liberate cytotoxic proteins such as eosinophil peroxidase (EPO), aggravating allergic inflammation. Therefore, it may be useful for the treatment of allergic diseases to determine the mechanism of eosinophil degranulation and to identify drugs that can inhibit the release of cytotoxic proteins from eosinophils. In the present study, the effects of several drugs on A23187-induced EPO release were investigated

2. MATERIAL AND METHODS

Male Hartly strain guinea pigs were injected intraperitoneally once a week with 1 mg/animal of polymyxin B sulfate. Six weeks later, the peritoneal exudate cells were collected, and the eosinophils were purified to greater than 95% of purity by centrifugation through a gradient of isotonic Percoll [1, 2].

Various concentrations of test compounds were added to eosinophils, and then various concentrations of A23187 were added followed by incubation for 60 min at 37°C. Thereafter, the eosinophils were centrifuged, and then both supernatant and cell pellet were assayed for EPO enzyme activity [1, 2].

3. RESULTS

Ca ionophore A23187 stimulated EPO release from guinea pig eosinophils. Isoproterenol, salbutamol, and fenoterol inhibited A23187-induced EPO release (Table 1). Both propranolol and ICI 118,551, a selective β_2-antagonist, antagonized the inhibitory effects of β-agonists on A23187-induced EPO release. Theophylline, rolipram, and db-cAMP also inhibited A23187-induced EPO release. The inhibition of EPO release caused by db-cAMP was attenuated by KT5720, a protein kinase A inhibitor. Moreover, calphostin C, a protein kinase C inhibitor, and cytochalasin D inhibited A23187-induced EPO release.

Table 1. Effects of β-agonists on A23187-induced EPO release from eosinophils

β-Agonists	0	10^{-8}	10^{-7}	10^{-6}	10^{-5} (M)
Isoproterenol	21.2 ± 1.5	15.6 ± 2.6	$13.0 \pm 2.9^*$	$9.6 \pm 2.3^{**}$	$5.5 \pm 1.0^{**}$
Salbutamol	23.7 ± 1.0	21.7 ± 2.8	20.4 ± 1.9	16.8 ± 2.5	$13.7 \pm 1.9^{**}$
Fenoterol	21.0 ± 2.0	20.1 ± 1.8	18.1 ± 2.4	$13.2 \pm 2.1^*$	$7.9 \pm 1.7^{**}$

Eosinophils were preincubated with β-agonists for 5 min, and then the cells were stimulated with 5×10^{-7} M A23187 for 60 min. Each value represents the mean of % EPO release $\pm$ S.E.M. * and ** indicate significant differences from the groups treated with A23187 alone at $p<0.05$ and $p<0.01$, respectively (n=6).

4. DISCUSSION

From these findings, it is concluded that an increase in intracellular Ca concentration may lead to exocytosis of eosinophil granules through activation of protein kinase C and microfilaments. Intracellular cAMP-elevating agents may be responsible for the inhibition of eosinophil degranulation through activation of protein kinase A.

REFERENCES

1. Y. Kirino, M. Mio and C. Kamei, Jpn. J. Pharmacol. 83 (2000) 293.
2. M. Mio, Y. Kirino and C. Kamei, J. Allergy Clin. Immunol. 106 (2000) 896.

© 2001 Elsevier Science B.V. All rights reserved.
Histamine Research in the New Millennium
T. Watanabe, H. Timmerman and K. Yanai (Editors)

Induction of VEGF expression by histamine in the granulation tissue in rats

A. K. Ghosh, N. Hirasawa and K. Ohuchi

Laboratory of Pathophysiological Biochemistry, Graduate School of Pharmaceutical Sciences, Tohoku University, Sendai, Miyagi 980-8578, Japan.

Roles of histamine in vascular endothelial growth factor (VEGF) expression and angiogenesis in carrageenin-induced granulation tissue in rats were analyzed. Incubation of the minced granulation tissue in the presence of histamine (0.1 - 10 μM) increased VEGF protein and its mRNA expression in a time- and concentration-dependent manner. The histamine-induced VEGF production was suppressed by the H2 receptor antagonist cimetidine (10 μM), the cAMP antagonist Rp-cAMP (100 μM), and the protein kinase A inhibitor H-89 (50 μM). Intra-pouch injection of cimetidine (400 μg) and indomethacin (100 μg) additively suppressed the carrageenin-induced increase in the pouch fluid accumulation, the granulation tissue formation, VEGF protein levels both in the granulation tissue and in the pouch fluid, and angiogenesis in the granulation tissue. These findings indicate that histamine has an activity to induce VEGF production via the H2 receptor - cAMP - protein kinase A pathway and augments angiogenesis in the granulation tissue.

1. INTRODUCTION

Histamine is produced in the rapidly growing tissue, and suggested to promote neoplastic growth and neovascularization. In a carrageenin-induced air pouch-type inflammation model in rats, we found that the angiogenesis markedly occurs during the formation of the granulation tissue, which produces VEGF [1] , and histamine level in the pouch fluid increases time-dependently after the carrageenin injection [2]. Therefore, we analyzed the roles of histamine in the induction of VEGF and angiogenesis in the granulation tissue in rats *in vitro* and *in vivo*.

2. MATERIALS AND METHODS

Air pouch-type inflammation was induced in male Sprague-Dawley rats, specific pathogen-free, weighing 160-170 g (Charles River Japan, Inc., Kanagawa, Japan), by injecting the carrageenin solution into the air pouch on the dorsum [1]. *In vitro* and *in vivo* studies were carried out as described previously [1]. VEGF protein levels in the conditioned medium and in the supernatant fractions of the granulation tissue homogenate and the pouch fluid were determined by Western blot analysis. VEGF mRNA levels in the minced granulation tissue were determined by RT-PCR, and angiogenesis in the granulation tissue was assessed by carmine dye method

[1]. VEGF-producing cells in the minced granulation tissue were analyzed by immunostaining.

3. RESULTS

Histamine (0.1 - 10 μM) increased VEGF content in the conditioned medium in a time- and concentration-dependent manner. mRNA levels for the three isoforms of VEGF in the granulation tissue were also increased by histamine in a concentration-dependent manner with a maximum at 1 h. VEGF levels in the minced granulation tissue reached a maximum at 3 h and then declined. The upregulation of VEGF expression by histamine was suppressed by the H2 receptor antagonist cimetidine (10 μM), but not by the H1 receptor antagonist pyrilamine (100 μM), the H3 receptor antagonist thioperamide (100 μM) or the cyclooxygenase inhibitor indomethacin (1 μM). The histamine-induced VEGF production was inhibited by the cAMP antagonist Rp-cAMP (100 μM) and the protein kinase A inhibitor H-89 (50 μM). In contrast, the protein kinase C inhibitors Ro 31-8425 and calphostin C or the tyrosine kinase inhibitor genistein showed no effect. Injection of cimetidine (400 μg) into the air pouch decreased the pouch fluid volume, the granulation tissue weight, VEGF levels both in the granulation tissue and in the pouch fluid, and angiogenesis in the granulation tissue. Combined local treatment with cimetidine (400 μg) and indomethacin (100 μg) showed additive effects. Histochemical analysis demonstrated that histamine increased the number of cells stained by anti-VEGF, and the VEGF-positive cells were macrophages, endothelial cells and fibroblast-like cells.

4. DISCUSSION

The histamine-induced VEGF expression was inhibited by the H2 receptor antagonist cimetidine but not by the H1 receptor antagonist pyrilamine or the H3 receptor antagonist thioperamide. The possibility that histamine induces VEGF by increasing PGE2 production [1] by the minced granulation tissue was excluded because indomethacin did not inhibit the histamine-induced VEGF production. Although there are several reports describing that cimetidine delays wound healing, the mechanism of action has not been clarified. The inhibition of the histamine-induced angiogenesis by cimetidine might contribute to the delay of the wound healing. The cAMP antagonist Rp-cAMP and the PKA inhibitor H-89 markedly inhibited VEGF production. In conclusion, our study demonstrated that histamine plays a significant role in the angiogenesis in the granulation tissue in rats by inducing VEGF expression through the H2 receptor - cAMP - PKA pathway.

REFERENCES

1. A.K. Ghosh, N. Hirasawa, H. Niki and K. Ohuchi, J . Pharmacol. Exp. Ther., 295 (2000) 802.
2. N. Hirasawa, M. Watanabe, S. Mue, S. Tsurufuji and K. Ohuchi, Inflammation, 15 (1991) 117.

© 2001 Elsevier Science B.V. All rights reserved.
Histamine Research in the New Millennium
T. Watanabe, H. Timmerman and K. Yanai (Editors)

Induction of histidine decarboxylase in the neointimal smooth muscle cells of balloon-injured porcine coronary arteries

Yang-Il Fang, Eriko Tsunoda, Takeharu Niioka, Kazutaka Momose

Department of Pharmacology, Showa University, School of Pharmaceutical Sciences, 1-5-8 Hatanodai, Shinagawa-ku, Tokyo 142-8555, Japan

Formation of neointima due to the proliferation of vascular smooth muscle cells is a common characteristic of the response of arterial wall to injury. To investigate the role of histamine in the formation of neointima, immunohistochemical changes of L-histidine decarboxylase (HDC), a histamine-forming enzyme, were examined in the balloon-injured porcine coronary artery. Intense immunostaining of HDC was observed in the neointimal smooth muscle cells. Western blot analysis revealed a 3.6-fold increase of 53 kDa HDC in the injured artery as compared to the uninjured artery. These results indicate a marked upregulation of HDC in the neointimal smooth muscle cells.

1. INTRODUCTION

Proliferation of vascular smooth muscle cells is a critical event in intimal thickening of the vascular wall accompanying restenosis after coronary angioplasty. In response to the clinical or experimental angioplasty, multiple peptide growth factors activate a fraction of medial smooth muscle cells to bring about the synthetic phenotype of smooth muscle cells which proliferate in the intima after the migration of the cells through the internal elastic lamina [1]. On the other hand, it has been reported that the induction of HDC, a histamine-forming enzyme, is implicated in the proliferation of cells in a number of growing tissues [2]. However, little is known about the role of histamine in the formation of neointima due to the proliferation of vascular smooth muscle cells. In the present study, we examined HDC immunoreactivity in the porcine coronary artery after exprimental balloon injury.

2. MATERIALS AND METHODS

The left circumflex coronary arteries of male pigs were injured using a clinical balloon catheter. Seven days after injury, the segments of balloon-injured arteries were removed in a block fashion and fixed with 2% paraformaldehyde. Transverse frozen sections (10 μm) were incubated with a 1:4000 dilution of rabbit antiserum against HDC (Euro-Diagnostica, Malmö, Sweden), followed by immunostaining using the avidin-biotin complex (ABC) method. Subsequently, they were developed with 3, 3'-diaminobenzidine tetrahydrochloride (DAB).

For western blot analysis of HDC in the coronary arteries, the neointima and media were mechanically stripped together from the adventitia with a pair of forceps. The protein extracts from the strips were fractionated in 10% SDS-polyacrylamide gels and electroblotted onto nitrocellulose membranes. The membranes were incubated with a 1:1500 dilution of rabbit antiserum against HDC and subsequently developed by the ABC method using DAB.

3. RESULTS

We examined the localization of HDC in the porcine coronary arteries with or without the inflation of balloon inserted in the vessel to give injury. Control coronary arteries which were not subjected to the balloon injury had no intimal cells between the endothelium and internal elastic lamina. When the balloon injury was performed, the luminal surface of the vessel was denuded of endothelium (not shown). Seven days after the injury, the formation of neointima was clearly noticeable, and the intense immunostaining for HDC was observed in the neointimal smooth

404

muscle cells (Fig. 1). In contrast, the staining in the medial layer was diffused and was much faint compared with that in the neointima. When the antibody against HDC was replaced with non-immuno rabbit serum, no immunostaining was observed in the coronary vessels tested.

Mammalian HDC is a homodimer containing two subunits with a molecular mass of approximately 53 kDa [2] and shows a single polypeptide band on SDS-polyacrylamide gels. To confirm the expression of HDC molecules in the neointima, those were extracted from porcine coronary artery at 7 days after the injury. Western-blot analysis revealed that 53 Kd protein, which is immunoreactive against HDC, increased 3.6-fold in the injured artery as compared with that in the control artery (Fig. 2).

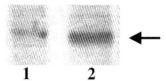

1   2

Fig. 2 Western blot analysis of HDC in balloon-injured porcine coronary artery. Lane 1, media from uninjured artery (control). lane 2, neointima / media from injured artery at 7 days after the operation. Arrows indicates the specific immunoreactive 53 kDa proteins for HDC

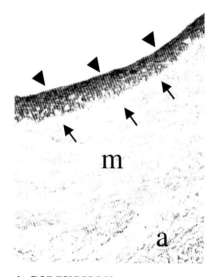

Fig. 1 Immunohistochemical detection of HDC in porcine coronary artery at 7 days after balloon-injury. A strong immunoreactive signal was seen in neointimal SMCs (arrowheads). Arrows indicates the internal elastic lamina; a, adventitia; m, media. Magnification X 400.

4. DISCUSSION

The major finding of the present study is the localization of intensive immunoreactivity for HDC in the neointimal smooth muscle cells of balloon-injured porcine coronary artery. Our results also demonstrated the increase in 53 kDa HDC in the injured artery. Previous ultrastructural studies have shown that most of the smooth muscle cells in the neointima have a synthetic phenotype during the formation of neointima [3]. These results indicate that a marked upregulation of HDC occurs in the synthetic smooth muscle cells of neointima after the balloon injury.

Histamine has been shown to be inducible by induction of HDC. The induced histamine has been suggested to play an important role in cell growth [2]. The activity of HDC has been reported to be high in a number of growing tissues such as healing of wound, embryogenesis, tissue transplantation, and malignant growth. In vitro studies, histamine is revealed to be a mitogen for fibroblast cells, airway smooth muscle cells, and carcinoma cells. In addition, histamine stimulates both migration and proliferation of vascular smooth muscle cells [4], and histamine receptor antagonists abolish the effect of histamine. Taken these reported facts into consideration, the upregulation of HDC in the neointimal smooth muscle cells may play a significant role in the formation of neointima.

REFERENCES
[1] C. Bauters, et al., Cardiovasc. Res., 31 (1996) 835.
[2] M. Hocker, Z. Zhang, T.J. Koh and T.C. Wang, Yale. J. Biol. Med., 69 (1996) 21.
[3] J. Thyberg, K.Blomgren, U. Hedin, M. Dryjski, Cell Tissue Res., 281 (1995) 421.
[4] L. Bell and J.A. Madri, Circ. Res., 65 (1989) 1057.

Histamine Research in the New Millennium
T. Watanabe, H. Timmerman and K. Yanai (Editors)

Localization of histamine N-methyltransferase in guinea pig tissues: an immunohistochemical study

A. Tahara, M. Nishibori, A. Ohtsuka, K. Sawada, J. Sakiyama, H. Kohka, N. Nakaya and K. Saeki

Departments of Pharmacology and Anatomy, and School of Health Sciences, Okayama University Medical School, 2-5-1 Shikata-cho, Okayama 700, Japan

Histamine plays very important roles in gastric acid secretion, inflammation or allergic response. Histamine N-methyltransferase (HMT)(EC 2.1.1.8) is crucial for the inactivation of histamine in the tissues. In the present study, we investigated the immunohistochemical localization of this enzyme in the guinea pig tissues using rabbit polyclonal antibody against bovine HMT and found the widespread distribution of strong HMT-like immunoreactivities (HMT-LI) in the alimentary, respiratory and genitourinary tracts. The widespread distribution of HMT-LI suggests that histamine plays many roles in different tissues.

1. Introduction

Histamine is stored in mast cells, basophils, enterochromaffin cells in the gastrointestinal tract, and histaminergic neurons in the central nervous system. The histamine released from storage or producing cells into extracellular space must be removed to terminate the effect of histamine on target cells. Although there are two main catabolic pathways of histamine in the tissues, methylation by HMT and oxidative deamination by diamine oxidase (EC 1.4.3.6) , the knowledge about the relative importance of two pathways in the catabolism of histamine in each tissue as well as the cellular localization of these enzymes is limited. In the previous study, we purified HMT from bovine brain (1). Recently, we raised specific antibody against bovine HMT (2). The antibody cross-reacted with HMT from different mammals including guinea-pig. In the present study, we investigated the immunohistochemical localization of HMT in the guinea pig tissues to better understand the inactivation of histamine in the tissues.

2. Materials and methods

The male Hartley guinea pig, weighing 250 g, was anesthetized with an intraperitoneal injection of pentobarbital sodium and perfused through the left ventricle with 50 ml of ice-cold saline followed by 500 ml of 10 % formalin in 0.01 M phosphate-buffered saline. The fixed tissues were dehydrated, embedded in paraffin and cut into serial sections of 5-7 μm thick. After blocking, rabbit anti-HMT antiserum (diluted to 1: 1500) was applied to the sections for one night at 4

℃. After washing, the sections were incubated with biotinylated anti-rabbit IgG goat IgG, and streptoavidin-peroxidase. The peroxidation reaction was developed using diaminobenzidine as a substrate in the presence of $NiCl_2$. The preimmune serum and the immune serum preabsorbed with purified guinea pig HMT did not stain any structure.

3. Results

Anti-bovine HMT antiserum recognized a single band in the samples from different guinea pig tissues on western blotting, which had the same size (33KDa) of purified HMT from guinea-pig intestine and brain. This indicated that antiserum cross-reacted with guinea pig HMT and the recognition by the antibody was specific for HMT. Immunohistochemical studies revealed that HMT-LI was distributed widely throughout the peripheral guinea-pig tissues. There were strong HMT-LI in the epithelial cells in the gastrointestinal tract, especially in the gastric fundus, duodenum and jejunum. The columnar epithelium in the gall bladder was also strongly positive. Almost all the myenteric plexus from stomach to colon was stained whereas the submucous plexus was not. Other strongly immunoreactive cells included the ciliated cells in the trachea and the transitional epithelium of the bladder. Intermediately immunoreactive cells contained islets of Langerhans, epidermis of the skin, alveolar cells in the lung, urinary tubules in the kidney and epithelium of semiferous tubules.

4. Discussion

The specific cells in the mucosal epithelium in the gastrointestinal tract were not immunostained. These distribution suggested the role of epithelial HMT for the inactivation of histamine from food. The acid-producing cells are parietal cells which are present in the deeper and inner portion of glandular body and have histamine H2-receptors. The relatively diffuse localization of HMT in the gastric mucosa corresponds to disposition of enterochromaffin-like cells and parietal cells, and suggests that histamine released from enterochromaffin-like cells may be taken up and catabolized in neibouring cells of enterochromaffin-like cells, contributing to the removal of histamine from interstitial fluid. The localization of HMT-LI in the myenteric plexus together with the finding that the histamine-immunoreactive nerve fibers were observed in the rat and guinea pig gut strongly suggested that the histaminergic transmission may be present in the myenteric plexus in the guinea pig gut. Strong HMT-LI ciliated cells in the trachea indicated the importance of epithelial HMT for the catabolism of histamine in the trachea because the supersensitivity of airway smooth muscle and mucous secretion to histamine was demonstrated to occur in animals with lesioned epithelial cell layer.

REFERENCES

1. M. Nishibori, R. Oishi, Y. Itoh and K. Saeki, Neurochem. Int., 19 (1991) 135.
2. M. Nishibori, A. Tahara, K. Sawada, J. Sakiyama, N. Nakaya and K. Saeki, Eur. J. Neurosci., 12 (2000) 415.

Signal Transduction

© 2001 Elsevier Science B.V. All rights reserved.
Histamine Research in the New Millennium
T. Watanabe, H. Timmerman and K. Yanai (Editors)

Agonist-mediated regulation of histamine H_1 receptors and Ca^{2+} signaling: Ca^{2+}/calmodulin-mediated regulation of receptor function and distribution

Shigeru Hishinuma

Department of Pharmacodynamics, Meiji Pharmaceutical University, Tokyo 204-8588, Japan.

In human U373 MG astrocytoma cells, agonist-induced, clathrin-mediated internalization of histamine H_1 receptors (H_1Rs) was inhibited by activation of Ca^{2+}/calmodulin (CaM), where Ca^{2+}/CaM-dependent enzymes, such as CaM kinase II and calcineurin (PP2B), and protein kinase C (PKC) were not involved. In contrast, H_1Rs were promptly desensitized before initiation of receptor internalization, which was dually regulated by desensitizing CaM kinase II and resensitizing PP2B via regulation of the agonist affinity for the H_1Rs. As a result, desensitization in the H_1R-mediated Ca^{2+} responses developed in a complex manner with a transient interruption by resensitization at its early stage, which might modulate a rapid and excess progress of desensitization even for accepting next stimuli coming. Thus, Ca^{2+}/CaM activated in response to agonist keeps H_1Rs on the cell surface membrane via CaM kinase II- and PP2B-independent mechanisms, while CaM kinase II and PP2B regulate the agonist affinity for H_1Rs to induce desensitization and resensitization, respectively. These suggest that Ca^{2+}/CaM plays a crucial role in a feedback modulation of both function and distribution of the G_q protein-coupled receptors in a smart manner, depending on changes in the intracellular Ca^{2+} concentration.

KEY WORDS

Histamine H_1 receptor, desensitization and internalization, calmodulin, CaM kinase II, protein phosphatase 2B, G protein-coupled receptor kinase.

1. INTRODUCTION

Many G protein-coupled receptors (GPCRs) undergo functional and distributional changes upon stimulation with agonist, i.e. desensitization and internalization of receptors. Phosphorylation of agonist-occupied GPCRs by G protein-coupled receptor kinases (GRKs) is thought to be a key event for induction of receptor desensitization and the subsequent arrestin-mediated internalization and protein phosphatase 2A (PP2A)-mediated resensitization (Figure 1). However, desensitization and internalization mechanisms of Ca^{2+}-mobilizing receptors coupled to the G_q family of G proteins, such as H_1Rs, have been much less studied, in particular, with respect to feedback modulation of the desensitization and internalization processes via the Ca^{2+}/CaM. In this paper, our novel findings on roles of Ca^{2+}/CaM in receptor desensitization and internalization are summarized.

410

2. DISCUSSION

A hypothesis for regulation of H_1Rs in human U373 MG cells is shown in Figure 1. Stimulation of H_1Rs with histamine increases intracellular Ca^{2+} concentration, which activates CaM. Ca^{2+}/CaM is known to inhibit GRK-mediated receptor phosphorylation *in vitro*, which might be account for inhibition of GRK-mediated receptor internalization to keep receptors on the cell surface [1]. Neither CaM kinase II nor PP2B is involved in the H_1R internalization [1]. On the other hand, CaM kinase II and PP2B are involved in regulation of the affinity of H_1Rs for histamine, resulting in a complex process of desensitization and resensitization in H_1R-mediated Ca^{2+} responses, i.e. appearance of a transient resensitization at the early stage of desensitizing process [2]. The decrease in the intracellular Ca^{2+} concentration even in the presence of agonist allows H_1Rs to be desensitized and proceed to internalization by canceling the Ca^{2+}/CaM-mediated inhibition of GRK-mediated mechanisms [1, 2]. Thus, Ca^{2+}/CaM plays a crucial role in determining the early process of desensitization and internalization of G_q protein-coupled receptors by regulating CaM kinase II and PP2B as well as GRKs, depending on changes in the intracellular Ca^{2+} concentration.

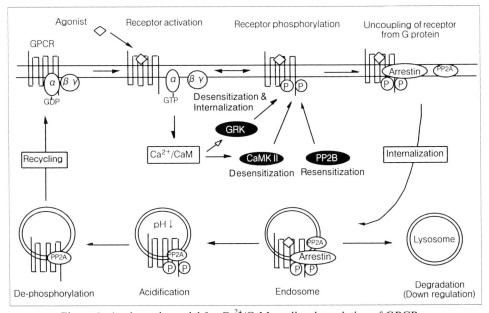

Figure 1. A schematic model for Ca^{2+}/CaM-mediated regulation of GPCRs.

ACKNOWLEDGMENTS
This work was supported by Grants-in-Aid for Scientific Research from the Ministry of Education, Science, Sports and Culture of Japan and from Meiji Pharmaceutical University.

REFERENCES
1. Hishinuma, S., Naiki, A., Tsuga, H. and Young, J.M. (1998). *J. Neurochem.*, **71**, 2626.
2. Hishinuma, S. and Ogura, K. (2000). *J. Neurochem.*, **75**, 772.

Histamine Research in the New Millennium
T. Watanabe, H. Timmerman and K. Yanai (Editors)

Involvement of protein kinase C in regulation of histamine H1 receptor expression in U373 astrocytoma cells.

Rumi Ishikawa, Kohji Kanayama, Maki Ogawa, Kumiko Saeki, Shuhei Horio and Hiroyuki Fukui.

Department of Pharmacology, Faculty of Pharmaceutical Sciences, University of Tokushima, Tokushima 770-8505, Japan.

1. Introduction

Histamine is a mediator of immune hypersensitivity in peripheral tissues and neurotransmitter in the central nervous system. Astrocytes express H1 receptors and are thought to function as target cells of histaminergic neurons [1]. U373 astrocytoma cells which express H1 receptors are useful for the study of H1 receptor-mediated histamine functions in astrocytes[2]. We observed that up-regulation of H1 receptors in U373 astrocytoma cells was induced by the treatment of 1 μ M phorbol-12-myristate-13acetate (PMA), a protein kinase C (PKC) activator.

The main role of H1 receptors is to transduce the histamine signal from outside to inside of cells. It is well known that signal transduction through H1 receptors is regulated by receptor desensitization. The onset of H1 receptor desensitization is very rapid, and its mechanism is thought to be involved in receptor phosphorylation [3]. On the other hand H1 receptors are synthesized through the receptor gene expression. The promoter of the H1 receptor gene possesses consensus sequences of inducer binding sites including AT-1, AT-2 and others [4]. The regulation of the H1 receptor gene expression has not been extensively investigated, and the effect of H1 receptor up-regulation on the receptor-mediated signaling has not been examined. We found that PMA induced H1 receptor up-regulation. In the present report, we describe that H1 receptor up-regulation is a regulatory mechanism of H1 receptor-mediated signaling.

keyword: hisatamine H1 receptor, protein kinase C (PKC), up-regulation, U373 astrocytoma

2. Materilas and Methods

Cell culture

U373 astrocytoma cells were cultured with DMEM/F12 containing 10 % fetal bovine serum and antibiotic-antimycotic (100 U/ml penicillin G sodium, 100 μ g/ml streptomycin sulfate, 0.25 μ g/ml fungizone in 85 % saline) under a humidified atomsphere of 5 % CO_2/95 % air at 37℃.

RT-PCR

Total RNA was converted to cDNA by reverse transcriptation and cDNA was subjected to PCR reaction. Denaturation was performed at 94℃ for 1 min, annealing was at 50℃ for 1 min and extention was at 72℃ for 2 min. Following H1 primers are used.

Sense   5'-AGC CAA TCC TTC TCT CGA-3'
Antisense   5'-TTA GGA GCG AAT ATG CAG-3'

Pyruvete kinase mRNA levels were determned simultaneously as the control.

Binding assay

Samples containing 4 nM [^{3}H]mepyramine with (non-specific) or without (total) 8 μM triprolidine were incubated at 25℃ for 1 hour. Bound and free radioligand in the sample was separated on a GR-B glassfiber filter under reduced pressure. GF-B fiters trapping bound radioligand were counted in a liquid scintilation counter.

Determination of inositol phosphates (IPs)

Myo-[^{3}H]inositol was incorporated into cells by culture with inositol-free DMEM containing 10 % dialyzed FBS for 24 hours. Then cells were stimulated by histamine. The stimulation was terminated by addition of 5 % TCA. TCA was neutralized, and [^{3}H]IPs was extracted by sonication. Samples were applied on AG1-x8 columns (Φ7.5 mm, volume of 0.5ml) and [^{3}H]IPs in samples were eluted by 5 ml solution of 1 M HCOONH4 and 0.1 M HCOOH. Then radioactivities were determined.

Statistical analysis

Data were analyzed by Student's unpaired t-test.

3. Results and Discussion

PMA-induced up-regulation of histamine H1 receptors

PMA, a PKC-activating phorbol ester, induced an increase in [^{3}H]mepyramine binding to membranes from U373 astrocytoma cells. [^{3}H]Mepyramine binding to U373 cell membranes treated by PMA for 20 hours was saturated by increasing concentrations of [^{3}H]mepyramine. Scatchard analysis showed that Bmax values for the control and PMA-treated membranes were 153.8 ± 3.5 fmol/mg protein and 308.4 ± 30.0 fmol/mg protein, respectively, and Kd values for control and PMA-treated membranes were 5.7 ± 1.4 nM and 5.7 ± 0.5 nM, respectively. The increase in [^{3}H]mepyramine binding was due to increased numbers of the binding site, i.e., up-regulation of the H1 receptor, and the affinity was not changed significantly. The up-regulation appeared 4 hours after the PMA treatment, and reached the maximal level 20 hours after PMA application (Fig 1. A). The PMA-induced up-regulation was suppressed to the level significantly below the control by the treatment of Ro 31-8220, a PKC inhibitor, 1 hour prior to PMA treatment. These results suggest that the PMA-induced up-regulation was mediated by the activation of PKC, and that in the cotrol cells H1 receptors are up-regulated a little by the activation of PKC to some extent.

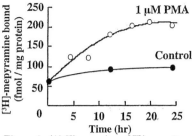
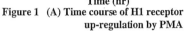
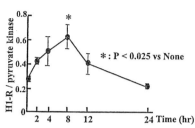

Figure 1 (A) Time course of H1 receptor
up-regulation by PMA

(B) Time course of H1 receptor mRNA level
by PMA

Preceding increase in H1 receptor mRNAs over the H1 receptor up-regulation

We examined whether increase in H1 receptor mRNAs was involved in this up-regulation.
As shown in Fig 1.B, the mRNA level also went time-dependently upword and reached maximum 8 hours after PMA treatment. The preceding increase in the receptor mRNAs over the
receptor up-regulation suggests the increased expression of the H1 receptor gene or the decreased degradation of the H1 receptor mRNAs. The mechanism remains to be elucidated.

Ro 31-8220 suppressed the PMA-induced increase in H1 receptor mRNAs to the level
below the control. This decrease in H1 receptor mRNAs is thought to precede over the
decrease in the level of H1 receptor by the PKC inhibitor.

Correlation between the number of expressed H1 receptors and H1 receptor-mediated signaling

We examined H1 receptor-mediated signaling by the accumulation of IPs. Histamine-
induced accumulation of IPs in U373 cells in which H1 receptors were up-regulated by PMA
was 1.5-fold that in the contol cells by the stimulation of histamine for 60 minutes. In
contrast, histamine-induced accumulation of IPs in PKC inhibitor-treated cells was 80 % that
in the control cells (Fig 2 .A). We found that there is a good correlation between the number
of expressed H1 receptors and H1 receptor-mediated signaling (Fig 2.B) In the present study
we revealed that the PKC activation-induced H1 receptor up-regulation is a novel regulatory
mechanism of H1 receptor signaling. Some bioactive substances were reported to induce H1
receptor up-regulation [5, 6] and H1 receptor up-regulation was observed in allergic diseases
[7]. The inhibition of this up-regulation mechanism will lead the development of new
therapeutic methods for H1 receptor-mediated pathological conditions.

414

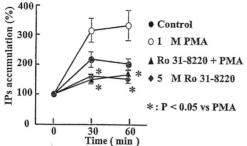
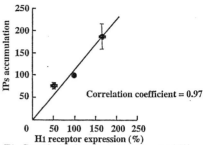

Figure 2 (A) Histamine induced accumulation of Ips
in U373 treated by PMA and / or Ro 31- 8220

Treatment of 1 µM PMA was carried out for 1hr and then
cells were cultured for 19 hr without PMA. Treatment of
5 µM Ro 31-8220 was carried out for 2 hrs and then cells
were cultured for 19 hrs without Ro 31-8220 (n = 3)

(B) Correlation between the amount of H1
receptor and H1 receptor signal transmission

In the horizontal axis H1 receptor expression of 132.2
fmol / mg protein was represented as 100 % . In the
vertical axis IPs accumulation of 0.5fmol / 105 cell /
hr was represented as 100 % .

References

[1] Inagaki N, Fukui H, Ito S, Yamatodani A, Wada H. Single type-2 astrocytes show
multiple independent sites of Ca^{2+} signaling in response to histamine. Proc. Natl. Acad.
Sci. USA. 88: 4215-4219 (1991)

[2] Hishinuma S, Young JM.. Characteristics of the binding of [^{3}H]-mepyramine to intact
human U373 MG astrocytoma cells: evidence for histamine-induced H1-receptor
internalisation. Br. J. Pharmacol 116: 2715-2723 (1995)

[3] Fujimoto K, Ohta K, Kanagawa K, Kikkawa U, Ogino S, Fukui H. Identification of
protein kinase C phosphorylation sites involved in phorbol ester-induced desensitization
of the histamine H1 receptor. Mol Pharmacol. 55: 735-742 (1999)

[4] De Backer MD, Loonen I, Verhasselt P, Neefs JM, Luyten WH. Structure of the human
histamine H1 receptor. Biochem. J. 335: 663-670 (1998)

[5] Takagishi T, Sasaguri Y, Nakano R, Arima N, Tanimoto A, Fukui H, Morimatsu M.
Expression of the histamine H1 receptor gene in relation to atherosclerosis. Am. J.
Pathol. 146: 981-988 (1995)

[6] Mak-JC, Roffel-AF, Katsunuma-T, Elzinga-CR, Zaagsma-J, Barnes-PJ. Up-regulation of
airway smooth muscle histamine H (1) receptor mRNA, protein, and function by beta (2)-
adrenoceptor activation. Mol.Pharmacol. 57: 857-864 (2000)

[7] N.Terada, N.Hamano, K.-I. Maesako, K. Hiruma, G.Hohki, K. Suzuki, K. Ishikawa, A.
Konno. Diesel exhaust particulates upregulate histamine receptor mRNA and increase
histamine-induced IL-8 and GM-CSF production in nasal epithelial cells and endothelial
cells. Cli. Exp. Allergy. 29: 52-59 (1999)

© 2001 Elsevier Science B.V. All rights reserved.
Histamine Research in the New Millennium
T. Watanabe, H. Timmerman and K. Yanai (Editors)

Glucose overload attenuates histamine H_2 receptor-mediated Ca^{2+} mobilization due to protein kinase C production in bovine cerebral endothelial cells.

M. Oike, C. Kimura and Y. Ito

Department of Pharmacology, Graduate School of Medical Sciences, Kyushu University, Fukuoka, 812-8582 Japan.

Intracellular Ca^{2+} concentration ($[Ca^{2+}]_i$) was measured in microvascular endothelial cells from bovine brain (BBEC). Effects of histamine on $[Ca^{2+}]_i$ was examined, and acute effect of changing extracellular glucose concentration on Ca^{2+} homeostasis was investigated. Application of 10µM histamine evoked an initial transient and following sustained increase in $[Ca^{2+}]_i$ in normal Krebs solution, but only the transient component in Ca^{2+} free solution, thereby indicating that histamine mobilizes Ca^{2+} both from intracellular store sites and extracellular space. The effects of histamine on $[Ca^{2+}]_i$ was inhibited by the H_2 antagonists, ranitidine and cimetidine, but not by the H_1 antagonist, pyrilamine. When histamine was applied to the cells pretreated with 23mM glucose for two hours, it failed to mobilize Ca^{2+} either from intracellular store site or extracellular space. Glucose overload-induced impairment of histamine action was reversed by pretreatment with staurosporine and calphostin C, and mimicked by phorbol-12,13-dibutyrate thereby suggesting the involvement of protein kinase C in the high glucose-induced inhibition of Ca^{2+} mobilization.
Keywords: calcium, endothelium, glucose, protein kinase C.

1. INTRODUCTION

In cerebral microvascular endothelial cells, only a few studies have been performed on the action of histamine on intracellular Ca^{2+} concentration ($[Ca^{2+}]_i$) (1,2), and characterization of the histamine receptor subtype is still controversial.

Cerebral endothelium of diabetic individuals is continuously exposed to high concentrations of glucose, and this has been supposed to cause diabetic cerebrovascular disorders (3). No study, however, has examined the acute effect of changing glucose concentration on cerebral endothelial Ca^{2+} homeostasis.

The aims of this study were firstly to characterize the subtype of histamine receptor that is involved in the regulation of $[Ca^{2+}]_i$ in bovine brain endothelial cells (BBEC), and secondarily to examine the acute effect of glucose overload on Ca^{2+} homeostasis in BBEC.

2. RESULTS AND DISCUSSION

2.1. Effects of histamine on $[Ca^{2+}]_i$ in BBEC.

BBEC was prepared from bovine brain gray matter by a Parcol gradient separation method (4). Collected endothelial cells were cultured in Dulbecco's modified Eagle medium.

Firstly we examined the effect of histamine on Ca^{2+} mobilization. On application of a submaximal concentration of histamine (10μM) in Ca^{2+} containing Krebs solution, a slowly developing transient elevation of $[Ca^{2+}]_i$ was observed. This declined to a new plateau level which was higher than the resting level of $[Ca^{2+}]_i$. The slowly occurring transient elevation of $[Ca^{2+}]_i$ was similarly observed on application of histamine (10μM) in Ca^{2+} free solution, but there was no sustained elevation.

When the cells were pretreated with pyrilamine, H_1 antagonist, subsequent application of 10μM histamine in Ca^{2+} free solution produced a similar increase in $[Ca^{2+}]_i$ as in the control. In contrast, in the presence of ranitidine or cimetidine, H_2 antagonists, histamine failed to increase $[Ca^{2+}]_i$ in Ca^{2+} free solution. These results indicate that, in BBEC, histamine mobilizes Ca^{2+} from intracellular store sites and the following Ca^{2+} entry by the activation of H_2 receptors.

2.2. Effects of glucose overload on histamine-induced Ca^{2+} transient in BBEC.

In an attempt to investigate the effects of glucose overload on Ca^{2+} homeostasis, we measured $[Ca^{2+}]_i$ with high concentrations of extracellular glucose (23mM; two times higher than normal) in Krebs. Cells were incubated with these solutions for two hours before each experiment. Histamine (10μM) failed to induce any change in $[Ca^{2+}]_i$ in high glucose-treated cells. These results indicate that acute glucose overload impairs histamine-induced Ca^{2+} mobilization in BBEC.

2.3. Restoration of high glucose-induced impairment of Ca^{2+} transient in BBEC.

It has been reported for vascular smooth muscle and endothelial cells that acute elevation of extracellular glucose activates protein kinase C (5). Therefore, we investigated the effects of staurosporine and calphostin C, protein kinase C inhibitors, and phorbol-12,13-dibutyrate (PDBu), a protein kinase C activator, on high glucose-induced impairment of histamine action. Staurosporine as well as calphostin C reversed the attenuation of histamine-induced Ca^{2+} transient in high glucose condition.   When cells were pretreated with PDBu in normal Krebs solution, histamine did not induce $[Ca^{2+}]_i$ elevation.   These indicate the involvement of protein kinase C in the high glucose-induced impairments of Ca^{2+} mobilization.

3. CONCLUSION

In conclusion, in BAEC, histamine mobilizes Ca^{2+} both from intracellular Ca^{2+} store sites and extracellular space through the activation of H_2 receptors. Acute glucose overload impairs histamine-induced Ca^{2+} homeostasis by the activation of protein kinase C. Such pathophysiological conditions in the endothelium would affect endothelium-dependent regulation of cerebral microcirculation, which may be involved in the pathogenesis of the acute phase of high glucose-induced cerebral disorders (6).

REFERENCES

1. P.A. Revest, N.J. Abbott and J.I. Gillespie, *Brain Res* 549:159-161, 1991.
2. G. Wiemer, R. Popp, B.A. Scholkens and H. Gogelein, *Brain Res* 638: 261-266, 1994.
3. N.B. Ruderman, J.R. Williamson and M. Brownlee, *FASEB J*   6: 2905-2914, 1992.
4. D.W. Miller, K.L. Audus and R.T. Borchardt, *J Tiss Cult Meth* 14: 217-224, 1992.
5. B. Tesfamariam, M.L. Brown and R.A. Cohen, *J Clin Invest* 87: 1643-1648, 1991.
6. C. Kimura, M.Oike, S.Kashiwagi and Y.Ito, Diabetes, 47:104-112, 1998.

Histamine Research in the New Millennium
T. Watanabe, H. Timmerman and K. Yanai (Editors)

Studies of histamine H_1 receptor down-regulation using mutant receptors lacking putative phosphorylation sites

Maki Ogawa[a], Shuhei Horio[a], Katsumi Fujimoto[b], Hiroyuki Fukui[a]

[a]Department of Pharmacology, Faculty of Pharmaceutical Sciences, University of Tokushima, Tokushima 770-8505, Japan

[b]Department of Biochemistry, School of Dentistry, Hiroshima University, Hiroshima 734-8553, Japan

1. Introduction

Receptor desensitization is thought to be a protection mechanism of receptor bearing cells against excessive stimuli of the receptor. Three steps of desensitization, (i) uncoupling of receptors with second messenger generating system, (ii) internalization of receptors and (iii) down-regulation of receptors, have been studied extensively. A down-regulation of H_1 receptors was reported by Smit et al. using Chinese hamster ovary (CHO) cells expressing recombinant receptors [1].

Fujimoto et al. reported that H_1 receptors lacking Ser^{398}, a putative phosphorylation site, showed a marked suppression of phorbol ester-induced receptor desensitization, suggesting that phosphorylation of receptors plays a major role in receptor desensitization [2].

In the present report, we describe complete abolishment of receptor down-regulation in the mutant H_1 receptor that lacks five putative phosphorylation sites. The participation of each site in the receptor down-regulation was also examined.

2. Materials and Methods

2.1. Cell culture

CHO cells expressing H_1 receptors, such as wild-type H_1 receptors (wild H_1-Rs), T140A H_1 receptors (T140A H_1-Rs), S396A H_1 receptors (S396A H_1-Rs), S398A H_1 receptors (S398A H_1-Rs), T478A H_1 receptors (T478A H_1-Rs), S396/398A H_1 receptors (S396/398A H_1-Rs) and T140A/T142A/S396A/S398A/T478A H_1 receptors (phospho.mutant H_1-Rs), were cultured with α-MEM medium containing 10% fetal bovine serum, antibiotic and antimycotic drug (100 U/ml penicillin D sodium, 100 μg/ml streptomycin sulfate, 0.25 mg/ml fungizone in 85% saline) under a humidified atmosphere of 5% CO_2 / 95% air at 37°C.

2.2. Binding assay

Samples containing 4 nM [³H]mepyramine with (non-specific) or without (total) 20 μM triprolidine were incubated at 25℃ for 1 hour. After incubation the sample was passed through a GR-B glassfiber filter under reduced pressure. GF-B filters trapping bound radioligand were counted in a lipid scintillation counter [3].

2.3. Determination of inositol phosphates (IPs)

Myo-[³H]inositol was incorporated into cells by culture with inositol-free DMEM medium containing 10% dialyzed FBS for 24 hours. Then cells were stimulated by 100 μM histamine in HEPES-buffered saline. The stimulation was terminated by addition of 5% TCA. After TCA was neutralized, [³H]IPs was extracted by centrifugalization (5000 rpm, 10min, 4°C). Samples were applied on AG1-✕8 columns (φ7.5 mm, volume of 0.5 ml) and [³H]IPs were eluted by 5 ml solution containing 1 M $HCOONH_4$ and 0.1 M HCOOH. Then radioactivities were determined.

2.4. Statistical analysis

Data were analyzed by Student's unpaired t-test.

3. Result

3.1. Histamine-induced down-regulation of wild H_1-Rs

Histamine induced receptor down-regulation time-dependently in CHO cells expressing wild H_1-Rs. H_1 receptors were decreased to $67.3 \pm 4.2\%$, $55.1 \pm 11.4\%$. and $39.1 \pm 2.3\%$ after the incubation with 100 μM histamine for 12,18 and 24 hours, respectively. This observation is comparable with the previous report [1].

3.2. Effect of five putative phosphorylation site elimination on H_1 receptor down-regulation

Using CHO cells expressing phospho.mutant H_1-Rs whose five putative phosphorylation sites; Thr^{140}, Thr^{142}, Ser^{396}, Ser^{398} and Thr^{478}, were replaced by alanine, levels of the receptor were determined (Fig.1). The level of the mutant H_1 receptor was not changed by the stimulation of 100 μM histamine at all.

3.3. Effect of each putative phosphorylation site elimination on H_1 receptor down-regulation

Histamine-induced down-regulation of each mutant H_1 receptor was examined using CHO cells expressing T140A H_1-Rs, S396A H_1-Rs, S398A H_1-Rs, T478A H_1-Rs and S396/398A H_1-Rs (Fig.2). Down-regulation was significantly suppressed in CHO cells expressing T140A H_1-Rs, S398A H_1-Rs and T478A H_1-Rs, compared with the wild receptor. Although down-regulation of S396A H_1-Rs was comparable with that of the wild H_1-Rs, S396A/S398A H_1-Rs showed larger decrease in down-regulation than S398A H_1-Rs.

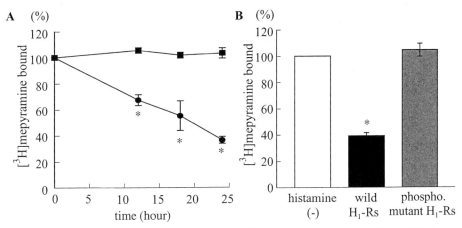

Fig. 2 (A) Time-course of levels of wild H$_1$-Rs (●) and phospho.mutant H$_1$-Rs (■) in the presence of 100 μM histamine. (B) Levels of the wild H$_1$-Rs and phospho.mutant H$_1$-Rs 24 hours after the stimulation by 100 μM histamine. The open bar indicates the level of receptors in the absence of histamine is represented as 100%. The filled bar indicates the level of the wild H$_1$-Rs and the shadowed bar indicates the level of the phospho.mutant H$_1$-Rs. Asterisk (＊) indicates p<0.001 (n=6).

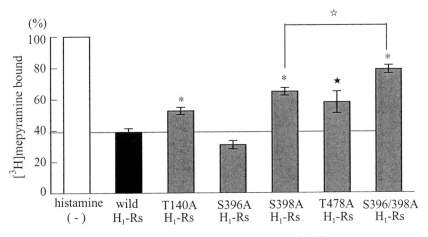

Fig. 3 Levels of wild H$_1$-Rs and mutant H$_1$ receptors lacking one or two putative phosphorylation site(s) by the treatment of 100 μM histamine for 24 hours. The level of the wild H$_1$-Rs was 39.1 ± 2.3% of that of non-treatment, and was indicated by the horizontal line. ＊indicates p<0.001 versus wild H$_1$-Rs (n=8). ★indicates p<0.05 versus wild H$_1$-Rs (n=10). ☆indicates p<0.005 between two mutant H$_1$ receptors (n=8).

3.3. Accumulation of IPs mediated by mutant H_1 receptors lacking putative phosphorylation site(s)

Ca^{++} dependent protein kinases including PKC and Ca^{++} / calmodulin-dependent protein kinase II are activated through H_1 receptor signaling, and candidates to induce down-regulation [4,5]. Then accumulation of IP_3 mediated by the mutant H_1 receptor lacking putative phosphorylation sites was determined. IP_3 were accumulated to comparable levels in any CHO cells expressing each mutant H_1 receptor by the stimulation of 100μ M histamine for 1 hour (data not shown).

4. Discussion

Here we showed that histamine induced down-regulation of CHO cells expressing wild H_1-Rs. This down-regulation was abolished in the cells expressing mutant H_1 receptor lacking five putative phosphorylation sites (phospho.mutant H_1-Rs). These results strongly suggest that down-regulation of H_1 receptors is exclusively induced by the receptor phosphorylation.

Further, we examined the participation in each phosphorylation site on down-regulation. Mutant receptors lacking each phosphorylation site showed various degree of down-regulation. These results suggest that each phosphorylation site participates to induce H_1 receptor down-regulation to some degree, and several sites are reguired for full down-regulation.

REFERENCES

1. M.J.Smit, H.Timmerman, J.C.Hijzelendoorn, H.Fukui and R.Leurs. Regulation of the human histamine H_1 receptor stably expressed in Chinese hamster ovary cells. Br.J.Pharmacol., 117, 1071-80 (1996)
2. K.Fujimoto, K.Ohta, K.Kanagawa, U.Kikkawa, S.Ogino and H.Fukui. Identification of protein kinase C phosphorylation sites involved phorbol ester-induced desensitization of the histamine H_1 receptor. Mol.Pharmacol., 55, 735-42 (1999)
3. H.Mizuguchi, H.Fukui, M.Yabumoto and H.Wada. Synaptic and extra-synaptic distribution of histamine H_1 receptors in rat and guinea pig brains. Biochem.Biophys Res. Commun., 174, 1043-47 (1991)
4. A.Warashina. Involvement of protein kinase C in homologous desensitization of histamine-evoked secretory responses in rat chromaffin cells. Brain. Res., 762, 40-6 (1997)
5. M.R.Zamani, D.R.Bristow. The histamine H_1 receptor in GT1-7 neuronal cells is regulated by calcium influx and KN-62, a putative inhibitor of calcium/calmodulin protein kinase II. Br.J.Pharmacol., 118, 1119-26 (1996)

Histamine Research in the New Millennium
T. Watanabe, H. Timmerman and K. Yanai (Editors)

Mechanism underlying histamine-induced desensitization of amylase secretion in rat parotid glands

H. Ishida[1], Y. Ishikawa[1], M. T. Skowronski[2] and N. Inoue[1]

[1]Dept. of Pharmacol., Tokushima Univ. School of Dentist., Tokushima 770-8504, Japan.
[2]Dept. of Animal Physiol., Warmia and Masuria Univ., Olsztyn 10-752, Poland

ABSTRACT   Short-term exposure of H_2 histamine (HIST) receptors (H_2Rs) on rat parotid glands to HIST induced desensitization of amylase (AMY) secretion. This desensitization was accompanied by decreases in H_2R density and in H_2R affinity for HIST as well as by an increase $Gi2\alpha$ function mediated by inhibition of protein kinase A (PKA) and activation of protein phosphatase (PP) 2A.
KEY WORDS   Desensitization, H_2 HIST receptor, Gi protein, PKA, PP2A

INTRODUCTION   We previously showed that changes in $Gi2\alpha$ function were associated with isoproterenol(IPR)-induced desensitization and supersensitivity of salivary secretion (1-2). The mechanism responsible for HIST-induced changes in the secretory response of parotid tissue was investigated.

METHODS   Rat parotid slices were incubated for 10 min with HIST (first incubation), allowed to recover for 10 min and again incubated for 10 min with 1 mM HIST (second incubation). Soluble and membrane fractions were then prepared and subjected to analysis.

RESULTS AND DISCUSSION   HIST, acting at H_2Rs, induced AMY secretion with an EC_{50} value of 60.3 $\pm$ 1.3 μM. Short-term treatment with HIST resulted in desensitization of AMY secretion that was mediated by H_2Rs (Table 1). Measurement of [³H]tiotidine binding to membranes revealed that the Bmax increased by ~34% after the first incubation with HIST and then decreased by ~53% after the second incubation. The second incubation also induced an approximately sixfold increase in the IC_{50} value for histamine but had no effect on that for ranitidine. The cyclic AMP content of the tissue increased threefold after the first incubation with HIST, but it was decreased by ~20% after the second   incubation (data not shown). HIST induced ~35% increase in the extent of ADP-ribosylation of Gs after the first incubation, but it induced ~28% decrease after the second incubation. In contrast, HIST triggered ~58% increase in the extent of ADP-ribosylation of Gi after the second incubation. Immunoblot analysis with antibodies AS/7 and RM/1 demonstrated that HIST did not affect the abundance of $Gi2\alpha$ or $Gs\alpha$ during the second incubation. Labeling of tissue with [³²P]orthophosphate and immunoprecipitation with AS/7 or RM/1 indicated that the extent of $Gi2\alpha$ phosphorylation was reduced by ~36% during the second incubation with HIST but did not change during the first incubation (Fig. 1). In contrast, the extent of Gsα phosphorylation increased during the first incubation with HIST but was unaffected during the second incubation (2). PKA activity increased by ~67% during the first incubation with HIST and then decreased by ~21% during the second incubation (Table 1), suggesting that PKA might phosphorylate Gsα during the first incubation with HIST. PP2A activity did not change during the first incubation with HIST, but increased by ~56% during the second incubation. The activity of PP1 was not affected by the first or second incubation with HIST. Pretreatment with okadaic acid prevented HIST-induced desensitization of AMY secretion (Table 1) as well as the increase in ADP-ribosylation of Gi2α (data not shown). These results indicate that the decrease in the phosphorylation of Gi2α during the second incubation with histamine is mediated by the inhibition of PKA and the activation of PP2A, and that this effect triggers the increase in the ADP-ribosylation of Gi2α.

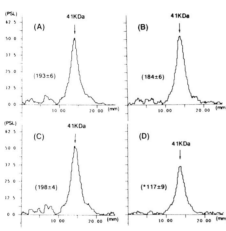

Fig.1 Effect of HIST-treatment on the stoichiometry of phosphorylation of Gi2α.
Parotid gland tissue was labeled with [³²P]orthophosphate and then incubated in the absence (A and C) or presence (B and D) of HIST for the first (A and B) and second (C and D) treatments. Tissues was lysed and subjected to immunoprecipitation with AS/7, and the precipitates were analyzed by SDS-PAGE, autoradiography and Bio-Imaging Analyzer(3). Peak height, and peak area shown in parenthesis are expressed as PSL and mm² per 100μg protein analyzed, respectively. Number in parenthesis is a mean of three experiments ± s.e.

Table 1. Effects of HIST-treatment on AMY secretion, [³H]tiotidine bindings, ADP-ribosylation of G proteins and PKA and PP activities.

Parameter	First incubation		Second incubation	
	Cont	HIST	Cont	HIST
Amylase secretion (mg maltose /100 mg tissue)				
without okadaic acid	16.1±1.3	25.6±2.2	16.2±1.2	15.5±1.7
with okadaic acid	17.6±0.8	29.8±2.5	16.5±2.1	28.0±3.4
Bmax value (f mol/mg protein)	177± 7	237 ±13	178± 8	111± 8
IC50 values (nM)				
for histamine	0.38±0.04	0.27±0.02	0.41±0.01	1.49±0.11
for ranitidine	0.43±0.03	0.42±0.02	0.37±0.03	0.41±0.01
ADP-ribosylation (PSL/100 μg protein)				
of Gs protein	164.8±14.9	223.1±16.1	158.5±9.0	161.5±16.9
of Gi protein	14.7±1.7	13.0±1.3	14.7±1.8	20.6±0.3
PKA activity (p mol/min /mg protein)	70.5±2.3	117.9 ±8.7	70.7±2.6	92.7±1.3
PP activity (n mol/min /mg protein)				
of PP1	2.72±0.02	2.60±0.01	2.66±0.11	2.83±0.13
of PP2A	0.87±0.05	1.00±0.04	1.00±0.05	1.56±0.1

Parotid gland tissue was subjected to two connective incubations in the absence (Cont) or presence of (HIST) of 1mM HIST, after which the indicated parameters were measured. Data are means of three to five separate experiments ± s.e.

REFERENCES

1. F. Hata, H. Ishida, K. Kagawa, E. Kondo, S. Kondo, and Y. Noguchi, J. Physiol., 341(1983) 185.
2. T. Eguchi, Y. Ishikawa and H. Ishida, Br. J. Pharmacol., 124 (1998) 1523.

Histamine Research in the New Millennium
T. Watanabe, H. Timmerman and K. Yanai (Editors)

Regulation of histidine decarboxylase protein expression in macrophages: Involvement of MAP kinases and inhibition by dexamethasone

Akira Murakami, Noriyasu Hirasawa, Muneshige Shiraishi, and Kazuo Ohuchi

Laboratory of Pathophysiological Biochemistry, Graduate School of Pharmaceutical Sciences, Tohoku University, Aoba Aramaki, Aoba-ku, Sendai, Miyagi 980-8578, Japan

Stimulation of RAW 264.7 cells with the Ca^{2+}-ATPase inhibitor thapsigargin increased histamine production and the expression of 74 kD histidine decarboxylase (HDC) protein. The MEK inhibitor U0126 and the p38 MAP kinase inhibitor SB203580 suppressed the thapsigargin-induced histamine production in parallel with the inhibition of the 74 kD HDC protein expression. The synthetic glucocorticoid dexamethasone inhibited the thapsigargin-induced histamine production and 74 kD HDC protein expression. The thapsigargin-induced activation of p42/p44 MAP kinase and p38 MAP kinase were also inhibited by dexamethasone. These findings indicate that the induction of histamine production by thapsigargin in RAW 264.7 cells is due to the increased expression of 74 kD HDC protein, and the inhibition by dexamethasone of the thapsigargin-induced HDC protein expression and histamine production is due to the inhibition of MAP kinase activation.

KEYWORDS: Histamine, Histidine decarboxylase (HDC) , Dexamethasone, p42/p44 MAP kinase

1. INTRODUCTION

Histamine is produced by mast cells, basophils, macrophages, neutrophils and lymphocytes. Mast cells and basophils constitutively express histidine decarboxylase (HDC) at 74 and 53 kD molecular mass. In an air pouch-type allergic inflammation model in rats, we demonstrated that the steroidal anti-inflammatory drug dexamethasone inhibits histamine production by non-mast cells at the late phase of inflammation [1]. However, the regulation mechanism of histamine production by non-mast cells has not been fully clarified. Recently, we found that the stimulation of the murine macrophage-like cell line RAW 264.7 cells by thapsigargin, a Ca^{2+}-ATPase inhibitor, increases HDC mRNA level and histamine production [2]. In the present study, we examined roles of MAP kinases in the induction of HDC protein expression by thapsigargin, and effects of dexamethasone on thapsigargin-induced histamine production in RAW 264.7 cells.

2. MATERIALS AND METHODS

RAW 264.7 cells were suspended at 5×10^5 cells/ml in Eagle's minimum essential medium (EMEM) containing 10% (v/v) heat-inactivated fetal bovine serum (EMEM (+)). The cells were preincubated at 37oC in EMEM (+) containing U0126 or SB203580 for 1 h or

424

dexamethasone for 24 h, then further incubated at 37oC in EMEM (+) containing thapsigargin (20 nM) in the presence of drugs for the period indicated. Histamine contents in the supernatant fraction of the conditioned medium and phosphorylation of MAP kinases were determined as described previously [1]. HDC in the cell lysate was immunoblotted by using the rabbit polyclonal antibody to rat HDC (Euro-diagnostica, Malmo, Sweden).

3. RESULTS

Although the level of 74 kD HDC protein in unstimulated RAW 264.7 cells was very low, the stimulation by thapsigargin increased 74 kD HDC protein expression in the cells and histamine contents in the conditioned medium. In contrast, 53 kD HDC protein was not detected. The MEK inhibitor U0126 inhibited the thapsigargin-induced histamine production and HDC protein expression. In addition, the p38 MAP kinase inhibitor SB203580 reduced partially but significantly the thapsigargin-induced HDC protein expression and histamine production. Pretreatment of RAW 264.7 cells with dexamethasone (10-1000 nM) for 24 h inhibited the thapsigargin-induced expression of 74 kD HDC protein and histamine production in a concentration-dependent manner. To clarify the mechanism by which dexamethasone inhibits histamine production, effects of dexamethasone on the thapsigargin-induced activation of MAP kinases were examined. It was demonstrated that dexamethasone inhibits the thapsigargin-induced phosphorylation of p42/p44 MAP kinase and p38 MAP kinase in a concentration-dependent manner.

4. DISCUSSION

The present study disclosed that thapsigargin-induced histamine production in RAW 264.7 cells is correlated with the expression of 74 kD HDC protein, which is regulated by p42/p44 MAP kinase and partially by 38 MAP kinase. In addition, it is indicated that the inhibition by dexamethasone of the thapsigargin-induced expression of 74 kD HDC protein and histamine production is due to the inhibition of thapsigargin-induced MAP kinase activation.

REFERENCES
1. Shiraishi, M ., Hirasawa, N ., Kobayashi, Y ., Oikawa, S ., Murakami, A ., Ohuchi, K . Participation of mitogen-activated protein kinase in thapsigargin- and TPA-induced histamine production in murine macrophage RAW 264.7 cells. *Br. J. Pharmacol., 129, 515-524 (2000)*
2. Hirasawa, N ., Funaba, Y ., Hirano, Y ., Kawarasaki, K ., Omata, M ., Watanabe, M ., Mue, S ., Tsurufuji, S ., Ohuchi, K. Inhibition by dexamethasone of histamine production in allergic inflammation in rats. *J. Immunol., 145, 3041-3046 (1990)*

Mast Cells

Histamine Research in the New Millennium
T. Watanabe, H. Timmerman and K. Yanai (Editors)

Functional maturation of mouse cultured mast cells to a connective tissue mast cell-like phenotype *in vitro*

Y. Taketomi, T. Saito, R. Kikuchi-Yanoshita, M. Murakami, and I. Kudo

Department of Health Chemistry, School of Pharmaceutical Sciences,
Showa University, 1-5-8 Hatanodai, Shinagawa-ku, Tokyo 142-8555, Japan

We developed a unique *in vitro* culture system to obtain a population of mouse mast cells that are similar, both morphologically and functionally, to connective tissue mast cells (CTMC). This method enabled us to identify a number of genes whose expression levels are dramatically changed during mast cell maturation.

1. Maturation of mouse immature mast cells to CTMC *in vitro*

Mast cells in different anatomical microenvironments show variation in multiple aspects of their phenotypes, including the amounts and types of preformed mediators, lipid mediators and cytokines that they produce, and their sensitivity to various agents that can influence their functions (1, 2). Rodent mast cells have been subdivided into two major subpopulations, CTMC and mucosal mast cells (MMC), which rapidly alter their phenotypes depending on the current microenvironment in which they reside. CTMC possess several remarkable features that are not shared with MMC or IL-3-dependent mouse bone marrow-derived mast cells (BMMC), which represent an *in vitro* culture-derived, relatively immature population of mast cells. Thus, only CTMC synthesize heparin, contain high concentrations of granule histamine, express CTMC-specific serine proteases, produce prostaglandin D_2 (PGD_2) in marked preference to leukotrienes immediately after $Fc_\varepsilon RI$-dependent activation, and respond to polycationic secretagogues that activate heterotrimeric G proteins, presumably by interacting directly with them (2). The growth and development of mast cells are crucially affected by the tissue-derived cytokine, stem cell factor (SCF), a ligand for the c-*kit* receptor tyrosine kinase (2, 3). The ability of mesenchymal cells to support survival and, in certain cases, maturation of mast cells *in vitro* depends on the membrane-bound form of SCF on their surface, even though SCF alone is insufficient for mast cells to undergo full maturation.

Coculture of IL-3-dependent immature BMMC with fibroblasts is a useful system for the analysis of some aspects of phenotypic change into a CTMC-like phenotype *in vitro* (2, 4). We modified this coculture system by adding soluble SCF to the medium such that a large number of CTMC-like cells were obtained *in vitro* in a short period (5). Following changes in BMMC occurred only after 4 days of coculture.

1.1. Granule maturation

Reflecting the difference in proteoglycan moieties, secretory granules of BMMC, which contain condroitin sulfate, are stained with alcian blue, whereas those of CTMC, which contain heparin, are stained with safranin (1). BMMC cocultured with Swiss 3T3 in the presence of SCF became larger in size and their granules were largely safranin-

428

positive, indicaticative of heparin biosynthesis (manuscript in preparation). Histamine content of BMMC increased ~4-fold during coculture (Figure 1), which was accompanied by a marked increase in the expression of histidine decarboxylase (HDC), a rate-limiting enzyme for histamine synthesis. Adddition of IL-3, IL-4, and IL-10 to the coculture increased HDC and histamine further (Figure 1). Secretory granules of cocultured BMMC also contained the CTMC-specific serine protease, MMCP-4.

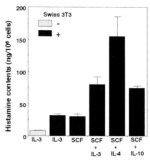

Figure 1. Changes in histamine content of BMMC after coculture in the presence of various cytokines

1.2. Functional maturation

Following crosslinking of $Fc_\varepsilon RI$, cocultured BMMC produced more PGD_2 than did those without coculture (5). This increased PGD_2 generation resulted from SCF-induced increase in cyclooxygenase-1 expression (6). Although BMMC did not respond to polycationic secretagogues (compound 48/80 and substance P), those after coculture fully responded to them, releasing more granule contents, generating PGD_2, and producing cytokines (5). IL-3 showed no effect on, and IL-4 and IL-10 inhibited, the SCF- and 3T3-deriven acquisition of compound 48/80 sensitivity, contrasting with their effect on histamine biosynthesis shown above. As that of rat CTMC, compound 48/80-induced degranulation of coclutured BMMC was suppressed by pertussis toxin (5) and several plant lectins (unpublished observation). 3T3-conditioned medium supported this functional maturation only minimally, indicating that mast cell-fibroblast contact is essential. Unaltered $G_{i3\alpha}$ protein expression during coculture raises the possibility that a putative compound 48/80 acceptor molecule might be induced in cocultured BMMC.

2. Identification of inducible genes in mast cells during the maturation process

In an effort to elucidate the regulatory mechanisms for mast cell maturation, we employed cDNA subtraction strategy to identify a series of genes that are highly upregulated in BMMC during coculture (manuscript in preparation). Of nearly 100 clones sequenced, about half corresponded to mouse chromosome 14-associated serine proteases, including the apoptosis-inducing protease granzyme B and the CTMC-specific protease MMCP-4. Besides them, a number of genes present in the EST data bases and those that had not been listed before were identified. The entire structures and possible cellular functions of these novel genes are under investigation.

REFERENCES
1. R.L. Stevens and K.F. Austen, Immunol. Today, 10 (1989) 381.
2. E. Razin and J. Rivera (eds.), Signal Transduction in Mast Cells and Basophils, Springer-Verlag, New York (1999)
3. S.J. Galli et al, Adv. Immunol., 55 (1994) 1.
4. F. Levi-Schaffer, F. et al, J. Immunol., 135 (1985) 3454.
5. T. Ogasawara et al, J. Immunol., 158 (1997) 393.
6. M. Murakami et al, J. Biol. Chem., 270 (1995) 3239.

Histamine Research in the New Millennium
T. Watanabe, H. Timmerman and K. Yanai (Editors)

Functional differences between the connective tissue and mucosal mast cells on the contraction of isolated rat trachea

Zullies Ikawati[a], Yoshinori Oka[a], Masato Nose[b], Kazutaka Maeyama[a]

[a]Department of Pharmacology Ehime University School of Medicine, Shigenobu-cho, Onsengun, Ehime 791-0295 Japan. [b]Department of Pathology II, Ehime University School of Medicine, Shigenobu-cho, Onsengun, Ehime 791-0295 Japan

In the rat trachea, two types of mast cells have been identified, connective tissue mast cells (CTMCs) and mucosal mast cells (MMCs). We have previously reported that CTMCs contributed to tracheal contraction that was induced non-immunologically by compound 48/80, via 5-HT release. This present study addressed whether MMCs also play a role in tracheal contraction, by employing mast cell-deficient *(Ws/Ws)* rats and their congenic *(+/+)* rats. MMCs were immunologically activated using ovalbumin sensitization followed by antigen challenge 12 to 14 days later. To exclude the influence of CTMCs, rats were pretreated for 7 days with i.p. injection of compound 48/80 in increasing doses. Histamine levels in trachea decreased, whereas histological examination showed that the degranulation occurred in CTMCs, but not in MMCs. Ovalbumin-specific IgE production was increased time-dependently both in *Ws/Ws* and *+/+* rats after sensitization with no significantly difference in values between the two groups. Nevertheless, ovalbumin challenge induced tracheal contraction only in sensitized control (*+/+*) rats, whereas *Ws/Ws* and compound 48/80-pretreated *+/+* rats gave no response. These findings suggest that there are functional differences between CTMCs and MMCs. CTMCs play more significant role in the tracheal contraction, both in immunologic and non-immunological conditions, whereas MMCs may have contributed to other features of asthma. In addition, *Ws/Ws* rats provide a good tool to study the mast cells role in airway system.

1. INTRODUCTION

Mast cells are implicated in the pathogenesis of airway, especially in the immediate type hypersensitivity reaction in a number of immunologic and non-immunological disorders. However, much controversy and confusion concerning mast cells has arisen because of their heterogeneity. Two types of mast cells has been observed in rat trachea, mucosal mast cells (MMCs) and connective tissue mast cells (CTMCs), respectively. We have previously reported that CTMCs play a significant role in tracheal contraction induced by compound 48/80 via 5-HT released during degranulation (1).

The discovery of mast cell-deficient rats (*Ws/Ws*) by Kitamura and colleagues (2) made it possible to make more direct study of the role of mast cells in various regions and, furthermore, the individual role of the different types of mast cells.

The present study addressed whether or not MMCs also play significant role, as do CTMCs, on tracheal contraction. Recognition of the functional difference between CTMC and MMC would be helpful in treatment of mast cell-associated disorder.

430

2. MATERIALS AND METHODS

Male *Ws/Ws* and *+/+* rats, 250-300 g weight and 3-4 months age, were used. Rats were sensitized with 1.0 ml of 1.0 mg/ml ovalbumin (OA) mixed with 10% Al(OH)$_3$ suspension in saline (s.c.) and *Bordetella pertussis* with 1.0 x 10^9 organism/ml (i.p). Serum samples were collected from tail vein at day 0, 3,7, 10, 14 to measure IgE titer. Rats were studied for contractile response on day 14, either with or without drugs (ketanserin, a 5-HT$_{2A}$ receptor antagonist, and ONO-1078, a leukotriene antagonist). In another series of experiment, rats received i.p. injection of compound 48/80 for 7 days with increasing doses to deplete CTMCs. Measurement of histamine tissue content and histochemical study were also carried out to confirm the depletion of CTMCs.

3. RESULTS AND DISCUSSION

After chronic treatment with compound 48/80, MMCs remained intact. It made us possible to study MMC function in the absence of CTMC. No contraction was observed both in compound 48/80-pretreated *+/+* and *Ws/Ws* rats, suggesting that MMCs contribute little to tracheal contraction. Ketanserin inhibited the ovalbumin-induced contraction in *+/+* rat tracheas, while ONO-1078 failed to do so, indicating that contraction is due to 5-HT, whereas leukotriene, a mediator specific derived from MMCs, has minimal, if any, contribution.

The above findings suggest that it is CTMCs playing a significant role, both in immunologic and non-immunologic stimulation. These studies do not rule out a function for MMCs in other airway responses such as airway inflammation or defense mechanism (Fig.1).

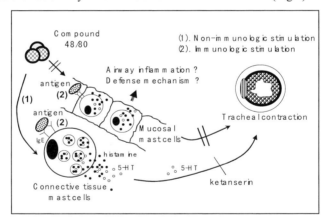

Fig.1. The model for the functional difference of two types of mast cells in rat airways. CTMCs play significant role on tracheal contraction, both in immunologic and non-immunological stimuli, whereas MMCs may contribute to airway inflammation or host defense mechanism. The function of MMCs in asthma response still remains to be elucidated.

REFERENCES

1. Ikawati Z, Hayashi M, Nose M, Maeyama K: The lack of compound 48/80-induced contraction on isolated trachea of mast cells deficient *Ws/Ws* rats in vitro: The role of connective tissue mast cells. Eur. J. Pharmacol., 402 (2000), 297-306
2. Niwa Y, Kasugai T, Ohno K, Morimoto M, Yamazaki M, Dohmae K, Nishimune Y, Kondo K, Kitamura Y: Anemia and mast cell depletion in mutant rats that are homozygous at 'white spotting (Ws)' locus. Blood, 78 (1991), 1936-1941

© 2001 Elsevier Science B.V. All rights reserved.
Histamine Research in the New Millennium
T. Watanabe, H. Timmerman and K. Yanai (Editors)

Rho GTPases regulate degranulation and cytokine release from RBL-2H3 cells

I. Hide[a], Y. Itoh[a], T. Hisahara[a], K. Ido[a], A. Inoue[a], T. Fujiwara[b], K. Aktories[c], M. Sugai[b], and Y. Nakata[a]

[a]Department of Pharmacology, Institute of Pharmaceutical Sciences, Hiroshima University School of Medicine, Hiroshima 734-8551, Japan
[b]Department of Microbiology, Hiroshima University School of Dentistry, Hiroshima 734-8553, Japan
[c]Institut für Pharmakologie und Toxikologie der Universität Freiburg, D-79104 Freiburg, Germany

Clostridium difficile Toxin B (toxin B), which inactivates Rho GTPases, Rho, Rac, and Cdc42, inhibited the release of TNF-α as well as degranulation from antigen-stimulated RBL-2H3 cells, independently of reorganization of actin microfilaments. Rho-associated kinase (ROCK), one of the downstream effectors of Rho, was selectively involved in the release of TNF-α, but not in degranulation. Toxin B inhibited the translocation of Ca^{2+}-dependent protein kinase C (α and β isozymes), which plays an important role in the release of TNF-α as well as degranulation. These results indicated that Rho GTPases regulate the release of TNF-α and degranulation by regulating at least the activation of Ca^{2+}-dependent PKC in antigen-stimulated RBL-2H3 cells.

1. Introduction

Mast cells secrete not only preformed mediators such as histamine by degranulation, but also various cytokines including TNF-α, in response to allergic and non-allergic stimuli. Recently, increasing evidence suggests that Rho GTPases, well-known regulators of actin cytoskeleton, is also a key regulator of degranulation in mast cells (1, 2, 3). However, their role in cytokine release is not clear. In the present study, we investigated whether Rho GTPases can regulate the release of TNF-α from cultured (RBL-2H3) mast cell line by using *Clostridium difficile* toxin B (toxin B), which inactivates Rho GTPases, Rho, Rac and Cdc42 by monoglucosylation (4).

2. Methods

RBL-2H3 cells were cultured in RPMI-1640 supplemented with 10 % fetal calf serum. The cells were plated in 24-well plates, sensitized overnight with 0.25 µg/ml DNP-specific IgE, and stimulated by 10 ng/ml DNP-BSA. The cells were also stimulated with 1 µM ionomycin. Released TNF-α was measured using an ELISA kit, and degranulation was assessed by the release of β-hexosaminidase (5). PKC translocation was detected by Western blotting using specific antibodies against PKC-α and β isozymes. Measurement of intracellular Ca^{2+} concentration was measured by fura-2 fluorescence.

432

3. Results and Discussion

Treatment of RBL-2H3 cells with toxin B caused a marked cell rounding, and inhibited degranulation and the release of TNF-α more potently from antigen-stimulated cells than from ionomycin-stimulated cells. Y-27632, ROCK inhibitor, inhibited only the release of TNF-α, but not degranulation. Inhibition by toxin B of the release of TNF-α was not likely to be related to the actin disassembly, because actin depolymerizing agents, cytochalasin D and mycalolide B, significantly enhanced the release of TNF-α as well as degranulation. Gö6976, a specific inhibitor of Ca^{2+}-dependent PKC, strongly suppressed the release of TNF-α in antigen-stimulated cells in a similar manner to toxin B. Toxin B strongly inhibited antigen-induced translocation of Ca^{2+}-dependent PKC isozymes α and β, which are expressed in RBL-2H3 cells (6). Furthermore, toxin B suppressed antigen-induced intracellular Ca^{2+} response in a concentration-dependent manner.

In conclusion, these results indicate that Rho GTPases are critical not only for degranulation, but also for the release of TNF-α especially in antigen-stimulated RBL-2H3 cells. It is also suggested that Rho GTPases may regulate these mast cell functions by activating Ca^{2+}-dependent PKC, which plays an important role in antigen-generating signals leading degranulation and the release of TNF-α.

REFERENCES

1. M.A. Brown, A.J. O' Sullivan and B.D. Gomperts, Mol. Biol. Cell, 9 (1998) 1053.
2. U. Prepens, I. Just, C. von Eichel-Streiber and K.Aktories, J. Biol. Chem. 271 (1996) 7324.
3. R. Sullivant, L.S. Price and A. Koffer, J. Biol. Chem. 274 (1999) 38140.
4. K. Aktories, Trends Microbiol. 5 (1997) 282.
5. I. Hide, N. Toriu, T. Nuibe, A. Inoue, M. Hide, S. Yamamoto and Y. Nakata, J. Immunol. 159 (1997) 2932.
6. K. Ozawa, Z. Szallasi, M.G. Kazanietz, P.M. Blumberg, H. Mischak, J.F. Mushinski and M.A. Beaven, J. Biol. Chem. 268 (1993) 1749.

Histamine Research in the New Millennium
T. Watanabe, H. Timmerman and K. Yanai (Editors)

Effect of lipid peroxide on histamine release from rat peritoneal mast cells

Masaaki Akagi, Eri Akashi-Nishioka, Reiko Kanoh, Habumi Tansei and Yoshitaka Katakuse

Department of Pharmacology, Faculty of Pharmaceutical Sciences, Tokushima Bunri University, Tokushima, 770-8514, Japan

Abstract
    t-butylhydroperoxide (TBHP), an analogue of lipid peroxide or hydrogen peroxide dose-dependently inhibited antigen- and 48/80-induced histamine release. It was suggested that the inhibitory effects may be due to the membrane stabilizing.

Key words: Lipid peroxide, Mast cell, Histamine release, Membrane stabilization

Mast cells play an important role in initiating allergic inflammation. In inflamed tissues, many kinds of phagocyotic cells generate superoxide anion (O_2^-), and O_2^- releases histamine from rat peritoneal mast cells (1). O_2^- in and around cell membranes can facilitate lipid peroxidation reactions that gradually destroy cell membrane structure, interfere with cell function, and lead to changes in gene expression. In the present study, we examined the effects of lipid peroxide and hydrogen peroxide on histamine release from rat peritoneal mast cells.
    Sensitized and non-sensitized male Wistar rats (250-300 g) were used. Peritoneal mast cells were collected from the abdominal cavity of rats, and purified to a level higher than 95% according to the method described previously (1). The purified mast cells were preincubated with different amounts of t-butylhydroperoxide (TBHP), an analogue of lipid peroxide, or hydrogen peroxide for 15 min at 37℃, and then antigen or compound 48/80 (48/80) was added. The reactions were allowed to proceed for 10 min and were terminated by chilling the test tubes in an ice bath. After centrifugation, the amount of histamine in the supernatants and the residual histamine content were determined fluorometrically. The viability of the cells was determined by the dye-exclusion test, and the content of peroxidized lipid in cell membrane was measured using TBA method. ^{45}Ca uptake into mast cells was measured according to the method of Spataro (2). Phospholipid metabolites in mast cells were measured using $H_3^{32}PO_4$-loading cells.
    TBHP alone slightly elicited histamine release from mast cells as well as hydrogen peroxide (Fig. 1). However, TBHP and hydrogen peroxide dose-dependently inhibited antigen- (Fig. 1, 2) and 48/80-induced histamine release, when mast cells were pretreated for 15 min with those. TBHP and hydrogen peroxide dose-dependently inhibited the hypotonic hemolysis and increased the amount of peroxidized lipid. When rat peritoneal mast cells were exposed to 48/80 (0.5 μ g/ml), ^{45}Ca uptake increased about 2 times more than that of control cells. Hydrogen peroxide prevented the increase of ^{45}Ca uptake induced by 48/80, dose-

dependently. TBHP and hydrogen peroxide did not increase the number of dying cells. Hydrogen peroxide increased the production of lysophosphatidylcholine and prevented the decrease of phosphatidylinositol 4,5-diphosphate in mast cells.

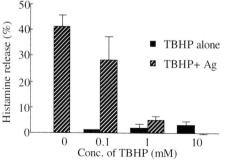

Fig. 1. Effect of TBHP on antigen-induced histamine release from sensitized rat mast cells

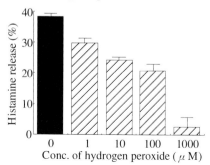

Fig. 2. Effect of hydrogen peroxide on antigen-induced histamine release from sensitized rat mast cells

In the previous study, we reported that O_2^- elicited histamine release from rat mast cells (1). O_2^- is rapidly dismutated to hydrogen peroxide catalysed by SOD. O_2^- in and around cell membranes can facilitate lipid peroxidation reactions. Therefore, we have considered that TBHP and hydrogen peroxide may elicit histamine release. However, TBHP and hydrogen peroxide inhibited histamine release induced by stimulants without cell damages, dose-dependently. Those inhibited the hypotonic hemolysis and prevented the increase of ^{45}Ca uptake. And hydrogen peroxide increased the production of lysophosphatidylcholine and prevented the decrease of phosphatidylinositol 4,5-diphosphate (PIP_2) in mast cells. Lysophosphatidylcholine (LPC) inhibits histamine release from mast cells induced by antigen and 48/80 (3), and the membrane stabilizing effect of LPC contributes to the inhibitory effect. 48/80 increases the amount of inositol 1,4,5-trisphosphate (IP_3), a product of PIP_2, and elicits histamine release from mast cells (4). The prevention of IP_3 generation results in the inhibition of histamine release. In conclusion, these findings suggested that the inhibitory effects on histamine release may be due to the membrane stabilizing.

REFERENCES

1. M. Akagi, Y. Katakuse, N. Fukuishi, T. Kan and R. Akagi, Biol. Pharm. Bull. 17 (1994) 732-734.
2. A.C. Spataro and H.B. Bosmann, Biochem. Pharmac., 25 (1976) 505-510.
3. M. Mio, A. Ikeda, M. Akagi and K. Tasaka, Agents and Actions 16 (1985) 113-117.
4. K. Izushi, T. Shirasaka, M. Chokki and K. Tasaka, FEBS Lett. 314 (1992) 241-245.

© 2001 Elsevier Science B.V. All rights reserved.
Histamine Research in the New Millennium
T. Watanabe, H. Timmerman and K. Yanai (Editors)

Effects of ultraviolet light (UV) on histamine release from rat peritoneal mast cells

M. Mio, M. Yabuta, K. Utsugi and C. Kamei

Department of Pharmacology, Faculty of Pharmaceutical Sciences, Okayama University, Okayama, 700-8530, Japan

Ultraviolet (UV) B, at doses higher than 7.8 kJ/m^2, induced histamine release from rat peritoneal mast cells even at 4°C. The UVB-induced histamine release was enhanced by some phenothiazine compounds. Ascorbic acid at concentrations higher than 500 µM inhibited the UVB-induced histamine release as well as that evoked by a combination of UVB and chlorpromazine. On the other hand, pretreatment with low doses of UVB (less than 5.6 kJ/m^2) to mast cells resulted in an inhibition of compound 48/80-induced histamine release but not that induced by either A23187 or TPA.

Keywords: Mast cell; Histamine release; Ultraviolet light; Compound 48/80

1. INTRODUCTION

Ultraviolet light (UV) is known to induce acute inflammation of the skin. On the other hand, low dose irradiation of UV is used for the treatment of atopic eczema. In either case, mast cell is considered as one of the target cells, though the mechanism of action is not clear. In this study, effects of UV on histamine release from rat mast cells were investigated.

2. MATERIALS AND METHODS

Rat mast cells were collected from the abdominal cavity of male Wistar rats (300 to 450 g), and purified by Percoll density gradient centrifugation. The cells were suspended in a HEPES-buffered Tyrode solution (in mM: NaCl 137, KCl 2.7, $CaCl_2$ 1.0, NaH_2PO_4 0.285, HEPES 10, glucose 5.6, pH 7,4) and added to each well of the 24-well culture plate (5×10^4 cells/ml/well). The plate was placed in a UV-lighting box which contained an ultraviolet light source in a light-tight box and irradiation was carried out for various periods of time at either 25°C or 4°C. The intensity (µW/cm²) of each UV light at the bottom of each well of the culture plate was measured by means of a UVX Digital Radiometer (UVP Inc., San Gabriel, CA, USA). The intensity was multiplied by the time of exposure to obtain the UV dose (J/m^2). Histamine in the supernatant and histamine remaining in the cells were determined separately by a fluorometric assay.

3. RESULTS AND DISCUSSION

When rat peritoneal mast cells were exposed to UV light (UVA, UVB and UVC), histamine release was evoked in a dose (intensity x time) dependent manner. The potency order of UV light in inducing the histamine release was UVC > UVB >> UVA. In this study, we focused on the effect of UVB on histamine release from rat mast cells. The UVB-induced histamine release occurred at doses higher than 7.8 kJ/m^2, even at 4°C. At a UVB dose of 18.8 kJ/m^2, where a $51.9 \pm 4.8\%$ histamine release and a $58.8 \pm 6.8\%$ degranulation took place, Trypan blue-stained cells accounted for $14.4 \pm 1.3\%$ of the cells, and the lactate dehydrogenase release was about $4.9 \pm 2.8\%$. This suggests that the membrane permeability to low molecular weight substances was increased by UVB exposure. The UVB-induced histamine release was enhanced by some phenothiazine compounds, i.e., promethazine, trimeprazine, mequitazine, chlorpromazine, trifluoperazine, ethopropazine and thioridazine [1]. Ascorbic acid at concentrations higher than 500 μM inhibited the histamine release induced by UVB as well as that evoked by a combination of UVB and chlorpromazine, suggesting an involvement of oxidative radical(s) in UVB-induced histamine release.

On the other hand, pretreatment with low doses of UVB (less than 5.6 kJ/m^2) to mast cells resulted in an inhibition of compound-48/80-induced histamine release (Figure 1) but not that induced by either A23187 or TPA (Figure 2). These results may suggest that an exposure to low dose of UVB cause an inhibition of early events in intracellular signal transduction.

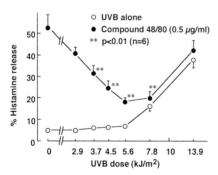

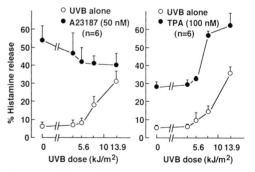

Figure 1. Effect of UVB-pretreatment on compound 48/80-induced histamine release from rat peritoneal mast cells.

Figure 2. Effect of UVB-pretreatment on A23187- or TPA-induced histamine release from rat peritoneal mast cells.

REFERENCES

1. Mio M., Yabuta M. and Kamei C. Immunopharmacology, 41 (1999) 55.

© 2001 Elsevier Science B.V. All rights reserved.
Histamine Research in the New Millennium
T. Watanabe, H. Timmerman and K. Yanai (Editors)

Placental mast cells and histamine in pregnancy complicated by intrauterine growth retardation (IUGR) – relation to the development of villous microvessels

D. Szukiewicz[a,b], M. Gujski[a], D. Maslinska[c], K. Wypych[b], G. Szewczyk[a], S. Maslinski[a]

[a] Laboratory of Placental Research, Department of General and Experimental Pathology, University School of Medicine, ul.Krakowskie Przedmiescie 26/28, 00-928 Warsaw, Poland

[b] First Department of Obstetrics and Gynaecology, Second Faculty of Medicine, University School of Medicine, ul. Kondratowicza 8, 03-242 Warsaw, Poland

[c] Institute of Medical Research Centre, Polish Academy of Sciences, Warsaw, Poland

1. INTRODUCTION

The formation of new capillary vessels is associated with some physiological circumstances and several pathological conditions. Numerous angiogenic factors, among them histamine (HA) and other mast cells (MC) mediators, have been identified, but the mechanism of tube formation is still poorly understood [1]. The placenta undergoes extensive angiogenesis and cellular proliferation to establish adequate blood supply to the fetus. It has been reported, that in many cases of intrauterine growth retardation (IUGR) fetal ischaemia may be caused by altered placental vascularization [2]. In our previous preliminary study [3] we found the correlation between mast cell number, HA levels, and development of villous microvessels. Now, when we are more experienced with the methods of placental angiogenesis assessment as well as obtained material is more sufficient for statistical analysis we have been continued this investigation.

The aim of study was to find the correlation between MC number, HA concentration and density of the network of placental vessels in IUGR-complicated pregnancy.

2. MATERIALS AND METHODS

Eleven placentae obtained from nulliparas after single pregnancies complicated by IUGR (Group I; mean gestational age 267 ± 9 days) were compared with eleven placentae obtained from gestationally matched controls (Group II; 270 ± 5 days). All newborns in group I and II were delivered by elective cesarean sections in fetal interest. HA concentrations were estimated fluorimetrically in placental cuts collected from the maternal surface. Five specimens of placental tissue were excised in a standardized manner [4]. Simultaneously, further samples were fixed in formalin, embedded in paraffin wax or frozen and cut at 6 μm, before staining with hematoxylin/eosin, toluidine blue or alcian blue. MC in tissue sections were also stained with tryptase and chymase antibodies. For each placenta the total number of stained MC was cal-

438

culated. Using light microscopy, with computed morphometry the vascular/extravascular tissulat index (V/EVTI) was measured in calibrated areas of the placental sections. For statistical analysis of V/EVTI and total number of MC Mann-Whitney's U test was applied. Differences between groups I and II were deemed statistically significant if $p < 0.05$.

3. RESULTS AND CONCLUSIONS

The results showed that in IUGR complicated pregnancy decreased density of the villous network of vessels (V/EVTI: 0.20 ± 0.022 vs 0.28 ± 0.033 in control; see Table 1) correlates with lower HA concentration (210.9 ± 21.2 ng/g of wet weight vs 267.3 ± 23.7 ng/g of wet weight in control; see Table 2) and decreased total number of MC (2784 vs 3814 in control; see Table 2).

Table 1
Vascular/extravascular tissular index (V/EVTI) in placental sections

Group	Number of specimens	V/EVTI (mean value)	± SD
I. IUGR	275	0.20 *	0.022
II. Control	275	0.28	0.033

* p < 0.05

Table 2
IUGR-complicated versus normal pregnancy: mean concentration of histamine (HA) and the total number of placental mast cells (TMCN).

Group	HA (ng/g of wet tissue; ± SD)	TMCN	TMCN(%)
I. IUGR	210.9 ± 21.2	2784	72.99
II. Control	267.3 ± 23.7	3814	100.0*

* mean value of TMCN obtained for control group (3814) was taken as 100%

REFERENCES
1. K. Norrby. Int. J. Exp. Pathol. No. 76 (1995) 87.
2. G. Altshuler, Pediatr. Pathol. Lab. Med. No. 16 (1996) 207.
3. D. Szukiewicz, A. Szukiewicz, D. Maslinska, P. Poppe, M. Gujski and M. Olszewski, Inflamm. Res. No 48 (Suppl. 1; 1999) 41.
4. D. Szukiewicz, A. Szukiewicz, D. Maslinska and M.W. Markowski, Trophoblast Res. No. 13 (1999) 503.

© 2001 Elsevier Science B.V. All rights reserved.
Histamine Research in the New Millennium
T. Watanabe, H. Timmerman and K. Yanai (Editors)

Involvement of mast cells in inflammation sites of colitis induced by dextran sulfate sodium

Y. Iba, Y. Sugimoto and C. Kamei
Department of Pharmacology, Faculty of Pharmaceutical Sciences, Okayama University, Okayama 700-8530, Japan

We investigated the role of mast cells in the sites of inflammation in colitis induced by dextran sulfate sodium (DSS).   Haematoxylin and eosin staining revealed a marked infiltration of inflammatory cells and oedematous changes in mucosa and submucosa after drinking of 4% DSS.   And, toluidine blue staining also revealed that the number of mast cells was increased after free drinking of 4% DSS.   These results suggest that mast cells may modulate the disorder of DSS-induced colitis.

KEY WORDS: colitis; dextran sulfate; inflammation; mast cells

1. INTRODUCTION

The number of mast cells is increased in the sites of inflammation or at the demarcation line in patients with ulcerative colitis.   In animal models of colitis, however, there have been few studies of the alterations in mast cell distribution in the sites of inflammation.   Oral administration of dextran sulfate sodium (DSS) results in colitis in animals, which is histologically similar to human ulcerative colitis.   Mucosal mast cells (MMCs) are present in the mucosa and connective tissue mast cells (CTMCs) are present in the submucosa and muscularis of the large intestine in rats. Therefore, the present study was performed to clarify the roles of mast cells in colitis induced by DSS in rats.

2. MATERIALS AND METHODS

Male SD rats weighing 220-270 g were used.   Rats were administered 4% DSS (mol wt. 5,000) by free drinking for 11 days.   On day 0, 3, 7 and 11, animals were anesthetized with diethyl ether and decapitated.   The rectums of 1-2 cm from the anal verge were removed, fixed in Carnoy's fixative for 2 h, and then embedded in paraffin.   The histological samples were cut into 4 μm thick sections, and were stained with haematoxylin and eosin (H-E) or toluidine blue (pH 0.5).

3. RESULTS AND DISCUSSION

H-E staining revealed a marked infiltration of inflammatory cells into the mucosa and submucosa on day 11 (Figure 1 (b)). The oedematous changes in mucosa and submucosa were also evident. And, toluidine blue staining revealed some mast cells in the mucosa and submucosa. The number of mast cells was increased after free drinking of 4% DSS (Figure 2 (b)).

At present, we do not know why the number of mast cells was increased. However, chronic degranulation of mast cells and inflammatory cytokines may result in the proliferation of mast cells in the inflammation sites of DSS-induced colitis, because the proliferation of mast cells requires interleukin (IL)-3 and IL-4 produced from T cells and mast cells themselves.

These results suggest that mast cells may modulate the disorder of DSS-induced colitis.

(a)   (b)

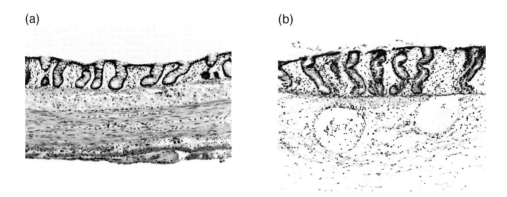

Figure 1. Microscopic findings (H-E staining). (a) Control (day 0) and (b) DSS-induced colitis (day 11).

(a)   (b)

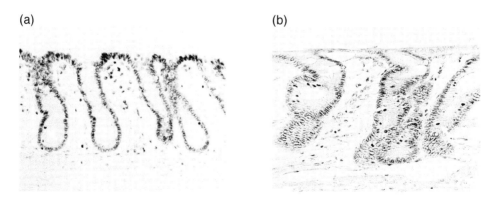

Figure 2. Microscopic findings (toluidine blue staining). (a) Control (day 0) and (b) DSS-induced colitis (day 11).

Histamine Research in the New Millennium
T. Watanabe, H. Timmerman and K. Yanai (Editors)

Development of histamine sensor using recombinant histamine oxidase

Shoko Iwaki[1,2], Yuichi Ohashi[2], Kazutaka Maeyama[1], Ryoji Kurita[3], Osamu Niwa[3] and Katsuyuki Tanizawa[4].

Department of [1]Pharmacology and [2]Ophthalmology, Ehime University School of Medicine, Ehime, 791-0295, Japan

[3]NTT Lifestyle and Environmental Technology Laboratories, Kanagawa, 243-0198, Japan

[4]Institute of Scientific and Industrial Research, Osaka University, Osaka, 567-0047, Japan

For microassay of histamine, we developed a microfabricated histamine sensor using recombinant histamine oxidase (HAO) which shows high catalytic activity on histamine. To detect the histamine level quantitatively, we used the electrochemical reaction by HAO and a carbon-based electrode modified with osmium-polyvinylpyridine containing horseradish peroxidase (Os-gel-HRP).

Using this sensor, we can monitor the histamine release from rat peritoneal mast cells in real time.

1. INTRODUCTION

Histamine has important roles in allergic reaction and as a neurotransmitter and so on. Determination of histamine released from a few mast cells and neurons provides the insight into its functions. The enzyme-modified electrode is useful for detecting current changes continuously but it is difficult to detect histamine itself amperometrically. However, using HAO which has higher sensitivity to histamine than diamines, we can determine histamine by the amperometric method. As shown in Figure 1, HAO oxidizes histamine to imidazole acetaldehyde and hydrogen peroxide. Hydrogen peroxide is subsequently reduced by HRP and the oxidized form of HRP is supplied an electron mediated by Os polymer. This reducing current is detected amperometrically.

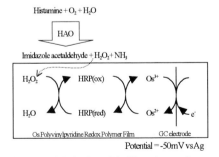

Figure 1.   Mechanism of the histamine sensing.

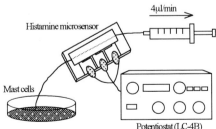

Figure 2.   System of the on-line histamine sensor.

2. MATERIALS AND METHODS

The recombinant HAO from *Arthrobacter globiformis* was overexpressed in *E. coli* (1) and purified using DE52 and Phenyl-Toyopearl column chromatography.

The microfabricated sensor consists of two glass plates connected with inlet and outlet silica capillaries (2). Three carbon film electrodes on one of the plates were modified with HAO, Os-gel-HRP and Ag paste as counter, working and reference electrodes, respectively. Histamine solution was aspirated via a sampling capillary at a flow rate of 4μl/min by a syringe pump (Fig.2). During the flow through the electrodes, hydrogen peroxide was generated and the reducing current was detected with the potentiostat (LC-4B, BAS).

We collected peritoneal mast cells from Wistar rats using Ficoll gradient and measured the histamine release from them stimulated by compound 48/80.

3. RESULTS AND DISCUSSION

HAO was purified 75-fold and its specific activity was 13.3μmol/min/mg protein.

When the standard solution of histamine was aspirated, the current was proportional to the histamine concentration from 0.1 to 100 μM. The lower limit of detection of histamine was 8nM.

Figure 3 shows the change in the histamine concentration when rat peritoneal mast cells were stimulated by compound 48/80. When 10 μl of compound 48/80 (10mg/ml) was added to the culture dish (1ml of PBS solution), the reducing current started to increase 100 seconds after compound 48/80 administration. This increase meant the increase in the histamine concentration by the histamine release from the peritoneal mast cells. The increase of 1nA current was equivalent to about 1μM of the histamine concentration.

By using this microfabricated histamine sensor, we can monitor the small changes in the histamine concentration in real time. This technique will be useful for measuring the histamine release from a few mast cells and histaminergic neurons. Furthermore, *in vivo* experiments, it will also be useful for monitoring the histamine concentration in tissues in combination with a microdialysis probe.

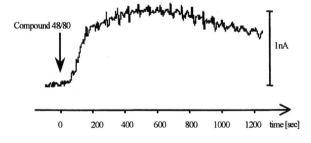

Figure 3. Continuous measurement of histamine from rat peritoneal mast cells. The increase of 1nA current was equivalent to about 1μM of the histamine concentration.

REFERENCES

1. Y-H. Choi et al., J. Biol. Chem. (1995) 270, 4712-20
2. O. Niwa et al., Sensors and Actuators B 67 (2000) 43-51

H3 Receptors and ligands

Histamine Research in the New Millennium
T. Watanabe, H. Timmerman and K. Yanai (Editors)

Histamine H_3 receptor mRNA expression in adult rat brain - cloning of receptor isoforms with differential expression patterns

K. Karlstedt[a], N. Peitsaro[a], G. Drutel[b], K. Wieland[b], M. J. Smit[b], H. Timmerman[b], R. Leurs[b] and P. Panula[a,c]

[a]Department of Biology, Åbo Akademi University, BioCity 2nd floor, Artillerigatan 6A, FIN-20520, Turku, Finland
[b]Leiden/Amsterdam Center for Drug Research, Division of Medical Chemistry, Faculty of Chemistry, Vrije Universiteit, De Boelelaan 1083, 1081 HV Amsterdam, the Netherlands
[c]Institute of Biomedicine, Department of Anatomy, University of Helsinki, POB 9, FIN-00014 University of Helsinki, Finland

We have identified three functional rat H_3 receptor isoforms (H_{3A}, H_{3B} and H_{3C}). The expression pattern of these H_3 receptor isoforms have been characterized by *in situ* hybridization. We have used isoform specific oligonucleotides as hybridization probes and shown a isoform-specific expression pattern in the rat brain.

INTRODUCTION

Histamine (HA) acts as a neurotransmitter through at least four distinct receptors, named H_1-, H_2-, H_3-, and H_4 receptors. They have distinct pharmacological characteristics, and they are all identified by molecular cloning and sequencing as members of the G-protein coupled receptor superfamily.[1,2,3]

The H_3 receptor was originally identified as a HA autoreceptor on the histaminergic neurons extending from the tuberomammillary nucleus to most parts of the brain. The H_3 receptor is also a heteroreceptor postsynaptically in respect to the histaminergic neurons. Pharmacological profiles for both H_3 receptor antagonists and agonists indicate that there may be more than one type of HA H_3 receptors. Using the human H_3 receptor sequence information[4] we set up this study to clone the rat H_3 receptor and to verify the existence of HA H_3 receptor isoforms.

METHODS

Total RNA isolated from adult rat brain was used as a template for cDNA preparation. RT-PCR amplification with human and mouse histamine H_3 specific primers resulted in a specific amplification of rat mRNA sequences. To be able to characterize the expression patterns for the isolated H_3 transcripts in rat tissue we prepared transcript specific oligonucleotides that were used as probes for *in situ* hybridizations.[2]

RESULTS AND DISCUSSION

Cloning and subsequent sequencing of isolated cDNA products revealed a sequence, rat H_{3A}, with over 90% identity with the human H_3 receptor cDNA.[4] We also isolated two clones identical to the H_{3A} clone but with deletions of 96 and 144 bp, respectively. The deletions are in-frame and the deleted 32 and 48 amino acids are located in the 3rd intracellular loop of the H_3 receptor.

In situ hybridization showed that the transcripts are differentially expressed in the brain. Based on our results the hippocampal expression of HA H_3 receptors mainly occurs in pyramidal neurons of CA1-3, dentate granule cells and multiple long-axon afferent pathways. The expression levels in the basal CA1 and CA3 areas are clearly more prominent than the expression in the dorsal parts of the hippocampus (Fig. 1). Binding studies with [^{3}H]-NAMH,[5] and histaminergic innervation[6] data also supports our data that the ventral hippocampal areas are regulated by tuberomammillary histaminergic neurons through HA H_3 receptors, and probably through H_{3A} and H_{3C} receptor isoforms.

These data indicate that the histaminergic signaling is complex, and that one regulatory level can be differential expression of HA H_3 receptor isoforms.

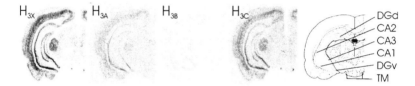

Figure 1. H_3 receptor expression in rat brain. Micrograph H_{3X} shows a hybridization detecting all receptor isoforms, and H_{3A}, H_{3B} and H_{3C}, the specific isoform expression, respectively (Bregma level –4.80). DGd, dorsal dentate gyrus; DGv, ventral DG; CA1-CA3, CA1-CA3 pyramidale layer of hippocampus; TM, tuberomammillary area.

REFERENCES

1. R. Leurs, M.J. Smit and H. Timmerman, Pharmacol. Ther. (1995) 66:413-463.
2. G. Drutel, N. Peitsaro, K. Karlstedt, K. Wieland, M.J. Smit, H. Timmerman, P. Panula and R. Leurs, Mol. Pharmacol. (2001) In press.
3. T. Oda, N. Morikawa, Y. Saito, Y. Masuho and S.I. Matsumoto, J. Biol. Chem. (2000) In Press.
4. T.W. Lovenberg, B.L. Roland, S.J. Wilson, X. Jiang, J. Pyati, A.Huvar, M.R. Jackson and M. G. Erlander, Mol. Pharmacol. (1999) 55:1101-1107.
5. P. Cumming, C. Shaw and S.R. Vincent, Synapse (1991) 8:144-151.
6. P. Panula, U. Pirvola, S. Auvinen and M. Airaksinen, Neuroscience (1989) 28:585-610.

Histamine Research in the New Millennium
T. Watanabe, H. Timmerman and K. Yanai (Editors)

Histamine H₃ receptor - mediated regulation of glutamatergic synaptic transmission in the hippocampus and striatum

Ritchie E. Brown, Nanuli Doreulee, Yevgeni Yanovsky and Helmut L. Haas

Department of Neuro- and Sensory Physiology, Heinrich-Heine Universität, POB 101007, D-40001, Düsseldorf, Germany.

1. INTRODUCTION

The hippocampus and striatum are brain regions which play a critical role in declarative and non-declarative memory respectively. Both regions receive an histaminergic input from the tuberomammillary nucleus[1] which modulates their activity across the sleep-wake cycle. We have studied the effects of histamine on synaptic potentials in these two regions using extracellular and intracellular recording techniques in brain slices maintained *in vitro*[2-4].

2. MATERIALS AND METHODS

400-500 μm thick slices containing the hippocampus or striatum were prepared from male, Wistar rats (3-7 weeks) according to standard procedures. Slices were maintained in a submerged type recording chamber and synaptic potentials/currents were elicited by the delivery of constant-voltage steps through stimulating electrodes placed within the slice. Glass microelectrodes were used to record the evoked field potentials (extracellular recording) or intracellular potentials/currents.

3. RESULTS

3.1. Effects of histamine on different synaptic pathways

In both regions, bath-applied histamine (0.1 – 20 μM) dose-dependently depressed synaptic transmission at the major afferent input – in the hippocampal formation the perforant path input from the entorhinal cortex and in the striatum the corticostriatal pathway. Synaptic potentials in the CA3 or CA1 regions of the hippocampus were not depressed by histamine. In the striatum histamine depressed field potentials in both the dorsal (neostriatum) and ventral (nucleus accumbens) parts. Synaptic potentials were never completely abolished by histamine – the maximum depression was between 30 and 40 %.

3.2. Analysis of the mechanism of histaminergic depression

Several different lines of evidence suggested that histamine depressed glutamatergic synaptic transmission via a presynaptic mechanism: 1) histamine had only small or no effects on postsynaptic membrane properties below threshold and still depressed synaptic transmission in voltage-clamp experiments; 2) histamine enhanced paired-pulse facilitation – a presynaptically mediated form of short-term plasticity; 3) histamine did not affect responses produced by pressure ejection of the glutamate receptor agonist AMPA into the slice; 4) histamine did not affect the amplitude of miniature synaptic potentials.

The magnitude of the histaminergic depression was not affected by inhibitors of serine/threonine or tyrosine kinases. The frequency of miniature synaptic potentials was unaffected, making a direct action on the release machinery unlikely. Experiments with antagonists of potassium and calcium channels suggested that histamine inhibits multiple types of presynaptic calcium channels.

3.3. Pharmacology

Histamine H_3 receptors have been shown to inhibit the release of many other neurotransmitters aside from histamine itself. Accordingly, we investigated a role for these receptors in the histaminergic depression. In both hippocampus and striatum the selective histamine H_3 receptor agonist R-α-methylhistamine (0.1 – 10 μM) mimicked the effects of histamine whereas the selective H_3 receptor antagonist, thioperamide (1 or 10 μM) completely blocked the effect of histamine.

4. CONCLUSIONS

Presynaptic histamine H_3 receptors modulate glutamatergic synaptic transmission at important pathways in the hippocampus and striatum. H_3 receptors probably act by a direct G-protein mediated inhibition of multiple presynaptic calcium channels.

REFERENCES

1. Inagaki, N., Yamotodani, A., Ando-Yamamoto, M., Tohyama, M., Watanabe, T., & Wada, H. (1988). Organization of histaminergic fibres in the rat brain. *The Journal of Comparative Neurology* **273**, 283-300.
2. Brown, R. E. & Reymann, K. G. (1996). Histamine H_3 receptor-mediated depression of synaptic transmission in the dentate gyrus of the rat in vitro. *Journal of Physiology* **496**, 175- 184.
3. Brown, R. E. & Haas, H. L. (1999). On the mechanism of histaminergic inhibition of glutamate release in the rat dentate gyrus. *Journal of Physiology* **515**, 777-786.
4. Doreulee, N., Yanovsky, Y., Flagmeyer, I., Stevens, D. R. Haas, H. L. & Brown, R. E. (2000). Histamine H_3 receptors depress synaptic transmission in the corticostriatal pathway. *Neuropharmacology* **40**, 106-113.
5. Takeshita, Y., Watanabe, T., Sakata, T., Munakata, M., Ishibashi, H & Akaike, N. (1998). Histamine modulates high-voltage-activated calcium channels in neurons dissociated from the rat tuberomammillary nucleus. *Neuroscience* **87**, 797-805.

Histamine Research in the New Millennium
T. Watanabe, H. Timmerman and K. Yanai (Editors)

Peripherally administered Ciproxifan elevates Hypothalamic Histamine Levels and Potently Reduces Food intake in the Sprague Dawley rat.

Christina Bjenning, Anne-Grethe Juul, Karina Z. Lange and Karin Rimvall. Novo Nordisk A/S, Health Care Discovery, Novo Nordisk Park, DK-2760 Måløv, Denmark

1. INTRODUCTION

The prevalence of obesity in the western world is increasing rapidly, and along with it major chronic debilitating diseases. Indeed, it is generally accepted that obesity, impaired glucose tolerance, hyperinsulinemia and insulin resistance *precede* frank type 2 diabetes. Fortunately, a relatively modest weight-loss will improve diabetic control, but dietary and exercise programs very rarely have any effect. Therefore it is important to identify compounds with appetite-reducing properties.

Histamine-H3 antagonists decrease food intake, presumably by increasing hypothalamic histamine levels. The aim of this study was to investigate the effect on food intake and hypothalamic histamine levels in the awake animal after peripheral administration of Ciproxifan, a histamine-H3 antagonist.

2. MATERIAL AND METHODS

2.1 Feeding assay

Male Sprague-Dawley (SD) rats were single-housed and adapted to a schedule-fed regime where food was available for 3h, between 9 am to noon, seven days a week. Water was available ad libitum 24h/day. The animals were given a diet with a high content of dietary fat (D12451, 44 kcal% fat from Research Diets, Inc. NJ, USA) to ensure that they achieved sufficient nutrition to gain bodyweight.

After 7-9 feeding sessions, the animals had a stable food intake, and were administered ip with 15 or 30 mg/kg of the histamine H3 antagonist Ciproxifan 30 minutes before schedule feeding. Food intake was monitored 1,2 and 3 hrs after food was presented.

2.2 Microdialysis

Effect on hypothalamic histamine levels: Guide-cannulae were implanted into the skull of male SD rats. The animals were allowed to recover for seven days before a microdialysis probe was introduced through the guide cannula into the hypothalamic region of the brain. The cannula was inserted 1.9 mm posterior to bregma and 1.5 mm lateral to bregma at angle of 10 degrees. The probe membrane area of dialysis (2 mm) thereby reached the paraventricular nucleus but did not enter the 3rd ventricle. After finished experiment each brain was sectioned in order to verify position of membrane. The probe was constantly perfused with a buffer solution (flow rate 2.3 μl/min) and fractions of 46 μl were collected by an auto-sampler every 20 minutes. Subsequently to a 2h stabilization period the rats were injected *ip* with either Ciproxifan (15 or 30 mg/kg) or vehicle and fractions of the hypothalamic perfusate were collected during an additional 200 minutes. Histamine levels were measured by an ELISA-kit from Bioconcepts.

450

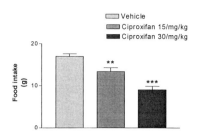

Figure 1. Ciproxifan dose-dependently inhibits 3h food intake in schedule-fed Sprague Dawley rats (n=9-11 animals / treatment, ip administration).

3. RESULTS AND CONCLUSION

In the 3-hour schedule fed rat model, Ciproxifan decreased food intake in a dose dependent fashion; 15 mg/kg reduced food intake with 21% and 30mg/kg reduced food intake with 46% compared to vehicle (Fig.1).

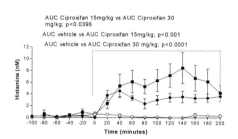

Figure 2. Ciproxifan dose-dependently increases hypothalamic histamine release in the awake, freely moving Sprague Dawley rat (?= vehicle; ?= 15 mg/kg; |= 30 mg/kg. n= 6 animals/treatment, ip administration).

Microdialysis revealed that Ciproxifan, 15 mg/kg, increased histamine AUC during 200 minutes from 64 nM to 676 nM p<0.001, whereas 30 mg/kg of Ciproxifan increased histamine AUC to 1170 nM; p<0.0001 (Fig. 2). Indeed, histamine output was significantly different between the 15 and 30mg/kg doses (p< 0.05).

We conclude that peripheral administration of the histamine-H3 antagonist Ciproxifan in doses that dose-dependently depresse appetite in the schedule-fed male SD rat significantly and dose-dependently augment hypothalamic histamine levels

Histamine Research in the New Millennium
T. Watanabe, H. Timmerman and K. Yanai (Editors)

Peripherally administered Histamine H3 Antagonist Potently Reduces Snacking Behavior in the Obese Zucker Rat.

Christina Bjenning, Wei Liu and Karin Rimvall. Novo Nordisk A/S, Health Care Discovery, Novo Nordisk Park, DK-2760 Måløv, Denmark

1. INTRODUCTION

An increase in sedentary lifestyles combined with excessive caloric consumption, in particular of dietary fat, has clearly increased the prevalence of obesity, a major factor in type 2 diabetes. Ciproxifan, a histamine-H3 antagonist [1] (Ligneau et al., 1998), decreases food intake in the schedule-fed rat and concomitantly increase hypothalamic histamine levels (see accompanying abstract). The aim of this study was to investigate the effect of ciproxifan on food intake in a fed-rat model. We utilized the rat snacking model in order to specifically measure alterations in preference for a very palatable high-fat or high-carbohydrate snack in the male obese Zucker rat.

2. MATERIAL AND METHODS

Male Obese Zucker rats, aged 4-5 months were single-housed and adapted to the substituting of their chow for a palatable high-carbohydrate (D12450b, 70 kcal% carbohydrates and 10 kcal% fat from Research Diets, Inc. NJ, USA) or a high fat (D12451, 44 kcal% fat, 35 kcal% carbohydrates from Research Diets, Inc. NJ, USA) snack during 4h two times weekly. Water was present ad libitum at all times. As the consumption of the palatable snack stabilized, after 7-9 sessions, the rats were considered habituated (Figure 1). Prior to testing with test compound the response to an appetite reducing compound, D-fenfluramine, was recorded (Fig. 2)

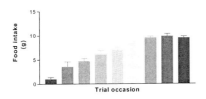

Figure 1. Habituation in the male Obese Zucker rat to the presence of a palatable snack during 4h twice weekly (n=8 animals).

452

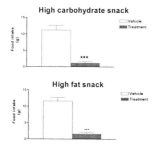

Figure 2. D-fenfluramine reduces snacking equally in Obese Zucker rats habituated to a high-carbohydrate snack and rats habituated to a high-fat snack (n=8 animals/treatment).

3. RESULTS AND CONCLUSION

We found that Ciproxifan dose-dependently reduced snacking behavior; the effect on a high carbohydrate snack was more potent than the effect on the high-fat snack. 30 mg/kg reduced the consumption of a high-fat snack with 95% and a high carbohydrate snack with 100%. 15mg/kg reduced high fat snack with 71% and high-carbohydrate snack with 100% and 5 mg/kg produced the consumption of the high-fat snack with 23% and of the low fat/high carbohydrate snack with 54% (Fig. 3).

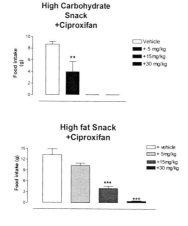

Figure 3. Ciproxifan dose-dependently reduces the intake of a palatable snack, the effect being more profound on the high-carbohydrate snack than on the high-fat snack (n=8 animals/treatement).

We conclude that the histamine H3 antagonist ciproxifan potently reduces excess feeding in the obese Zucker rat and, in particular, the consumption of a palatable high-carbohydrate snake.

[1] X. Ligneau, J. Pharmacol. Exp. Ther. 287:658-666, 1998.

Histamine Research in the New Millennium
T. Watanabe, H. Timmerman and K. Yanai (Editors)   453

Auditory evoked potentials in rats: effect of anticonvulsants and thioperamide

S. Lensu[1], A. Valjakka[1], H. Olkkonen[2], J. Vartiainen[3], G. De Siena[1,4] and Leena Tuomisto[1]

[1]Department of Pharmacology and Toxicology, University of Kuopio, Finland; [2]Department of Applied Physics, University of Kuopio, Finland; [3]NOKIA Research Center, Tampere, Finland; [4]Department of Preclinical and Clinical Pharmacology, University of Florence, Italy

Earlier studies have proposed that histaminergic neurons are involved in anticonvulsive mechanisms. Both inhibitory and excitatory effects of histamine on different neurons have been found in electrophysiological studies [1] while auditory evoked potentials (AEPs) have been used to study neuronal functions. We measured AEPs from the amygdala and frontal cortex of amygdala-kindled male Wistar-rats. Rats were treated with gabapentin, phenytoin, thioperamide or NaCl 0.9% and the effect on AEPs and convulsions was assessed. Brain histamine levels of non-operated rats were measured after treatment of antiepileptic drugs. Used antiepileptics did not change histamine levels, but they reduced analogously seizure severity and AEPs. Kindling as such did not have significant effect on AEPs, and responses after H₃-receptor antagonist thioperamide treatment were not consistent.

1. INTRODUCTION

Previous studies implicate histaminergic neurons in anticonvulsive mechanisms [2]. They also interact with the inhibitory gabaergic system [3]. One way to evaluate the level of neuronal inhibition e.g. during anaesthesia is to study AEPs [4]. The purpose of this study was to determine the effect of kindling, anticonvulsants and histaminergic compounds on AEPs. We also studied the effect of anticonvulsants on brain histamine levels.

2. MATERIAL AND METHODS

Male Wistar-rats (National Animal Centre of Kuopio; n=38, weight ca. 250g) were operated under chloral hydrate anaesthesia (350 mg/kg i.p.). A bipolar electrode was implanted in the amygdala and stainless steel screws were driven above the frontal cortex. The recovery period was at least one week.

For each rat afterdischarge (AD) threshold (lowest electrical intensity producing AD with a duration of at least 3s) was quantified. Development of kindling was assessed by recording ADs following the stimulation (duration 3s, intensity 150-300uA). Both the seizure score and duration of ADs were recorded. Controls had similar electrodes but were not stimulated. AEPs were measured from the amygdala and frontal cortex. Tone-pip stimuli (1.5ms; 8kHz) varied from 74 to 104 dB in 5 dB-steps. Peak energy of 30-200Hz oscillations of the responses were computed to characterize the intensity-responses. The effects of anticonvulsants and thioperamide on seizure severity, AD duration and AEPs were studied.

To measure the brain histamine levels non-operated male Wistar-rats (n=28) were used. Rats were given antiepileptic drug (gabapentine 100 mg/kg i.p. or phenytoin 45 mg/kg i.p.) or saline (NaCl 0.9% 2ml/kg i.p.), decapitated after one hour and eight different areas of the brain were taken to the analysis. Histamine levels were quantified using HPLC-method [5]. Results were statistically tested using t-test or one-way ANOVA with Tukey's post hoc -test.

3. RESULTS

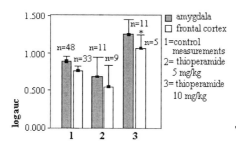 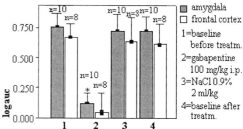

Figure 1. Effect of thioperamide on AEPs. *p<0.05; thioperamide 10mg/kg vs. control and vs. thioperamide 5 mg/kg (fr. cortex).

Figure 2. Effect of gabapentine on AEPs. *p<0.05; gabapentine 100mg/kg vs. baselines and vs. NaCl (amygdala).

There were no differences in AEPs between untreated control and kindled animals. Effect of gabapentine and thioperamide on AEPs is shown in the figures 1 and 2. Gabapentine decreased significantly (p<0.001) the duration of AD and seizures. Phenytoin had a tendency to increase AD duration (ns.), though it alleviated seizures dose-dependently (Pearson's corr. -0.766; p<0.001), which effect was also seen in AEPs. Thioperamide had no significant effect on AD duration or seizures. Brain histamine levels were not significantly diffenrent between control and drug treated groups.

4. CONCLUSIONS
Antiepileptic drugs did not affect brain histamine concentrations, but their effect was detectable analogously in seizure severity and AEPs. Kindling as such did not have significant effect on AEPs. Responses to H_3-receptor antagonist thioperamide were not dose-dependent.

REFERENCES
1. Haas, H.L., Reiner, P.B., Greene, R.W. *In*: Watanabe, T., Wada, H. (eds.) Histaminergic Neurons: Morphology and Function. CRC Press, 1991, 195.
2. Tuomisto, L. & Tacke, U. Neuropharmacology, Vol. 25 (1986) No.8: 955
3. Okakura-Mochizuki, K., Mochizuki, T., Yamamoto, Y., Horii, A., Yamatodani, A. J. Neurochem. 67 (1996) 171.
4. Haberham,Z.L., van den Brom, W.E., Venker-van Haagen, A.J., de Groot, H.N. Baumans, V., Hellebrekers, L.J. Brain Res. Vol. 11 (2000) 873(2) 287.
5. Yamatodani, A., Fukuda, H., Wada, H., Iwaeda, T., Watanabe, T. J. Cromatography 344 (1985) 115.

Histamine Research in the New Millennium
T. Watanabe, H. Timmerman and K. Yanai (Editors)

Histamine H₃ receptor activation modulates glutamate release from rat striatal synaptosomes.

A. Molina-Hernández, A. Nuñez and J.-A. Arias-Montaño.

Departamento de Fisiología, Biofísica y Neurociencias, Centro de Investigación y de Estudios Avanzados (CINVESTAV), Apdo. Postal 14-740, 07000 México, D.F., México.

1. Introduction

The striatum possesses a high density of histamine H_3 receptors (1,2,6,8) and lesioning studies have shown that the major portion is located on GABAergic projection neurones (8,9). However, in other brain areas H_3 receptors are mainly found on nerve terminals and we have recently shown that striatal synaptosomes are endowed with H_3 receptors (7). The major synaptic input to striatum is provided by nigro-striatal (dopaminergic) and cortico-striatal (glutamatergic) pathways (3) and lesion to dopaminergic neurones indicate that ~20% of presynaptic H_3 receptors are located on nigro-striatal terminals where they modulate dopamine synthesis and release (7,11). The remaining portion of presynaptic H_3 receptors could thus be located on cortico-striatal afferents and we present herein data indicating that H_3 receptor activation modulates glutamate release.

2. Methods

Striatal synaptosomes were prepared from adult male rats (Wistar strain, 280-300 g) by homogenisation and centrifugation (4). The synaptosome pellet was resuspended in Krebs-HEPES solution and glutamate release was assessed by a fluorimetric method (10). Briefly, striatal synaptosomes were incubated with glutamate dehydrogenase (50 U.ml^{-1}) and NADP+ (1 mM). The rate of conversion of NADP+ to NADPH due to glutamate release was followed at 460 nM (excitation set at 340 nM). Neurotransmitter release was evoked by 4-aminopyridine (4-AP; 4 mM) and drugs under test were present 5 min before depolarisation. Intracellular free Ca^{2+} ($[Ca^{2+}]_i$) was determined in fura 2-loaded synaptosomes according to Grynkiewicz et al. (5). Drugs under study were added 5 min before depolarisation with 4-AP.

3. Results

The Ca^{2+}-dependent release of glutamate evoked by 4-AP-induced depolarisation was inhibited in a concentration-dependent manner by the selective H_3 agonist immepip (60 ± 10% inhibition, IC_{50} 70 ± 10 nM, n_H 1.4 ± 0.3). The effect of 300 nM immepip (45 ± 5% inhibition) was reversed by 100 nM thioperamide, a selective H_3 antagonist (96 ± 3% of control values).

In fura-2-loaded striatal synaptosomes depolarisation-induced increase in $[Ca^{2+}]_i$ (resting level ~100 nM; $\Delta[Ca^{2+}]i$ ~ 100 nM) was modestly, but significantly, reduced (28 ± 5% inhibition) by 300 nM immepip.

The effect of the agonist was also reversed by 100 nM thioperamide.

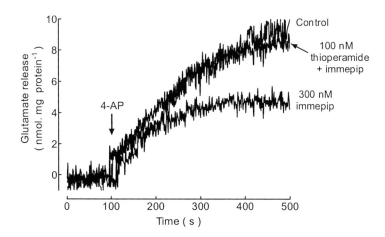

Figure 1. The selective H_3 agonist immepip inhibits depolarisation-evoked glutamate release and this effect is blocked by the H_3 antagonist thioperamide. A representative trace is depicted.

4. Conclusions
These observations indicate that H_3 receptor activation modulates glutamate release from cortico-striatal projections. Our data also suggest that H_3 receptor-mediated inhibition of Ca^{2+} entry underlies the reduction in neurotransmitter release. Since the striatum is the main input nucleus of the basal ganglia and processes synaptic information relevant for motor control, our results provide an additional mechanism for histamine to influence motor behaviour.

References
1. Arrang J.M. et al. *Nature* 327, 117-123 (1987).
2. Cumming P., Shaw C., Vincent S.R. *Synapse* 8, 144-151 (1991).
3. Gerfen C.R., Wilson C.J. The basal ganglia. (Handbook of Chemical Neuroanatomy, Vol. 12), pp. 369-466 (1996).
4. Gray E.G., Whittaker V.P. *J. Anat.* 96, 79-84 (1962).
5. Grynkiewicz G. et al. *J. Biol. Chem.* 260, 3440-3450 (1985).
6. Ligneau X. et al. *J. Pharmacol. Exp. Ther.* 271, 452-459 (1994).
7. Molina-Hernandez A. et al. *Neuroreport* 11, 163-166 (2000).
8. Pollard H. et al. *Neuroscience* 52, 169-189 (1993).
9. Ryu J.H. et al. *Neuroreport* 5, 621-624 (1994).
10. Sánchez-Prieto J. et al. *J. Neurochem.* 49, 50-57 (1987).
11. Schlicker E. et al. *J. Neural Transm.* 93, 1-10 (1993).

© 2001 Elsevier Science B.V. All rights reserved.
Histamine Research in the New Millennium
T. Watanabe, H. Timmerman and K. Yanai (Editors)

Mechanism for the inhibition of amygdaloid kindled seizures induced by histamine in rats

Chihiro Okuma , Tadashi Hirai and Chiaki Kamei

Department of Pharmacology, Faculty of Pharmaceutical Sciences, Okayama University, Okayama 700-8530, Japan

The mechanism for inhibitory effect of histamine on amygdaloid kindled seizures was investigated.   Intracerebroventricular (i.c.v.) injection of histamine resulted in inhibition of amygdaloid kindled seizures.   I.c.v. injection of $CaCl_2$ and A23187 caused dose-dependent inhibition of kindled seizures. $CaCl_2$ and A23187 significantly potentiated the effect of histamine. The inhibition of kindled seizures induced by histamine was antagonized by calcium chelators (EGTA and EGTA/AM). Furthermore, the inhibition of kindled seizures induced by histamine was antagonized by calcium calmodulin dependent protein kinase II (CaM kinase II) inhibitor (KN62).   These results support the hypothesis that histamine-induced inhibition of amygdaloid kindled seizures is closely associated with CaM kinase II activated pathway.

Keywords: histamine, amygdaloid kindling, calcium, CaM kinase

1. Introduction

It has been recognized that histaminergic neuron system is important for epileptic seizures.   Histidine and metoprine inhibited maximal electroshock seizure at a dose causing an increase in brain histamine content (1,2).   On the other hand, we have reported that histidine, metoprine and H3-antagonists, thioperamide and clobenpropit, caused an inhibition of amygdaloid kindled seizures through H1 receptors (3,4).   However, inhibitory mechanism of histamine on kindled seizures is still unclear.   The present study was performed to clarify the mechanism for inhibitory effect of histamine via H1-receptors on amygdaloid kindled seizures.

2. MATERIAL AND METHODS

Under pentobarbital anesthesia (35 mg/kg, i.p.), rats were fixed to a stereotaxic apparatus and bipolar electrodes were implanted into the right amygdala (A:5.0, L:5.0, H:-2.5) according to the atlas of de Groot.   A guide cannula made of stainless steel tubing was implanted into the right lateral ventricle (A: 5.4, L: 1.5, H: 3.0).   Electrodes were connected to a miniature receptacle, which was embedded in the skull with dental cement.   EEG was recorded with an electroencephalograph; stimulation was applied bipolarly every day by a constant current stimulator and continued until a generalized convulsion was obtained. Stimulation parameters were 1.0 ms pulse duration, 60 Hz frequency and 1.0 s train duration at intensity just sufficient to induce after discharge (AD).

3. RESULTS AND DISCUSSION

Intracerebroventricular injection of histamine at doses of 2-10 µg/site resulted in a dose-related inhibition of amygdaloid kindled seizures. I.c.v. injection of H1-agonists (2-methylhistamine and 2-thiazolylethylamine) also caused an inhibition of kindled seizures. However, H2-agonists (4-methylhistamine and dimaprit) exhibited no significant inhibition of kindled seizures. In addition, although H1-antagonists (diphenhydramine and chlorpheniramine) attenuated histamine induced inhibition of amygdaloid kindled seizures, H2-antagonist (zolantidine) was no effect on the inhibition of amygdaloid kindled seizures induced by histamine even at a dose of 50 mg/kg. These results confirmed that histamine plays a suppressive role in amygdaloid kindled seizures through H1-receptors.

On the other hand, i.c.v. injection of $CaCl_2$ at doses of 10-50 µg/site and A23187 at doses of 2-10 µg/site caused dose-dependent inhibition of kindled seizures. $CaCl_2$ at doses of 10 and 20 µg/site, which showed no significant effect on kindled seizures when used alone, significantly potentiated the effect of histamine (Table 1). Similar findings were observed with A23187 at doses of 2 and 5 µg/site (Table 1). Furthermore, calcium chelators (EGTA and EGTA/AM) antagonized the inhibition of kindled seizures induced by histamine. Moreover, the inhibition of kindled seizures induced by histamine was antagonized by calcium calmodulin dependent protein kinase II (CaM kinase II) inhibitor (KN62) (Table 1). However, no antagonism was observed with protein kinase C (PKC) inhibitor (calphostin C) on the inhibitory effect of histamine (Table 1). These results support the hypothesis that histamine-induced inhibition of amygdaloid kindled seizures is closely associated with CaM kinase II activated pathway.

Table 1 Effects of EGTA, EGTA/AM, KN62 and Calphostin C on amygdaloid kindled seizures induced by histamine.

Drugs	Dose (µg/site)	Seizure Stage	AD duration (sec)
Histamine	2	4.5±0.3	44.6± 2.6
+CaCl2	20	2.1±0.7 *	23.1± 3.7 **
+A23187	5	1.9±0.5 **	21.7± 4.0 **
Histamine	10	2.4±0.4	24.4± 3.6
+KN62	10	4.6±0.4#	68.6±12.7# #
+Calphostin C	20	2.8±0.9	36.3± 8.7

Each value represents the mean ±S.E.M. of 8 rats. *, **: Significantly different from histamine treated (2 µg/site) group (P<0.05 and P<0.01, respectively). #,# #: Significantly different from histamine treated (10 µg/site) group (P<0.05 and P<0.01, respectively).

REFERENCES

1. L. Tuomisto and U. Tacke, Neuropharmacology., 25 (1986) 955.
2. H. Yokoyama, K. Onodera, K.Maeyama, K. Yanai, K. Iinuma, L. Tuomisto and T. Watanabe, Naunyn-Schmiedeberg's. Arch. Pharmacol., 346 (1992) 40.
3. C. Kamei, K. Ishizawa, H. Kakinoki and M. Fukunaga, Epilepsy Res., 30 (1998) 187.
4. H. Kakinoki, K. Ishizawa, M. Fukunaga and C. Kamei, Brain Res Bull., 46, (1998) 461.

© 2001 Elsevier Science B.V. All rights reserved.
Histamine Research in the New Millennium
T. Watanabe, H. Timmerman and K. Yanai (Editors)

The role of endogenous histamine in learning and memory in rats

C. Kamei, Y. Sugimoto and Z. Chen

Department of Pharmacology, Faculty of Pharmaceutical Sciences, Okayama University, Okayama 700-8530, Japan

To clarify the role of endogenous histamine in learning and memory, the effects of α-fluoromethylhistidine (FMH) on active avoidance response and spatial cognition were investigated in rats. Both intraperitoneal (i.p.) and intracerebroventricular (i.c.v.) injection of FMH caused a significant prolongation of the response latency in active avoidance response. FMH also showed spatial memory deficits characterized by an increase in the number of total errors and a decrease in the number of initial correct response. There was high correlation between the memory deficit and a decrease in the brain histamine content.

Keywords: α-fluoromethylhistidine, active avoidance response, spatial cognition

1. INTRODUCTION

Since its discovery by Kollonitsch et al. [1] and Duggan et al. [2], FMH, a potent inhibitor of histidine decarboxylase, has been used for in vitro and in vivo studies of brain histaminergic mechanisms [3]. On the other hand, we have demonstrated that histamine plays some crucial role in learning and in memory recollection [4, 5]. In relation to the effect of histamine applied by i.c.v. injection, it has been suggested that externally applied histamine may not truly reflect the histamine action exerted in the brain. To clarify the role of endogenous histamine in learning and memory, the effects of FMH on active avoidance response and spatial cognition were investigated in rats.

2. MATERIALS AND METHODS

Male Wistar rats 7-8 weeks old and weighing 200-280 g were used, and under sodium pentobarbital anesthesia, guide cannula was implanted into the right lateral ventricle. One-way active avoidance response and eight-arm radial maze performance were used. The histamine content of the brain was determined by means of the method of Oishi et al. [6].

3. RESULTS AND CONCLUSION

FMH significantly prolonged the response latency in active avoidance response when administered by either i.p. or i.c.v. When FMH was injected i.c.v. there was a high correlation between a prolongation of response latency in the active avoidance response and a decrease in the brain histamine content [7]. I.c.v. injection of FMH also resulted in spatial memory deficit characterized by an increase in the number of total error and decrease in the number of initial correct response. There was a strong correlation between increases in the number of total error and decreases in histamine contents of the cortex and hippocampus of the brain. Both histamine and thioperamide, a H_3-antagonist significantly ameliorated the memory deficit induced by FMH, however, metoprine, an inhibitor of N-methyltransferase showed no significant effect on the FMH-induced memory deficit. Pyrilamine, a H_1-antagonist, and [R]- α-methyl-histamine, a H_3-agonist, enhanced the memory deficit induced by FMH, at doses that had no appreciable effect when administered alone. No significant influence on FMH-induced memory deficit was observed with zolantidine, a H_2-antagonist [8].

From these results, endogenous histamine may play an important role in learning and memory both in active avoidance response and spatial cognition of eight-arm radial maze task.

REFERENCES

1. J. Kollonitsch, A. A. Patchett, S. Marburg, A.L. Maycock, L.M. Perkins, G. A. Doldouras, D.E. Duggan and S.D. Aster, Nature, 274 (1978) 906.
2. D. E. Duggan, K. F. Hooke and A. L. Maycock, Biochem. Pharmacol., 33 (1984) 4003.
3. M. Garbarg, G. Babrin, E. Rodergas and J. C. Schwartz, J. Neurochem., 35 (1980) 1045.
4. C. Kamei and K. Tasaka, Biol. Pharm. Bull., 16 (1993) 128.
5. C. Kamei, Z. Chen, S. Nakamura and Y. Sugimoto. Meth. Find. Exp. Clin. Pharmacol., 19 (1997) 253.
6. R. Oishi, M. Baba, M. Nishibori, M. Itoh, K. Saeki, Naunyn-Schmiedeberg's Arch. Pharmacol., 339 (1989) 159.
7. C. Kamei, Y. Okumura and K. Tasaka, Psychopharmacology 111 (1993) 376.
8. Z. Chen, Y. Sugimoto and C. Kamei, Pharmacol. Biochem. Behav., 64 (1999) 5.

Histamine Research in the New Millennium
T. Watanabe, H. Timmerman and K. Yanai (Editors)
463

Effects of immunosuppressive drugs on food and kaolin intakes, and hypothalamic histamine turnover in rats

R. Oishi, K. Sunada, T. Nakao, A. Yamauchi, H. Shuto and Y. Kataoka

Department of Hospital Pharmacy, Faculty of Medicine, Kyushu University, Fukuoka 812-8582, Japan

Cyclosporine and taclorimus induced a decrease in food intake, an increase in kaolin intake and an inhibition of hypothalamic histamine turnover in rats. The anorexia may be partly due to nausea, and the decreased histamine turnover may be a compensatory response.

1. INTRODUCTION

Cyclosporine and taclorimus are widely used for the prevention of graft rejection of organ and tissue implantation. But various adverse reactions including renal, cardiovascular, central nervous system, hepatic and gastrointestinal effects are frequently observed during the therapy. Anorexia is one of these adverse effects, but the mechanism is still unclear. In this study, we examined the effects of these drugs on body weight, food intake and histamine (HA) turnover of hypothalamus in rats. The kaolin intake was also measured as the model of nausea[1].

2. METHODS

Male Wistar rats were treated with cyclosporine 50 mg/kg (Sandimmun Injection, Novartis), taclorimus 2 mg/kg (Prograf Injection, Fujisawa) or vehicle (a mixture of cremophor EL and ethanol), i.p., once a day at 12:00 for 3 days. Body weight, food intake and kaolin intake were measured everyday. Kaolin (500g) was mixed with gum arabic (5g) in water (300mL), put into the disposable syringe, and dried. On Day 1 and Day 3, the weight of retroperitoneal and epifdidymal fat pad was measured, and the HA turnover in the hypothalamus was estimated from the accumulation of tele-methylhistamine (t-MH) for 90 min after pargyline treatment (65 mg/kg, i.p.). cyclosporine and taclorimus were injected 15min before pargyline treatment. t-MH was determined by HPLC with fluorometric detection. Ten rats were used in each experimental group.

Table 1

Effects of Cyclosporine (Cyclo) and Taclorimus (Taclo) on body weight, food and kaolin intakes in rats

	Weight gain (g)		Food intake (g/day)		Kaolin intake (g/day)	
	Day 1	Day 3	Day 1	Day 3	Day 1	Day 3
Vehicle	6.2 ± 0.6	22.4 ± 0.8	17.2 ± 0.5	20.1 ± 0.5	1.1 ± 0.4	1.1 ± 0.3
Cyclo	$-3.0 \pm 1.8^{**}$	$-4.3 \pm 2.7^{**}$	$8.5 \pm 1.8^{**}$	$9.3 \pm 2.5^{**}$	0.8 ± 0.4	$2.8 \pm 0.7^{*}$
Vehicle	4.9 ± 0.8	21.6 ± 1.1	17.3 ± 1.4	21.3 ± 1.0	0.6 ± 0.2	0.4 ± 0.2
Taclo	$-0.3 \pm 2.3^{*}$	$3.5 \pm 1.4^{**}$	12.4 ± 4.4	17.2 ± 2.3	0.8 ± 0.4	$1.4 \pm 0.4^{*}$

$^{*}p < 0.05$, $^{**}p < 0.01$ (Student's t-test)

3. RESULTS

Cyclosporine and taclorimus, at the doses examined, markedly inhibited the gain of body weight and food intake (Table 1). The kaolin intake was not affected on Day 1, but significantly increased by both drugs on Day 3. The weight of fat pad was also decresed by both drugs by 20 % on Day 3.

In the vehicle-treated control group, the pargyline-induced t-MH accumulation in the hypothalamus for 90 min was 177.6 ± 7.7 or 159.8 ± 22.8 µg/g on Day 1 or Day 3, respectively. Cyclosporine decreased the t-MH accumulation to 91.3% and 57.3% of the control on Day 1 and Day 3, and taclorimus also decreased to 88.9% and 37.3%, respectively.

4. DISCUSSION

The present study clearly showed that cyclosporine and taclorimus inhibit the food intake and gain of body weight. Since the increase in kaolin intake is considered to be a result from nausea[1], the anorexia induced by these drugs may be due to nausea at least in part. As brain HA is an inhibitory substance for appetite, the decreased HA turnover by these drugs may be a compensatory response to the decreased body weight or nausea.

REFERENCES

1. D. Mitchell et al., Physiol. Behav., 17 (1976) 691.

© 2001 Elsevier Science B.V. All rights reserved.
Histamine Research in the New Millennium
T. Watanabe, H. Timmerman and K. Yanai (Editors)

Glucagon-like peptide 1 modulates histaminergic action in the central regulation of food intake in rats

Yohei Kurose, Akihiko Suzuki, Naoyoshi Tamura, Masaki Tamura, Takahisa Nakao, Tomoko Noguchi, Tohru Hasemi, Yoshiaki Terashima

Department of Animal Nutrition, Faculty of Animal Science, Kitasato University, Towada, 034-8628, Japan

We investigated whether central histamine is responsible for the reduction in food intake by GLP-1. The inhibitory effect of GLP-1 on eating was attenuated by histamine depletion and the blockade of histamine H1-receptors. These results suggests that activation of histamine H1-receptors may contribute to the inhibitory effect of GLP-1 on feeding. Histamine levels were unexpectedly decreased by GLP-1 infusion in the hypothalamus. The local injection of GLP-1 into the hypothalamus might cause feeding-stimulatory processes that reduce histamine release.

Keywords: histamine, glucagon-like peptide 1, food intake, brain, microdialysis

1.Introduction

Glucagon-like peptide 1 (GLP-1) has been known to powerfully inhibit feeding when given intracerebroventricularly [1]. However the inhibitory effect of GLP-1 on food intake has not been fully elucidated. Histamine acts as a satiety signal in the brain. So we hypothesized that the inhibitory effect of GLP-1 on eating might be modulated by histamine. In the present study, we determined whether histamine is responsible for the reduction in food intake by GLP-1 and reduces food intake through the activation of histamine H1-receptors in the brain. In addition, we investigated the interactions of GLP-1 and histamine in the hypothalamus.

2.Materials and Methods

Male rats of Wistar strain (300 g BW) were used for experimental animals. In all experiments, rats were deprived of food 24 hours before drug administrations. In experiment 1, the animals were intracerebroventricularly injected with 500 μg of S(+)-alpha-fluoromethylhisti dine hydrochloride (alpha-FMH, histidine decarboxylase inhibitor), and 60 min later were intracerebroventricularly injected with 3 μg of GLP-1(7-36) amide. In experiment 2, the animals were intracerebroventricularly injected with 82 μg of triprolidine (histamine H1-receptor antagonist) and 3 μg of GLP-1(7-36) amide. Soon after the drug administration, food intake during 2 hours was measured. In experiment 3, we administered GLP-1(7-36) amide and collected histamine simultaneously in the para-ventricular nucleus (PVN) by microdialysis technique. Each sample was analyzed for histamine by RIA. Ninety minutes after the start of dialysis, GLP-1(7-36) amide dissolved in Ringer's solution (20 ng/3 μl) was continuously injected into the PVN at a rate of 3 μl/min for 60 min. Data were analyzed by ANOVA and differences between two values were tested using Fisher's PLSD.

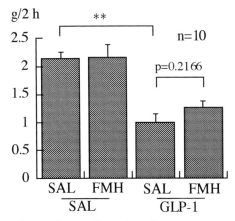

Figure1. Food intake after i.c.v. injection of alpha-FMH and/or GLP-1

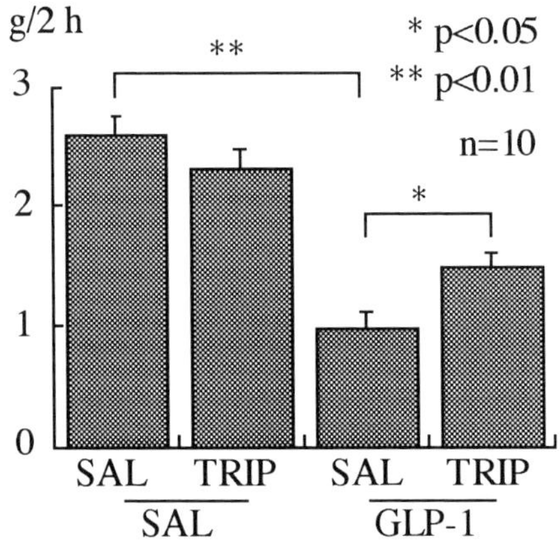

Figure 2. Food intake after i.c.v. injection of triprolidine and/or GLP-1

3.Results

Food intake in rats given both alpha-FMH and GLP-1(7-36) amide was a little greater than that in rats given GLP-1(7-36) amide alone (Figure 1). Triprolidine significantly ($p<0.05$) attenuated the inhibitory effect of GLP-1(7-36) amide on food intake (Figure 2). The reduction rate of histamine levels in rats given GLP-1(7-36) amide was significantly ($p<0.01$) greater than that in rats given saline alone at 30 min (Figure 3).

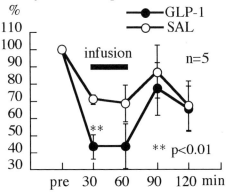

Figure 3. Changes of histamine levels in the hypothalamus during GLP-1 infusion

4.Discussion

GLP-1 may decrease food intake partly through histaminergic activity. In addition, activation of histamine H1-receptors may contribute to the inhibitory effect of GLP-1 on feeding. It has been reported that GLP-1 produces a biphasic effect on food intake [2]. Therefore the local injection of GLP-1 into the hypothalamus might cause feeding-stimulatory processes that reduce histamine release. Further research must be focused on glucose metabolism to clarify the relationship between histamine and GLP-1 in the brain.

References

1. M.D.Turton, D.O'Shea, I.Gunn, S.A.Beak, C.M.B.Edwards, K.Meeran, S.J.Choi, G. M.Taylor, M.M.Heath, P.D.Lambert, J.P.H.Wilding, D.M.Smith, M.A.Ghatei J.Herbert and S.R.Bloom, Nature, 379 (1996) 69.
2. M.Navarro, F.R.de Fonseca, E.Alvarez, J.A.Chowen, J.A.Zueco, R.Gomez, J.Eng and E.Blázquez, J. Neurochem., 67 (1996) 1982.

© 2001 Elsevier Science B.V. All rights reserved.
Histamine Research in the New Millennium
T. Watanabe, H. Timmerman and K. Yanai (Editors)

Histamine-induced itch-scratch response and cutaneous nerve firing in mice: comparison with serotonin

H. Nojima, T. Maekawa and Y. Kuraishi

Department of Applied Pharmacology, Faculty of Pharmaceutical Sciences, Toyama Medical and Pharmaceutical University, 2630 Sugitani, Toyama 930-0194, Japan

To assess the itch-associated response of primary afferents innervating the murine skin *in vivo*, dose-response curves and time-courses for itch-scratching and cutaneous nerve firing responses to intradermal injections of pruritogens (histamine and serotonin) were compared in ICR and ddY mice. Histamine increased itch-scratch response and cutaneous nerve firing in ICR, but not ddY, mice. Serotonin increased these two responses in either ICR or ddY mice. The dose-response curves and time-courses for histamine- and serotonin-induced nerve firing were similar to those for the itch-scratch response. The results suggest that histamine does not necessarily act as a pruritogen in mice, and raise the possibility that strain difference in the pruritogenic action of histamine is at least partly due to the difference in responsiveness of cutaneous nerve to this biogenic amine.

1. Introduction

Pruritus is produced primarily near the dermal-epidermal junction, and then the itch signal is conveyed through the excitation of primary afferents to dorsal horn. In the sense, it is important to measure the activity of cutaneous nerve evoked by application of known pruritogens. Although recording of the activity of afferent nerve innervating the skin is indispensable for the study of itch, such a method has not been established yet in animals. Therefore, we attempted to record the itch-associated response of afferent nerve innervating the skin of mice *in vivo*. Histamine and serotonin, which are inflammatory chemical mediators, are appreciable to act as pruritogens not only in human subjects but also in mice. However, there is an obvious strain difference in itch-scratch response to histamine between ICR and ddY mice and there are a few lines of evidence against the role of histamine as common itch mediator in mice. Hence, we compared the effects of histamine and serotonin on the nerve activity with the effects on itch-scratch response in these strains of mice.

2. Methods

In behavioral experiments, immediately after intradermal (i.d.) injection of each pruritogen into the rostral part of the back, the mice were put into a cage for the behavioral observation. The behaviors were videotaped. The scratching of the injected site by the hind paws was counted by the playing back. In electrophysiological experiments, under urethane anesthesia the skin of the rostral back (about 1.5 cm in mediolateral width and about 2.5 cm in rostrocaudal length) was turned inside out. The cutaneous nerve branch was then exposed and maintained in a pool of mineral oil. The cutaneous nerve firing was recorded extracellularly using bipolar electrodes of silver wire. Each pruritogen was injected intradermally into the receptive region after a stable nerve activity was obtained.

468

3. Results and Discussion

In ICR mice, histamine dose-dependently increased scratch responses at i.d. doses up to 1,000 nmol/site. The effect of histamine on cutaneous nerve activity reached a low ceiling at doses of 100–300 nmol/site. In ddY mice, histamine did not significantly increase scratch response and cutaneous nerve activity. In either ICR or ddY strain, serotonin dose-dependently increased scratch responses at i.d. doses up to 100 nmol/site. The cutaneous nerve activity was also increased by serotonin at doses up to 100 nmol/site. Scratch response and cutaneous nerve firing following pruritogen injection were similar to each other in the time-course and dose-response relationship. Comparison between them elicited by i.d. injection of histamine and serotonin at a dose of 100 nmol/site was shown in figure 1. In mice, cutaneous injection of serotonin elicits itch-related rather than pain-related behavioral responses (1,2), suggesting that serotonin is pruritogenic rather than algogenic in mice. With regard to histamine, there are apparent strain differences in pruritogenic potency. With these findings taken into account, the present results suggest that cutaneous nerve activity reflects the pruritic stimulation of the skin.

Histamine increased the firing of cutaneous nerves as well as itch-scratch response in ICR mice, but not in ddY mice. The simplest explanation of this strain difference is that H_1 histamine receptors are expressed on itch-signaling sensory neurons in ICR mice but not in ddY mice. However, in our preliminary experiments, the expression level of H_1 receptor mRNA in the dorsal root ganglia of ddY mouse was similar to that of ICR mouse. Thus, further experiments are needed to elucidate the cause of the strain differences.

In summary, we found that the dose-response curves and time-courses for cutaneous nerve firing to pruritogens were similar to those for the itch-scratch responses, and histamine did not significantly increase itch-scratch response and cutaneous nerve activity in ddY mice. The results suggest that histamine does not necessarily act as a pruritogen in mice and raise the possibility that strain difference in the pruritogenic action of histamine is at least partly due to the difference in responsiveness of cutaneous nerve to this biogenic amine.

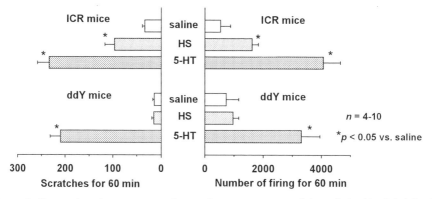

Figure 1. Comparison between scratches and cutaneous nerve firing elicited by i.d. injection of histamine (HS, 100 nmol) and serotonin (5-HT, 100 nmol) in ICR and ddY mice

References
1. T. Yamaguchi, T. Nagasawa, M. Satoh and Y. Kuraishi, Neurosci. Res., 35 (1999) 77–83.
2. K. Hagiwara, H. Nojima and Y. Kuraishi, Pain Res., 14 (1999) 53–59.

Histamine Research in the New Millennium
T. Watanabe, H. Timmerman and K. Yanai (Editors)

Intrathecal histamine elicits a scratching, biting and licking behavior in mice

Tohru Orito[1], Akihiko Yonezawa[1], Takafumi Hayashi[1], Jalal Izadi Mobarakeh[2], Kazuhiko Yanai[2], Takehiko Watanabe[2], Tsukasa Sakurada[3], and Shinobu Sakurada[1]

[1]Department of Physiology and Anatomy, Tohoku Pharmaceutical University, Sendai, Japan. [2]Department of Pharmacology, Tohoku University School of Medicine, Sendai, Japan. [3]Department of Biochemistry, Daiichi College of Pharmaceutical Sciences, Fukuoka, Japan.

keywords: Histamine; *d*-Chlorpheniramine; Cimetidine; Substance P; N-methyl-D-asparate

Histamine (HA) H_1 receptors have been detected within the guinea-pig spinal cord, and the role of histamine is proposed as a mediator of cutaneous pain. The projections of descending histaminergic neurons originate from the hypothalamus, and terminate at the periaqueductal gray and dorsal horn of the spinal cord, which are considered to be an important site for pain modulation. In the present study, we have found histamine, injected intrathecally (i.t.) into conscious mice, can elicit a characteristic behavioural response of scratching, biting and licking (SBL) similar to that seen after i.t. injection of substance P (SP) or N-methyl-D-asparate (NMDA). The involvement of spinal neuronal systems containing not only HA, but also SP and glutamate was examined by determining the ability of each receptor antagonist to modify HA-induced behavioural response.

1. Methods

Male ddY mice weighing 20-22 g were used. Immediately after the i.t. injection, the behavioural response was measured in 5 min intervals for 20 min except in the time course experiment. These behaviours included caudally directed biting and licking along with reciprocal hindlimb scratching. All these different behaviours were pooled as a single value for each animal.

For antagonist studies, the substances were tested for ability to inhibit the behavioural response produced by i.t. injection of HA. All antagonists for H_1, H_2, tackykinin NK_1, NK_2 and NMDA receptors were co-administered i.t. with HA in a volume of 5 µL

2. Results

The i.t. administration of HA resulted in a characteristic behavioural response consisting of vigorous SBL, which peaked at 10-15 min and had disappeared at 20-

25 min post-injection (Fig. 1). A dose-dependent increase in total time of SBL was observed following i.t. administration of HA in doses ranging from 200-800 pmol (Fig. 2). The maximum effect of HA was evoked at 800-1200 pmol. Relative to the most effective dose (800-1200 pmol) of HA, 1600 and 3200 pmol of HA were less potent in inducing the behavioural response. In further experiments, 800 pmol of HA was therefore used in combination with various drugs to test their inhibitory actions.

The H_1 receptor antagonist, d-chlorpheniramine, and the H_2 receptor antagonist, cimetidine, inhibited the HA-induced SBL response. When co-administered with HA (800 pmol), all tachykinin NK_1 antagonists (CP-96,345, CP-99,994, [D-Phe^7, D-His^9]SP(6-11), sendide and RP-67580) produced a dose-related inhibition of the induced behavioural response. The behavioural response to HA was also inhibited by D-APV, a competitive NMDA receptor antagonist and MK-801, a non-competitive NMDA receptor antagonist.

3. Discussion

The present data clearly show that i.t. administered HA resulted in behavioural syndrome indicative of a nociceptive behavioural response such as SBL. This behavioural response was reduced dose-dependently by i.t. co-administration of d-chlorpheniramine, a H_1 receptor antagonist, and cimetidine, a H_2 receptor antagonist, suggesting an involvement of H_1 and H_2 receptors in spinally mediated HA-induced response. It should be noted that the peak time effect of HA was much later than that of SP-induced behavioural response, which peaked at 0-5 min following i.t. injection. It is, therefore, speculated by this phenomenon that HA-induced SBL response may be elicited indirectly, possibly through the release of excitatory neurotransmitters in the dorsal spinal cord. This speculation is supported by the results that HA-induced response was reduced by co-administration of peptidic ([D-Phe^7, D-His^9]SP(6-11) and sendide) and non-peptidic (CP-96,345, CP-99,994 and RP-67580) antagonists for NK_1 receptors, D-APV, a competitive NMDA antagonist and MK-801, a NMDA ion-channel blocker. These results suggest that not only H_1 and H_2 receptors, but also NK_1 and NMDA receptors in the mouse spinal cord may be involved in elictation of the behavioural response following i.t. injection of HA.

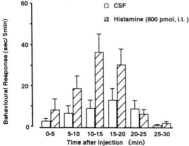

Fig. 1 Time courses of the SBL response induced by i.t. injection of histamine (800 pmol) or artificial CSF. These data are given as the mean ± S.E.M. for groups of 10 mice.

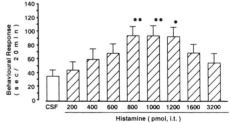

Fig. 2 Effects of varying doses (200-3200 pmol) of i.t. histamine administered in mice. The duration of SBL induced by histamine was determined over a 20 min period starting immediately after injection. Each value represents the mean ± S.E.M. of ten mice in each group. **$P<0.01$, *$P<0.05$, when compared with CSF-controls by the Dunnett's test.

© 2001 Elsevier Science B.V. All rights reserved.
Histamine Research in the New Millennium
T. Watanabe, H. Timmerman and K. Yanai (Editors)

The role of brain histamine in visceral pain and emotion: Analysis through functional neuroimaging in human barins

M. Kano[1,2], S. Fukudo[2,3], T. Watanabe[1], M. Hongo[2,4], and K. Yanai[1]

[1]Departments of Pharmacology, [2]Psychosomatic Medicine, [3]Behavioral Medicine, [4]Comprehensive Medicine, Tohoku University School of Medicine, Sendai 980-8575, Japan

To study the participation of the histaminergic neuron system in pain perception, H1 receptor occupancy by released histamine and regional cerebral blood flow were examined by positron emission tomography (PET). Our activation study using [^{11}C]doxepin suggested that endogenous histamine could be released by colonic distention. In accordance with this, the treatment of d-chlorpheniramine, an H_1 antagonist, significantly decreased the changes of rCBF accompanied with visceral perception. From both studies, histaminergic projections are suggested to play a functionally crucial role in human visceral perception.

1. Introduction

The exact mechanism of visceral pain perception has not been clearly elucidated. We previously reported the participation of H_1 receptors in pain perception with H_1 receptor knockout mice[1]. In order to reveal the role of histaminergic neuron system in pain perception, we investigated whether histamine could be released in relation to pain perception and whether the blocking of H1 receptors could modify the change of regional cerebral blood flow (rCBF) by colonic distention.

2. Methods and Subjects

In the first study, seven healthy male volunteers (right handed) were intravenously given twice with [^{11}C]-doxepin (a potent H_1-antagonist): One PET scan was obtained during the repetitive colonic distention with intracolonic barostat bag and the other was without colonic distention. The binding of [^{11}C]-doxepin were compared between the two PET scans to demonstrate the endogenous histamine release by colonic stimulation. Parametric images of the binding potential (Bmax/KD) were analyzed using statistical parametric mapping (SPM96). Next, [^{15}O]H$_2$O-PET scans were performed in nineteen normal right-handed volunteers (male) to detect the rCBF changes by mild (20mmHg) and severe (40mmHg) colonic distention. In order to examine the effects of H_1 antagonists on the rCBF changes, the same procedures were repeated after injection of 5mg d-chlorpheniramine or saline (5ml) as placebo. Visceral perception and emotion were also assessed with graded ordinate scale.

3. Results

Colonic distention significantly decreased [^{11}C]-doxepin binding in human brains. The reduction of the bindings was probably due to the endogenous histamine release in the brain.

472

SPM96 analysis revealed endogenous histamine release in the anterior cingulate cortex (ACC), hippocampus, prefrontal cortex, and precuneus. The activated regions are consistent with the encoding of perceived unpleasantness and high-order sensory integrations[2]. The rCBF was increased during visceral pain perception in prefrontal cortex, ACC, thalamus, parietal cortex. These changes were significantly attenuated after injection of 5mg d-chlorpheniramine, but not by placebo. The effects of H_1 antagonist were the most potent in ACC (Fig. 1). The effects of antihistamine are more effective at the mild stimulus (20 mmHg) than the severe one (40 mmHg). Abdominal discomforts by colon stimulation were also reduced with an H_1 antagonist at the mild stimulus.

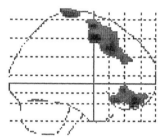

Fig 1 Brain regions where rCBF activation by the mild colonic distention was decreased with 5mg d-chlorpheniramine. The image was obtained by means of subtraction of the rCBF activation images under 20mmHg colon stimulation between 5mg d-chlorpheniramine and placebo condition.

4. Discussion

These data clearly indicated that endogenous histamine was released by colonic distention and that the visceral perception and subjective discomfort were modified through H_1 receptors in humans. The H_1 receptor knockout mice showed behavioral change relating to their emotions [3] and decreased nociceptive sensitivity [1]. Our human studies are almost consistent with the previous data obtained by the knockout mice. In conclusion, histaminergic projections play a functionally crucial role in visceral pain and consequence of stimulation-evoked emotion in human.

REFERENCES

1) J. I. Mobarakeh, et al. Eur. J. Pharmacol. 391, 81-89, 2000
2) P. Rainville, et al. Science 277, 968-971, 1998
3) K. Yanai K et al. Neuroscience 87(2): 479-87, 1998

Histamine Research in the New Millennium
T. Watanabe, H. Timmerman and K. Yanai (Editors)

Involvement of histamine receptors in p-hydroxyamphetamine-induced head-twitch behavior

T. Tadano[a], M. Hozumi[a], R. Oka[a], Y. Agatsuma[a], O. Nakagawasai[a], K. Tan-No[a], F. Niijima[a], Y. Arai[b], T. Aiuchi[b], H. Yasuhara[b], H. Kinemuchi[c], K. Yanai[d], J.I. Mobarakeh[d], T. Watanabe[d] and K. Kisara[a]

[a]Department of Pharmacology, Tohoku Pharmaceutical University, Sendai 981-8558, Japan*

[b]Department of Pharmacology, School of Medicine, Showa University, Tokyo 142-8555, Japan

[c]Laboratory of Biological Chemistry, Faculty of Science and Engineering, Ishinomaki 986-8580, Japan

[d]Department of Pharmacology, Tohoku University School of Medicine, Sendai 980-8575, Japan

Involvement of either the histamine H1- or H2 receptor on the head-twitches (HT) induced by i.c.v. administration of p-hydroxyamphetamine (p-OHA) in mice, has been studied. Simultaneous injection of histamine (HA), which could not induce this response alone, increased the total number of HT by about 2~3 folds, as compared to those using p-OHA alone . Pretreatment with α-fluoromethylhistidine, an inhibitor of HA biosynthesis, and H1 receptor antagonists, diphenhydramine, chlorpheniramine or promethazine, reduced the response induced by p-OHA. In contrast, cimetidine, an H2 receptor antagonist, did not alter the results from that of using p-OHA alone. p-OHA showed a low number of HT in the mutant mice lacking H1 receptors. These results indicate that H1 receptor may be involved in the p-OHA-induced HT in mice.

*Department of Pharmacology, Tohoku Pharmaceutical University, 4-4-1 Komatsushima, Aoba-ku, Sendai 981-8558, Japan

476

1. INTRODUCTION

The amphetamine metabolite, p-OHA, induces HT which has been regarded as an experimental model for hallucinatory conditions. We previously have reported that p-OHA in mice when administered directly into the mouse brain, markedly induces this response (1,2,3). This p-OHA-induced HT is mainly due to activation of central 5-HT neuronal system, since the HT was potentiated by simultaneous administration of 5-HT in small dose and MAO-A inhibitor, clorgyline, but suppressed by 5-HT biosynthesis inhibitor, p-chlorophenylalanine and 5-HT receptor antagonists, dimethothiazine or cyproheptadine. Furthermore, this p-OHA-induced HT was increased by pretreatment with yohimbine but reduced by it with prazosin (2), suggesting the hypothesis of the participation of α_1 or α_2 adrenoceptors by modulating noradrenergic neurons into this behavior. It has been recently demonstrated that histaminergic neurons receive afferent input from fibers containing various substances including norepinephrine and 5-HT (4). In this study, we performed some experiments to clarify the involvement of HA neurons in the HT- induced by p-OHA.

2. MATERIALS AND METHODS

Groups of ten male ddY mice were used in this study. The mutant mice the lacking H1 receptor subtype were generated by homologous recombination as previously described (5). The number of head-twitches was counted for 2 min at 10 min intervals from 10 to 90 min after i.c.v. administration of p-OHA. The techniques used for unilateral i.c.v. injection of p-OHA was the same as Brittain and Handley (6).

3. RESULTS AND DISCUSSION

The i.c.v. administration of p-OHA (20, 40, 80 and 160 μg/mouse) alone dose-dependently increased the total number of HT in mice. HT induced by p-OHA continued for 20~80 min and peak time of the head-twitch activity was approximately 30 min after i.c.v. adminstration of p-OHA. Simultaneous injection of HA (20, 40 and 80 μg/mouse), which could not induce this response alone, increased the total number of HT by about 2~3 folds of p-OHA alone (Fig. 1). Thus, p-OHA-induced HT was potentiated by co-administration with

HA. In addition, α-fluoromethylhistidine (200 mg/kg, i.p.), a suicide

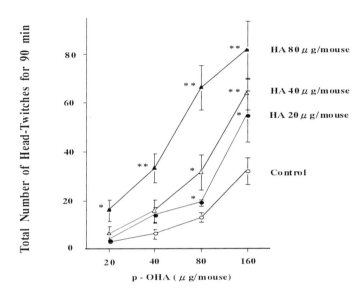

Figure 1. Dose-response curve of intracerebroventricularly injected histamine (HA) and p-OHA. HA and p-OHA were simultaneously injected.
Each point shows total number of head-twitches for 90 min. ○:control (20, 40, 80 and 160 μg/mouse), ●:HA (20 μg/mouse) and p-OHA (20, 40, 80 and 160 μg/mouse), △:HA (40 μg/mouse) and p-OHA (20, 40, 80 and 160 μg/mouse), ▲:HA (80 μg/mouse) and p-OHA (20, 40, 80 and 160 μg/mouse). *:$p<0.05$, **:$p<0.01$, Significantly different from the controls treated by p-OHA alone.

inhibitor of l-histidine decarboxylase, suppressed the number of HT induced by p-OHA. In this study, it might be suggested that the potentiated effect is due to inhibition of brain MAO activity, since HA-induced HT is only developed after the MAO inhibitor treatment (7) and p-OHA selectively inhibits MAO-A activity. In contrast, it appears that the potentiated effect by HA does not relate to inhibition of DAO activity since p-OHA did not cause a significant change of DAO activity (data not shown). H_1 receptor antagonists, diphenhydramine, chlorpheniramine or promethazine, reduced the number of HT induced by p-OHA, but not by H_2-receptor antagonist, cimetidine (40 and 80 μg/mouse, i.c.v.) (Table 1). Moreover, p-OHA (80 and 160 μg/mouse, i.c.v.) produced a low frequency of HT in the mutant mice lacking H_1 receptor (Table 1). These results indicate that the effect of HA on p-OHA-induced HT may involve in H_1 receptor via modulation of histaminergic neuron function in the brain.

Table 1

Effect of histaminergic drugs and mutant mice on head-twitches induced by p-OHA

	p-OHA 20 µg	p-OHA 40 µg	p-OHA 80 µg	p-OHA 160 µg
p-OHA control	3.0 ± 1.1	6.5 ± 1.4	13.2 ± 2.1	28.6 ± 8.9
p-OHA + HA 20 µg	3.8 ± 0.8	13.9 ± 3.3	$19.2 \pm 1.4^*$	$54.6 \pm 10.5^*$
p-OHA + HA 40 µg	6.5 ± 2.8	15.9 ± 4.6	$31.6 \pm 7.1^*$	$63.8 \pm 6.6^{**}$
p-OHA + HA 80 µg	$16.2 \pm 4.4^*$	$33.2 \pm 5.9^{**}$	$66.2 \pm 9.3^{**}$	$81.8 \pm 12.0^{**}$
p-OHA + α-FMH 200 mg/kg			$4.2 \pm 0.8^{**}$	$7.8 \pm 1.1^{**}$
p-OHA + DPH 10 mg/kg			$5.5 \pm 1.2^*$	
p-OHA + PMA 10 mg/kg			$3.0 \pm 0.9^{**}$	
p-OHA + CPA 8 mg/kg			$6.2 \pm 1.7^*$	
p-OHA + CMD 80 µg (i.c.v.)			8.1 ± 2.1	
H1 receptor-deficient mouse		2.9 ± 1.0	$4.1 \pm 1.4^*$	$3.0 \pm 1.2^{**}$

HA : Histamine, α-FMH : α-Fluoromethylhistidine, DPH : Diphenhydramine, PMA : Promethazine, CPA : Chlorpheniramine, CMD : Cimetidine
*:$p<0.05$, **:$p<0.01$ significant different from p-OHA alone.

4. REFERENCES

1. T. Tadano, S. Satoh and K. Kisara, Japan J. Pharmacol., 41 (1986) 519.
2. T. Tadano, S. Satoh, K. Kisara, Y. Arai and H. Kinemuchi, Neuropharmacol., 26 (1987) 1463.
3. T. Tadano, S. Satoh, N. Satoh, K. Kisara, Y. Arai, S.K. Kim and H. Kinemuchi, J. Pharmacolo. Exp. Ther., 250 (1989) 254.
4. H. Ericson, A. Blomqvist and C. Kohler, J. Comp. Neurol., 281 (1989) 169.
5. I. Inoue, K. Yanai, D. Kitamura, I. Taniuchi, T. Kobayashi, T. Watanabe and T. Watanabe, Proc. Nat. Acd. Sci. U.S.A. 93 (1996) 316.
6. R.T. Brittain and S.L. Handley, J. Physiol., 192 (1967) 805.
7. A. Pilc and J.Z. Nowak, Eur. J. Pharmacol., 55 (1979) 269.

Histamine Research in the New Millennium
T. Watanabe, H. Timmerman and K. Yanai (Editors)

The role of histaminergic neuron system in the methamphetamine induced behavioral sensitization: A study using histamine related gene knockout mice.

Y. Kubota[a,b], C. Ito[b], K. Yanai[a], K. Iwabuchi[a,b], H. Ohtsu[a], T. Watanabe[c], T. Watanabe[a] and M. Sato[b]

Departments of [a]Pharmacology and [b]Psychiatry, Tohoku University School of Medicine, Sendai, 980-8575, Japan.   [c]Medical Institute of Bioregulation, Kyushu University. Fukuoka, 812-8582, Japan.

To investigate the role of brain histaminergic neuron system in acute and chronic behavioral effects of methamphetamine (METH), we administrated METH repeatedly on L-histidine decarboxylase (HDC) -, histamine H1 receptor - and histamine H2 receptor - gene knockout (-/-) mice, and wild type (+/+) mice corresponding to each of them, and measured the increases of locomotion during the acute and chronic administration of METH.   The increases of locomotor activity were more exaggerated in the HDC gene -/- mice, but not in the H1 or H2 gene -/- mice in either acute behavioral effect or the development of behavioral sensitization.   These results indicate that brain histamine has an inhibitory effect on the acute and chronic behavioral effects of the METH.

Keywords: Methamphetamine; Histamine; Histidine decarboxylase; H1 receptor; H2 receptor; behavioral sensitization

1. INTRODUCTION

Histamine (HA) has recently been suggested to be a neurotransmitter or neuromodulator[1, 2].   Synthesis of HA involves a single step decarboxylation of L-histidine by HDC.   The HA neuron system has been shown to be involved in diverse brain functions and behaviors through H_1, H_2, and H_3 receptors[1, 2].

A psychostimulant, METH induces increase of locomotor activity and stereotyped behavior[3].   Repeated administration of METH causes a progressive and lasting augmentation of locomotion and stereotyped behavior called behavioral sensitization[3].   We have previously showed that brain HA has an inhibitory role in acute and chronic behavioral responses to METH by pharmacological studies[4, 5].   Recently, the mutant mice lacking HDC, H1 or H2 receptor were generated by homologous recombination, using gene-targeting technique[6-8].   To further investigate the role of brain HA neuron system in acute and chronic behavioral effects of METH, we administrated METH repeatedly on HDC -, histamine H1 receptor - and histamine H2 receptor - gene -/- mice, and +/+ mice corresponding to each of them, and measured the increases of locomotion during the acute and chronic administration of METH.

2. MATERIALS and METHODS

2.1. Animals and drug treatments

Male -/- mice of HDC, H1 receptor, H2receptor and +/+ mice corresponding to each of them weighing 30-40 g were group-housed (3-4 mice per cage) with free access to food and water in a room maintained at 22 ±2 ℃ and 65±5 % humidity under a 12-h light-12-h dark cycle (light on at 6.00 a.m.). These mice were bred in our laboratory and were produced using usual gene-targeting methods. All experiments were performed in animals at ages of 9-15 weeks old. This study was conducted in accord with a guide for the case and use of laboratory animals regulated by Tohoku University School of Medicine, and NIH guidelines on animal care. In the acute treatment with METH, mice were injected with METH (1mg/kg i.p.) in the light period. In the chronic treatment with METH, they were injected METH (1mg/kg i.p.) once daily in the light period for 7 consecutive days. METH (Dainippon Pharmaceut. Co., Japan) was dissolved in saline (0.9 % w/v NaCl).

2.2. Measurements of locomotor activity

Locomotor activity of mice was monitored under an infrared ray passive sensor system (Muromachi, Tokyo, Japan) and the activity was integrated every 5 min. An apparatus with the infrared beam-sensor was set on the top of conventional polypropylene cage in which each mouse was put and number of movements was counted and relayed to a computer. In the acute treatment study, locomotor activity has been measured for 2-h after the first injection of METH. In the chronic treatment study, locomotor activity was counted for 2-h after the 7th administration of METH.

2.3 Statistical analyses

The statistical analysis of data was carried out using ANOVA. In all cases, a P value less than 0.05 was considered statistically significant.

3. RESULTS

3.1 The effects of acute and chronic treatment of METH on the locomotor activity of HDC gene -/- mice

Acute administration of METH (1 mg/kg i.p.) induced the hyperlocomotion both in the HDC gene -/- and +/+ mice. But in the -/- mice, the increases of locomotor activity were significantly more exaggerated than in the +/+ mice. It was 166.2 % ± 62.4 % (mean ± S.E.M., n = 11 for +/+ mice, n = 9 for -/- mice) of the locomotor activity of the +/+ mice. In the chronic treatment study, the locomotor activities after the last administration of METH were increased compared with the acute treatment of METH, and behavioral sensitization was developed in both +/+ and -/- mice. But the locomotor activity of the -/- mice was significantly more exaggerated than in the +/+ mice. It was 151.7 % ± 88.5 % (mean ± S.E.M., n = 8 for +/+ mice, n = 6 for -/- mice) of the locomotor activity of the +/+ mice (Table. 1).

3.2. The effects of acute and chronic treatment of METH on the locomotor activity of H1 receptor gene -/- mice

Acute administration of METH (1 mg/kg i.p.) induced the hyperlocomotion both in the H1 receptor gene +/+ and -/- mice. There was no significant change of the locomotor activity in between the -/- and +/+ mice. Chronic treatment of METH induced the behavioral sensitization in both +/+ and -/- mice, but there was no significant change between two genotypes (Table. 1).

3.3. The effects of acute and chronic treatment of METH on the locomotor activity of H2 receptor gene -/- mice

As well as the result of the H1 receptor knockout mice study, although both +/+ and -/- mice showed the increase of locomotion by the acute administration of METH and the development of behavioral sensitization by the chronic administration of METH, there was no significant change of locomotion between +/+ and -/- mice in either acute behavioral effect or the development of behavioral sensitization (Table. 1).

Table 1. Effects of acute and chronic treatment of METH on the locomotor activities of histamine related gene knockout mice ($\times 10^3$ counts / 2-h)

genotype	acute		chronic	
	+/+	-/-	+/+	-/-
HDC	15.50 ± 2.90	25.75 ± 1.81 *	23.30 ± 3.49	35.35 ± 3.09 *
H1	10.33 ± 2.19	9.40 ± 2.19	20.88 ± 1.66	20.56 ± 1.49
H2	13.15 ± 2.70	12.21 ± 3.54	15.09 ± 1.35	17.59 ± 2.95

Results are mean values $\pm$ S.E.M., n = 11 for the acute treatment of HDC +/+ mice, n = 9 for the acute treatment of HDC -/- mice, n = 8 for the chronic treatment of HDC +/+ mice, n = 6 for the chronic treatment of HDC -/- mice, n = 12 for the H1 +/+ and -/- mice, n = 10 for the H2 +/+ mice, n = 6 for the H2 -/- mice. Statistical analysis was performed by means of ANOVA (* P < .05 vs. -/- mice).

4. DISCUSSION

It is well known that METH increases dopamine release by inhibiting the dopamine transporter and thus causes hyperlocomotion and stereotyped behavior[3]. Recently, it has been reported that L-histidine, which increases contents of HA in the brain, inhibited METH-induced stereotyped behavior, and α-fluoromethylhistidine, which is an inhibitor of the HDC, enhanced METH-induced stereotyped behavior in rats[4]. Thus, it is suggested that the brain HA neuron system has an inhibitory effect on acute and chronic effects of METH. In the present study, we found that increase of locomotor activity by the acute administration of METH was more exaggerated in the HDC -/- mice. Moreover, behavioral sensitization induced by the chronic treatment of METH was more promoted in the HDC -/- mice. Because there is no significant change in spontaneous locomotion and the effect of saline treatment on locomotor activity in HDC -/- mice compared with +/+ mice (data not shown) and -/- mice lack for HA in the brain, it seems like by that the exaggerated METH-induced hyperlocomotion is due to the lack of HA in the brain. On the other hand, we found that there are no significant changes of locomotion between wild type mice and H1 or H2 gene -/- mice in either acute behavioral effect or the development of behavioral sensitization. In the previous study, pretreatment of an H_1 antagonist pyrilamine or an H_2 antagonist zolantidine enhanced the development of METH-induced behavioral sensitization[4]. Thus, it seems like by that the inhibitory effect of HA on the METH-induced behavioral sensitization is mediated by the H1 receptor and H2 receptor. In other word, the potency of the H1 receptor's inhibitory effect on the METH-induced behavioral sensitization is similar to the H2 receptor, or these two receptors participate the inhibitory effect in cooperation. From our present study, it may be that the lack of H1 receptor is compensated by the H2 receptor in H1 receptor -/- mice, and the lack of H2 receptor is compensated by the H1 receptor in H2 receptor -/- mice. It may be interesting to examine the effects of METH in H1- and H2-receptor double knockout mice.

In conclusion, our study shows that the brain HA has an inhibitory effect on both acute behavioral effect of METH and behavioral sensitization induced by the chronic treatment of METH. And it may be that both H1 and H2 receptors participate this inhibitory effect in cooperated manner, and the lack of one receptor is compensated by the other.

REFERENCES

1. Watanabe T, Wada H: Histaminergic Neurons: Morphology and Function. . Boca Raton, Florida: CRC Press, 1991.
2. Onodera K, Yamatodani A, Watanabe T, Wada H: Neuropharmacology of the histaminergic neuron system in the brain and its relationship with behavioral disorders. Prog Neurobiol 1994; 42(6): 685-702.
3. Segal DS, Kuczenski R: Behavioral pharmacology of amphetamine. In: Cho AK, Segal DS, eds. Amphetamine and its analogs. New York: Academic Press, 1994; 115-150.
4. Ito C, Onodera K, Watanabe T, Sato M: Effects of histamine agents on methamphetamine-induced stereotyped behavior and behavioral sensitization in rats. Psychopharmacology (Berl) 1997; 130(4): 362-7.
5. Ito C, Sato M, Onodera K, Watanabe T: The role of the brain histaminergic neuron system in methamphetamine- induced behavioral sensitization in rats. Ann N Y Acad Sci 1996; 801: 353-60.
6. Ohtsu H, Suzuki S, Watanabe T: Assessment of in vivo effect of histamine using histidine decarboxylase (HDC) gene disrupted mice. Naunyn Schmiedebergs Arch Pharmacol 1998; 358(Suppl. 2): R 762.
7. Inoue I, Yanai K, Kitamura D, et al.: Impaired locomotor activity and exploratory behavior in mice lacking histamine H1 receptors. Proc Natl Acad Sci U S A 1996; 93(23): 13316-20.
8. Kobayashi T, Tonai S, Ishihara Y, Koga R, Okabe S, Watanabe T: Abnormal functional and morphological regulation of the gastric mucosa in histamine H2 receptor-deficient mice. J Clin Invest 2000; 105(12): 1741-9.

Histamine Research in the New Millennium
T. Watanabe, H. Timmerman and K. Yanai (Editors)

Brain histamine as protective system for the formation of neural sensitization

Chihiro Ito[a], Mitsumoto Sato[a] and Takehiko Watanabe[b]

Department of [a]Psychiatry and [b]Pharmacology, Tohoku University School of Medicine, 1-1, Seiryo-machi, Aoba-ku, Sendai 980-8574, Japan.

The long-term behavioral sensitization (LBS) and kindling are related to neural sensitization. Meanwhile, histamine (HA) was recently suggested to be a neurotransmitter in the mammalian brain, which regulates many brain functions. In this study, the roles of central HA neurons in LBS and kindling were investigated. As the results, the central HA have the role of preventing the formation of neural sensitization, although central HA after the completion of LBS and kindling has the opposite role each other. The drugs acting to the central HA may be develop as the drug protecting the acquired vulnerability of mental diseases, which regulates the central dopamine and exicitatory amino acid.

Key Words: Central histamine, Neuronal sensitization, Methamphetamine, Long-term behavioral sensitization, Kindling

1. INTRODUCTION

A biogenic amine HA, was recently suggested a neurotransmitter or neuromodulator in the mammalian brain. The cell bodies of the HA neurons are localized in the tuberomammillary nucleus in the posterior hypothalamic region, while their varicose fibers are found in almost all regions of the brain. HA is synthesized from L-histidine (HIS) by histidine decarboxylase (HDC) and is inactivated by histamine N-methyltransferase to N-tele-methylhistamine. The HA neuron system has three different receptors; H_1, H_2 and H_3 receptors [1].

The central HA is known to be responsive to various stimuli, which has the protective role to them. Psychostimulants such as methamphetamine (MAP) and cocaine, restraint stress or electrical stimulus increased the central HA turnovers in the limbic system, diencephalon and so on. Treatments with agents that activate the central HA inhibited the psychostimulant-induced locomotor, stereotyped behavior and reiforcing effect, and the electrical stimulus-induced convulsions in the rodents. On the other hand, those that inhibit the central HA potentiated them [1].

Repeated administration of a psychostimulant such as metamphetamine causes the progressive and lasting augmentations of locomotion, which is called LBS. [2]. In the kindling paradigm, repeated electrical stimuli also induce progressively increasing and lasting epileptiform response [3]. It is said that these 2 phenomena are related to neural sensitization in general, which is known to vulnerability of mental disorders. The mechanisms between the development of neural sensitizaion, and the states after the completions of it are likely to be different.

In our study, the role of central HA in stimuli-induced neuronal sensitization such as LBS and kindling in the behavioral pharmacological and neurochemical methods.

2. DISCUSSION

2.1. Roles of central HA in the formation of neural sensitization

LBS have been well established as the models of drug abuse, drug-induced psychosis and schizophrenia. A key finding to explain LBS is presumed to the central dopamine neuron system, but the detailed mechanism is unclear [2]. In our study, repeated treatments with MAP and an HA agonist HIS inhibited the development of LBS, whereas those with MAP and a H_1 antagonist pyrilamine (PYR) or a H_2 antagonist zolantidine (ZOL) enhanced it [4]. Moreover, this finding was also consistent with our results in HDC gene knock-out mice (to be submitted). These findings suggest that the central HA has an inhibitory role in the development of LBS. The combination of tripelennamine and an opioid pentazocine having a very strong interaction with the dopamine neuron system is commonly used by addicts, and increases drug dependence, which is called "T's and Blues" [5]. Therefore, the central HA is likely to protect the formation of drug dependence, and the appearance of drug-induced psychosis or schizophrenia.

The kindling is well known as an adequate model for complex partial seizures with secondary generalization and temporal lobe epilepsy. The central exicitatory amino acid is thought to be a key finding to explain kindling, but the kindling mechanism is also unclear in detail [3]. Yokoyama et al. [6] reported that PYR accelerate the kindling development in rats. Furthermore, Kamei et al. [7] reported that repeated HIS administration, causing central HA increment, retarded kindling development, indicating the inhibitory role in the kindling development of HA. There are many case reports that anti-histamine agents caused convulsion and epileptic discharges, especially in children of pre-school age [8]. An epidemic of self-administration of a narcotic antihistaminic combination sometimes causes major motor seizures [9]. These lines of evidence indicate the inhibitory role of the central HA through H_1 receptors in the kindling development, and in generalization of complex partial seizures.

From these finding, it is suggested that the central HA has the protective role in the formation of neural sensitization such as LBS and kindling, and in acquiring vulnerability of mental disorders (Figure 1.).

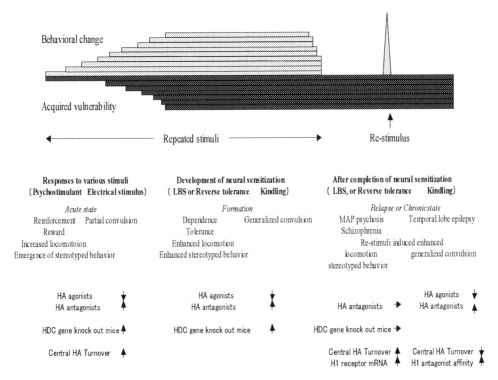

Figure 1. The relationship with the central HA and neural sensitization

2.2. Roles of central HA after the completion of neural sensitization

From the present study, the role of central HA after the completion of LBS is on the contrary to that after the completion of kindling.

Our study showed that HA turnovers in the striatum, cortex and diencephalon were enhanced at the rechallenge of MAP after the completion of LBS [10,11], and that the striatal H_1 and H_2 receptor mRNAs were also increased after the completion of LBS [12]. But HA antagonists did not longer enhance the stereotyped behavior induced by the rechallenge of MAP after the completion of LBS, and there is no difference of locomotor induced by the rechallenge of MAP after the completion of LBS between HDC gene knock-out and wild typed mice (data not shown). Crow [13] reported that type 1 schizophrenia responsive to D_2 antagonists might move to the type 2 schizophrenia resistant to them. In fact, Prell et al. [14] recently showed that the levels of N-tele-methylhistamine were elevated in the cerebrospinal fluid of patients with chronic schizophrenia. Atypical antipsychotics such as risperidone, olanzapine and clozapine strongly antagonize the bindings of H_1 receptors [15]. A H_1 receptor gene variant was related to schizophrenic patients (to be submitted). Meanwhile, Kaminsky et al. [16] reported a case in which the high dose of administration of an H2 antagonist famotidine, was associated with improvement in the deficit symptoms of schizophrenia, although in our study, neither three H_2 receptor gene variants had the relation to schizophrenia [17]. Therefore, it may be suggested that activated central HA and excessive H1 receptor-mediated neurotransmission after the completion of LBS may be related to the relapse and chronic state of drug-induced psychosis and schizophrenia (Figure 1.).

After the completion of kindling, decreased HA turnovers in the bilateral amygdalas and diencepahlon [18], and increased binding affinity of H1 antagonist in the right amygdala was present in our study [19]. It is known to a positive transfer effect that prior kindling through one electrode would facilitate subsequent kindling through a second electrode located elsewhere in the limbic system. The contra-lateral amygdala required a fewer stimulation to reach a full kindled seizure following prior amygdaloid kindling [3]. Kamei et al. [7] also reported that histidine and metoprine inhibited kindled seizure and that these effects were antagonized by PYR but not ZOL. And Kakinoki et al. [20] reported that H3 antagonists inhibited kindled seizure dose dependently. In clinical study, Iinuma et al [21] reported an increased histamine H_1 receptor antagonist binding levels in epileptic foci and surrounding regions in brains of patients with complex partial seizure by positron emission tomography. Therefore, the decreased central HA and increased the affinity of H_1 receptor antagonist may be related to resistant temporal lobe epilepsy (Figure 1.).

REFERENCES

1. K. Onodera, A. Yamatodani et al., Prog. Neurobiol., 42 (1994) 685.
2. L.S. Seiden, K.E. Sabol et al., Ann. Rev. Pharmacol. Toxicol., 32 (1993) 639.
3. M. Sato, R.J. Racine et al., Electroenceph. Clin. Neurophysiol., 76 (1990), 459.
4. C. Ito, K. Onodera et al., Psychopharmacology, 130 (1997) 362.
5. W.R. Lange and D.R. Jasinski, Adv. Alchol. Subst. Abuse, 5 (1984) 71.
6. H. Yokoyama, M. Sato et al., Neurosci. Lett., 217 (1996) 194.
7. C. Kamei, C. Ishizawa, H et al., Epilepsy Res., 30 (1998) 187.
8. M.S. Mueller, New Engl. J. Med., 308 (1983) 653.
9. A. Poklis, P.L. Whyatt et al., Sci., 25 (1980) 72.
10. C. Ito, K. Onodera et al., Brain Res., 734 (1996) 98.
11. C. Ito, K. Onodera et al., J. Pharmacol. Exp. Ther., 279 (1996) 271.
12. Y. Kubota, C. Ito et al., Neurosci. Lett., 275 (1999), 37.
13. T.I. Crow, Br. J. Psychiatry, 139 (1981) 251.
14. G.D. Prell, J.P. Green et al., Schizophr. Res., 14 (1995) 93.
15. J.M. Vanelle, J.P. Olie et al., Acta Psychiatr. Scand., 380 (1994) 59.
16. R. Kaminsky, T.M. Moriarty et al., Lancet, 335 (1990) 1351.
17. C. Ito, S. Morisset et al., Mol. Psychiatry, 5 (2000) 159.
18. H. Toyota, C. Ito, M et al., Brain Res., 802 (1998) 241.
19. H. Toyota, C Ito et al., J. Neurochem. 72 (1999) 2177.
20. H. Kakinoki, K. Ishizawa, M et al., Brain Res. Bul., 46 (1998) 461.
21. K. Iinuma, H. Yokoyama et al., Lancet, 341 (1993) 238.

Histamine Research in the New Millennium
T. Watanabe, H. Timmerman and K. Yanai (Editors)

The changes of histamine concentrations in the plasma and brain in response to acute stress

Zhi-Bo Yang[1], Takaharu Tanaka[1], Yoshinobu Kiso[1], Eiko Sakurai[2], Takehiko Watanabe[2] and Kazuhiko Yanai[2]

[1]Research Center, Suntory Ltd., 1-1-1 Wakayamadai, Shimamoto-cho, Mishima-gun, Osaka, Japan, and [2]Department of Pharmacology, Tohoku University School of Medicine, Seiryo-machi 2-1, Aoba-Ku, Sendai, Japan

It is well known that the central histaminergic system has been shown to be involved in various physiological functions through the H_1, H_2 and H_3 receptor. A large volume of experimental evidence supports the theory that histaminergic neurons play important roles such as maintenance of energy metabolism, internal homeostasis, sleep-awake cycle, locomotor activity, appetite and drinking, convulsion, learning-memory and so on. Recent studies indicated that the activity of the histaminergic system increased when mice were exposed to stress. The activated histaminergic neural system also seems to prevent stress-induced vicious cycles. In the present study, we used the histamine concentration in the brain and plasma as an index of stress, and examined the effects of acute stress on histaminergic system.

Seven-week old male ICR, WBB6F$_1$-W/W^v and WBB6F$_1$-W+/W+ mice were purchased from Funabashi Animal Farm. Blood was collected from the carotid arteries of conscious or diethyl ether-anesthetized mice, and centrifuged at 2,000 rpm for 15 min at 4°C. The plasma was treated with 1/20 volume of 60% perchloric acid, and then centrifuged at 13,000 rpm for 5 min at 4°C. The supernatants were stored at 4°C until histamine analysis. Mice were sacrificed by decapitation. The brain was rapidly removed and dissected on ice into four parts consisting of cortex, midbrain, cerebellum and brain stem. The brain parts were homogenized in 5 volumes of 30% perchloric acid containing 5mM Na$_2$-EDTA with a Polytron homogenized at the maximal setting for 10 seconds in an ice bath, and then the homogenate was centrifuged at 13,000 rpm for 20 min at 4°C The supernatants were stored at 4°Cuntil histamine analysis. Histamine was measured by a sensitive HPLC-fluorometric method described by Yamatodani et al [1].

In the present experiment, we investigated the effects of acute stress on plasma histamine levels. Fig,1 shows the basal histamine concentration in plasma taken from ICR mice anesthetized with diethylether was 4.9±0.6 pmol/ml, while it increased to 94.5±11.8 pmol/ml after mice were exposed to restraint stress for 3 hrs.

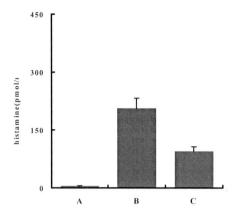
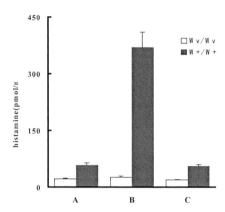

Fig.1. The changes in histamine concentrations in Plasma obtained from ICR mice loaded with stress.

The results represent the mean ±SE obtained from seven ICR mice respectively. (A) non-stressed control mice. (B) stressed mice with taken blood under conscious conditions. (C) restraint stressed mice fixed in a restraint cage for 3 hours.

Fig.2. The changes in histamine concentrations in plasma obtained from W/Wv and W+/W+ mice loaded with stress.

The results represent the mean ±SE was obtained from seven mice of mast cell- deficient WBB6F1-W/Wv mice and wil d type W+/W+ normal counterpart mice respectively. (A) non-stressed control mice. (B) stressed mice with blood taken under conscious conditions. (C) restraint stress mice fixed in a restraint cage for 3 hours.

When the blood samples were obtained from conscious conditions, the plasma histamine concentration also markedly increased to 206.0±27.2 pmol/ml in the basal conditions. The histamine contents in the midbrain also increased after the exposure to restraint stress for 3 hours. To reveal the origin of increased histamine in the plasma and brain, the effects of acute stress on the histamine levels were examined in mast cell-deficient $WBB6F_1$-W/W^v (W/W^v) and their wild type $WBB6F_1$-W^+/W^+ (W^+/W^+) control mice. The basal plasma histamine level was significantly increased in conscious W^+/W^+ mice, but the increase was not observed in conscious mast cell-deficient W/W^v mice as shown in Fig.2. From these results, increased basal levels of plasma histamine observed during consciousness of the control mice would be due to the histamine released from mast cells. However, we also investigated the relationship between the histamine level and acute stress in the brain regions, similarly, restraint stress decreased the midbrain histamine contents of the W/W^v mice while it increased the histamine contents of the control (+/+) mice. Since brain histamine in mast cell-deficient mice was exclusively derived from histaminergic neurons, the neuronal histamine was released in response to stress and the concentration of histamine decreased. However, the stress could increase the histamine concentration from mast cells in the brain.

It is well known that histamine is mainly stored in mast cells, basophils and enterochromaffin-like cells. Our experimental results suggest that acute stress-induced increase in plasma histamine concentration mainly derived from mast cells. Although we are unable to understand the mechanism of this stress-induced histamine response. Our results suggest that the activity of histaminergic neuron and plasma histamine concentration markedly increased during exposure to stress. This result is implicated in host stress response and may play an important role in improvement of stress-induced physiological changes.

Reference

1. A.Yamatodani,H.Fukuda,H.Wada,T.Iwaeda,T.Watanabe, J.Chromatogr.344(1985).115-123.

Histamine Research in the New Millennium
T. Watanabe, H. Timmerman and K. Yanai (Editors)

Anti-stress effects of chicken essence in food-deprived activity stress: Possible involvement of histaminergic neurons

Zhi-Bo Yang[1], Takaharu Tanaka[1], Yoshinobu Kiso[1], Eiko Sakurai[2], Takehiko Watanabe[2] and Kazuhiko Yanai[2]

[1]Research Center, Suntory Ltd., 1-1-1 Wakayamadai, Shimamoto-cho, Mishima-gun, Osaka, Japan, and [2]Department of Pharmacology, Tohoku University School of Medicine, Seiryo-machi 2-1, Aoba-Ku, Sendai, Japan

It has been widely reported that stress is involved in various diseases. It is important to alleviate the adverse effects of stress maintain health. Several studies demonstrated that the activity of histaminergic neurons likely increased in response to stress. Recently, we reported that food-deprived active stress decreased the activity of the histaminergic neural system in rats. The enhancements of the histaminergic neural system could significantly reduce the hyperactivity caused by food-deprived activity stress [1].

Chicken essence contains high concentrations of histidine and glutamic acid. It is widely used in Chinese communities as a traditional remedy for several diseases. It is believed, for example, to help recovery from physical and mental fatigue and from anemia during childbirth and menstruation. Similar meat extracts were also commonly used in these regions at the beginning of the century. Since chicken essence is invigorating without causing addiction, it is recommended to use as stimulants for appetite and digestion. In the present study, the effects of chicken essence on food-deprived active stress were examined in order to determine whether the histaminergic system is involved in its effects.

Seven-week-old male Sprague-Dawley rats were purchased from Charles River Japan Inc. (Tokyo, Japan). These animals were housed in standard laboratory cages under controlled conditions of room temperature ($24\pm1°C$) and kept on a 12:12 light-dark cycle (lights on at 0600 and off at 1800h), and were fed a normal diet and tap water. The animals were acclimated for 1 week before experiment. Running-wheel activity cages were used in the experiments, and rats were subjected to food-deprived active stress for 22 hours per day, and were permitted to take food and water for 2 hours per day in the lateral ventricle of the activity wheel. In the placebo-treated group (7.5% gelatin; 1ml/100g/p.o.), and chicken essence-treated group (1ml/100g/p.o.), rats were treated daily. The histamine concentrations in plasma and brain tissues were measured with a sensitive HPLC-fluorometric method described by Yamatodani et al [2].

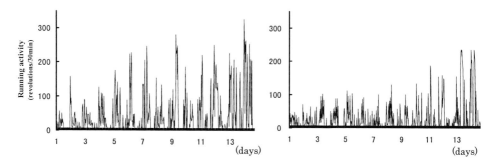

Fig.1 Chronological change in running activity under active stress after gelatin administration

The results represent the average value obtained from five SD rats in each experimental group.

Fig.2 Chronological change in running activity under active stress after BEC administration

The results represent the average value obtained from five SD rats in each experimental group.

In this study, we investigated anti-stress effects of chicken essence during food-deprived activity stress. Our results indicated that in the placebo-treated group, the circadian rhythm of the wheel running disappeared 4 days after exposure to active stress as shown in Fig.1 and stress-induced hyperactivity was observed. Fig. 2 shows in the chicken essence-treated group, the rotation number did not significantly increase until 9 days after the exposure to active stress. The histamine concentrations in plasma, cortex and midbrain tissues markedly increased after exposure to active stress, and stress-induced hyperactivity of histaminergic neurons was eased by the chicken essence administration. As extensive exercise and restricted feeding are thought to be associated with anorexia nervosa, chicken essence might be useful for treating of the appetite disorders. Possible involvement of histaminergic neurons in its effects also discussed.

Recently, several studies have indicated that histamine may be related not only to allergic disorders, but also to physiological homeostasis. This study showed that histaminergic neural activity markedly increased during exposure to stress. Our data suggest that the activity of histaminergic neurons may play an important role in controling stress stimulation.

1) Endou M, Yanai K. et al. Abstracts for this meeting (HA2000)

2) A.Yamatodani,H.Fukuda,H.Wada,T.Iwaeda,T.Watanabe, J.Chromatogr.344(1985).115-123.

Histamine Research in the New Millennium
T. Watanabe, H. Timmerman and K. Yanai (Editors)
493

Decreased histamine H_1 receptors in the rat brain subjected to food-deprived activity stress.

Masatoshi Endou [a,b], Kazuhiko Yanai [a], Eiko Sakurai [a], and Takehiko Watanabe [a]

[a] Department of Pharmacology, Tohoku University School of Medicine, Seiryou-machi 2-1, Sendai 980-8575, and Division of [b]Nuclear Medicine, Tohoku University, Aramaki 2-1, Sendai 980-8578, Japan.

Abstract: We investigated the changes of histamine content and histamine H_1 and H_3 receptors in the rat brains subjected to food-deprived activity stress. For purposes of comparison, we also examined the stressful effects of forced swimming on the histaminergic neuron system of rats. The H_3 receptor density rapidly declined in the acute phase of stress but gradually returned to the control level in the chronic phase. On the other hand, the H_1 receptor slowly decreased and remained at a low level during the chronic phase. These results reveal that there is a discrepancy between the levels of H_1 and H_3 receptors in the acute and chronic phases of stress. These changes resulted in the inhibition of histaminergic neuronal activity in the chronic stress condition.

Key words: food-deprived activity stress, forced swimming, histamine, H_1 receptor, H_3 receptor, microdialysis, reward, hypothalamus

1. Introduction
Food-deprived activity stress gradually increased hyperactivity on the running wheel and actually resulted in decreased food consumption. Food-deprived activity stress reduces food consumption, changes the daily cycle of locomotor activity and induces hyperactivity of wheel-running, such evidence suggests that the histaminergic neuron system plays an important role on the pathophysiology of food-deprived activity stress. In this study, we examined the effects of food-deprived activity stress on the histaminergic neuron. The important feature of the food-deprived activity stress is the self-induced hyperactivity and the decline of food consumption; such a phenomenon was not observed in forced swimming stress. We intended to discover the changes of the histaminergic neuron system specifically induced by food-deprived activity stress.

2. Materials and methods

2.1. activity stress
Male SD rats were individually housed in activity wheel(the food-deprived activity stress group; divided into two subgroups, short activity stress group and long activity stress group); others were isolated in plastic cages(the control group). Rats in the food-deprived activity stress group were forced to run on an activity wheel and were subjected to food deprivation for 22.5 hours per day, and the rotation number of the wheel was measured.

2.2. Forced swimming

Male SD rats were subjected to forced swimming for 1 hour daily for 1, 4, and 14 days. In another experiment, rats were implanted with a microdialysis probe in the anterior hypothalamus. Rats were forced to swim for one 1 and the histamine release was measured.

2.3. Binding assay of histamine H_1 and H_3 receptors

After the experiment, rats were sacrificed and their brains were removed and divided into three parts. The amounts of H_1 and H_3 receptor bindings were measured.

24. Measurements of brain histamine content

The histamine content was determined fluorometrically with o-phthalaldehyde by HPLC.

2.5. Intracerebroventricular administration of histamine to the lateral ventricle

Rats were received an administration of histamine. The rotation number of the running wheel was measured. The locomotor activity was also measured in an open field for 30 minutes and home cages for two consecutive days.

3. Results

The H_1 receptors density was not statistically changed by short-term activity stress while it was significantly less after exposure to long-term activity stress. The H_3 receptors density was significantly reduced by the short-term activity stress. H_1-receptor bindings in all brain regions did not change by forced. The H_3-receptor bindings were significantly reduced after 1-day exposure to forced swimming. The amounts of H_3 receptors were not significantly different by the 14th day of forced swimming in any region. The concentration of histamine was not significantly changed by the short-term activity stress. After long-term exposure to activity stress, brain histamine content significantly increased. Histamine release increased significantly up to 170% of the baseline during forced swimming stress.

The activity of wheel running was significantly inhibited in the dark phase by the intracerebroventricular injection of histamine. The locomotor activities were not affected by the injection of histamine.

4. Discussion

It is speculated that hyperactivity of the activity wheel occurred when the histaminergic neuron system was inhibited. Since the activation of the histaminergic neurotransmission may inhibit the reward system, the attenuated histaminergic neuron system might cause the activation of the reward system and then the hyper-running would be conditioned. In accordance with this hypothesis, our behavioral studies clearly demonstrate that the intracerebroventricular treatment of histamine can attenuate the hyperactivity of wheel running in the late phase. In conclusion, the differential changes between the levels of H_1 and H_3 receptors in the chronic phase would result in the inhibition of histaminergic neuronal activity. The hyperactivity induced by food-deprived activity stress was partially reversible by the injection of histamine into the lateral ventricle.

References

[1] Masatoshi Endou [a,b], Kazuhiko Yanai [a], Eiko Sakurai [a], Shin Fukudo [b], Michio Hongo [c], and Takehiko Watanabe, Food-deprived activity stress decreased the activity of the histaminergic neuron system in rats, Brain Res. in press.

[2] P. F. Aravich, T. S. Rieg, I. Ahmed, T. J. Lauterio, Fluoxetine induces vasopressin and oxytocin abnormalities in food-restricted rats given voluntary exercise: relationship to anorexia nervosa, Brain Res. 612(1-2) (1993) 180-189.

[3] W. M. Beneke, S. E. Schulte, J. G. vander Tuig, An analysis of excessive running in the development of activity anorexia. Physiol. Behav. 58(3) (1995) 451-457.

[4] P. Ghi, C. Ferretti, M. Blengio, Effects of different types of stress on histamine-H_3 receptors in the rat cortex, Brain Res. 690(1) (1995) 104-107.

Histamine Research in the New Millennium
T. Watanabe, H. Timmerman and K. Yanai (Editors)

Central histamine influences respiration in the POA/AH

M. Iwase, M. Izumizaki, M. Kanamaru and I. Homma

Department of 2nd Physiology, Showa University School of Medicine, Tokyo 142-8555 Japan

Effects of central histamine and the preoptic area/anterior hypothalamus (POA/AH) neurons on respiration were examined in rats. Electrical and chemical stimulation of the POA/AH neurons and histamine given to the same sites increased respiratory frequency (f). The increase by histamine was prevented by injection of pyrilamine into the POA/AH. The results suggest that central histamine causes polypnea through H1 receptors in the POA/AH presumably contributing to hyperthermia.

Key words: Central histamine, Preoptic area / anterior hypothalamus, Respiration, H1 receptors.

1. INTRODUCTION

Breathing pattern is affected by hyperthermia with inputs from the hypothalamic thermoceptive structure. It is reported that thermal stimulation of the ventral hypothalamus causes polypnea [1]; however the exact site concerning thermal polypnea and the mediator are unknown. Central histamine activates heat loss mechanisms in the central thermoregulatory pathway [2]; therefore, central histamine may have some effects on respiration at thermal condition. In this study we examined roles of central histamine and POA/AH neurons on respiration in rats.

2. METHODS

Male Wister rats were anesthetized with urethane-α-chloralose i.p., paralyzed with gallamine, vagotomized and artificially ventilated. Phrenic nerve activity, P_{ETCO2} and arterial blood pressure were monitored. Rats were administered histamine, electrically stimulated by a monopolar electrode and chemically stimulated by injection of DL-homocysteic acid in the POA/AH. Each rat body was warmed with a heating pad and a heating lamp causing the body temperature to rise from $37^{o}C$ to $39^{o}C$.

3. RESULTS

Respiration increased in frequency by shortening both inspiratory and expiratory time (TI, TE) at the raised body temperature. Electrical and chemical stimulation of the POA/AH neurons and administration of 100 nmol-histamine into the POA/AH increased f with a shortening of TE (Figure 1). This increase by histamine was prevented by injection of 200 nmol-pyrilamine, histamine H1 receptor antagonist into the POA/AH.

Figure 1. Effects of 100 nmol/µl-histamine administered into the POA/AH on respiratory frequency (A), inspiratory time (B, TI), expiratory time (B, TE) and C. The traces of integrated phrenic nerve activity before (control) and after (HA 100 nmol) administration of histamine. n = 5, mean ±SE.

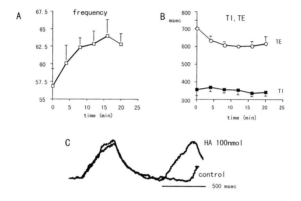

4. DISCUSSION

Facilitation of f induced by chemical and electrical stimulation in the POA/AH indicates that there is an excitatory pathway from the POA/AH to the respiratory center in the medulla oblongata. Histamine also increased f through H1 receptors in the POA/AH. Thermal polypnea is reduced by pyrilamine given in the POA/AH, or S(+)α-fluoromethylhistidine given into the lateral ventricle in rabbits [3]. We have also reported that hyperthermia causes the c-Jun expression of histaminergic neurons in the tuberomammillary nucleus of rats [4]. The histaminergic neuron is probably activated at the hyperthermia and influences the POA/AH neurons to increase f and contributes to the generation of thermal polypnea through H1 receptors.

REFERENCES

1. C. von Euler, F. Herrero, I. Wexler, Control mechanisms determining rate and depth of respiratory movements, Respr. Physiol., 10 (1970) 93.
2. M. D. Green, B. Cox, P. Lomax, Sites and mechanisms of action of histamine in the central thermoregulatory pathways of the rat, Neuropharmacology, 15 (1976) 321.
3. M. Iwase, M. Izumizaki, M. Kanamaru, I. Homma, Involvement of central histaminergic neurons in polypnea induced by hyperthermia in rabbits, Neurosci. Lett., In press.
4. M. Iwase, M. Kanamaru, I. Homma, Fos and Jun expression after raising the body temperature in the hypothalamus and the medulla oblongata, Jpn.J. Physiol., 47 (1997) s96.

© 2001 Elsevier Science B.V. All rights reserved.
Histamine Research in the New Millennium
T. Watanabe, H. Timmerman and K. Yanai (Editors)

Central histamine is a contributory factor in temperature-induced polypnea in conscious mice

Masahiko Izumizaki[a], Michiko Iwase[a], Kazuhiko Yanai[b], Takehiko Watanabe[b], Takeshi Watanabe[c], and Ikuo Homma[a]

[a]Department of Physiology, School of Medicine, Showa University, Shinagawa-ku, Tokyo 142-8555, Japan
[b]Department of Pharmacology, School of Medicine, Tohoku University, Aoba-ku, Sendai, 980-8575, Japan
[c]Department of Molecular Immunology, Medical Institute of Bioregulation, Kyushu University, Fukuoka 812-8582, Japan

ABSTRACT

Little is known about histamine's effect on breathing pattern. Since central histamine activates the heat loss mechanisms according to behavioral studies, central histamine may influence breathing pattern to increase evaporation through the respiratory tract. We first examined the effect of body temperature on breathing pattern. Mice were positioned in a plethysmograph and were inhaled three levels of hypercapnic gas mixture (5,7,and 9% CO_2 in O_2) at <37°C and 39°C. A raised body temperature increased respiratory frequency (f) with reductions in inspiratory (TI) and expiratory time (TE). We then studied the effect of central histamine on respiration with S-α-fluoromethylhistidine hydrochloride in a similar way. The depletion of central histamine inhibited the reduction in TE at 39°C, resulting in lowered f; whereas at <37°C, no difference were detected. Finally, we studied the role of H1 receptors in thermal polypnea by using mutant mice lacking histamine H_1 receptors. Breathing pattern was characterized during a comparable challenge. In wild mice a raised body temperature increased f mainly due to a reduction in TE, whereas in mutant mice f did not increase even though body temperature was elevated. In conclusion, central histamine contributed to temperature-induced polypnea with a reduction in T_E through histamine H_1 receptors.

Key words: Histamine H1 receptors; Respiration; Body temperature; Heat loss

1. INTRODUCTION

It is well known that a raised body temperature augments respiratory frequency (f). However, the underlying mechanisms of temperature-induced polypnea remain poorly understood. Central histamine activates heat loss mechanisms according to behavioral studies, but it is uncertain whether central histamine changes breathing pattern. Therefore, we investigated the role of central histamine in thermal polypnea in conscious mice.

2. MATERIALS AND METHODS

2.1. Effects of body temperature Mice were exposed to three different hypercapnic gas mixtures (5, 7, and 9% CO_2 in O_2) in a double chamber plethysmograph. Measurements of respiratory variables were made at a normal and an elevated body temperature ($39^{\circ}C$).

2.2. Effects of S-α-fluoromethylhistidine hydrochloride (FMH) Respiratory variables were measured with the hypercapnic gas mixtures at the two body temperatures after the intraperitoneal injection of 100 mg/kg of FMH or sterilized saline.

2.3. Histamine H_1 receptor-deficient mice We characterized breathing patterns in mutant mice lacking histamine H_1 receptors and in wild-type mice at the two different body temperatures in a similar way.

3. RESULTS

3.1. Effects of body temperature A raised body temperature increased f with reductions in inspiratory time (T_I) and expiratory time (T_E).

3.2. Effects of FMH FMH attenuated an increase in f at $39^{\circ}C$ because of a prolongation of T_E, but at a normal temperature FMH had no significant effects on breathing pattern.

3.3. Histamine H_1 receptor-deficient mice In mutant mice f did not increase even though the body temperature was elevated, whereas in the wild-type mice a raised body temperature increased f mainly due to a reduction in T_E.

4. DISCUSSION

We first characterized the effect of body temperature on breathing pattern. A raised body temperature reduced in both T_I and T_E, resulting in an increase in f. The next experiment using FMH showed that central histamine contributed to thermal polypnea with a reduction in T_E. Furthermore, we used the mutant mice to advance our investigation. This study supported this results and found that histamine H_1 receptors played an important role in thermal polypnea. In conclusion, central histamine contributed to temperature-induced polypnea with a reduction in T_E through histamine H_1 receptors.

REFERENCES

1. M. Izumizaki et al. Neurosci. Lett., 284 (2000) 139-142.
2. M. Izumizaki et al. J. Appl. Physiol., 89 (2000) 770-776.

Histamine Research in the New Millennium
T. Watanabe, H. Timmerman and K. Yanai (Editors)

Histamine release in the medulla oblongata influences tracheal tone and blood pressure

M. Kanamaru, M. Iwase and I. Homma

Department of Physiology, Showa University School of Medicine, Tokyo, 142-8555, Japan

Histamine release in three areas (RVL:the rostral ventrolateral medulla, nR:the raphe nuclei and nTS:the solitary nucleus) of the medulla oblongata was measured in the anesthetized rabbit using microdialysis and HPLC with fluorescence detection. Tracheal tone and blood pressure were measured through the rostral trachea and the femoral artery, respectively. Histamine release in the three areas was increased by electrical stimulation in the posterior hypothalamus or hyperthermia. Tracheal dilation and pressor response caused by the stimulation was significantly suppressed by perfusion of pyrilamine or (+)-chlorpheniramine in the RVL. These results suggest that histamine release in the medulla oblongata originated from histaminergic neurons in the posterior hypothalamus and is activated by hyperthermia. Brain histaminergic neurons play an important role in adjustments of airway and peripheral vascular tone via H_1 receptors in the RVL.

Key words: Brain, Histamine, Microdialysis, Trachea, Blood pressure, H_1 receptors

1. INTRODUCTION

In brain histaminergic neurons, the cell bodies are restrictedly localized in the tuberomammillary nucleus of the posterior hypothalamus and the fibers are widely distributed in the brain [1]. The medulla oblongata is important for respiration and cardiovascular regulation, however, studies on histamine in the medulla oblongata are very few. Administration of histamine into the fourth ventricle (histamine i.c.v.) decreased tracheal pressure dose-dependently; the decrease was almost completely and significantly suppressed only in the group of animals pretreated by an H_1 receptor antagonist, pyrilamine and not by an H_2 receptor antagonist, cimetidine [3]. Tracheal dilation induced by electrical stimulation in the posterior hypothalamus was partially but significantly suppressed only after administration of pyrilamine into the fourth ventricle [4]. Histamine release from the RVL, nR and nTS in the medulla oblongata was induced by electrical stimulation in the posterior hypothalamus and autoregulated via H_3 receptors [5]. The aim of this study is to define physiologic responses influenced by histamine release in the medulla oblongata.

2. METHODS

Japanese white rabbits were anesthetized by urethane (450 mg/kg) i.v. and α-chloralose (45 mg/kg) i.v., underwent a tracheotomy 3 cm caudal to the cricoid cartilage, and were artificially ventilated and paralyzed by 1.3 mg/0.3 ml per kg gallamine triethiodide i.v. A balloon was inserted into the rostral trachea through the incision of tracheotomy. Saline including 5% glucose and gallamine triethiodide was infused through the femoral vein. A canula was inserted in the femoral artery to measure blood pressure. The rabbit brain was stereotaxically mounted according to the method of Sawyer et al [2]. Histamine release was collected by microdialysis; probes were inserted from the dorsal surface of the medulla oblongata. Histamine concentration was analyzed by HPLC with fluorescence detection of o-phthalaldehyde post-column derivatization. Electrical stimulation was applied with a stainless-steel monopolar electrode. After each experiment, the brain was removed, fixed, cut and stained with neutral red. The sites of microdialysis probes and the electrode were verified by light microscopic examination. Statistical significance of effects was determined by one-way repeated-measurement ANOVA with the Greenhouse-Geisser correction.

3. RESULTS

Histamine release from the RVL, nR and nTS was significantly increased by unilateral electrical stimulation (500μA, 50 Hz, 0.5 msec pulses, 15 sec) in the posterior hypothalamus and by hyperthermia (ca. 39.5 - 41℃ as rectal temperature) induced by body heating for 25 minutes. Tracheal pressure decrease and pressor response were caused by the stimulation. The tracheal and pressor responses induced by electrical stimulation were significantly suppressed after perfusion of pyrilamine for 25 minutes (1.25×10^{-6} mol/50μl/25 minutes) in the ipsilateral RVL and those by hyperthermia were also suppressed during perfusion of (+)-chlorpheniramine (5×10^{-6} M) in the bilateral RVL [7].

4. DISCUSSION

Histamine release from the RVL, nR and nTS in the medulla oblongata originated from the posterior hypothalamus and was enhanced by hyperthermia. Histamine increase from the RVL caused tracheal dilation and pressor response via H_1 receptors in the RVL.

Tracheal pressure decreased by histamine i.c.v. or electrical stimulation in the posterior hypothalamus is significantly suppressed by phentolamine i.v. or both phentolamine and propranolol i.v.; decreased tracheal pressure is not suppressed by either atropine i.v. or bilateral transection of the cervical vagus nerves and the superior laryngeal nerves [3, 4]. Histamine i.c.v. or chemical stimulation in the posterior hypothalamus enhances activities of the cervical sympathetic nerve and decreases tracheal pressure; these responses are suppressed by microinjection of an H_1 receptor antagonist in the bilateral RVL [6]. Taken together, histamine release in the medulla oblongata originated from hypothalamic histaminergic neurons and is activated by hyperthermia; brain histaminergic neurons play an important role in the adjustments of airway and peripheral vascular tone via H_1 receptors in the RVL and the sympathetic nervous system.

REFERENCES

1. J.-C. Schwartz, J.-M. Arrang, M.Garbarg, H. Pollard, M. Ruat, Physiol. Rev., 71 (1991) 1.
2. C.H Sawyer, J.W. Everett, J.D. Green, J. Comp. Neurol. 101. (1954) 801.
3. M. Kanamaru, M. Iwase, I. Homma, Neurosci. Lett. 169 (1994) 35.
4. M. Iwase, M. Kanamaru, I. Homma, J. Auton. Nerv. Syst. 53 (1995) 69.
5. M. Kanamaru, M. Iwase, I. Homma, Neurosci. Res. 31 (1998) 53.
6. M. Iwase, M. Kanamaru, A. Kanamaru, I. Homma, J. Auton. Nerv. Syst. 74 (1998) 23.
7. M. Kanamaru, M. Iwase, I. Homma, Am J Physiol Regulatory Integrative Comp Physiol, submitted.

© 2001 Elsevier Science B.V. All rights reserved.
Histamine Research in the New Millennium
T. Watanabe, H. Timmerman and K. Yanai (Editors)

The effects of histamine receptor antagonists on the induction of metallothionein mRNA after lipopolysaccharide injection in the mouse spleen

N. Sogawa[a], C.A. Sogawa[a], T. Inoue[b], N. Oda[a], K. Onodera[a], H. Furuta[a]

[a]Department of Dental Pharmacology,
[b]Department of Oral Microbiology,
Okayama University Dental School, 2-5-1 Shikata-cho, Okayama, 700-8525, Japan

1. ABSTRACT

Metallothioneins (MTs) are low molecular weight and metal-binding proteins, and can be induced in several mouse tissues including the spleen by lipopolysaccharide (LPS). However, the physiological role of MT in the immune system remains unclear. On the other hand, LPS also induces histamine via histidine decarboxylase (HDC) in the mouse spleen. Histamine is reported to produce immunomodulatory effects. Therefore, as an approach to clarifying the physiological function of MT, we investigated the relation between histamine and MT mRNA induction in the mouse spleen after LPS injection (100μg/kg, *i.v.*) using histamine antagonists and HDC inhibitor by the reverse transcriptase-polymerase chain reaction (RT-PCR) method and Northern blot analysis. Induction of MT mRNA was reduced by cimetidine (10, 50mg/kg) and α-methylhistidine (25mg/kg), but it was unchanged by diphenhydramine (10, 25 mg/kg). The findings in this study suggest that histamine may play a role via H_2 receptors on the mechanism of MT mRNA induction by LPS in the mouse spleen.

2. INTRODUCTION

Metallothioneins (MTs) are low molecular weight and metal-binding proteins that are rich in cysteine residue, and are induced by many different types of inducers including heavy metals, some chemicals, hormones, stress, and immunostimulatory substances, such as bacterial lipopolysaccharide (LPS) and cytokines *in vivo* [1-3]. It has been demonstrated that there are four major isoforms of MT in mammals, generally designated MT-I, MT-II, MT-III and MT-IV. Whereas MT-III expression is virtually brain-specific and MT-IV expression is squamous epithelium cell-specific, MT-I and MT-II genes are expressed in many tissues including the brain, liver, kidney and spleen [4-7]. It is generally agreed that MTs play an important role in the detoxification of heavy metals, in the homeostasis of essential metals and in the scavenging of free radicals [8-10]. But the exact physiological functions of MT have not yet been defined.

On the other hand, LPS also induces histamine via histidine decarboxylase (HDC) in several mouse tissues and cells, such as spleen, liver, kidney and macrophage [11,12]. It has been reported that histamine has a function to modulate some cytokine synthesis such as interleukin-1 (IL-1) and interleukin-6 (IL-6) [13,14]. These findings are very interesting considering MT induction is mediated through the above cytokines [3]. Therefore, we think that histamine may be related to MT induction by LPS. To our knowledge no report has previously investigated the relation with histamine and MT induction. To clarify MT physiological function, it is important to investigate the mechanism involved in MT induction.

In this study, we investigated the effects of histamine antagonists and HDC inhibitor on MT mRNA induction in the mouse spleen after LPS injection by analyzing the level of MT mRNA expression and the mode of its regulation using the reverse transcriptase-polymerase chain reaction (RT-PCR) method and Northern blot analysis.

MT mRNA induction by LPS

Fig.1A shows quantitative RT-PCR amplification at various concentrations (0.063- 1.0μg) of DNase I -pretreated total RNA from spleen with MT-I and G3PDH primers [15]. The nucleotide sequences of the PCR product were identical to that of MT-I reported from mouse MT-I cDNA [16]. Simultaneous amplification of MT-I and G3PDH mRNA sequences had no effect on the amplification efficiency of the individual sequences. The intensity of MT-I and G3PDH product increased linearly with the amount of RNA from 0.125 to 0.5 μg. Therefore, in PT-PCR experiments, 0.4 μg DNase I -pretreated total RNA was used with 20 cycle PCR.

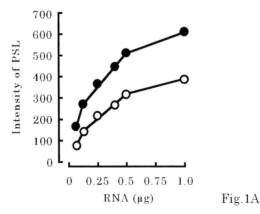

Fig.1A

Fig. 1 (A): Quantitative analysis by RT-PCR of MT-I and G3PDH mRNAs. Amplification curves for MT-I (closed circles) and G3PDH (open circles) mRNAs at various concentrations (0.063-1.0μg) of DNase I-pretreated total RNA from spleen.

To examine whether LPS (100µg/kg, *i.v.*) can induce MT in spleen, a time-course study was conducted with ddY mice (male, 9 weeks old). Relative MT-I mRNA induction increased following *i.v.* injection with LPS in a time dependent manner. The increase was rapid and achieved maximum at 3 hours after Cd injection. At that time, the value of relative induction was an approximate 9-fold increase compared to the induction at 0 hour (Fig.1B).

And, Northern blots of RNA isolated from spleen also showed the peak of MT mRNA accumulation at 2~3 hours after LPS injection (Fig.1C).

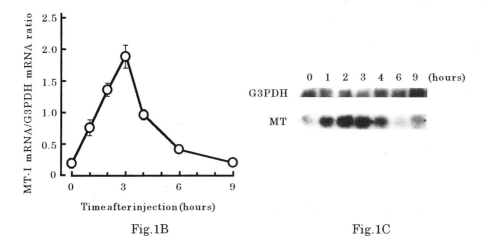

Fig.1B   Fig.1C

Time course of induction of MT mRNA by LPS in the mouse spleen. (B): Relative MT-I mRNA levels were determined by RT-PCR method. Each value was expressed relative to G3PDH mRNA value. Results are mean ± S.D. of four mice. (C): Northern blot analysis was performed using mouse MT-I cDNA (335bp fragment : which has approximately 80% homology to mouse MT-II mRNA coding region) [17] probe at 65°C for 18 hours. Total RNA pretreated with DNase I was hybridized sequentially to ^{32}P-labeled probes detecting MT and G3PDH.

In this study, the induction of MT mRNA reached maximum level at 3 hours after LPS injection. The induction by LPS is transitory, so it is assumed that certain kinds of cells are activated temporarily. According to the previous studies, MT can be induced in immunocytes including monocytes, T lymphocytes and B lymphocytes [18]. On the other hand, MT mRNA was induced directly in monocytes by LPS and reached maximum level at 30 minutes, and this high activation remained for the following 90 minutes *in vitro* [19]. So, the substances relating to induction of MT *in vivo* are different from those *in vitro*.

LPS is an immunostimulant that can activate monocytes/macrophages, leading to the induction of various inflammatory agents, such as cytokines and histamine. It is reported that MT was induced directly in monocytes by LPS *in vitro* [19] and suggested that the induction of MT by LPS may be mediated through some cytokines including IL-1, IL-6 and tumor necrosis factor-α (TNF-α) *in vivo* [3]. LPS and these cytokines can also induce HDC activity in macrophages or mouse tissues including spleen [12,20]. Macrophages regulate IL-1 synthesis by histamine produced by macrophages *per se* and enterogenous histamine via H_2 receptor [21]. Furthermore, it is reported that histamine enhances IL-1 induced IL-1 and IL-6 gene expression and protein synthesis via H_2 receptors in peripheral blood mononuclear cells [13,14]. Therefore, it is very interesting to investigate the effects of histamine antagonists on LPS-induced MT synthesis.

Effect of Histamine Antagonists and HDC Inhibitor with MT mRNA Induction

As MT mRNA induction in the mouse spleen peaked at 3 hours after LPS injection, the following study was performed at this interval time. Pretreatment with cimetidine (Cim : 10, 50mg/kg) and α-methylhistidine (α-MH : 25mg/kg)

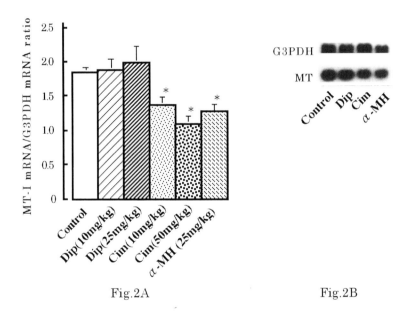

Fig.2A   Fig.2B

Effects of H_1, H_2 antagonists (diphenhydramine : Dip and cimetidine : Cim respectively) and HDC inhibitor (α-methylhistidine : α-MH) on the LPS-induced MT mRNA expression in spleens. (A): Relative MT-I mRNA levels were determined by RT-PCR method. Each value was expressed relative to G3PDH mRNA value. Results are mean ± S.D. of five mice. Experimental data was evaluated for statistical significance by ANOVA followed by Fisher's PLSD test. *p<0.01 vs control. (B): Northern blot analysis of MT and G3PDH mRNAs. Total RNA pretreated with DNase I was hybridized sequentially to ^{32}P-labeled probes detecting MT and G3PDH.

significantly diminished relative MT-I mRNA induction (p<0.01). The decrease in induction by Cim pretreatment occurred in a dose dependent manner. But diphenhydramine (Dip: 10, 25mg/kg) pretreatment did not change relative MT-I mRNA induction (Fig.2A). Fig.2B shows the results of Northern blot analysis for MT and G3PDH. Both RT-PCR and Northern blots showed similar results.

In our results, H_2 receptor antagonist, Cim suppressed MT mRNA expression by LPS in the mouse spleen. It is reported that the single administration of Cim fails to influence the tissue concentration of some trace elements and minerals (Cu, Zn, Fe, Mn, Ca, Mg) in spleen and MT induction in liver and kidney [22]. In our study, Cim, Dip and α-MH alone failed to influence MT-I mRNA induction in spleen (control : 0.144±0.051, Cim 10mg/kg : 0.127±0.036, Cim 50mg/kg : 0.163±0.038, Dip 10mg/kg : 0.155±0.042, Dip 25mg/kg : 0.136±0.023, α-MH : 0.119±0.036). Accordingly, it is thought that the suppressive effect of Cim on MT induction in this study is due to the block of histamine action via H_2 receptor. Activation of H_2 receptors results in an increased level of cyclic adenosine monophosphate [23]. It has been reported that both histamine and prostaglandin E_2, another activator of adenylate cyclase, are able to enhance IL-1 induced IL-1 and IL-6 synthesis in peripheral blood mononuclear cells [13,14]. Therefore, it may need a similar mechanism in MT induction by LPS.

In conclusion, the findings in this study suggest that histamine may play a role via H_2 receptors on the mechanism of MT mRNA induction by LPS in the mouse spleen.

REFERENCES

1. S. Onosaka and M.G. Cherian, Toxicology, 22 (1981) 91.
2. S.H. Oh, J.T. Deagen, P.D. Whanger and P.H. Weswig, Am. J. Physiol. 234 (1978) E282.
3. J. Liu, Y.P. Liu, L.E. Sendelbach and C.D. Klassen, Toxicol. Appl. Pharm. 109 (1991) 235.
4. S. Choudhuri, K.K. Kramer, N.E.J. Berman, T.P. Dalton, G.K. Andrews and C.D. Klassen, Toxicol. Appl. Pharmacol. 131 (1995) 144.
5. R.D. Palmiter, S.D. Findley, T.E.Whitmore and D.M. Durnam, Proc. Natl. Acad. Sci. USA 89 (1992) 6333.
6. R.K. Mehra and I. Bremner, EXS 52 (1987) 565.
7. C.J. Quaife, S.D. Findley, J.C. Erickson, G.J. Froelick, E.J. Kelly, B.P. Zambrowicz, and R.D. Palmiter, Biochemistry 33 (1994) 7250.
8. W.S. Din and J.M. Frazier, Biochem. J. 230 (1985) 395.
9. M.Webb and K. Cain, Biochem. Pharmacol. 31 (1982) 137.
10. P.J.Thornalley and M.Vasak, Biochim. Biophs. Acta. 827 (1985)36.
11. Y. Endo, Biochem. Pharmacol. 31 (1982) 1643.
12. C. Oh, S. Suzuki, I. Nakashima, K. Yamashita and K. Nakano, Immunology 65 (1988) 143.

13. E. Vannier and C.A. Dinarello, J. Clin. Invest. 92 (1993) 281.

14. E. Vannier and C.A. Dinarello, J. Biol. Chem. 269 (1994) 9952.

15. N. Sogawa, C. A. Sogawa, N. Oda, T. Fujioka, K. Onodera and H. Furuta, Methods Find Exp. Clin. Pharmacol. *in press.*

16. D.M. Durnam, F. Perrin, F. Gannon, and R.D. Palmiter, Proc. Natl. Acad. Sci. U.S.A. 77 (1980) 6511.

17. N. Glanville, D.M. Durnam, R.D. Palmiter, Nature 292 (1981) 267.

18. O.J. Mesna, I.L. Steffensen, H. Hjertholm and R.A. Andersen, Chemico-Biological Interactions 94 (1995) 225.

19. M.E. Leibbrandt and J. Koropatnick, Toxicol. Appl. Pharm. 124 (1994) 72.

20. Y. Endo, Biochem. Pharmacol. 38 (1989) 1287.

21. H. Okamoto and K. Nakano, Immunology 69 (1990) 162.

22. Y. Naveh, P. Weis, H.R. Chung and J.D. Bogden, J.Nutr. 117 (1987) 1576.

23. W. Roszkowski, M. Plaut and L. LichtensteinI, Science 195 (1977)683.

Histamine Research in the New Millennium
T. Watanabe, H. Timmerman and K. Yanai (Editors)
511

Evidence for the presence of histamine reuptake system in the brain and its characterization

Eiko Sakurai[1], Eiichi Sakurai[2], Lars Oreland[3], Takehiko Watanabe[1], Kazuhiko Yanai[1]

[1]Department of Pharmacology, Tohoku University School of Medicine, [2]Department of Pharmaceutics I, Tohoku Pharmaceutical University, [3]Department of Medical Pharmacology, Uppsala University.

Abstracts

We examined whether or not there is a histamine reuptake system in the brain using *in vitro* assay technique of uptake of other neurotransmitters. In addition, the uptake of histamine into human astrocytoma cells (1321N1) was examined under intact cell conditions. There was two types histamine reuptake system in the brain. Na^+, Cl and HCO_3 ions were essential for the uptake of histamine into P2 fractions of brain homogenates. These results further support the existence of specific histamine re-uptake system in the brain.

Key words: Histamine, brain, uptake, astrocytoma cell

1. Introduction

Histamine has many physiological roles in the brain and periphery. Neuronal histamine is metabolized almost exclusively by histamine *N*-methyltransferase. Although several neurotransmitter systems such as dopamine and 5-hydroxytryptamine have their specific re-uptake system in their neurons and glial cells, the primary mechanism of inactivation of histamine, a specific histamine re-uptake system into the corresponding nerve terminals or glial cells, has not yet been well elucidated. Recently, it was reported that a specific uptake mechanism replenishes histamine stores in the photoreceptor in an activity-dependent fashion[1]. In this report, we characterized the uptake of histamine into the P2 fractions of rat forebrain homogenized in 0.32 M sucrose using *in vitro* uptake assay techniques. In addition, the uptake of histamine into human astrocytoma cells (1321N1) was examined under intact cell conditions.

2. Material and Method

Adult male rats of Sprague-Dawley strain (Funabashi Farm, Funabashi, Japan) weighting 190-200g were used. The brains were rapidly removed and dissected on ice into forebrain and others. The rats forebrain were homogenized in 0.32M sucrose, and separated into fraction P1 and P2.

512

The localization of histamine uptake system in subcellular fractions from the rat brain was examined using the established methods dopamine and serotonine[2].

The human astrocytoma cells (1321N1) were cultured in Dulbecco's modified Eagle's medium (DMEM) with 5% fetal bovine serum (FBS). The cells were incubated with histamine in Krebs-Henselei't bicarbonate buffer at 4 and 37°C. The uptakes of histamine into the cells were measured by HPLC-fluorometry[3] and the difference in histamine level between those at 37°C and 4°C was defined as the uptake.

Results and discussion

The uptakes of [³H]-histamine into the P2 fractions of rat brain homogenate were increased with the increment of added protein amount. Fig.1 shows that [³H]-Histamine uptakes were also temperature- and time-dependent. Carrying protein of histamine in the brain would be activating in body temperature.

Fig. 1 Effects of the incubation time and temperature on [³H]-histamine uptake into P2 fraction of brain

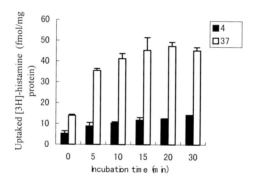

The total amount of [³H]-histamine uptake into the P2 fractions was 42.3 ± 2.9 fmol/mg protein/15min. Na^+, Cl and HCO_3 ions were essential for the uptake of histamine in P2 fractions. When chloride ion was replace with isocyanate, [³H]-histamine uptake was decreased to 24% of total uptake in normal buffer condition. By removal of sodium and bicarbonate ions from Krebs-Henseleit bicarbonate buffer, [³H]-histamine uptake was almost half that in normal buffer.

[³H]-Histamine uptake was significantly inhibited in the presence of several tricyclic antidepressants. In addition, we examined whether imipramine could affect the K^+-evoked histamine release from perfused brain slices. The release of histamine from brain slices evoked by 100 mM K^+ was augmented in the presence of 20μ M imipramine. Imipramine may inhibit histamine reuptake system.

All histamine H1, H2 and H3 receptor ligands had no effect on the histamine uptake.

The subcellular localization of histamine uptake system in the brain homogenate was examined.

The apparent capacity for [³H]-histamine uptake was high in the synaptosomal fraction (B), as shown in Fig.2.

Fig.2 [³H]-Histamine uptake into fractions of rat forebrain homogenate divided by sucrose separation. A, B and C fractions were obtained using sucrose-density centrifugation of P2 fractions of rat forebrain

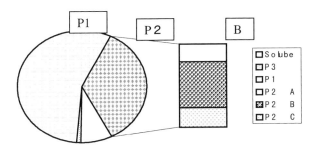

Similar results were obtained in human astrocytoma 1321 cells. Cultured astrocytoma cells in 6 well plates were preincubated for 5 min with Krebs-Henseleit bicarbonate buffer containing 20 μM SKF-91488 as histamine N-methyltransferase inhibitor at 4 or 37°C. After preincubation, cold histamine added to final concentration of 1, 10 and 100 μM and the mixture were incubated for 15 min at 4 or 37°C. The cells were washed 5 times with cold buffer and then corrected for a measurement of histamine by HPLC-fluolometric method. Fig. 3 shows that histamine was trapped dose-dependently into astrocytoma cells.

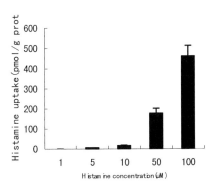
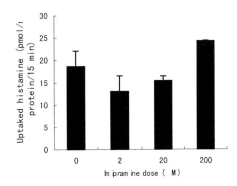

Fig.3 Histamine uptake into astrocytoma cells. **Fig.4** Effects of Imipramine concentration on astrocytoma cells

Histamine was added to astrocytoma cells and the cells were incubated for 15 min at 4 or 37°C. The uptaked histamine into the cells was the value of uptaked histamine on 37°C minus 4°C.

Imipramine was also inhibited histamine uptake in human astrocytoma cells, as shown in Fig. 4. From these results further support was obtained for the existence of specific histamine re-uptake system in the brain.

REFERENCES

1. Stuart AE. From fruit flies to barnacles, histamine is the neurotransmitter of arthropod photoreceptors. Neuron. 22(3):431-3, 1999
2. Jossan SS. Sakurai E. Oreland L. MPTP toxicity in relation to age, dopamine uptake and MAO-B activity in two rodent species. Pharmacology & Toxicology. 64(3):314-8, 1989.
3. Yamatodani A. Fukuda H. Wada H. Iwaeda T. Watanabe T. High-performance liquid chromatographic determination of plasma and brain histamine without previous purification of biological samples: cation-exchange chromatography coupled with post-column derivatization fluorometry. Journal of Chromatography. 344:115-23, 1985.

© 2001 Elsevier Science B.V. All rights reserved.
Histamine Research in the New Millennium
T. Watanabe, H. Timmerman and K. Yanai (Editors)   515

The effects of "sleepiness" on the brain activity during spatial cognition tasks: A human PET study

H. Mochizuki[1], M. Tagawa[2], M. Kano[1], M. Itoh[3], N. Okamura[1], T. Watanabe[1] and K. Yanai[1]

[1]Department of Pharmacology, Tohoku University School of Medicine, Sendai, 980-8575, [2]Dainippon Pharmaceutical Co., Ltd, [3]Cyclotron and Radioisotope Center, Tohoku University, Japan

The aim of this study was to visualize the effects of sleepiness on the brain activity during choice reaction time task (CRT) using positron emission tomography (PET). In this study, "sleepiness" could be induced by the oral administration of 6 mg d-chlorpheniramine (Chl), an H1 antagonist. This study suggested that Chl-induced deterioration of spatial discrimination would contribute to the decreased activity in right parietal cortex that participates spatial cognition. Activities in the right cingulate cortex were also increased in proportion to impaired spatial cognition, suggesting increasing attentional demands for the task performance.

1. INTRODUCTION

First generation antihistamines are well known to induce sleepiness and to impair various brain functions such as psychomotor and verbal learning. These impairments are due to occupy H1 receptors in the brain. However, there are few reports focused on functional neuroimaging of antihistamines-induced impaired cognition in humans. The aim of this study was to visualize the effects of "sleepiness" on brain activities during a spatial discrimination task using PET and $[^{15}O]$-H_2O.

2. MATERIALS AND METHODS

Sixteen healthy men participated in this study. Subjects were orally administrated with placebo (Biofermin-R), 2mg or 6mg Chl on a single blind procedure. Subjects were instructed to perform choice reaction time task (CRT), which was to discriminate left or right stimulus against the center of the display. Reaction time (RT) and subjective sleepiness were measured during CRT. Statistic parametric mapping (SPM) imaging software was used to create statistical maps of significant rCBF changes.

3. RESULTS

Subjective sleepiness tended to increase and RT was significantly prolonged when orally administrated 6mg Chl. To identify brain regions related to the prolonged RT, images when administrated 6mg *d*-chlorpheniramine were compared to those of placebo and 2mg *d*-chlorpheniramine.

SPM analyses demonstrated that the rCBF in right parietal cortex (Brodmann area 40; BA 40) was decreased and that in cingulate cortex (BA 24) was increased significantly by treatment of 6mg Chl (Table1)

Table 1

Brain region	BA	axis (x,y,z)	change of rCBF	Z score
right cingulate cortex	24	22,-16,38	increase	2.98
right parietal cortex	40	62,-60,38	decrease	3.50

Brain regions in which the rCBF were significantly changed after administration of 6mg *d*-chlorpheniramine.

4. DISCUSSION

In this study, we visualized the effect of orally administered Chl on brain activity during CRT. The prolonged PR would contribute to the decrease of rCBF in right parietal cortex, since right parietal cortex is involved in spatial discrimination (1). It was previously reported that the activity of cingulate cortex was related to attention (2) and that its activity had a positive correlation with task difficulty (3,4). The previous works indicated that the enhanced activity in right cingulate cortex would represent increasing attentional demands for the task.

5. CONCLUSION

These findings suggested that the Chl-induced spatial cognitive impairment would result in the decreased activity in right parietal cortex. The enhanced activity in right cingulate cortex might be associated with subjective feelings of sleepiness, because sleepiness was actually recognized when attentional demands for the task were subjectively increasing.

REFERENCES

1. M. Corbetta, F.M. Miezin, G.L. Shulman and S.E. Petersen, J Neurosci (1993) 13 (3).
2. M. Corbetta, F.M. Miezin, S. Dobmeyer, et al. Science (2000) 2 248 (4962).
3. M.I. Posner and S.E. Petersen, Annu Rev Neurosci (1990) 13.
4. N. Okamura, K. Yanai, M. Higuchi, et al. Br J Pharmacol 129 (2000) 115

Index of authors